Advanced Practice Nursing with Older Adults

Clinical Guidelines

Notice

Advanced Practice Nursing with Older Adults

Clinical Guidelines

Valerie T. Cotter, MSN, RN, CS

Associate Director
Adult Health and Gerontology Nurse Practitioner Programs
School of Nursing
Nurse Practitioner and Education Director, Alzheimer's Disease Center
University of Pennsylvania
Philadelphia, Pennsylvania

Neville E. Strumpf, PhD, RN, C, FAAN

Edith Clemmer Steinbright Professor in Gerontology
School of Nursing
University of Pennsylvania
Philadelphia, Pennsylvania

with 30 contributors

McGraw-Hill
Medical Publishing Division
New York • Chicago • San Francisco • Lisbon • London • Madrid • Mexico City
Milan • New Delhi • San Juan • Seoul • Singapore • Sydney • Toronto

McGraw-Hill

A Division of The McGraw-Hill Companies

Advanced Practice Nursing with Older Adults: Clinical Guidelines

1234567890 DOC/DOC 0987654321

ISBN 0-07-134157-9

This book was set in Sabon by V&M Graphics, Inc.
The editor was Sally J. Barhydt.
The production supervisor was Lisa Mendez.
Project management was provided by Roundhouse Editorial Services.
The index was prepared by Fred Leise.
R. R. Donnelley & Sons was printer and binder.

This book is printed on acid-free paper.

Library of Congress Cataloging-in-Publication Data

Advanced practice nursing with older adults : clinical guidelines / [edited by] Valerie Cotter,
Neville E. Strumpf.
   p. ; cm.
   Includes bibliographical references and index.
   ISBN 0-07-134157-9
   1. Geriatric nursing. 2. Nurse practitioners. 3. Aged—Medical care. I. Cotter, Valerie.
II. Strumpf, Neville E.
   [DNLM: 1. Geriatric Nursing. 2. Nurse Practitioners. 3. Nursing Diagnosis. WY 152
A244 2001]
RC954 .A32 2001
610.73′65—dc21

                                                              00-054888

This book is dedicated to our physician colleague, Barbara Bates, MD, who has mentored us and thousands of advanced practice nurses at the University of Pennsylvania and across the United States.

CONTENTS

CONTRIBUTORS

Valerie T. Cotter, MSN, RN, CS
Associate Director
Adult Health and Gerontology Nurse Practitioner Programs
School of Nursing
Nurse Practitioner and Education Director, Alzheimer's Disease Center
University of Pennsylvania
Philadelphia, Pennsylvania

Neville E. Strumpf, PhD, RN, C, FAAN
Edith Clemmer Steinbright Professor in Gerontology
School of Nursing, University of Pennsylvania
Philadelphia, Pennsylvania

Joseph Adler, MS, PT
Senior Physical Therapist
Department of Occupational and Physical Therapy
Hospital of the University of Pennsylvania
Philadelphia, Pennsylvania

Tim Baum, MSN, RN, CS
Nurse Practitioner
Lancaster Veteran's Affairs Medical Center
Lancaster, Pennsylvania

Anna S. Beeber, MSN, RN
John A. Hartford Foundation Predoctoral Scholar
School of Nursing, University of Pennsylvania
Philadelphia, Pennsylvania

Marie Boltz, MSN, CRNP
Gerontologic Nurse Practitioner
Elkins Park, Pennsylvania

Patricia Katheder Bourne, MSN, RN, CDE
Landenberg, Pennsylvania

Christine Wanich Bradway, MSN, RN, CS
Gerontologic Nurse Practitioner and Doctoral Candidate
School of Nursing, University of Pennsylvania
Philadelphia, Pennsylvania

Izzie Brown-Gordon, MS, RD
Dietetic Technician
Clinical Nutrition Support Service
Hospital of the University of Pennsylvania
Philadelphia, Pennsylvania

Elizabeth Capezuti, PhD, RN, CS, FAAN
Associate Professor
Independence Foundation–Wesley Woods
Chair in Gerontological Nursing
Emory University
Atlanta, Georgia

Ara A. Chalian, MD, FACS
Assistant Professor, School of Medicine
Chief, Reconstructive and Microvascular Surgery
Department of Otorhinolaryngology
Head and Neck Surgery
University of Pennsylvania
Philadelphia, Pennsylvania

Gerald Driscoll, MSN, RN, CS
Primary Home Care, LLC
Philadelphia, Pennsylvania

William F. Edwards, MSN, RN, CS, CRNP
Project Manager, Center for Clinical
    Epidemiology and Biostatistics
University of Pennsylvania
Philadelphia, Pennsylvania

Michelle A. Feil, MSN, CRNP
Hospital of the University of Pennsylvania
Philadelphia, Pennsylvania

Mechele Fillman, MSN, RN
Staff Nurse, St. Joseph's Hospital
Denver, Colorado

Sherry Greenberg, MSN, RN, CS
Clinical Assistant Professor
Gerontological Nurse Practitioner and Coordinator
Advanced Practice Nursing: Geriatric Program
Division of Nursing, School of Education
New York University
New York, New York

Kathleen A. Hill-O'Neill, MSN, RN, CS, NHA
Gerontological Nurse Practitioner and Administrator
Rydal Park
Rydal Park, Pennsylvania

Sarah H. Kagan, PhD, RN
Assistant Professor of Gerontological Nursing
School of Nursing, University of Pennsylvania
Philadelphia, Pennsylvania

Mary F. Kelley, MSN, RN, CS
Geriatric Nurse Practitioner
Center for Senior Health Care
Cherry Hill, New Jersey

Lenore H. Kurlowicz, PhD, RN
Assistant Professor of Geropsychiatric Nursing
School of Nursing, University of Pennsylvania
Philadelphia, Pennsylvania

Barbara J. Maschak-Carey, MSN, RN
Diabetes Clinical Nurse Specialist
University of Pennsylvania
Philadelphia, Pennsylvania

Rosemary C. Polomano, PhD, RN, FAAN
Senior Researcher
Outcomes, Research, and Informatics
Assistant Professor, Department of Anesthesiology
The Pennsylvania State Milton S. Hershey Medical Center and
Pennsylvania State University College of Medicine
Hershey, Pennsylvania

Alicia A. Puppione, MSN, RN
Santa Monica, California

Diane Schretzman, MSN, RN, CS
Neurosurgery Research Coordinator
Hennepin County Medical Center
Minneapolis, Minnesota

Marianne Shaughnessy, PhD, RN, CS
Assistant Professor
School of Nursing, University of Maryland
Baltimore, Maryland

Sara Lisa Sheiman, MSN, RN, CS
Geriatric Nurse Practitioner
Philadelphia, Pennsylvania

Howard Tuch, MD
Director of Palliative Care Services
Genesis ElderCare
Kennett Square, Pennsylvania

Kathleen C. Tully, MSN, RN, CS
Vice President of Health Services
Cadbury Senior Services
Cherry Hill, New Jersey

Laura Wagner, MSN, RN, CS
Gerontological Nurse Practitioner
Wexner Heritage Village
Columbus, Ohio

Gale Yetman, MSN, RN, CS
Gerontological Nurse Practitioner
Shore Continence Center
Toms River, New Jersey

Jean Yudin, MSN, RN, CS
In-Home Primary Care Program
School of Medicine, University of Pennsylvania
Philadelphia, Pennsylvania

Johanna Yurkow, MSN, RN, CS, CCM
Director of Health Services
Medford Leas Continuing Care Retirement Community
Medford, New Jersey

PREFACE

With the publication of *Advanced Practice Nursing with Older Adults* we begin a new century of thinking regarding the role of nurses in the primary care of elders in all settings. In 1900, when life expectancy was roughly 47 years of age, such care fell mainly to kind, hearty souls—often family members—to supply shelter and attention. The notion of specialty care for sick and aged persons was virtually unknown, although whispers concerning their needs were noted in several early 20th-century issues of the *American Journal of Nursing*. Occasionally, editorials were written about those aged who were left to deteriorate in the bleak, cheerless surroundings of the poorhouse. Gradually, with the expansion of the public health movement, Americans came to understand there were specific needs for modifications in diet, provision for regular exercise and fresh air, and recreational therapy. Virginia Henderson, in her Nursing Studies Index for 1900–1929, began citing scattered references to "Geriatrics and Nursing," but not until Kathleen Newton's text *Geriatric Nursing* in 1950 did nurses have any detailed guide for the care of an older adult. Newton's book clearly paved the way for the specialized role of advanced practice nurses in gerontology.

Over the past 30 years, we have witnessed the evolution of the Scope and Standards of Practice for Gerontological Nurses, the development of master's education for gerontological nurse practitioners and clinical specialists, the formation of numerous specialty organizations and interest groups, an ever-growing body of clinical research focused on older adults, a substantial evidence base for practice, and extraordinary opportunities for advanced practice with this population.

At the beginning of the 21st century, the average life expectancy for women is 79 years, and for men, 74 years with a rapidly growing population of 70-, 80-, and 90-year-olds, as well as centenarians. Despite these demographic changes, texts dedicated specifically to advanced practice with older adults are few in number. Thus, this is an appropriate time for nursing to claim its historic role: to make a significant contribution to the health and well-being of a major portion of society and to demonstrate, through careful assessment, treatment, and support, that a good old age is an achievable goal for all. We believe this book is an important foundation for such practice in the 21st century.

Advanced Practice Nursing with Older Adults

Clinical Guidelines

PART 1

Advanced Practice Nursing with Older Adults

1

The Role of Advanced Practice Nurses in Care of Older Adults

Valerie T. Cotter

Neville E. Strumpf

In *Advanced Practice Nursing with Older Adults*, we present state-of-the-art guidelines for geriatric care that are useful to any nurse practitioner who encounters aging persons in practice. The book is an outgrowth of our 15 years of experience educating advanced practice nurses in the Gerontology Nurse Practitioner Program at the University of Pennsylvania School of Nursing, a program ranked #1 by the *U.S. News and World Report* in its 2001 edition on Best Programs in Colleges and Universities. Although we continue to witness a rapid explosion of knowledge and profound changes in the delivery and reimbursement of health care, what remains constant is the need for expert response by advanced practice nurses (APNs) to the acute and chronic problems of older adults, regardless of setting.

The APN must possess a substantive background in the relevant pathophysiology, age-related issues, implications, and their impact on an older population; clinical presentation, history, physical examination, laboratory, and diagnostic workup; and interventions and clinical management. In particular, the most current research and evidence base are crucial in considering the goals of care, effects of coexisting conditions, prevention strategies, lifestyle modifications, patient and caregiver education, drug therapy, referral and consultation, and long-term follow-up. We have applied this framework to every chapter in the book, whether a discussion of disease or functional problem common to older adults. While the chapters are by no means exhaustive, we believe that, overall, the book covers the major problems likely to appear in primary-care practice with older adults.

We have kept in mind the *Scope and Standards of Gerontological Nursing Practice* developed by the American Nurses' Association, the National Gerontological Nursing Association, the National Association of Directors of Nursing Administration in Long Term Care, and the National Council of Geriatric Nurse Practitioners.[1] The standards clearly focus on assessment, diagnosis, outcome identification, planning, implementation, and evaluation, all of which are thoroughly covered in this text. As was noted so well by one of the pioneers of geriatric nursing, Doris Schwartz, in 1969: practice must emphasize the identification of patient problems requiring nursing attention, core knowledge to address those problems, and solutions directed toward "incipient ailments and manageable chronic conditions before they reach crisis proportions."[2]

We view primary care very broadly, from community-based practice to nursing home care, and much in between. Clearly, primary care is as much about the sick as the well, and certainly, given the nature of an aging population, must encompass chronicity, loss of function, frailty, and death. The first text in geriatric nursing did not appear until 1950, and the specialty truly came into its own only during the past 20 years. Although we have now many more texts in gerontological nursing, this one is unique in its focus on actions germane to the practice characteristics of gerontologic APNs in acute care, ambulatory care, home care, and long-term care. It illustrates implementation of the principles of primary care as identified in the current statement of Standards and Scope of Practice, as well as underscores the depth and breadth of knowledge needed to engage in accountable and ethical practice.

The covenant between APN and patient is rooted in the profession's moral and ethical foundations and its abiding commitment to persons in need. As health care changes and science constantly advances, the boundaries of nursing practice continuously expand. This is quite apparent in a book where the knowledge, skills, and performance expectations of APNs working with older adults and their families are very high, requiring both independence in clinical judgement and knowledgeable collaboration with other health providers. Embedded within accountable practice is responsibility for excellent care, a caring relationship, and commitment to the most appropriate outcomes. Advanced practice nurses are challenged daily both by the complexities of patient care and the parameters of ever-evolving systems of care. Nevertheless, the rewards and satisfactions remain when one is intellectually and emotionally outfitted to care *for* and *about* people in the later portions of their lives. For advanced practice nurses taking that journey, this book is meant to provide one such reference point.

References

1. American Nurses Association. *Scope and Standards of Gerontological Clinical Nursing Practice*. Washington, DC: American Nurses Association, 1995.
2. Schwartz D. Aging and the field of nursing. In: Riley M, Riley J, Johnson M, eds. *Aging and Society: Vol 2: Aging and the Professions*. New York: Russell Sage Foundation, 1969: 79–113.

CHAPTER **2**

Principles Guiding Care of Older Adults

Diane Schretzman
Neville E. Strumpf

Introduction

This chapter begins our exploration into basic tenets of advanced practice gerontological nursing. Although older adults are as diverse and heterogeneous as younger people, and must be considered and treated as individuals, certain factors distinguish the health care of older adults. Nurse practitioners are guided by universal principles when encountering complex age-specific issues, from utilizing age-appropriate physical assessment techniques to dealing with the many ethical questions surrounding the care of cognitively impaired older people.

This chapter's goal is to review the principles guiding advanced practice nursing care of older adults. These focus on special considerations in gerontological assessment, differentiation between normal age-related changes and pathology, issues concerning medication management, and health promotion and disease prevention in older adults. The content that follows can be applied in almost any clinical situation.

Background and Overview

Advanced Practice Gerontological Nurses

Nurse practitioners provide individualized, holistic care to a heterogeneous population of older adults. Roles vary by practice setting, specialty, and regional needs. Nurse practitioners function as members of interdisciplinary teams that provide interrelated services along the wellness–illness continuum. Addressing physical, psychosocial, cultural, and family concerns, these health-care providers go beyond focusing on illness and disease alone to promoting health and emphasizing successful aging.[1, 2, 3]

The American Nurses Association's *Scope and Standards of Gerontological Clinical Nursing Practice* lists health promotion, health maintenance, disease prevention, and facilitation of self-care as critical functions for nurse practitioners. This document also describes essential aspects of practice and is summarized in Table 2–1.[4]

Table 2–1 Advanced Practice Gerontological Nursing[4]

Gerontological Nurse Practitioners have the knowledge and skills to:

1. Demonstrate in-depth understanding of interacting pathophysiologic and psychosocial changes of aging as well as interventions necessary for management of these alterations in health status.

2. Employ clinical reasoning as a basis for distinctions between customary and unusual findings, with emphasis on changes in functional status.

3. Provide comprehensive services independently, with caregivers, or with members of the interdisciplinary team.

4. Promote healthy aging.

5. Define, explore, and resolve ethical dilemmas.

6. Provide consultation and education.

7. Provide leadership and advocacy.

8. Collaborate in, use, and disseminate research.

9. Provide leadership in developing and maintaining standards of practice.

10. Participate in continuing education and certification.

Table 2–2   Top Eight Most Prevalent Chronic Conditions Among Older Adults[8]

1. Arthritis
2. Hypertension
3. Heart disease
4. Respiratory disease
5. Diabetes mellitus
6. Cancer
7. Cerebrovascular disease
8. Atherosclerosis

Table 2–4   Top Twelve Causes of Death Among Older Adults[8]

1. Heart disease
2. Cancer
3. Cerebrovascular disease
4. Chronic obstructive pulmonary disease (COPD) and associated conditions
5. Pneumonia and influenza
6. Diabetes mellitus
7. Accidents
8. Alzheimer's disease
9. Kidney disease
10. Septicemia
11. Atherosclerosis
12. Hypertension

Gerontological nurse practitioners provide high-quality care in the midst of complex and dynamic health-care systems. Health care for older adults is significantly affected by shifts in public policy, including changes in Medicare and Medicaid, and evolution toward managed care in most sectors of health care.[5,6] Nurse practitioners are trained to provide high-quality and cost-effective care, and to facilitate access to services by older people who must navigate systems and services.[2]

Nurse practitioners utilize a comprehensive approach that can provide older adults with coordinated care. It is especially valuable to those older adults who suffer from multiple concomitant conditions, require a variety of diverse services, and utilize numerous resources. This comprehensive approach best suits nurse practitioners who address problems that are common in an older population.[2,7] Tables 2–2, 2-3, and 2–4 list common chronic conditions, causes of hospitalization, and causes of death among this group.

Demographic Issues

The number and proportion of older Americans is rising sharply, leading to the graying of America. This increase is projected to continue into at least the middle of the 21st century and will likely have a huge impact on the national health-care system.[8,9,10]

Growing Numbers of Older Americans

The number of older adults, defined as persons aged 65 and older, grew from three million in 1900, or 4% of the total population, to more than 34.5 million in 1999, nearly 13% of the population.[9] This group's older (and frailer) cohort, people aged 85 and older, is projected to increase the fastest, from 3.6 million in 1995 to more than 8.5 million in 2030.[8] Estimates for 2050 project that this over-85 group will include more than 18 million, nearly 5% of the total population.[9]

This demographic trend, summarized in Table 2–5, has multiple causes. Members of the large Baby Boom Generation, born between 1946 and

Table 2–3   Top Ten Leading Causes of Hospitalization Among Older Adults[8]

1. Heart disease
2. Cancer
3. Cerebrovascular disease
4. Pneumonia
5. Fractures
6. Bronchitis
7. Osteoarthritis
8. Diabetes mellitus
9. Disease of the nervous system or sense organs
10. Prostate hyperplasia

Table 2–5   Older American Population, 1994–2050 (in thousands)[9]

Year	1994	1999	2000	2025	2050
Total population	260,289	273,000	274,634	335,050	393,931
65 and over	33,618	34,517	34,709	61,952	78,859
85 and over	3,684	4,259	4,899	7,046	18,223
100 and over	48	59	72	274	834

*projected

1964, are becoming older adults at a time of much greater longevity.[10] Women have tended to outlive men, so the greatest expansion is occurring in the proportion of women aged 85 and older.[11]

Utilization of Health-Care Resources

Older Americans utilize health-care services at rates that are disproportionate to their overall representation in the population. They are hospitalized more frequently, suffer from more chronic diseases, and use more medications than any other group. In 1995, older adults made up 13% of the U.S. population, but accounted for 35% of health-care expenditures.[8] Medications alone cost more than $3 billion a year.[12]

Substantial increases are predicted for the coming years. It is estimated that by 2020, older adults will comprise 20% of the population, but will use more than 70% of the country's health-care resources.[5,8] These data are consistent across practice settings. Use of primary, acute care, home care, and long-term nursing care services all rise steeply as individuals age.[8]

The impact of aging on health-care systems and other caregiving structures is likely to be extensive. Older adults receive health care in a variety of settings along the continuum of care, from primary-care clinics to critical-care units. Older people are also seen in other clinics, adult day care, home care, additional hospital areas, rehabilitation settings, hospices, and nursing homes. Transitional services, such as subacute care, are also used. In all of these settings, nurse practitioners collaborate with other team members to provide care to the growing numbers of older adults.[2,13]

The heavy burden also will likely be borne by social institutions and family structures, which provide both formal and informal home-care services.[13] Most older adults live at home, and some are frail or dependent due to chronic or acute illnesses. Nearly 30% of people 65 to 74, over 40% of people 75 to 84, and more than 60% of people 85 and older experience some functional impairment and therefore require assistance.[14] Since older people, particularly older women, tend to live alone, external caregivers may be needed. Services are often provided or coordinated by younger relatives.[15]

Other Demographic Issues

Older Americans are becoming increasingly diverse, ethnically, racially, and culturally. In 1994, 10% of older adults were other than white. By 2050, racial and ethnic diversity among older adults is projected to double to at least 20% of the total older population. The proportion of older people who are Hispanic is expected to grow from 4% to nearly 16% over that period.[11] Nurse practitioners must provide culturally sensitive care and maintain cultural competence to minimize race-based inequalities in health care[16,17,18] that have been noted among older adults.[10,19–22]

The current cohort of older adults also contains a significant percentage of poor individuals. Poverty is a significant consideration, because it affects health, the use of health-care services, and the outcome of some diseases and illnesses.[21] Some 11% of people aged 65 to 74, and 16% of those aged 75 and older, live below the poverty line; 16% of older women and 9% of older men live in poverty; and 33% of older African Americans, 22% of older Hispanic Americans, and 11% of older Caucasians are poor.[11] Income disparities among older people depend on many factors, including age, gender, race, ethnicity, marital status, living arrangements, education, and present or former occupation.[23]

Ethical Issues

Ethical issues are significant for gerontological advanced practice nurses. Many commonly encountered situations, from driving cessation to terminal care, bring dilemmas for patients, family members, and providers. Knowledge regarding basic ethical principles must be applied thoughtfully to specific clinical situations.[24]

Ethical Principles

The principles of autonomy, veracity, beneficence, and justice help guide ethical decision making. Older adults have the right to make personal choices regarding health care and treatment, after receiving complete and true information in understandable terms.[25] Older adults must be treated in ways that are of benefit and do no harm, or as little harm as possible, and are consistent with high-quality health care.[24,26] In a just society, age-based rationing of health care is inappropriate, because any necessary health care should be available regardless of age.[27] Confidentiality must be maintained while health-care providers handle health information, computer data, or genetic information.[26]

End-of-Life Issues

Issues surrounding death and dying are of great consequence in the care of older adults, because at least 74% of annual deaths occur in this population.[8] Advance directives, health-care power of attorney, and living wills can facilitate end-of-life decision making.[28]

Advance directives, documents containing decisions about initiating, terminating, or continuing life-sustaining treatments, are used to communicate an individual's wishes for end-of-life care.

Advance directives also designate an individual to make treatment decisions for patients who lack decision-making capability.[28,29]

Living wills and durable power of attorney for health care are types of advance directives. Through living wills, individuals provide concrete, specific instructions about desired treatments. These instructions are followed if individuals are unable to communicate. Durable power of attorney for health care, or health-care proxy, allows individuals to appoint surrogate decision makers. The decision makers are called on if individuals are unable to guide their own care.[28,29]

The use of advance directives has been mandated by federal law. The Patient Self Determination Act (PSDA) of 1991 requires that all facilities receiving federal Medicare and Medicaid funds provide patients with information regarding advance directives. While implementation varies among states and facilities, PSDA has encouraged patients and family members to discuss wishes and treatment goals with staff members. It has also provided a method by which practitioners can facilitate individual autonomy in medical decision making.[25,30]

Despite the widespread availability of advance directives, they are not always put to use, and ethical dilemmas regarding prolongation of life and dignified death are common. Decisions are complicated when individuals become critically ill or unable to communicate. In those cases, decisions regarding the provision of life-sustaining treatments are left largely to the health-care team and family members.[31]

Decisions surrounding the withholding or withdrawing of care are often complex. Further, a peaceful death is no longer easy to achieve. It is important for nurse practitioners to provide and coordinate end-of-life care that is both compassionate and consistent with individuals' wishes.[32] Palliative care, which strives to meet these goals, is addressed in more detail later in this book.

Principles of Assessment in Older Adults

Older adults generally require health assessments that are multidimensional and interdisciplinary.

These comprehensive assessments yield important information about multiple, complex, and interrelated problems. Data regarding biomedical, functional, psychological, and social issues are obtained. This information can be used during the planning and implementation of individualized health care.[33,34]

Issues in Physical Assessment

When obtaining health histories and conducting physical assessments of older adults, nurse practitioners should employ an age-appropriate approach, with special attention to older adults' unique and individualized needs. Eliciting a complete history from an older person may take longer than for a younger person. In most cases, multiple sessions accomplish more and are less fatiguing to older adults than a single, longer visit.[35]

The environment should be comfortable and of moderate temperature. Interviewing and examination areas should adjust for sensory deficits, with as little glare, direct light, and background noise as possible. Nurse practitioners should be attentive to older adults' body language, which may signify fatigue, anxiety, some degree of cognitive impairment, or a need to void.[35]

Social Assessment

Assessment of an older adult's social functioning yields information regarding family relationships, support systems, and available social and financial resources.[36] A caregiver assessment, to elicit the potential burdens and needs of family caregivers, should be conducted as part of social assessment.[15,37] Intervention is warranted when social isolation is occurring, resources are inadequate and health endangered, or domestic violence or abuse is suspected.[38]

Individualized Assessments and Care

Individualized care acknowledges that older individuals are unique people, and strives to provide assessments, services, and care in ways that are consistent with personal preferences. This is dependent on a thorough knowledge of people as individuals as well as members of families and communities. Further, older people are encouraged to maintain their identities and relationships.[39]

Individualized care, which is inherently culturally sensitive, provides older adults with opportunities to participate in the direction and implementation of their care. Preferences on issues ranging from physical environment to food choices should be elicited and observed. Choice is also important as older individuals decide how they choose to relate to other people, including caregivers.[39,40]

Individualized care is especially beneficial in nursing homes and other institutional settings. Individualized care has been shown to relieve anxiety, increase activity levels, promote a sense of normalcy, decrease the use of physical restraints, and increase satisfaction among staff and family members.[39]

Functional Assessment

Assessment of functional status is a key part of comprehensive geriatric assessment.[33] Change in an older adult's ability to function is often associated with significant change in general health, and has enormous implications for the achievement and maintenance of independence.[41,42]

Functional assessment is itself multifaceted. It explores physical and mental health, cognitive status, and social and economic resources. Examining older adults' ability to complete specific activities and tasks provides insight into their overall functional status.[43] Assessments are conducted serially over time, so changes in function can be noted.[42]

Activities of Daily Living

Activities of daily living (ADLs) are basic self-care activities. These activities include mobility, dressing, personal hygiene, eating, and continence. Older adults with deficits in these realms are unable to meet their most basic needs.[43] Older adults' ADL abilities are also important predictors of major events such as nursing home admission and mortality. For example, older people who become incontinent may face institutionalization;[44]

Table 2–6   Activities of Daily Living (ADLs) [33,43]

Mobility
Dressing
Personal hygiene
Eating
Toileting/continence

and refusal to eat may be a harbinger of death[45] (Table 2–6).

Instrumental Activities of Daily Living

Instrumental activities of daily living (IADLs) are the activities that contribute to independent functioning. IADLs require a higher level of physical and/or cognitive ability to complete than ADLs. IADLs include shopping, household maintenance, use of telephone and other appliances, paying bills, cooking, and washing laundry. Assessment of IADL ability yields information regarding an older person's ability to live and function independently[33,43] (see Table 2–7).

IADL Clinical Example   Changes in social situation may have critical implications for IADL ability and for overall functional status.[36] For example, an older man with no significant health problems may experience a sharp decrease in functional status when his wife dies. Although he is basically healthy, if he has never cooked or done housework, he may find these tasks difficult.

Table 2–7   Instrumental Activities of Daily Living (IADL)[33,43]

Shopping
Household maintenance
Using telephone
Paying bills/managing financial matters
Administering medications
Cooking
Laundry

External assistance, such as home health services, may be needed to maintain independence.

Advanced Activities of Daily Living

Advanced Activities of Daily Living (AADLs) are a more complex measure of functional status. AADLs include voluntary social, occupational, and recreational activities. Losing the ability to engage in these activities may signal a significant decline in an older adult's overall health[43] (see Table 2–8).

AADL Clinical Example   An older person who experiences functional decline related to decreased visual acuity may no longer be able to drive. Mobility is affected, along with the potential for travel to recreational activities. Increasingly, these needs, if met, require the intervention of formal or informal support services. In this case, maintenance of maximal function depends on continued participation in activities, despite a decline in vision and ability to drive.[46]

Standardized Assessment Tools

Assessment of functional status may be facilitated by standardized tools, which are particularly useful during the screening of older people who are frail or who have multiple interrelated problems. These tools have reasonable objectivity, employ a common language, and are useful when establishing baseline assessments. Over time, such tools can play an important role in detecting subtle alterations in function, tracking changes over time, and guiding interventions.[47]

A huge array of assessment tools exists. Instruments should be chosen with the purpose and time limitations of the assessment in mind, along with validity, reliability, and clinical rele-

Table 2–8   Advanced Activities of Daily Living (AADLs) [43]

Voluntary social activities
Occupational activities
Recreational activities

vance. Gender and cultural issues should also be considered[43,47] (see Table 2–9).

Standardized measures do not take the place of other, nonstandardized clinical assessments, which at times are more useful. For example, nurse prac-

titioners may make direct clinical observations that provide important information about an older adult's health and functional status. An approach utilizing both standard and other assessments is warranted.[48]

Table 2–9   Instruments Used to Assess Functional Status[47]

Assessing Physical Function	
Instrument	**Function Assessed**
Katz ADL Scale	Basic self-care
Barthel Index	Self-care and ambulation
Kenny Self-Care Scale	Self-care and ambulation
IADL Scale	Complex activities including food preparation, shopping, housekeeping
Timed Manual Performance	Timed assessment of performance of structured manual tasks
Performance Test of ADL	Self-care, mobility, and transfers
Framingham Disability Scale	Self-care and physical activities
Lawton Scale	IADL ability

Assessing Cognitive Function	
Instrument	**Function Assessed**
Short Portable Mental Status Questionnaire	Memory, attention, and orientation
Folstein Mini-Mental State Examination	Memory, orientation, attention, constructional ability
Wechsler Memory Scale	Broader categories of memory
Dementia Rating Scale	Memory and behavior
Short Care Scale	Cognitive impairment
CERAD battery of tests	Dementia

Assessing Emotional State	
Instrument	**Function Assessed**
Beck Depression Inventory	Symptoms of depression
Zung Self-Rating Depression Scale	Symptoms of depression
Hamilton Depression Inventory	Symptoms of depression
Center for Epidemiologic Studies Depression Scale	Symptoms of depression
Profile of Mood States	Broad array of mood states
Geriatric Depression Scale	Symptoms of depression
Short Care Scale	Symptoms of depression
Cornell Scale	Symptoms of depression

Atypical Presentation of Illness

It is often difficult to determine which aspects of disease presentation are due to age-related change and which result from pathology. In older adults, atypical symptoms are common and normal age-related changes may cloud disease presentation.[49]

Atypical Symptoms

Atypical presentation, rather than the classic signs and symptoms of a particular illness, is often the rule with older adults. Nonspecific, vague complaints may signify serious disease, and older adults may exhibit milder symptoms than younger people.[49] For example, older people with acute traumatic injuries, including perforated bowels, do not normally develop fevers and may report only mild pain.[50] The onset of these nonspecific symptoms may be less clear than in younger people, making diagnosis quite challenging.[51]

Older people may present with altered radiographic studies and laboratory values, which need to be interpreted in light of the aging process.[52] In addition, older people may underreport symptoms, or attribute serious symptoms to "old age."[49,53] Nurse practitioners must be alert for atypical presentations of common illnesses. The underlying problem must be identified and treated, if possible, because vague symptomatology is often associated with serious illness. In older people this includes cognitive changes, feelings of weakness or loss of appetite, loss of bladder control, and change in activity pattern[49,52] (see Table 2–10).

Case Study 1: Atypical Presentation of Pneumonia   A 72-year-old man presents with slight dyspnea at rest and during activity. His family reports a decrease in appetite and activity level. He is observed having a dry, nonproductive cough, but no discolored copious sputum. On examination, he is afebrile. Lung sounds are slightly diminished in one base, but not absent. Serum studies show no increase in white blood cell count and only a slight increase in erythrocyte sedimentation rate. Chest x-ray shows a bronchopneumatic pattern of consolidation. Despite its atypical presentation, this man has pneumonia and needs treatment.[49,50,52]

Case Study 2: Atypical Presentation of Myocardial Infarction   An 85-year-old woman presents with nonspecific symptoms, including a right frontal headache for the past 12 hours. The headache is rated 3 on a 0–10 pain scale, and has not been relieved with over-the-counter analgesics. The woman has a decreased appetite, but no nausea or vomiting. She feels generally weak, and has not participated in her normal activities today. She has no chest pain or shortness of breath. She looks pale. Oxygen saturation level is low, ECG shows ischemic changes, and cardiac enzyme serum studies confirm a diagnosis of myocardial infarction. Although her symptoms are vague, a life-threatening condition is present and requires immediate treatment.[49,51]

Case Study 3: Atypical Presentation of Severe Infection   An 82-year-old woman with no history of cognitive impairment presents with cellulitis on her lower left leg. She was seen scratching the area during the previous week, but did not seek medical care. Today she is brought by family members who have noted mental status changes and increasing lethargy. She is mumbling inco-

Table 2–10   Examples of Atypical Symptoms Reported by Older Adults[33,49]

Cognitive changes

Vague complaints (feelings of discomfort, not feeling well)

Feelings of weakness

Decreased or lost appetite

Recurrent falls

Change in activity pattern

Loss of bladder control

Change in ADL, IADL, AADL abilities

herently, occasionally crying out, and unable to answer questions correctly. She has a low-grade fever and slightly increased white blood cell count. Her lower left leg is reddened and swollen. Although her symptoms are atypical, she is presenting with a serious infection and delirium, and needs treatment. Intravenous antibiotics and fluids are started. Pain medication is also administered. Two days later, her mental status returns to baseline.[49,50,54]

 Understanding Age-Related Physiology

It is important to distinguish changes associated with normal aging from changes attributable to pathophysiology. The aging process results in observable and measurable molecular, cellular, organic, and systemic changes, so certain age-related changes are considered normal. Other changes, even those that may commonly occur among older people, are classified as pathological and abnormal. Older people who experience pathological symptoms require evaluation and treatment.[6,52]

Age-related changes have many clinical implications. A summary of these changes is presented in Table 2–11. Alterations in the structure and function of multiple body systems may affect an older person's appearance, mobility, and capacity to ward off infections.[50,55] In addition, changes in muscle mass and body fluid composition affect the disposition of medications.[56]

Table 2–11   Age-Related Alterations in Physiology

Dermatologic[52]		
Structural Change	**Functional Change**	**Clinical Implication**
Thinning of epidermis	Increased skin fragility Increased cell irregularity Decreased epidermal proliferation Decreased capacity for repair	Increased wrinkling Dry appearance Uneven pigmentation Susceptible to infection when break occurs
Thinning of dermis	Decreased collagen flexibility Changes in the elastic fiber network	Decreased elasticity Increased wrinkling Vulnerable to trauma Vulnerable to irritant dermatitis
Decrease in amount of subcutaneous fat		Sagging of skin Decreased fat pads on soles of feet, which may impair ambulation
Changes in adnexal structures	Decreased sebaceous gland activity Decreased eccrine gland function Decreased rate of nail growth Thinning of hair	Decreased sweating Decreased growth of hair Decreased nail growth Thinning and graying of hair Susceptibility to infection
Changes in neurosensory function	Increased threshold for pressure and touch Decreased vibratory sense in toes Decreased thermal sense	Potential for injury because of decreased sensation

(text continues on page 18)

Table 2–11   Age-Related Alterations in Physiology *(continued)*

Ocular[52]

Structure	Structural Change	Clinical Implication
Cornea	Increased translucency Flattening of curvature	Increased scattering of light rays, causing a blurring effect Increased refractive power
Choroid	Thickens Becomes less elastic	Decreased quality of image reaching retina, causing acuity changes
Iris	Becomes more rigid	Pupil size becomes less refractive to light Decreased ability to accommodate to different light intensities Decreased night vision acuity
Ciliary body	Decreased production of aqueous humor	Decreased nourishment and cleansing of lens and cornea Increased eye dryness Vulnerable to infection
Ciliary muscle	Decreased mass and size	May change flexibility of lens Can cause acuity changes Decreased peripheral vision Decreased accommodation
Retina	Decreased number of rods, cones, and ganglion cells	Change in visual acuity may occur Night vision is altered
Lens	Increased density Decreased elasticity Increased yellow pigmentation	Decreased accommodation Blurred vision Impaired color discrimination
Vitreous body	Liquefaction occurs	Floaters and light flashes possible

Auditory[52]

Structural Change	Clinical Implication
Tympanic membrane becomes thinner, less resilient, and may be affected by sclerotic changes	Possible impairment in auditory function
Ossicular chain may become calcified	Decreased sensitivity to high-frequency tones (presbycusis)
Pinna (external ear) becomes wider, longer, and less flexible	Changes in appearance of ear

Gustatory and Olfactory[52]

Change	Clinical Implication
Decreased salivation Decreased number of olfactory cells Decreased thirst	Decreased sensitivity to tastes Decreased sensitivity to smells May impair hydration and nutrition

Table 2–11   *(continued)*

Endocrine[52,57]	
Hormone	**Alteration**
Thyroxine (T_4)	Decreased secretion
Thyroid-stimulating hormone (TSH)	Secretion may decrease slightly, or may remain at previous levels
	Decreased response to thyrotropin-releasing hormone (TRH)
Insulin	Decreased secretion
	Adipocytes have decreased sensitivity to insulin
Renin	Decreased secretion
	Decreased response to adrenocorticotropic hormone (ACTH)
Aldosterone	Decreased secretion
	Decreased response to ACTH in presence of sodium restriction
	Vulnerability to extreme hypernatremia
Growth hormone	Decreased secretion
Glucocorticoid hormone	Clearance may be slightly decreased
Parathyroid hormone	Secretion slightly increased
Cortisol	Decreased responses to ACTH
Glucagon	No alteration
Decreased cellular response to many hormones	Laboratory values must be interpreted carefully
Decreased stress hormone secretion	Decreased response to stressors (internal and external)

Cardiovascular[51,52]	
Structural Change	**Functional Change**
Increased weight of heart and vessels	Decreased cardiac output at rest and exercise
	Decreased myocardial contractile efficiency
Increased left ventricular posterior wall thickness (not greater than upper limits of normal)	Increased systolic pressure
Decreased early diastolic closure rates of mitral valve	Increased left ventricular ejection time and pre-ejection period
Replacement of pacemaker cells by fibrous and connective tissue in SA and AV nodes	Decreased responsiveness to catecholamines
	Increased ectopic activity
Increased thickness of aorta and peripheral arteries (occurs independently of arteriosclerotic disease)	Decreased maximal oxygen uptake
Valves become more sclerotic	Increased stroke volume with progressive exercise
	May cause murmurs
	S_4 heart sound may be present
Decreased response to beta adrenergic stimulation	Decreased heart rate at rest and exercise
	Orthostatic blood pressure changes may occur

(continues)

Table 2–11   Age-Related Alterations in Physiology *(continued)*

Pulmonary[52]	
Structural Change	**Clinical Implication**
Enlargement of alveolar duct	Alteration in pulmonary function
Decreased elastic recoil	Decreased sensitivity to changes in levels of oxygen and carbon dioxide
Increased closing volume	Alteration in pulmonary function
Loss of cilia	Alteration in pulmonary function
Increased size and stiffening of trachea and central airways	Alteration in pulmonary function
Calcification of chest wall	Leads to loss of alveoli
Decreased cough reflex	Decreased ability to clear infections and environmental stimulants

Alteration in Pulmonary Function with Age[52]
Decrease in forced vital capacity
Increase in residual volume
Increase in functional residual capacity
Decrease in forced expiratory volume per second
Decrease in forced expiratory flow
Increase in residual volume / total lung capacity

Gastrointestinal[52]	
Alteration	**Clinical Implication**
Mouth: Decreased saliva	Decreased protection of teeth and tongue from bacteria Decreased taste sensation Difficulty talking and chewing
Stomach: Decreased gastric juice secretion, including decreased intrinsic factor, peptic, and hydrochloric acid Decreased gastric motility	Decreased vitamin B_{12} absorption Decreased protein digestion Decreased iron and folic acid digestion (may lead to anemia) Delayed emptying and maldigestion
Small intestine: Decreased mucosal surface area Changes in secretion of hydrochloric acid, peptin, and gastric juices	Decreased carbohydrate absorption Calcium malabsorption (may lead to osteoporosis) Decreased vitamin D absorption Impaired fat absorption

Table 2–11 *(continued)*

Colon:

Mucosal atrophy	Function remains intact
Atrophy of muscle layer	
Changes in mucosal glands	

Liver:

Decreased size	Decreased drug metabolism
Decreased activity of drug-metabolizing enzymes	Decreased hepatic protein synthesis
Increased size of hepatocytes with decreased proliferative activity	
Decreased splanchnic blood flow	

Pancreas:

Decreased number of secretory acini and islets of Langerhans	Decline in glucose tolerance (independent of diabetes)

Renal[52,67]

Structure	Structural Change	Manifestation
Glomeruli	Decreased number Increased surface area	Decreased filtration of blood Decreased glomerular filtration rate (GFR) by up to 30–40% May contribute to decreased clearance of medications
Tubules	Thickened membrane Fatty degeneration Shortening	Decreased tubule transport Decreased urine-concentrating capacity Decreased sodium conservation Decreased concentrating mechanism in Henle's loop Decreased renal acidification
Renal vasculature	Stiffening Narrowing	Decreased blood flow Decreased efficiency in removal of waste products
Connective tissue	Decreased expandability and compressibility of bladder Decreased sensation	Decreased bladder capacity Increased residual urine volume after voiding

Musculoskeletal[52]

Age-Related Change	Clinical Implication
Decreased bone volume	Increased incidence of microfractures (especially hip, wrist, forearm, and vertebrae) Causes balance and gait problems
Decreased size, number of muscle fibers Lean body mass replaced by fat	Decreased lean body mass Decreased total body water Impaired ability to compensate for fluid and electrolyte changes

Table 2–12   Laboratory Values that Do Not Change with Normal Aging

Value	Implication
Red blood cell (RBC) Hemoglobin Hematocrit	Anemia is not normal in older adults.[60]
Blood urea nitrogen (BUN) Creatinine	These measures of renal function do not generally change, although renal function does change with aging. These measures are generally not an accurate reflection of renal function. Individualized estimates of creatinine clearance are more accurate.[67]
Liver function tests	Generally do not change, although total protein may decrease slightly.[66]
Thyroxine (T_4)	Thyroxine levels do not generally change with aging, despite decreasing production of thyroid hormone. The interaction between T_4, T_3, and TSH should be evaluated.

Interpretation of Laboratory Values

Interpretation of laboratory data in older adults requires careful consideration. Abnormal values may either signify normal age-related physiologic changes or reflect illness.[57] Lab values may also be affected by medication and disease. Furthermore, values in older adults commonly differ from normal ranges, and there is scant information about age-related standard values.[58,59] Age-adjusted confidence intervals or reference ranges may be helpful, and each clinical situation should be considered individually.[58]

Certain abnormal values suggest underlying pathology. Attributing these values to aging alone could lead to misdiagnosis and undertreatment.[58] For example, the lab values associated with anemia, although common among older people, are not normal in older adults, and such findings

require thorough investigation and treatment when discovered.[60] Table 2–12 lists the laboratory values that do not change with normal aging.

On the other hand, some laboratory values consistently fall outside normal ranges and do not necessarily reflect disease in older people. Hyperglycemia, for example, may frequently occur as a result of normal age-related endocrine changes. Understanding age-related changes helps clinicians avoid overtreating patients in similar situations.[61] Table 2–13 reviews the lab values that commonly change with normal aging.

Still other laboratory results are more equivocal. Older adults' abnormal levels need to be evaluated thoroughly and carefully, and their relationship to the clinical situation determined. Elevation in erythrocyte sedimentation rate (ESR) level, for example, may be considered pathological

Table 2–13   Laboratory Values that Change with Normal Aging

Laboratory Value	Age-Related Change
Glucose	Slight increase[61]
Creatinine clearance	Decreased
Serum uric acid	Slight increase[67]
Lactic dehydrogenase (LDH)	No change or slight increase
Alkaline phosphatase	Gradual increase
Total protein	No change or slight decrease[66]
Total cholesterol	Slight increase or decrease possible
Low-density lipoproteins (LDL)	Increased
High-density lipoproteins (HDL)	Slight increase or decrease possible
Triglycerides	Slight increase[57]
Triiodothyronine (T_3) thyroid hormone	Decreased
Thyroid stimulating hormone (TSH)	No change or slight increase[57]

in a patient with other symptoms of disease, but reflect normal age-related changes in an older person without additional clinical findings.[59]

Medication Management

Nurse practitioners should provide meticulous medication management to minimize drug-related problems in this vulnerable population.[62,63] Older adults, who take more medications than any other group, are at high risk for drug-related problems and toxicities. Older people receive nearly 40% of all prescriptions written in the United States each year,[56] which is about three times the number dispensed to younger patients.[64] At the same time, older people are very susceptible to adverse drug reactions (ADRs).[63]

Polypharmacy

Polypharmacy, the simultaneous use of multiple medications, can cause a variety of ADRs and deleterious drug interactions in older people. Primary drug reactions occur when one drug causes one side effect; secondary drug reactions occur when one medication interacts with another. Secondary reactions often result in potentiation of drugs, which can lead to serious toxicities. Additional ADRs, involving drug–drug and drug–nutrient interactions, may also occur.[65]

Polypharmacy is prevalent in this group. Older individuals receive an average of 13 to 15 prescriptions per year and take an average of 4.5 prescription medications per day.[62] These medicines, which can be essential parts of the treatment of complex acute and chronic illnesses,[64] are often prescribed by multiple providers.[56] Plus, nearly 90% of older adults take over-the-counter medications, at least intermittently.[6] Nurse practitioners can facilitate safe medication management by coordinating care.[62]

Changes in Drug Disposition

Changes in drug disposition, which are associated with both age-related changes and disease states,

can significantly affect drug levels and dosages.[63] These changes can affect the pharmacokinetics and pharmacodynamics associated with many drugs.[65] Drug dosages often need to be adjusted and levels watched closely in light of these changes.[63]

Pharmacokinetic changes, including altered absorption, distribution, metabolism, and excretion of medications, have important clinical implications.[56] Absorption of medications generally is unimpaired in older adults, but may be affected by gastrointestinal disorders or the effects of polypharmacy. Drug distribution is usually altered in older people because of characteristic age-related decreases in lean muscle mass and increases in body fat.[65] Metabolism of many medications is affected by age-related hepatic changes.[66] Excretion can be affected by changes in renal function, including glomerular filtration rate decreases of at least 30% by age 70.[67] Pharmocokinetic changes may result in concomitant changes in the metabolism of drugs in older adults. Smaller doses given to older people may achieve results comparable to larger doses for younger adults.[62,63]

Alterations in pharmacodynamics, drug actions, and side effects, are also noteworthy.[63] Pharmacodynamics can be affected by age-related changes, disease states, alcohol use, or other medications.[56] These changes can be especially significant, and may cause harm in older adults taking multiple medications for concomitant illnesses.[63] Changes in pharmacodynamics explain why normal serum drug levels (calculated using young, healthy adults) are often inaccurate predictors of the amount of active drug available in older people.[62]

Drug levels may also be clouded by age-related alterations in serum creatinine levels. Serum creatinine, which tends to increase as muscle mass decreases, both interferes with drug metabolism and leads to inaccuracies of drug levels. The levels are most often inaccurate when drugs are renally excreted and when excretion is affected by concomitant medications or illnesses.[62] Nurse practitioners can utilize an estimated creatinine clearance, taking body mass and age into account, while interpreting such levels.[67] The formula for this is presented in Table 2–14.

Table 2–14   Formula for Estimated Creatinine Clearance in Older Adults[67]

$$\text{creatinine clearance (ml/min)} = \frac{(140 - \text{age in years}) \times (\text{body weight in kg})}{72 \times (\text{serum creatinine, mg/dL})}$$

For women, the calculated value is multiplied by 0.85

Case Study 1: Fall and Hip Fracture Secondary to a Drug Reaction   An 85-year-old woman with heart failure and hypertension takes two daily medications: an anticholinesterase inhibitor and a potassium-sparing diuretic. She has a stable course until she experiences lower-extremity edema and shortness of breath. She calls her health-care provider and a loop diuretic is prescribed. That night, she takes both diuretics at bedtime. She wakes in the middle of the night to urinate, falls on the way to the bathroom, and breaks her hip. This fall and fracture are adverse drug reactions related to the double dose of diuretic at bedtime.[65]

Case Study 2: Drug Toxicity with Normal Serum Drug Level   A 75-year-old man is treated with digoxin and serum digoxin levels are maintained at the high end of normal. Following complaints of nausea, he is sent by his primary physician to a gastroenterologist, who orders multiple diagnostic tests. The results are unremarkable; however, two weeks later, the man is admitted to the hospital after he begins vomiting every few hours. At this point, the digoxin level is dangerously high, and there is some evidence to support that earlier serum drug levels were inaccurate.[68] In this case, as with many other older adults on medications where even subtle changes in serum levels merit careful observation, more frequent monitoring and assessment could have avoided this adverse drug reaction.[62]

Medication Management

The first step in medication management is comprehensive assessment of all drugs, both prescription and over-the-counter, for purpose, effect, dose, level, and potential interactions. Unnecessary drugs should be discontinued and inappropriate dosages adjusted, yielding regimens and dosing schedules that are as simple as possible.[56]

Medication dosages should be carefully contemplated, because dosages for older adults may differ markedly from those used in the general adult population. While relatively little clinical data is available concerning optimal dosages for older adults on specific medications,[69] it is clear that, for most medications, a small starting dose and slow dose increase is appropriate.[62] Older people require close observation when medications or dosages are adjusted because responses to such adjustments are often unpredictable.[69]

Newer drugs should not replace established therapies in older adults unless the older treatments are ineffective. These newer medications are usually tested on younger people and appropriate dosages for older adults are not readily established. The potential for unforeseen side effects or medication interactions with these newer drugs can make them quite dangerous for older people.[6]

Nurse practitioners should therefore use a cautious approach when prescribing medications to older people.[63] Table 2–15 provides recommendations for successful medication prescription and management.

 Health Promotion and Disease Prevention

Health promotion and disease prevention are critical components of the care of older adults. Goals include both preventing disease and delaying morbidity if disease occurs. Preventive care is also relevant in the presence of chronic disease, where goals include enhancing functional capacity and optimizing quality of life.[12]

Notably, although at least half of all older adults report at least one chronic illness, approximately three-quarters of older people rate their

Table 2–15 Basic Tenets of Prescribing Drugs to Older Adults

1. **Evaluate the need for drug therapy.** Avoid drugs if at all possible, but use drugs if they would enhance quality of life.[64]
2. **Remember that drugs may cause illness.**[65]
3. **Conduct careful history of medication use and personal habits.** Know that patients may be receiving prescriptions from several providers. Be aware of the effects of smoking, alcohol, and caffeine on the response of specific drugs.[33]
4. **Know the pharmacology of the drugs prescribed.** Use a few drugs well, rather than many drugs poorly. Maintain an awareness of age-related alterations in drug disposition and drug response.[56]
5. **Prescribe smaller doses for older people.** Remember that the "standard" dose is often too large for older people. Also know that hepatic metabolism of drugs may be unpredictable and that renal excretion of drugs and metabolites declines with age.[63]
6. **Titrate slowly and carefully.** Titrate drug dosage on the basis of the patient's response. [63]
7. **Avoid newly approved medications.** New drugs may pose significant risks for older people, who are not necessarily included in clinical trials. Newer drugs may have unexpected toxicities, which may have disastrous effects on older people. Only use newer medications after more standard drugs have been tried and failed.[6]
8. **Simplify therapeutic regimen and encourage adherence.**
   - avoid intermittent schedules
   - select simplest dosage form[64]
   - ensure that drug containers are clearly labeled
   - give careful instructions
   - utilize assistive devices if appropriate. These can include medication calendar, diary, and pillboxes.[56]
9. **Review medication regimen regularly.** [63]
10. **Discontinue drugs when they are no longer necessary.**[63]
11. **Encourage the destruction of expired or discontinued medications.**[56]

Health Promotion   Health-promotion activities are appropriate for older people with or without disease. Activities such as improving nutrition, cessation of smoking, and exercising regularly, can decrease symptom intensity in certain diseases.[13] For example, the effects of hypertension, a chronic disease, can be reduced with a limitation of sodium intake.[70] For people without disease, health-promotion activities can both counteract age-related changes and prevent illnesses.[71]

Focus on Function   Interventions geared toward maintaining or improving functional abilities are important because decreased function has detrimental consequences. Older adults are said to become frail when they experience declines in function, specifically in strength, endurance, balance, and mobility.[72] Older people may experience falls, injuries, diminished independence, and may even face institutionalization when increases in frailty occur.[41,72] Optimizing function, then, is a major goal of care.[73]

Physical Activity   Regular exercise has many benefits for older people, including reducing cardiovascular disease, reducing or preventing obesity, reducing the risk of osteoporosis, controlling stress, and lessening depression. Sedentary lifestyles, on the other hand, have been associated with early mortality.[74] Notably, older adults who engage in less activity become deconditioned and are often less able to remain active (leading to the often-quoted statement "if you don't use it, you'll lose it").[72]

Nurse practitioners can assess older individuals' physical abilities and then help design appropriate activity programs. Supervised activity programs, consisting of some combination of strength, balance, and endurance training, are beneficial in many older people. Other individualized regimens, including targeted exercises to prevent falls, can also be valuable. Clearly, programs are most effective when they consist of activities that older individuals find enjoyable.[72]

Nutrition Issues   Health promotion also includes screening older adults' nutritional status.[13] Nutritional excesses, deficits, and imbalances may

health as "good."[14] Disease itself does not appear to determine health rating, especially if function is intact and disability minimized.[12]

Table 2–16   Factors that Determine Nutritional Health in Older Adults[75]

Disease

Eating difficulty

Tooth loss/mouth pain

Economic hardship

Reduced social contact

Multiple medicines

Involuntary weight loss or gain

Needs assistance with self-care

Age above 80 (because this may be associated with increased fraility)

be caused by diseases or medications; the presence of physical disabilities or difficulty tasting, chewing, or swallowing food; social isolation; or poverty.[33,75] These problems are especially common with cognitive impairment.[45,76] Table 2–16 provides a list of factors that can affect older adults' nutrition.

Nurse practitioners work with an interdisciplinary team, particularly with nutritionists and dietitians, to address these issues.[75] Individualized plans for dietary modification[70] or nutritional rehabilitation can be implemented,[45] for example, decreasing consumption of saturated fats.[70] In cases where older adults become malnourished related to a refusal to eat, food substitutions or other interventions can be instituted.[45]

Disease Prevention

Disease prevention is particularly germane to the older adult population. Prevention activities, which are divided into primary, secondary, and tertiary levels, are aimed at reducing premature morbidity and mortality. Among older adults, where presence of disease can herald functional decline, prevention of disease can limit associated decreases in independence and quality of life.[77,78]

Primary prevention focuses on the identification and possible reversal of risk factors for disease. Activities of this type are implemented for individuals who are asymptomatic and free of clinical evidence of the targeted disease. Primary preventive activities include immunizations, smok-

Table 2–17   Disease Prevention Activities in Older Adults[79]

Primary Prevention
Update immunizations (e.g., yearly flu shot)
Encourage chemoprophylaxis (e.g., aspirin for heart disease, estrogen replacement therapy for osteoporosis)
Encourage smoking cessation
Address alcohol use or abuse
Maintain adequate nutrition
Encourage exercise
Advise on use of sunscreen
Review safety factors to prevent accidents (including accidental burns)
Encourage safe driving (wear seatbelts, test vision and hearing periodically, advise additional evaluation for people with cognitive impairment)
Encourage good dental health
Review all prescription and nonprescription medications periodically and carefully
Secondary Prevention
Targeted Screening for:
Hypertension
Cancer (breast, colon, prostate, cervical)
Obesity or undernourishment
Diabetes mellitus
Thyroid disease
Hearing and visual impairment
Tertiary Prevention
Screening for :
Early dementia
Depression
Urinary incontinence
Other illnesses (common to older people but often overlooked)

ing cessation, improved nutrition, physical activity, skin protection, and safety.[12]

Secondary prevention activities, focusing on early disease detection and intervention, minimize the impact of preexisting disease. These activities can include checking for early signs of disease in asymptomatic people, as well as identifying and treating the presence of certain disease-specific modifiable risk factors.[71] Secondary prevention activities include blood pressure screening, cancer screening (particularly for breast, colon, prostate, and cervical cancers), management of obesity, identification and treatment of diabetes and thyroid disease, and screening for visual and hearing impairment.[12,79]

Tertiary prevention focuses on reducing the discomfort or disability caused by disease. It aims both to limit the progression of disease and to maximize function.[71] Even in irreversible disease states, prevention activities may be useful, for example, the benefits of exercise for persons with dementia.[72]

Specific disease prevention guidelines are provided by the U.S. Preventive Services Task Force (USPSTF).[79] This information is quite useful, but more research is needed into the timing and efficacy of specific prevention activities in this population.[80] Disease-prevention activities are reviewed in Table 2–17.

Conclusion

Every man desires to live long; but no man would be old.[81]

These words, written by 18th-century satirist Jonathan Swift, reflect the principles discussed in this chapter. Gerontological nurse practitioners are dedicated to the assessment, management, and maintenance of older adults in situations and circumstances that support the highest standards of clinical practice and environments dedicated to quality of life. This is echoed throughout this book.

The principles presented here help guide the care of older adults. Individualized, interdisciplinary, coordinated assessments and interventions yield much more than longer lives. Such care and consideration also adds, we hope, to a better life.

References

1. Burns-Tisdale S, Goff W. The geriatric nurse practitioner in home care: challenges, stressors, and rewards. *Nurs Clin N Am.* 1989;24(3):809–817.
2. Ruiz BA, Tabloski PA, Frazier SM. The role of gerontological nurse practitioners in geriatric care. *J Am Geriatr Soc.* 1995;43(9):1061–1064.
3. Strumpf N. Innovative gerontological practices as models for health care delivery. *Nurs Health Care.* 1994;15(10):522–527.
4. American Nurses Association. *Scope and Standards of Gerontological Clinical Nursing Practice.* Washington DC: American Nurses Association, 1995.
5. American Medical Association Council on Scientific Affairs. American Medical Association white paper on elderly health. *Arch Intern Med.* 1990;150:2459–2472.
6. Finucane TE. Geriatric medicine: special considerations. In: Barker LR, Burton JR, Zieve PD, eds. *Principles of Ambulatory Medicine.* 4th ed. Baltimore: Wilkins and Wilkins; 1994:82–98.
7. Kane RL, Garrard J, Skay CL, et al. Effects of a geriatric nurse practitioner on process and outcome of nursing home care. *Am J Public Health.* 1989;79(9):1271–1277.
8. Desai MM, Zhang P, Hennessy CH. Surveillance for morbidity and mortality among older adults—United States, 1995–1996. *MMWR Morb Mortal Wkly Rep.* 1999;48(SS-8):7–25.
9. US Bureau of the Census. Demographic data. 2000. Available at: www.census.gov.
10. Blackman DK, Kamimoto LA, Smith SM. Overview: surveillance for selected public health indicators affecting older adults—United States. *MMWR Morb Mortal Wkly Rep.* 1999;48(SS-8):1–6.
11. US Bureau of the Census: *Sixty-Five Plus in the United States.* Washington DC: US Department of Commerce; 1995.
12. Scheitel SM, Fleming KC, Chutka DS, et al. Geriatric health maintenance. *Mayo Clinic Proceedings.* 1996;71:289–302.
13. Janes GR, Blackman DK, Bolen JC, et al. Surveillance for use of preventive health care services by older adults. *MMWR Morb Mortal Wkly Rep.* 1999;48(SS-8):51–88.
14. Campbell VA, Crews JE, Moriarty DG, et al. Surveillance for sensory impairment, activity limitation, and health-related quality of life among older adults—United States, 1993–1997. *MMWR Morb Mortal Wkly Rep.* 1999;48(SS-8):131–156.
15. Faison KJ, Faria SH, Frank D. Caregivers of chronically ill elderly: perceived burden. *J Comm Health Nurs.* 1999;16(4):243–253.
16. Germain CP. Cultural care: a bridge between sickness, illness, and disease. *Holistic Nurs Pract.* 1992;6(3):1–9.
17. Lavizzo-Mourey RJ, Mackenzie E. Cultural competence: an essential hybrid for delivering high

quality care in the 1990s and beyond. *Trans Am Clin Climatol Assoc.* 1995;107:226–235.

18. Outlaw FH. A reformation of the meaning of culture and ethnicity for nurses delivering care. *Medsurg Nurs.* 1994;3(2):108–111.

19. Boult L, Boult C. Underuse of physician services by older Asian-Americans. *J Am Geriatr Soc.* 1995; 43(4):408–411.

20. Brangman SA. African-American elders: implications for health care providers. *Clin Geriatr Med.* 1995; 11(1):15–23.

21. Funkhouser SW, Moser DK. Is health care racist? *Adv Nurs Sci.* 1990;12(2):47–55.

22. Pousada L. Hispanic-American elders: implications for health care providers. *Clin Geriatr Med.* 1995; 11(1):39–51.

23. Perkins K. Recycling poverty: from the workplace to retirement. *J Women Aging.* 1993;5(1):5–23.

24. Beckel J. Resolving ethical problems in long-term care. *J Gerontol Nurs.* 1996;22(1):20–26.

25. Rice VH, Beck C, Stevenson JS. Ethical issues relative to autonomy and personal control in independent and cognitively impaired elders. *Nurs Outlook.* 1997;45(1):27–34.

26. American Nurses Association. *Code for Nurses with Interpretative Statements.* Washington DC: American Nurses Publishing; 1995.

27. American Geriatrics Society Ethics Committee. Rational allocation of medical care: a position statement from the American Geriatrics Society. *J Am Geriatr Soc.* 1997;45(7):884–885.

28. Johns JL. Advanced directives and opportunities for nurses. *Image: J Nurs Scholarship.* 1996;28(2):149–153.

29. Mezey M, Bottrell MM, Ramsey G. Advanced directives protocol: nurses helping to protect patient's rights. *Geriatr Nurs.* 1996;17(5):204–210.

30. Mezey M, Mitty E, Rappaport M, et al. Implementation of the Patient Self-Determination Act (PSDA) in nursing homes in New York City. *J Am Geriatr Soc.* 1997;45(1):45–49.

31. American Geriatrics Society Ethics Committee. Making treatment decisions for incapacitated older adults without advanced directives. *J Am Geriatr Soc.* 1996;44(8):986–987.

32. American Nurses Association Center for Ethics and Human Rights Task Force on the Nurse's Role in End-of-Life Decisions. *Compendium of Position Statements on the Nurse's Role in End-of-Life Decisions.* Washington DC: American Nurses Publishing; 1992.

33. Palmer RM. Geriatric assessment. *Med Clin N Am.* 1999;83(6):1503–1523.

34. Rubenstein LZ. An overview of comprehensive geriatric assessment: rationale, history, program models, basic components. In: Rubenstein LZ, Weiland D, Bernabei R, eds. *Geriatric Assessment Technology: The State of the Art.* New York: Springer Publishing; 1995:1–9.

35. Mezey MD, Rauckhorst LH, Stokes SA. Interviewing for the health history. In: Mezey MD, Rauckhorst LH, Stokes SA. *Health Assessment of the Older Individual.* 2nd ed. New York: Springer Publishing; 1993:15–30.

36. Kane RA. Assessment of social functioning: recommendations for comprehensive geriatric assessment. In: Rubenstein LZ, Weiland D, Bernabei R, eds. *Geriatric Assessment Technology: The State of the Art.* New York: Springer Publishing; 1995:91–110.

37. Medeiros MM, Ferraz MB. Quaresma MR: The effect of rheumatoid arthritis on the quality of life of primary caregivers. *J Rheumatol.* 2000;27(1):76–83.

38. Lachs MS, Pillemer K. Abuse and neglect of elderly persons. *N Engl J Med.* 1995;332:437–443.

39. Happ MB, Williams CC, Strumpf NE, et al. Individualized care for frail elders: theory and practice. *J Gerontol Nurs.* 1996;22(3):6–14.

40. Evans LK. Knowing the patient: the route to individualized care. *J Gerontol Nurs.* 1996;22(3):15–19.

41. Tinetti ME, Williams CS. Falls, injuries due to falls, and the risk of admission to a nursing home. *N Engl J Med.* 1997;337(18):1279–1284.

42. Wolinsky FD, Stump TE, Callahan CM, et al. Consistency and change in functional status among older adults over time. *J Aging Health.* 1996;8(2):155–182.

43. Hedrick SC. Assessment of functional status: activities of daily living. In: Rubenstein LZ, Weiland D, Bernabei R, eds. *Geriatric Assessment Technology: The State of the Art.* New York: Springer Publishing; 1995:51–58.

44. Cohen CA, Gold DP, Shulman KI, et al. Factors determining the decision to institutionalize dementing individuals: a prospective study. *Gerontologist* 1993;33(6):714–720.

45. Marcus EL, Berry EM. Refusal to eat in the elderly. *Nutr Rev.* 1998;56(6):163–171.

46. Burke M. Motor vehicle injury prevention for older adults. *Nurse Pract.* 1994;19(2):26–28.

47. Applegate WB, Blass JP, Williams TF. Instruments for the functional assessment of older patients. *N Engl J Med.* 1990;322(17):1207–1214.

48. Mezey MD, Rauckhorst LH, Stokes SA. Functional assessment. In: Mezey MD, Rauckhorst LH, Stokes SA. *Health Assessment of the Older Individual.* 2nd ed. New York: Springer Publishing; 1993:31–45.

49. Sexton RC. Unusual manifestations of disease in the aged. *Tenn Med.* 1998;Feb:61–64.

50. Frankenfield D, Cooney RN, Smith JS, et al. Age-related differences in the metabolic response to injury. *J Trauma.* 2000;48(1):49–57.

51. Wei JY. Age and the cardiovascular system. *N Engl J Med.* 1992;327(24):1735–1739.

52. Blair KA. Aging: physiological aspects and clinical implications. *Nurse Pract.* 1990:15(2):14–28.

53. Williamson JD, Fried LP. Characterization of older adults who attribute functional detriments to "old age." *J Am Geriatr Soc.* 1996;44(12):1429–1434.

54. Cole MG, Primeau FJ, Elie LM. Delirium: prevention, treatment, and outcome studies. *J Geriatr Psych Neurol.* 1998;11:126–137.

55. Mezey MD, Rauckhorst LH, Stokes SA. Assessment of general appearance, skin, hair, feet, nails, and endocrine status. In: Mezey MD, Rauckhorst LH, Stokes SA. *Health Assessment of the Older Individual.* 2nd ed. New York: Springer Publishing; 1993:46–59.

56. Walker MK, Foreman MD. Medication safety: a protocol for nursing action. *Geriatr Nurs.* 1999; 20(1):34–39.

57. Perry HM. The endocrinology of aging. *Clin Chem.* 1999;45(8):1369–1376.

58. Melillo KD. Interpretation of laboratory values in older adults. *Nurse Pract.* 1993;18(7):59–66.

59. Mezey MD, Rauckhorst LH, Stokes SA. Changes in laboratory values and their implications. In: Mezey MD, Rauckhorst LH, Stokes SA. *Health Assessment of the Older Individual.* 2nd ed. New York: Springer Publishing, 1993:207–231.

60. Izaks GJ, Westendorp RG, Knook DL. The definition of anemia in older persons. *JAMA* 1999;281(18): 1714–1717.

61. Morley JE. An overview of diabetes mellitus in older persons. *Clin Geriatr Med.* 1999;15(2):211–224.

62. French DG. Avoiding adverse drug reactions in the elderly patient: issues and strategies. *Nurse Pract.* 1996;21(9):90–105.

63. Hughes SG. Prescribing for the elderly patient: why do we need to exercise caution? *Br J Clin Pharmacol.* 1998;46:531–533.

64. Monane M, Monane S, Semla T. Optimal medication use in elders: key to successful aging. *West J Med.* 1997;167(4):233–237.

65. Bradway CW. Adverse drug reactions and drug toxicities. In: Bradway CB, ed. *Nursing Care of Geriatric Emergencies.* New York: Springer Publishing; 1996:130–153.

66. LeCouteur DG, McLean AJ. The aging liver: drug clearance and an oxygen diffusion barrier hypothesis. *Clin Pharmacokinet.* 1998;34(5):359–373.

67. Beck LH. Changes in renal function with aging. *Clin Geriatr Med.* 1998;14(2):199–209.

68. Gosselink AT, van Veldhuisen DJ, Crijns HJ. When,

and when not, to use digoxin in the elderly. *Drugs Aging.* 1997;10(6):411–420.

69. Turnheim K. Drug dosage in the elderly. *Drugs Aging.* 1998;13(5):357–379.

70. Whelton PK, Appel LJ, Espeland MA, et al. Sodium reduction and weight loss in the treatment of hypertension in older persons: a randomized controlled trial of nonpharmacologic interventions in the elderly. *JAMA* 1998;279(11):839–846.

71. Koltoff-Burrell E. Health promotion and disease prevention for the older adult: an overview of the current recommendations and a practical application. *Nurse Pract For.* 1992;3(4):195–209.

72. Chandler JM, Hadley EC. Exercise to improve physiologic and functional performance in old age. *Clin Geriatr Med.* 1996;12(4):761–784.

73. Wagner EH. Preventing decline in function: evidence from randomized trials around the world. *West J Med.* 1997;167(4):295–298.

74. Allison M, Keller C. Physical activity in the elderly: benefits and intervention strategies. *Nurs Pract.* 1997; 22(8):53–69.

75. Lipschitz DA, Ham RJ, White JV. An approach to nutrition screening for older Americans. *Am Fam Phys.* 1992;45(2):601–608.

76. Riviere S, Gillette-Guyonnet S, Nourhashemi F, et al. Nutrition and Alzheimer's disease. *Nutr Rev.* 1999; 57(12):363–367.

77. Applegate B, Pahor M. Geriatric medicine. *J Am Med Assoc.* 1997;277(23):1863–1864.

78. Hazzard WR. Ways to make "usual" and "successful" aging synonymous: preventive gerontology. *West J Med.* 1997;167(4):206–215.

79. US Public Health Service Office of Disease Prevention and Health Promotion: *The Clinician's Handbook of Preventive Services: Put Prevention into Practice.* 2nd ed. Alexandria, International Medical Publishing, Inc., 1998.

80. Goldberg TH, Chavin SI. Preventive medicine and screening in older adults. *J Am Geriatr Soc.* 1997; 45(3):344–354.

81. Swift J. Thoughts on various subjects. In: Ross A, Wooley D, eds. *Jonathan Swift.* New York: Oxford University Press; 1984:182.

PART 2

Evaluation and Management of Disease and Illness

3

Cardiovascular Disease in Older Adults

Kathleen C. Tully

Introduction

Despite recent advances in the field, and a declining death rate in older adults, cardiovascular disease continues to be the leading cause of morbidity and mortality in this population.[1,2,3] Because those 65 and older represent the fastest growing segment of the population, this presents a significant health problem. Nurse practitioners, in all settings, need to understand the significance of cardiovascular disease and be prepared to assess quickly and to treat appropriately those who present with symptoms. Since older adults often present with atypical symptoms of cardiovascular disease, they represent a unique challenge to the nurse practitioner.

Like their younger counterparts, older adults can experience a variety of cardiovascular disorders. Those disorders, commonly encountered in primary care and long-term care settings, are presented here. Hypertension, coronary artery disease, heart failure, and dysrhythmias are discussed in this chapter. For each disorder, problem definition, significance in the older population, and relevant pathophysiology are reviewed. Clinical presentations, including common atypical presentations, are discussed. A format for history taking and physical examination specific to the identification of cardiovascular disease is suggested. Differential diagnoses, diagnostic tests, and nursing and medical interventions are included for each entity.

Overview

Prevalence and Significance

Cardiovascular disease is present in 50% of the population over the age of 65 and it accounts for 40% of the mortality in this group.[4] Clearly, with the aging of America, cardiovascular disease will continue to be a major health problem into the 21st century.

All body organs and tissues are dependent on the cardiovascular system in order to maintain function. Any disruption in this system can have serious consequences for the individual. Because of the changes associated with normal aging, and some of the unique aspects of reporting and presentation in older adults, underestimation of the seriousness of cardiac disease often occurs. This can lead to misdiagnosis, undertreatment, and devastating consequences.

Increased Longevity and Cardiovascular Disease

While support can be found in the literature for the origins of cardiovascular disease early in life, the incidence increases with aging. Greater life expectancy has increased the likelihood of cardiovascular disease.

Pathophysiology of Cardiovascular Disease

Atherosclerosis and Arteriosclerosis

Cardiovascular disease is most commonly caused by a disruption in circulation, secondary to decreased vessel patency. Vessel patency may be compromised by a variety of factors including constriction, spasm, and occlusion. Arteriosclerosis and/or atherosclerosis is often the underlying pathology for diminished vessel patency.

Arteriosclerosis is a disease of the arteries characterized by abnormal thickening and hardening of vessel walls, resulting in loss of elasticity. Atherosclerosis is a disease of the arterial intima involving both atherosis and sclerosis. Atherosis is defined as soft fatty deposits on the arterial lining. Atherosclerosis is atherosis, accompanied by hardening and the presence of collagenous material on the intima.

Atherosclerosis is an insidious process that begins early in life. Atherosclerotic lesions are initiated by endothelial injury, which is then fol-

Table 3–1 Progression of Atherosclerotic Lesions[5]

Phase	Process
I	Lipid accumulation in atherosclerotic plaque
	Macrophage formation from monocytes
	Uptake of LDL by macrophages which then form foam cells
	Development of fatty streaks
	Proliferation of smooth muscle cells which produce collagens, elastins, and proteoglycans to form extracellular matrix
II	Plaque formation from:
	Accumulation of lipids on intima from:
	macrophage rupture
	debris from cell death
	Thin fibrous cap covers lipid accumulation
	Localized inflammatory process causes plaque to become unstable
	Foam cells release free radicals, proteolytic enzymes, and products of lipid oxidation
	Plaque ruptures
III	Platelet and coagulation activation secondary to intimal injury
	Thrombus formation which further develops into atheromatous lesion, or thrombus may rupture
IV	Ruptured plaque resealed by thrombus, increasing size of lesion
V	Formation of advanced sclerotic plaque consisting of collagen scar tissue

lowed by lipid infiltration and smooth muscle proliferation. Several mechanisms have been implicated in vessel-wall injury. Changing patterns of blood flow at areas of vessel branching and bending, vessel-wall stress associated with hypertension, or abnormal vasomotion related to increased levels of low-density lipoprotein (LDL) all may alter endothelial cells. These alterations increase cell permeability for lipoprotein particles. Increased cholesterol levels appear to stimulate endothelial production of oxygen-free radicals that participate in the oxidation of LDL, further increasing abnormal vasomotion. Likewise, diabetes, tobacco smoke, circulating vasoactive substances, immune responses, and certain infections are also implicated in intimal injury. Once intimal injury occurs, the progression of atherosclerotic lesions occurs during a five-phase process (Table 3–1).

Atherosclerotic disease is the major cause of cardiovascular disease in persons over the age of 65. This condition is highly influenced by lifestyle and may be partially reversed by changes in that lifestyle. For a variety of reasons, many older adults have not made these changes and thus atherosclerotic coronary vessels, resulting in cardiovascular disease, contribute to the high incidence of morbidity and mortality in the older population.[5]

Myocardial Injury and Necrosis

When coronary-artery blood flow is compromised, the myocardium is at risk for ischemia and necrosis. Angina and myocardial infarction may be the result. Myocardial contractility is impaired by ischemia, while necrotic myocardium loses its ability to contract. If the area of necrosis is large, and contractility is severely impaired, heart failure will likely occur. In addition, ischemic myocardium can become irritable and produce cardiac dysrhythmias. Dysrhythmias may also result from scar tissue that forms around necrotic myocardium.

Cardiovascular Changes of Aging

The cardiovascular changes of normal aging (Table 3–2) may also contribute to a high rate of cardiovascular disease in older adults. The athero-

Table 3–2   Cardiovascular Changes of Normal Aging

↑ Incidence of atherosclerosis and ↑ stiffness of the aorta and arteries resulting in:

   ↑ SVR/afterload

   ↑ Systolic blood pressure

   Left ventricular hypertrophy

   ↓ Baroreceptor sensitivity

Sclerosis of the fibrous skeleton/areas of calcification resulting in:

   Valvular dysfunction

   Conduction abnormalities

Altered cardiac output secondary to:

   ↓ Diastolic filling → ↓ preload

   ↓ Response to sympathetic stimulation

      ↓ Myocardial contractility

      ↓ Heart rate

↓ Secretion of neurohormones (renin, angiotensin II, vasopressin, & aldosterone)

   Inadequate CV compensatory mechanisms during stress

   ↓ Plasma volume

      ↑ Susceptibility to hypotensive effects of diuretics

      ↑ Risk of orthostatic hypotension

sclerotic process contributes to aortic and arterial stiffness (arteriosclerosis). This translates into decreased vessel compliance, which results in increased systemic vascular resistance. Elevated systolic blood pressure follows and left ventricular hypertrophy occurs as an adaptive mechanism. Aortic and arterial stiffness contributes to loss of baroreceptor sensitivity, which may further compromise blood flow. The aging process usually produces sclerosis of the fibrous skeleton of the heart and areas of patchy calcification throughout the heart. This process contributes to the thickening of the atrioventricular valves and the aortic cusp. The sclerosis and calcification processes also contribute to conduction abnormalities.

Many factors combine to alter cardiac output. Diastolic filling is impaired, secondary to calcification. The aging process results in a decrease in the sensitivity of beta receptors, rendering the older heart less able to respond to sympathetic stimulation. This, in turn, causes a decrease in myocardial contractility. While there is little or no change in the resting heart rate as people age, there is an impaired ability to increase heart rate during stress or in response to a change in plasma volume or position.

Older adults secrete lower levels of renin, angiotensin I, vasopressin, and aldosterone. These hormones are instrumental in maintaining cardiovascular homeostasis in the face of certain stressors. Lower levels of these substances, coupled with baroreceptor insensitivity, lower the capacity to cope with physiological or psychological stress. Low levels of these hormones also contribute to an increased risk for orthostatic hypotension, dehydration, and medication intolerance.

Risk Factors for Cardiovascular Disease

In addition to the physiological changes of aging that place the older adult at risk for cardiovascular disease, risk is increased in this population by a variety of other factors. Increased age, in and of itself, represents an increased risk for cardiovascular disease. This is particularly true for aging females, as postmenopausal women lose the cardioprotective effects of estrogen. As is also the case for their younger counterparts, hypertension, diabetes, stress, sedentary lifestyle, and obesity, particularly abdominal fat, increase the risk of cardiovascular disease in the elderly. Less clear is the role of cholesterol levels in heart disease in the older adult. Also of interest is the fact that the contribution of cigarette smoking to cardiovascular disease may present a lower risk with increasing age.[6,7]

While many risk factors may be modified to decrease one's risk for cardiovascular disease, because of educational, cognitive, or emotional factors, many older adults are not motivated to make necessary lifestyle changes. Consequently, identification and treatment of cardiovascular disease in this population continues to challenge nurse practitioners in all settings.

Hypertension

Definition/Classification (Stages)

Hypertension is defined as a systolic blood pressure (SBP) equal to or greater than 140 mm Hg, a diastolic blood pressure (DBP) equal to or greater than 90 mm Hg, or taking medication for the control of blood pressure.[8] Blood pressure is classified by three stages as defined in Table 3–3. If systolic and diastolic blood pressures fall into different classifications, the blood pressure is defined by the higher of the two numbers. Isolated systolic hypertension (ISH) is defined as a systolic pressure equal to or greater than 140 mm Hg with a diastolic pressure of less than 90 mm Hg.

Types

For purposes of identifying causes, and thus treatment options, hypertension (HTN) is usually classified as one of three types. Primary hypertension, also known as essential hypertension, occurs without evidence of causation. Conversely, secondary hypertension is usually the result of pathology elsewhere, such as in the endocrine or renal systems.[9] Isolated systolic hypertension, commonly seen in older adults, results from decreased vessel compliance and is usually related to arteriosclerosis of large arteries.

Prevalence and Significance

Hypertension is the most common cardiovascular disorder in the United States. It affects more than 50% of adults over the age of 65.[10] Hypertension presents a major risk factor for cardiovascular, cerebrovascular, peripheral vascular, and renal disease. It is a significant contibutor to myocardial infarction, heart failure, stroke, limb ischemia, and renal failure.

Pathophysiology

The pathophysiology of hypertension is multifactorial. The arteriosclerotic and atherosclerotic processes produce decreased arterial compliance and increased peripheral vascular resistance. This is the physiological basis for isolated systolic hypertension. The autonomic nervous system and renal mechanisms also play a role in the development of hypertension. Activation of renal mechanisms may be triggered by sympathetic stimulation and by low blood flow to the kidneys. In response to the decrease in renal artery pressure, the juxtaglomerular cells of the kidney increase secretion of renin. Renin is an enzyme that activates the plasma protein angiotensinogen and converts it to angiotensin I. Angiotensin I is an inactive compound that is converted, by a converting enzyme in the lung, to angiotensin II, a potent arteriolar vasoconstrictor. Angiotensin II stimulates the kidney to retain sodium and water. It also activates the adrenal cortex and promotes the release of aldosterone, which induces the distal tubule of the kidney to reabsorb sodium. Sodium retention ensues, followed by fluid retention, increased blood volume, and increased blood pressure.[11]

In the older adult, the normal changes of aging also contribute to the development of hypertension. In addition to vessel arteriosclerosis, sclerosis and calcification of the cardiac chambers occur and result in impaired diastolic filling. Cardiac output and renal blood flow may fall, triggering the renal adaptive mechanisms described above. Hypertension results, or is exacerbated, in response.

Regardless of causation, hypertension can initiate a series of physiological changes that serve to perpetuate the hypertensive state and increase the risk of end-organ damage. Increased pressure against vessel walls causes shear and, as previously described, intimal damage. Over time, increased

Table 3–3 Stages of Hypertension as Defined by JNC-VI[8]

	Systolic Pressure (mm Hg.)	Diastolic Pressure (mm Hg.)
Stage I	140–159	90–99
Stage II	160–179	100–109
Stage III	>180	>110

arterial pressure leads to further degenerative changes, including arteriosclerosis and further vessel constriction.

Clinical Presentation

Hypertension has long been known as "the silent killer." This is particularly true of primary/essential hypertension which is most often asymptomatic. It is frequently identified, for the first time, during a routine office visit for an unrelated condition. Occasionally, the client will complain of an occipital headache usually noted on awakening.[11] Other symptoms, such as epistaxis, tinnitus, fatigue, nervousness, and irritability, may also be reported. Symptoms of secondary hypertension are related to the system that is the primary cause of the hypertension.

History

The diagnostic workup for hypertension must include, at a minimum, a medical history, family history, a comprehensive review of risk factors for hypertension, and a review of systems, specifically as related to end-organ disease.

In reviewing the medical history with the patient, the nurse practitioner should question the onset and duration of the hypertension. It would also be important to ask whether this ever has been previously diagnosed and treated. Often the older adult does not fully comprehend the significance of a diagnosis of hypertension and, for a variety of reasons, has not complied with previously prescribed medical therapy. The nurse practitioner should ask about a history of kidney or abdominal trauma or the presence of symptoms such as headache, diaphoresis, dizziness, or palpitations, any of which might suggest secondary causes of hypertension. It is important to ask about the symptoms of target-organ damage as related to cardiovascular disease, cerebrovascular disease, peripheral vascular disease, and renal disease. The patient should also be questioned about a history, or symptoms, of diabetes, dyslipidemia, or gout. The nurse practitioner should explore the use of prescription medications, as well as

over-the-counter drugs. Decongestants, glucocorticoids, antacids that contain sodium, and nonsteroidal anti-inflammatory drugs may contribute to new onset hypertension.[10] The older adult should be questioned about dietary habits and lifestyle factors that may contribute to hypertension. It is important to identify the use and daily amounts of tobacco, alcohol, caffeine, and sodium. It is also important to ask about life stressors and leisure-time activities, including exercise.

Family history should be explored; specifically the patient should be asked if parents or siblings have ever been diagnosed with hypertension. This may be information that the older adult is not able to provide. The nurse practitioner can, however, ask questions regarding a history of hypertensive-related conditions in the family. If parents or siblings experienced premature heart disease or stroke, it is possible that hypertension may have been present.

Physical Examination

A diagnosis of hypertension is usually based on two blood pressure readings, separated by two minutes, and obtained on two different visits. In order to verify readings, blood pressure should be checked in both arms. Specific techniques to be used when assessing the older adult include:

- Check the blood pressure in the supine, sitting, and standing positions to identify orthostasis.
- Perform Osler's maneuver to identify pseudohypertension due to excessive vascular stiffness (see Table 3–4).

Table 3–4   Osler's Maneuver[10]

1. Palpate the radial or brachial artery
2. Inflate the BP cuff until pulsations can no longer be palpated
3. If the pulseless artery is still palpable, this is a positive Osler's and may indicate pseudohypertension
4. If the pulseless artery is not palpable, this is a negative Osler's

The phenomenon of "white coat hypertension" should be considered if the client reports that previous blood pressure measurements, taken out of the office environment, have not been elevated.

Weight should be checked and a multisystem examination conducted to identify causative factors and presence of target organ damage. While a complete physical examination must be performed, the following represents a guideline for the nurse practitioner who examines the older adult with possible hypertension.

Head and Neck Assessment   Perform an opthalmoscopic exam to identify signs of retinopathy. Look for:

- arteriolar constriction and arterial/venous nicking
- hemorrhages
- papilledema

Neck: to identify causes of secondary hypertension and signs of target organ damage.

- Check for distended neck veins which may be indicative of ventricular dysfunction.
- Auscultate for carotid bruits.
- Examine thyroid for evidence of thyromegaly.

Skin: identify symptoms of hypertension or causes of secondary hypertension.

- Check temperature, color, and moisture of the skin. Excess diaphoresis may be present with pheochromocytoma.
- Observe for cushingoid signs: truncal obesity, purple striae, bruising.

Cardiac Assessment   Identify cardiac compensation or presence of target organ damage.

- Palpate point of maximal impulse (PMI) to identify enlarged cardiac silhouette or precordial heave.
- Auscultate for presence of tachycardia, arrhythmia, murmur, S3/S4.

Pulmonary Assessment   Identify presence of target organ damage (cardiac).

- Auscultate for crackles or wheezing.

Abdominal Assessment   Identify causative factors or target organ damage.

- Auscultate for bruits over renal arteries and abdominal aorta.

Peripheral Vascular Assessment   Identify presence of peripheral vascular disease.

- Inspect lower extremities for color, temperature, presence/absence of pulses, hair distribution, edema.

Differential Diagnoses

Differential diagnoses of hypertension, in the older adult, must include consideration of the diagnoses of isolated systolic hypertension, essential hypertension, secondary hypertension, pseudohypertension, and the phenomenon of "white coat hypertension."

Diagnostic Tests

The diagnostic workup for hypertension should begin with basic laboratory tests including a urinalysis, complete blood count, fasting glucose, electrolytes, lipid panel, and creatinine. It is important to note that, because of decreased muscle mass in older adults, a serum creatinine may not accurately represent kidney function. In this population, creatinine clearance would be a more specific indicator of kidney disease. A chest x-ray should be obtained and a 12-lead electrocardiogram (ECG) should be performed. Additional tests to consider include blood urea nitrogen (BUN), triglycerides, calcium, and uric acid.[8,10] If "white coat" hypertension is suspected, ambulatory blood pressure monitoring may be utilized as a diagnostic tool. Pseudohypertension may be diagnosed by performance of Osler's maneuver, as previously discussed.

Interventions   The goal of hypertensive treatment is to reduce the morbidity and mortality associated with high blood pressure. While achieving and maintaining a SBP <140 and a DBP <90 represents the ultimate goal, this presents more of a challenge in the older adult than in their younger counterparts. Caution must also be exercised not to drop blood pressure too far too fast. Lowering DBP in clients with coronary artery disease (CAD) has the potential to decrease coronary perfusion pressure and increase the risk for coronary events. Reductions in cerebrovascular and renal disease, however, have been noted when DBP is reduced.[8] Although it is reported that treatment of HTN in men older than 75 should be directed at lowering the SBP without dramatically affecting the DBP,[10] recent evidence supports the reduction of DBP in all ages.[8]

While primary prevention of hypertension is a national goal, in older adults with a definite diagnosis of hypertension, it must be treated to prevent morbidity and mortality. Treatment always begins with lifestyle modifications, which may also require pharmacological interventions. Effective lifestyle modifications include:

- weight loss, if needed
- participation in an aerobic exercise program
- reduction of sodium intake and dietary fat
- alcohol limitation
- smoking cessation
- maintenance of adequate dietary intake of potassium, calcium, and magnesium

When lifestyle modifications are not sufficient to control blood pressure, or when blood pressure is markedly elevated and/or target organ damage or cardiovascular disease is present, pharmacological treatment must be initiated. Pharmacological treatment of hypertension in older adults has been shown to decrease cardiovascular morbidity and mortality. Protective effects against stroke, coronary events, heart failure, renal disease, and progression of hypertension have also been demonstrated.[8] Pharmacological treatment of hypertension follows the adage of all drug prescribing for older adults: "start low and go slow." Medications should be started with one-half the usual dose and titrated slowly to achieve desired

outcome. It is important to recognize that pharmacotherapy places the older adult at risk for hypotension secondary to volume depletion, which may result from the treatment. Additionally, decreased baroreceptor sensitivity predisposes the older adult to hypotension, particularly orthostatic hypotension.

First-line medical therapy for treatment of uncomplicated hypertension in older adults is usually a diuretic. Diuretics are particularly effective in the treatment of isolated systolic hypertension (ISH) because they exert a more profound effect on the SBP than the DBP.[10] Thiazide diuretics work well in those older adults who have a tendency toward sodium and fluid retention. Potassium-sparing diuretics, although generally weaker diuretics, may be used when hypokalemia would present a serious risk, as with concurrent digitalis use. Combination thiazide and potassium-sparing preparations are also available and deserve consideration. Loop diuretics are not appropriate as first-line therapy for primary hypertension in older adults. Because they result in large volume loss, they should be considered only in the presence of target organ disease or if thiazides are not successful in controlling the hypertension.

While beta blockers also have been recommended as first-line therapy for treatment of hypertension, their use in older adults recently has been brought into question.[12] The negative inotropic and chronotropic effects of beta blockers, along with a concommitant increase in peripheral vascular resistance, can place the older adult at increased risk for unpleasant side effects from beta blockers. Additionally, the central nervous system effects of beta blockers, such as depression and confusion, can exacerbate preexisting problems in the older adult. Because the normal aging process results in a decrease in the sensitivity of beta receptors,[13] it is also possible that the older adult will not realize the same benefit from this class of drugs as younger persons.

Calcium antagonists are also a treatment alternative for older adults with hypertension. Caution must be used when prescribing a dihydropyridine, as these are potent vasodilators and may cause orthostasis and reflex tachycardia. The nondihydropyridines frequently cause constipation, a problem particularly distressing to most elderly clients.

Finally, angiotensin converting enzyme (ACE) inhibitors, and the new angiotensin II receptor antagonists, present yet another option for treatment of hypertension. ACE inhibitors have been effective in lowering blood pressure and are well tolerated in older adults, but the common side effect of a dry cough can be distressing. Angiotensin II receptor blockers have been effective in controlling blood pressure without this annoying side effect.

Combination therapy is often most effective for treatment of hypertension in older adults. This approach allows for smaller doses of each drug and thus avoids unpleasant side effects common in older adults. Combinations most frequently utilized are:

- thiazide diuretic and potassium sparing diuretic
- thiazide diuretic and beta blocker
- thiazide diuretic and calcium antagonist

Other classes of drugs, such as alpha adrenergic antagonists, peripheral acting adrenergic antagonists, and central sympatholytics exhibit an unacceptable side effect profile for this population. While these drugs are not contraindicated for use in older adults, they should be used with extreme caution and only when other drugs have failed to control the hypertension.

Any time pharmacological treatment is utilized, the clinician needs to be mindful of issues affecting compliance. In an older population, financial constraints represent a barrier to compliance and must be a consideration when choosing a drug for treatment of hypertension. In general, thiazide diuretics are the least-expensive treatment option. Beta blockers and ACE inhibitors, depending on the specific product used, cost about the same, while calcium channel antagonists are more expensive.

Compliance can also be enhanced by prescribing a long-acting preparation that requires only once-a-day dosing. Most older adults lead active lives that may interfere with taking medication three or four times daily. Additionally, for those with some level of cognitive decline, a once-a-day medication can be taken routinely on arising, or retiring, and becomes part of a daily routine that is more easily remembered.

Management of Coexisting Morbidities   Coexisting morbidities also play a role in the treatment of hypertension and must be considered before prescribing medication. The presence of coronary artery disease, or history of myocardial infarction, should prompt the clinician to consider therapy with a beta blocker, while the presence of heart failure would be an indication for using a diuretic and an ACE inhibitor. Hypertension, in the presence of diabetes mellitus, is best managed by treatment with an ACE inhibitor.[8]

Education

Older adults present many unique challenges to the primary-care provider, not the least of which is teaching. Nurse practitioners must bear in mind that many older adults have not been active participants in health care. Historically, they have trusted medical personnel to act in their best interests and often they do not wish to assume responsibility for health-care needs. Additionally, belief systems may hold that to be old is to be ill, and such ideas may be difficult to change. Cognitive and sensory losses and physiological and psychological stress may individually or in combination impede the learning of new information. If disease or disability prevents participation in care, family members or others must then be included in any educational efforts.

In teaching about hypertension, the nurse practitioner must stress the importance of lifestyle modifications.

- Smokers must be encouraged to stop. Smoking cessation aids contain lower amounts of nicotine and therefore can be safely used, along with behavioral modifications.
- If obesity is a factor, the benefits of weight reduction must be stressed. Decreased caloric intake, coupled with increased physical activity, can be very successful in reducing weight, increasing energy, and reducing blood pressure.
- The importance of dietary sodium restriction must be emphasized. Older adults need to understand that sodium restriction goes

beyond putting away the salt shaker. They should be counseled to read product labels and avoid processed and packaged foods that contain high amounts of sodium, such as canned vegetables, frozen dinners, and prepared foods such as rice and pasta dishes.

- Alcohol intake should be limited and older adults should consume no more than 1 oz. of ethanol. This translates to 12 oz. of beer, 5 oz. of wine, or 1 oz. of 100-proof whiskey per day.[8]

- Unless contraindicated by medical therapy, the older adult should be counseled to consume foods that are high in potassium, calcium, and magnesium, as high dietary intake of these substances prevents hypertension and improves blood pressure control.[8]

In addition to educating the older adult about the importance of lifestyle changes for hypertension control, the clinician must stress the importance of medication use and the rationale for long-term therapy. Because most people with hypertension are asymptomatic, and may actually have more symptoms from medication side effects than from the disease itself, the concept of lifelong medical therapy is difficult for many to accept. A simple explanation of the changes of aging, which support the pathophysiology of hypertension, may be helpful in promoting an understanding of the condition and its treatment.

It is important to inform the older adult about signs and symptoms that need to be reported to the clinician. Side effects of the particular medication should be discussed. The symptoms of hypotension, or a worsening of hypertension, should be made clear. The older person should also be instructed regarding the potential for orthostatic hypotension and should be cautioned to change positions slowly in order to avoid this problem.

The rationale for compliance with the regimen and follow-up care must be discussed as well with the older adult. During subsequent visits, the clinician should question the older adult regarding the ability to implement lifestyle changes and assist, as needed, with providing resources for these changes. Blood pressure should be monitored monthly for three to six months in order to evaluate the effectiveness of nonpharmacologic management.[10] Likewise, the effectiveness of pharmacological therapy must be closely monitored.

Transportation and/or financial constraints may make it difficult for the older adult to be monitored frequently in the office setting. In this situation, the nurse practitioner must be prepared to offer alternatives that will ensure that blood pressure is routinely checked and reported. A list of community resources should be discussed and made available. At-home monitoring might also be a convenient option for assessing blood pressure, if finances permit and the individual, or a caregiver, is able to master this skill. Under these circumstances, it is important to stress that blood pressure needs to be reported on a scheduled basis to the clinician's office.

Anticipated Outcomes

Normalization and control of blood pressure, along with prevention of end-organ damage, are the anticipated outcomes of antihypertensive therapy. Achievement of these goals are dependent on the client's motivation to implement the recommended lifestyle changes and comply with a prescribed regimen.

Blood pressure readings represent the objective measure of adherence. Lack of a decrease in blood pressure should prompt the nurse practitioner to question the patient regarding areas of difficulty with the treatment plan. If adherence is not an issue, the clinician must revise the plan in order to achieve the desired outcome.

Hypertension is a chronic disease that requires ongoing evaluation in order to ensure that the goals of therapy are being met. This is particularly true for hypertension in older adults. The physiological changes of aging, the new onset of a chronic disease, or even the presence of an acute infection may render a previously effective treatment plan ineffective.

Referral

As a primary-care provider, educated in areas of health maintenance, the nurse practitioner is ideally suited to manage chronic health conditions such as hypertension. The nurse practitioner must also recognize those situations that require referral and be prepared to make this referral promptly. The following situations require consultation with or referral to either a physician or hospital:

Refractory hypertension:	refer to physician
SBP >180, DBP >110:	consult with physician
Target organ damage:	consult with/refer to physician
SBP >210, DBP >120:	refer to hospital ER

Any health situation that requires immediate reduction in blood pressure in order to limit or prevent target organ damage should be referred to the hospital emergency room. These include, but are not limited to, hypertensive encephalopathy, intracranial bleeding, unstable angina, myocardial infarction, pulmonary edema, or dissecting aneurysm.[8]

Coronary Artery Disease

Definition and Consequences

The term coronary artery disease (CAD) describes the disorder in which one or more of the coronary arteries are narrowed, compromising blood supply to the myocardium. Several factors play a role in the severity of CAD and its consequences, including the degree of obstruction, whether obstruction results from a chronic or acute situation, duration of a low-flow state, and the myocardial oxygen need during decreased perfusion.[5] Clinical sequellae of CAD are angina, myocardial infarction, heart failure, and dysrhythmias.

Prevalence and Significance

Because of the difficulty diagnosing coronary artery disease in older adults, prevalence may be understated. Recent estimates, however, suggest that it is the most frequent cause of heart disease in the older adult[6] and it remains the leading cause of death in those over the age of 65. With the projected population increase for those over the age of 65, and particularly those over the age of 85, CAD represents both a health and an economic priority.

Pathophysiology

As previously described in this chapter, the pathophysiology of CAD is related to the development of the atherosclerotic plaque in the coronary arteries. Once plaque formation has occurred, a variety of local and systemic factors contribute to the further development and severity of CAD.

Over time, the atherosclerotic process results in progressive narrowing of the coronary artery or arteries. In addition, development of the atherosclerotic plaque produces luminal irregularities and roughness, which attract platelets and fibrin deposits, increasing the degree of stenosis and producing the potential for thrombus formation. Concurrently, blood flow through the stenotic artery produces a high shear rate which may result in plaque disruption. Plaque disruption induces platelet aggregation, further increasing the likelihood of thrombus formation.[5]

Thrombus formation may also be enhanced in the presence of diabetes mellitus and elevated cholesterol levels, both of which increase coagulation and enhance platelet activity. High levels of sympathetic activity, such as that produced by smoking and stress, may also enhance platelet activation and production of thrombin. Other hemostatic components, specifically high levels of fibrinogen and factor VIII, are also associated with increased risk of thrombosis. Both of these substances are increased in the aging process, as well as with obesity, hyperlipidemia, diabetes, smoking, and during periods of emotional stress.[5]

Angina

Angina pectoris, also commonly referred to as ischemic heart disease, is the most common clinical consequence of CAD. Angina occurs when the oxygen supply to the myocardium is inadequate to meet myocardial demand. This imbalance between supply and demand may be the result of coronary arterial narrowing, thrombus formation within the vessel, coronary artery spasm, or any other condition that results in decreased blood flow to the myocardium or increased myocardial oxygen need.

Classification

Angina is frequently classified as stable or unstable. Stable angina, often referred to as exertional angina, occurs when the atherosclerotic coronary arteries are sufficiently narrowed to limit necessary oxygen to the myocardium. Stable angina occurs in response to situations that increase myocardial oxygen demand, such as exercise, stress, or cold weather.[14] The character, duration, intensity, and relieving factors of stable angina are usually the same.

Unstable angina is the term used to describe new onset angina, angina that occurs at rest, or a change in the character, intensity, frequency, or duration of previously stable angina. Variant angina, non-Q-wave MI, and post-infarction angina are included in the definition of unstable angina.[15] Variant angina, also known as Prinzmetal's angina, is a form of unstable angina and is thought to be related to coronary vasospasm. It occurs at rest, frequently at night during periods of REM sleep. Variant angina usually follows a pattern of occurrence at the same time each day. It is associated with ST segment elevation on the 12-lead ECG.[14]

Differentiation from Myocardial Infarction

While angina is often the presenting symptom of CAD, the nurse practitioner must be aware that the first symptom of coronary artery disease may be myocardial infarction (MI). Because of the morbidity and mortality associated with MI, it is imperative that the practitioner be able to assess the client quickly in order to differentiate angina from myocardial infarction. Although symptoms of angina and myocardial infarction are similar, angina is often brought on by exercise or stress and is alleviated by rest or nitroglycerin. Anginal pain is usually of shorter duration (less than five minutes) than that associated with MI. Whenever MI is suspected, a quick, brief history and physical, directed at identifying signs and symptoms of MI, should be conducted and a 12-lead ECG performed. Stable angina may be appropriately treated by a nurse practitioner in both inpatient and outpatient settings, while MI and some unstable angina require prompt activation of the emergency medical system and physician referral.

Clinical Presentation

The classic clinical presentation of agina pectoris is squeezing chest pain or pressure beneath the sternum. The pain often radiates to the left arm, neck, or jaw. Occasionally, anginal symptoms are epigastric and indigestion may be the chief complaint. Fatigue, shortness of breath, diaphoresis, nausea, palpitations, and weakness may all be associated with anginal episodes. For a variety of reasons, the older adult may present with vague complaints, or atypical symptoms, making it difficult for the clinician to diagnose angina correctly in this population.

Changes associated with the normal aging process may prevent the older adult from perceiving the pain associated with myocardial ischemia. Silent ischemia is common in older adults and diminished pain perception may result in pain that is less severe, prompting the practitioner to explore other diagnoses. Further complicating the diagnosis of angina is the fact that the clinician may attribute anginal symptoms to concomitant diseases, such as chronic obstructive pulmonary disease (COPD), arthritis, or gastroesophageal reflux.[6,16] Cognitive impairment can obscure the diagnosis by limiting recognition or description by older adults of the pain associated with angina. Additionally, sedentary lifestyle may eliminate any symptoms of exercise-induced angina, further complicating the diagnostic process.[6,16]

The first symptom of CAD in the older adult is usually angina. Instead of chest pain, however, the most common presenting symptom of angina in this population is dyspnea. Other common complaints include syncope or palpitations with exertion and episodic confusion.[17] Periods of confusion or increased confusion, weakness, falls, and difficulty performing activities of daily living (ADLs) also have been reported as anginal symptoms. When presented with any of these symptoms, angina should be immediately considered. If chest pain or dyspnea is the chief complaint, quickly conduct a brief, directed history to assess the possible implications of the complaint.

The nurse practitioner should ask questions about the onset, location, and duration of symptoms. If chest pain is present, ask for a description of pain and severity rating and identify if radiation occurs to the arm, neck, jaw, or back. Ask whether this pain has ever occurred before and if so, how the pain was relieved. It is important to determine if there is a pattern to the pain. For example, does it occur at the same time of day; does a specific activity produce the pain; is it influenced by temperature or emotional stress? Other questions, relevant to nonanginal pain, and thus to differential diagnoses, may be found in Table 3–5.[18]

The practitioner should also determine if other associated symptoms, such as dyspnea, weakness, palpitations, nausea, or diaphoresis are present. If yes, and MI is a possibility, postpone the remainder of the history. Vital signs should be taken and a 12-lead ECG obtained. Myocardial infarction requires immediate transfer to the hospital. Thrombolytic therapy, if administered early in the course of MI, significantly reduces the morbidity and mortality associated with MI. While awaiting the arrival of the EMTs, the following interventions should be implemented:

■ Keep patient at rest in a quiet environment.

Table 3–5   Questions to Determine Differential Diagnoses[18]

Question	If Answer is Yes, Consider:
Is there any relationship between the occurrence of the pain and meals?	Gastrointestinal
• Before meals	• Peptic ulcer disease
• After meals	• Gall bladder disease; GERD, esophageal spasm
Is the pain influenced by position?	Gastrointestinal
• Supine	• GERD
Is the pain brought on by eating a particular food, or type of food?	Gastrointestinal
• Fatty	• Gall bladder disease
• Spicy	• GERD; esophageal spasm
Has there been a recent upper-respiratory infection?	Pneumonia; pleurisy; pericarditis
Has the client been coughing?	Pneumonia, pleurisy
Is the cough productive?	Pneumonia; pulmonary embolus
• Sputum is green or yellow	• Pneumonia
• Hemoptysis is present	• Pulmonary embolus
Has the client recently performed activities that may have caused muscle strain?	Musculoskeletal
	• Costochondritis
Is there a history of varicella?	
• Itching or burning present	• Herpes zoster
Is the pain influenced by:	
• Movement	• Musculoskeletal; pleurisy
• Respiration	• Pleurisy; pericarditis
Is the pain reproduced by palpation?	Musculoskeletal; herpes zoster
• Sternal pressure	• Costochondritis
• Light touch	• Herpes zoster

- Provide supplemental oxygen and monitor for adequate oxygenation with pulse oximeter, if available.
- Give nitroglycerin (0.3–0.4 mg) sublingually q 5 minutes x 3. Vital signs must be carefully monitored as nitroglycerin is a potent vasodilator and results in decreased blood pressure.
- Give aspirin 80–324 mg PO if not contraindicated by allergy or recent history of peptic ulcer disease or gastrointestinal bleeding.
- Keep ECG electrodes on patient and monitor in lead II for dysrhythmias.

In a nonemergent situation, the nurse practitioner should continue with a complete history and physical examination.

History

Because a change in mental status may be the first indication of illness in the older adult, it is important to determine if the patient is confused or has had an increase in the level of confusion. Questions relevant to orientation, memory, and attention may be asked in order to assess possible changes in these areas (see Table 3–6).

In proceeding with the history, it is important to assess the general state of health as perceived by the older adult. Ask about ADLs, sleep and dietary habits, stressors, and exercise and leisure activities. Explore the use of both prescription and over the counter medications, including vitamins and herbal products, and ask about borrowing medications from a spouse, another family member, or friend. Finally, it is important to identify the use, and daily amounts, of tobacco, alcohol, and caffeine.

In addition to the history of presenting symptoms, the nurse practitioner should determine any past medical history of hypertension, diabetes, thyroid disorder, hyperlipidemia, or rheumatic fever, as well as any previous diagnosis of cardiac disease, palpitations, edema, orthopnea, or paroxysmal nocturnal dyspnea.

To the extent possible, the nurse practitioner should attempt to identify any family history of angina or MI. Often the older adult is not able to provide specific information regarding the cause of death of parents or siblings. It is nevertheless important to determine the approximate age at death of family members and anything that the patient can remember about those deaths (e.g., a sudden death versus a long illness).

Physical Examination

As previously described, accurate diagnosis of angina in the older adult may be difficult since the physical examination may be normal. Because the elderly often present with atypical symptoms, it is necessary to perform a complete physical in order to rule out other conditions and substantiate a diagnosis of angina. The following are components of the physical specific to the diagnosis of angina in older adults.

Vital signs: performed to identify risk factors for angina or signs of decreased cardiac output and low perfusion state.

- Check blood pressure to identify presence of hypertension or hypotension.
- Check pulse to identify rate, rhythm, and pulse amplitude.
- Check respiratory rate to identify tachypnea or other abnormal respiratory pattern.

Head and neck assessment: performed to identify evidence of, or causative factors for, angina.

Table 3–6 Questions to Determine Change in Mental Status

Determining orientation and memory
- What year is it?
- What is the month?
- What is the date?
- What is the day of the week?
- Where are you now?

Assessing attention
- Ask patient to spell a five-letter word and then spell it backwards (e.g., World)
- Ask patient to subtract 7 from 100 and to keep subtracting 7.

Face:

- Observe for facial grimacing which may be indicative of pain.
- Inspect for pallor, perioral cyanosis, or evidence of diaphoresis, which may be secondary to decreased cardiac output.

Eyes:

- Inspect palpebral conjunctiva for pallor, which may indicate anemia. Anemia may decrease myocardial oxygen supply, resulting in anginal symptoms.
- Perform opthalmoscopic exam to identify retinal vascular abnormalities which may be suggestive of generalized atherosclerosis.

Neck:

- Inspect for distended neck veins. Myocardial ischemia can impair ventricular contractility causing decreased cardiac output. This may result in increased jugular venous pressure.
- Auscultate for carotid bruits which, if present, suggests atherosclerotic disease.
- Examine thyroid for evidence of thyromegaly. Hyperthyroidism causes increased myocardial oxygen demand.

Skin assessment: performed to identify signs of decreased perfusion.

- Check temperature, color, and moisture of the skin. Skin may be cool, pale or cyanotic, and moist, indicating low perfusion.

Cardiac assessment: to identify signs of ischemic heart disease.

- Palpate for chest wall tenderness to rule out costochondritis.
- Auscultate for presence of:
  1. Tachycardia or bradycardia: may be response to or result of myocardial ischemia.
  2. Dysrhythmias: may be due to myocardial ischemia.
  3. Murmurs:
     (a) Transient systolic murmur of mitral regurgitation may be due to acute papillary muscle ischemia and dysfunction

     (b) Systolic murmur of aortic stenosis or sclerosis
     (c) Diastolic murmur of aortic regurgitation or mitral stenosis
  4. S3: may occur during acute anginal episode secondary to decreased myocardial contractility; usually associated with volume overload or heart failure.
  5. S4: may indicate coronary artery disease or obstruction to ventricular outflow.
  6. Pericardial friction rub: may rule out angina as a diagnosis.

Pulmonary assessment: to identify consequences of myocardial ischemia. Auscultate lungs for presence of:

- Crackles: myocardial ischemia may cause left ventricular dysfunction which results in pulmonary congestion.
- Wheezing: may indicate a more serious condition such as MI or pulmonary embolus.

Abdominal assessment: to identify signs of generalized atherosclerosis.

- Auscultate for bruits over renal arteries and abdominal aorta.

Peripheral vascular assessment: to identify additional signs of generalized atherosclerosis as well as consequences of cardiovascular disease.

- Inspect lower extremities for color, temperature, presence/absence of pulses, hair distribution, edema.

Mental-status assessment: as previously discussed, conducted to identify mental-status changes which may be related to decreased cerebral perfusion.

Differential Diagnoses

Because of the atypical clinical presentation of illness in the older adult, the differential diagnoses for angina must include consideration of multisystem diagnoses.[18]

- Cardiovascular: myocardial infarction, pericarditis
- Pulmonary: pneumonia, pleurisy, pulmonary embolus

■ Gastrointestinal: peptic ulcer disease, esophogeal spasm, gastroesophogeal reflux disease, gall bladder disease

■ Musculoskeletal: chest wall pain/costochondritis

■ Other: herpes zoster

Although aortic dissection may also present as chest pain, severity of the symptoms usually prompt an immediate call to the emergency medical system, rather than the primary-care practitioner.

Diagnostic Tests

If, after completing the history and physical examination, the practitioner believes angina is likely, a 12-lead ECG should be performed, noting that it is most useful if performed when anginal symptoms are present. Without symptoms, the specificity of the ECG in the diagnosis of angina is low. The ECG can provide useful information regarding prior or current cardiac conditions, confirming a diagnosis of angina. See Table 3–7 for possible ECG findings and etiologies.

While there are no laboratory tests specific to the diagnosis of angina, labs should be obtained to identify causative or contributing factors for symptoms, including complete blood count, chemistry screen, thyroid function studies, and a lipid profile. Other diagnostic tests to be considered include ambulatory Holter monitoring and referral for exercise or medical stress testing.

Interventions

Treatment of angina pectoris is dictated by the type and severity of the disease. A diagnosis of chronic stable angina may be treated in the outpatient setting, while unstable angina requires physician referral and hospitalization. The goal of anginal treatment is to ensure that myocardial oxygen supply is adequate to meet oxygen demand. This may be accomplished through nonpharmacological and pharmacological interventions directed at modifying both sides of the supply/demand ratio (see Table 3–8).

Lifestyle modifications such as weight loss, stress management, and reduction of caffeine intake contribute to decreasing myocardial workload and oxygen demand. Control of hypertension and correction of metabolic disorders such as hyperthyroidism also reduce cardiac work and oxygen requirements. Treatment of an underlying anemia or pulmonary disease improves myocardial oxygen supply. Oxygen supply may also be improved through smoking cessation and participation in a cardiac rehabilitation

Table 3–7   Possible ECG Findings and Etiologies

ECG Findings	Possible Etiologies
T wave inversion ST depression	Ischemia
ST segment elevation	Injury
Q waves	Previous myocardial infarction
Dysrhythmias	Chronic Ischemia Electrolyte imbalance

Table 3–8   Interventions Used to Modify Supply/Demand Ratio of Myocardial Oxygenation

Lifestyle interventions to decrease myocardial oxygen demand	Lifestyle interventions to increase myocardial oxygen supply
• Weight loss • Stress management • Limit caffeine intake	• Exercise program • Smoking cessation
Other interventions to decrease myocardial oxygen demand	Other interventions to increase myocardial oxygen supply
• Control of hypertension • Treatment of hyperthyroidism	• Correction of anemia
Pharmacological interventions to decrease myocardial oxygen demand	Pharmacological interventions to increase myocardial oxygen supply
• Beta blockers • Calcium channel blockers	• Nitrates • Calcium channel blockers

or other structured exercise program. Control of diabetes and dyslipidemia may decrease some of the morbidity and mortality associated with coronary artery disease.

Pharmacological agents may be used alone or in combination to balance oxygen supply and demand. Sublingual nitroglycerin (NTG) is the first-line treatment for acute anginal episodes. Nitroglycerin is a potent vasodilator affecting both the venous and coronary arterial systems, decreasing preload and oxygen demand, and increasing myocardial oxygen supply. Sublingual NTG may be the only drug required for the treatment of anginal symptoms in older adults. It is appropriate for those who have infrequent attacks; it may also be used prophylactically for situationally induced angina, such as prior to exercise or sexual activity.

Long-acting nitrates may be prescribed for stable or unstable angina and especially for those who experience more frequent anginal episodes. Long-acting nitrates are available in both oral or transdermal form and are usually well tolerated in the elderly.[17] Headache is the most common side effect, which may be relieved with acetaminophen and usually disappears within a week or two of initiation of treatment. Because nitrate tolerance may develop, continuous dosing with long-acting nitrates is not recommended. In a 24-hour period, a nitrate-free interval of 8 to 12 hours should be provided to maintain efficacy.[17,19] Because nitrates decrease preload and consequently cardiac output, long-term nitrate therapy should not be prescribed for patients who experience orthostatic hypotension. If nitrate therapy is not effective in controlling anginal symptoms, a beta blocker or a calcium channel blocker may be substituted or added to the regimen.

Beta blockers decrease myocardial oxygen demand through a reduction in heart rate, blood pressure, and myocardial contractility. Although beta blockers have been shown to decrease mortality, they should be used cautiously in older adults.[19] Because beta blockers exert both negative inotropic and chronotropic effects, symptomatic bradycardia, hypotension, and heart failure may occur. The vasoconstrictive peripheral vascular effects of beta blockers can exacerbate or cause claudication. Beta blockers are lipid soluble and thus may cross the blood–brain barrier, creating the potential for depression and increased confusion. As previously discussed, the normal aging process may result in decreased sensitivity of beta receptors, decreasing the effectiveness of these drugs.

Calcium channel blockers are a treatment alternative for older adults with stable angina; they are also indicated for treatment of variant or Prinzmetal's angina. Nondihydropyridines reduce myocardial oxygen demand by exerting a negative chronotropic effect. Dihydropyridines are potent vasodilators; as such, they increase oxygen supply while also decreasing demand. In the older adult, nondihydropyridines frequently cause constipation in older adults, while dihydropyridines may cause hypotension, orthostasis, and reflex tachycardia.

Currently, a daily dose of aspirin is recommended with a diagnosis of coronary artery disease. Because aspirin inhibits platelet aggregation, it may prevent unstable angina and myocardial infarction. Clients with a history of aspirin allergy, hematological disorders, or gastrointestinal or cerebrovascular bleeding are not candidates for this therapy. Specific recommendations for dosing are not available and a daily dose of 80–324 mg may be given.

Whenever prescribing pharmacological treatment in older adults, the practitioner must consider issues related to adherence. In general, it is well to keep the following principles in mind when treating the older adult:

- Since many older adults live on a fixed income, the cost of the drug must be considered.
- Because the elderly often experience adverse drug reactions, the initial prescription should be for a limited supply (no more than two weeks).
- Because of problems with cognitive impairment, the need to depend on others for assistance with medications, or an active lifestyle that may interfere with taking medication frequently during the day, adherence may be enhanced by prescribing a long-acting preparation that requires dosing once a day.

Finally, treatment of angina must include treatment of coexisting morbidities such as thyroid disorders, diabetes, hypertension, and dyslipidemia. Endocrine disorders such as hyper-/hypothyroidism and diabetes mellitus require intervention in order to prevent poor outcomes associated with coronary artery disease and improve quality of life. Treatment of these disorders is beyond the scope of this chapter; treatment of hypertension in the elderly is discussed elsewhere in this chapter.

Although hyperlipidemia is known to be a factor in the development of atherosclerosis, treatment in older adults is controversial. Total cholesterol level, in and of itself, does not appear to be predictive of coronary artery disease in older adults; however, levels of low-density lipoproteins and high-density lipoproteins is predictive.[6,20,21,22] At issue is the value of treatment. Despite numerous studies documenting the effect on cardiovascular mortality of lowering cholesterol, it is unclear at what age this intervention loses its benefit. Lifestyle modifications may be implemented with little risk and perhaps some benefit. Because of the potential for adverse effects, comorbid conditions requiring other drug therapies, and a limited life expectancy, pharmacological treatment should be prescribed only after a careful review of risk/benefit ratio.

■ Education

As previously discussed, teaching the older adult can be challenging. When the diagnosis is angina pectoris, it is critical that the patient, and/or a significant other, understand the meaning of the anginal symptoms and their appropriate management. A brief explanation of angina and its consequences may be helpful in promoting compliance with the plan of care. Other issues to be discussed include:

■ Smoking cessation, if applicable.

■ Activity: if appropriate, encourage participation in daily aerobic activity for at least 20 minutes per day. It must be stressed that activity should be gradually increased over a period of several weeks. For the most part, this activity should take place in a climate-controlled environment such as a mall or health club to avoid weather extremes. Activity should be immediately discontinued if anginal symptoms develop.

■ Diet: patients under the age of 80 with hyperlipidemia should be encouraged to consume a low-fat, low-cholesterol diet. A list of appropriate choices should be made available. Even those without elevated cholesterol levels should be encouraged to eat a balanced diet, including five servings of fruit and vegetables each day.

■ Stress reduction should be discussed. Encourage participation in enjoyable activities. The importance of adequate sleep and rest should also be discussed.

■ Use of medications: provide printed medication instructions that include the dose, frequency of administration, and side effects to be reported. If a beta blocker or a nondihydropyridine calcium channel blocker is prescribed, teach how to take a pulse rate. Parameters for withholding the drug and notification of the clinician should be given in writing.

■ Interventions for anginal symptoms: if symptoms develop, stop any activity and rest. Counsel on the use of one sublingual nitroglycerin every five minutes; if the symptoms are not relieved after three tablets, go to the nearest emergency room.

■ Signs and symptoms of unstable angina and MI (see Table 3–9). Make sure patients and family members know how to activate the EMS.

Table 3–9   Symptoms of Unstable Angina Versus MI

Symptoms of Unstable Angina	Symptoms of MI
• Chest pain, or anginal equivalent, usually lasting less than 5 minutes	• Chest pain, or anginal equivalent, lasting 30 minutes or more
• Marked limitations of ordinary physical activity	• Chest pain, or anginal equivalent, unrelieved by rest or NTG x 3
• Chest pain, or anginal equivalent, occurs at rest	• Sweating, nausea, vomiting, and apprehension in conjunction with angina

Follow-up care must also be discussed. Frequency of visits will depend on the severity of illness and protocols of the practice. Those who have had an MI or who have been hospitalized with unstable angina should be evaluated within two to four weeks after hospital discharge and require closer monitoring initially than persons with stable angina. Anyone with angina or a history of MI should have an ECG annually.

Anticipated Outcomes

Anticipated outcomes for persons with angina include absence or control of anginal symptoms, prevention of MI, increased exercise tolerance, and compliance with and verbalized understanding of the therapeutic regimen.

Referral

The nurse practitioner can provide comprehensive care to older clients with stable angina. Patients experiencing symptoms of unstable angina or myocardial infarction require hospitalization and physician notification. Additionally, hemodynamic compromise, with or without objective evidence of MI, must be referred to an acute-care setting for evaluation.

 ## Heart Failure

Definition and Classification

Heart failure is a clinical syndrome of impaired cardiac performance, with cardiac output inadequate to meet metabolic needs. It is characterized by signs and symptoms of volume overload and inadequate tissue perfusion.[23]

Heart failure can be classified in a variety of ways. Practitioners historically have referred to heart failure as high output versus low output, forward or backward failure, or right- or left-sided failure. These classifications may still be useful to the practitioner in the identification of assessment findings; however, they provide no guidance for treatment.[24] A more recent classification identifies heart failure in terms of either

systolic or diastolic dysfunction. The term systolic dysfunction refers to the inability of the heart to contract forcefully enough to eject its contents, while diastolic dysfunction refers to an inability of the left ventricle to fill during diastole. The ability to classify heart failure in this way gives the clinician clear guidelines for treatment decisions.

Prevalence and Significance

Heart failure is a major health problem in the United States. More than two million Americans have a diagnosis of heart failure, and 400,000 new cases are diagnosed each year.[23] The incidence of heart failure increases with age and is common in older adults.[25] Age-related changes in the cardiovascular system predispose older adults to the development of heart failure. This predisposition is compounded by the high prevalence of cardiovascular disease. Recent estimates indicate that 6–10% of older adults are affected.[26] As more people live into old age, it is likely that heart failure will become an even greater health concern.

Although advances have been made in the treatment of heart failure, mortality rates remain high and the diagnosis of heart failure carries a poor prognosis. Ten percent of all patients with heart failure die within the first year of diagnosis and only 50% survive more than five years.[23] Heart failure is the leading cause of death in older adults.[27]

Heart failure extracts a high economic cost to both society and individuals. Approximately $10 billion is spent each year on the treatment of heart failure. Heart failure is the leading cause of hospitalization in older adults.[24] Because of the discrepancy between actual cost of care in this population and Medicare payment, heart failure contributes significantly to uncompensated care.[23]

In addition to the economic burden imposed by the diagnosis of heart failure, the effect on quality of life for affected individuals can be devastating. Physical functioning, social interaction, and emotional well being can all be affected adversely by the diagnosis of heart failure.

Pathohysiology

As previously defined, heart failure is a syndrome, not a disease. It may be the result of other diseases or conditions that result in decreased cardiac output (see Table 3–10). In the older population, heart failure is often the result of cardiovascular aging, coupled with the high prevalence of cardiovascular disease. Coronary artery disease, hypertension, valvular heart disease, and cardiac dysrhythmias contribute to the propensity for older adults to develop heart failure. Additionally, reduced responsiveness to beta adrenergic stimuli may slow the heart rate and decrease myocardial contractility. Ventricular stiffness may adversely affect diastolic filling and preload, while changes in vascular compliance may increase afterload and myocardial work.[27] Medications, such as beta blockers, calcium channel blockers, and nonstereoidal anti-inflammatory drugs (NSAIDs) also have been implicated in the development of heart failure.

In order to understand heart failure and its management fully, it is important to review the components of cardiac output. Cardiac output (CO) is the amount of blood pumped by the heart in one minute and it is a factor of both heart rate (HR) and stroke volume (SV).

$$CO = HR \times SV$$

Stroke volume is defined as the amount of blood ejected from the ventricle with each contraction. Stroke volume is determined by preload, contractility, and afterload.

- Preload refers to the length of cardiac muscle fiber at the end of ventricular diastole and to the tension exerted on the walls of the chamber by the volume of blood in the chamber. Preload is the result of venous return and represents the amount of blood available to be pumped by the ventricle during systole.

- Contractility refers to the ability of the myocardial muscle fibers to shorten and eject the ventricular contents. As demonstrated by the Frank-Starling curve, the more ventricular fibers are stretched during diastole (preload), the more forceful myocardial contraction during systole will be.

- Afterload is the resistance against which the ventricle must pump to eject its contents. Afterload is a factor of systemic vascular resistance and ventricular wall tension. Mechanical resistance to flow, such as that encountered by aortic stenosis or sclerosis, may also be a component of afterload.

Changes in heart rate or any of the components of stroke volume affect cardiac output and can result in the development of acute or chronic heart failure. In response to decreased cardiac output, compensatory mechanisms intended to maintain perfusion are initiated. These compensatory mechanisms involve the autonomic nervous system and the renal/endocrine systems. Additionally, initiation of the Frank-Starling curve and the development of ventricular hypertrophy represent compensatory mechanisms.

Decreased cardiac output results in decreased blood pressure. In response to this, the sympathetic nervous system increases heart rate and myocardial contractility, and attempts to maintain

Table 3–10 Conditions That May Precipitate Heart Failure in the Older Adult[27]

Myocardial infarction or ischemia
Hypertension
Excess dietary sodium
Excess fluid intake
Alcohol use
Dysrhythmias
Noncompliance with prescribed medications
Drugs
• Beta blockers
• Calcium channel blockers
• Antiarrhythmics
• Nonsteroidal anti-inflammatory agents (NSAIDS)
Anemia
Infection
Thyroid disorders
Renal insufficiency
Hypoxemia

perfusion to vital organs through vasoconstriction. Decreased blood pressure results in decreased renal flow, intiating increased secretion of renin. Renin, in the presence of angiotensinogen, promotes the conversion of angiotensin I to angiotensin II. Angiotensin II is a powerful vasoconstrictor that raises blood pressure. It also stimulates the adrenal glands to produce aldosterone which, in turn, promotes reabsorption of sodium and water. The end result of these mechanisms is an increase in blood pressure and organ perfusion.

Age-related changes in the older adult often prevent the initiation of these compensatory mechanisms for decreased cardiac output. A decreased response to beta adrenergic stimulation may prevent the increase in heart rate and contractility necessary to increase cardiac output. Ventricular stiffness may not allow the initiation of the Frank-Starling curve, thus compromising both preload and contractility. Other age-related changes in both the nervous and renal systems may also interfere with the physiological adaptation to decreased cardiac output and precipitate heart failure. Treatment of heart failure is directed at the causative factors and includes augmentation of these compensatory mechanisms.

Clinical Presentation

Like their younger counterparts, the most common symptoms of heart failure in older adults are dyspnea on exertion, orthopnea, fatigue, exercise intolerance, and peripheral edema. As is often the case with the older adult, presenting symptoms may also be nonspecific or atypical. Sometimes the client only has vague complaints of malaise, decreased activity, anorexia, abdominal discomfort, nausea, and diarrhea. Often these symptoms are attributed to other conditions. Confusion, irritability, and sleep difficulty may also be symptoms of heart failure in the older adult, but may not be attributed to heart failure.[28]

History

The diagnosis of heart failure in the older adult may be complex and must be based on evidence gathered from a comprehensive history and physical examination. In reviewing the history of the illness, the nurse practitioner should ask about onset and duration of symptoms. Questions specific to the diagnosis of heart failure include:

- How many pillows do you sleep on?
- Do you ever awaken at night with difficulty breathing? If so, how is this relieved?
- Do you have a cough? Is it productive? Describe the sputum.
- Have you ever had swelling of your ankles?
- Have you had a recent weight gain?

In exploring the past medical history and family history, the practitioner should ask about any previous diagnoses of cardiac disease. Specifically, ask about a history of myocardial infarction, valvular heart disease, hypertension, cardiac dysrhythmias, anemia, renal disease, pulmonary disease, or thyroid disorders. It is also important to determine the reasons for any current medications.

In addition to the presence of cardiac and endocrine disease, the client should be assessed for the presence of other risk factors for heart failure. Questions should be asked regarding alcohol consumption, dietary sodium intake, medication use, and medication compliance.

Physical Examination

Accurate diagnosis of heart failure in the older adult may be difficult because of atypical symptoms or the presence of comorbid conditions. Often the physical examination provides objective evidence to substantiate the diagnosis of heart failure. The following are components of the physical examination specific to the identification of heart failure.

Weight: to identify fluid retention.

Vital signs: to identify signs of decreased cardiac output and low perfusion state.

- Check blood pressure to identify presence of hypertension or hypotension. Blood pressure should be taken in the supine, sitting, and standing positions to identify the presence of orthostasis.

- Check pulse to identify rate, rhythm, and pulse amplitude.
- Check respiratory rate to identify tachypnea or other abnormal respiratory pattern.

Head and neck assessment: to identify evidence of heart failure.

Face:

- Inspect for pallor, perioral cyanosis, or evidence of diaphoresis, which may be secondary to decreased cardiac output.

Eyes:

- Inspect palpebral conjunctiva for pallor, which may indicate anemia. Anemia may decrease myocardial oxygen supply, resulting in decreased contractility and heart failure.
- Perform opthalmoscopic exam to identify abnormalities that may be suggestive of atherosclerosis or hypertension.

Neck:

- Inspect for distended neck veins. Increased jugular venous pressure is indicative of heart failure.[23]
- Examine thyroid for evidence of thyromegaly. Hyperthyroidism causes increased heart rate and myocardial oxygen demand and may precipitate heart failure.

Skin assessment: to identify signs of decreased perfusion.

- Check temperature, color, and moisture of the skin. Skin may be cool, pale or cyanotic, and moist, indicating low perfusion.

Cardiac assessment: to identify signs of heart failure.

- Palpate PMI. Lateral displacement is indicative of heart failure.[23]
- Auscultate for presence of:
  1. Tachycardia: may be compensatory response to heart failure
  2. Bradycardia: may be etiology of heart failure
  3. Dysrhythmias: may be etiology of heart failure

4. Murmurs/heart sounds:
   (a) Systolic murmur of mitral regurgitation, aortic stenosis/sclerosis, or diastolic murmur of aortic regurgitation or mitral stenosis may indicate valvular heart disease as causative factor for heart failure
   (b) S3: diagnostic of volume overload or heart failure
   (c) S4: may indicate obstruction to ventricular outflow

Pulmonary assessment: to identify consequences of heart failure. Auscultate lungs for presence of:

- Crackles: may indicate pulmonary congestion secondary to left ventricular dysfunction.

Abdominal assessment: to identify signs of heart failure.

- Perform abdominojugular test for evidence of increased JVP

Peripheral vascular assessment: to identify signs of right-sided heart failure.

- Inspect lower extremities for peripheral edema

Mental status assessment: to identify change in mental status which may be secondary to decreased, and uncompensated, cardiac output.

Even positive findings on physical exam are not specific to heart failure. Elevated jugular venous pressure (JVP), presence of an S3, and displacement of the PMI are the most specific signs considered to be diagnostic, when accompanied by symptoms of heart failure.[23]

Differential Diagnoses

Differential diagnoses for heart failure in the older adult include consideration of acute heart failure versus chronic heart failure. Pulmonary diagnoses of pneumonia, chronic obstructive pulmonary disease, and pulmonary embolus must be taken into account. The practitioner must also consider renal disease, liver disease, or venous insufficiency as the cause of symptoms.

Diagnostic Tests

The diagnostic workup for heart failure begins with a 12-lead electrocardiogram to identify possible etiologies. Evidence of myocardial infarction, myocardial ischemia, cardiac dysrhythmias, and ventricular and/or atrial hypertrophy supports a diagnosis of heart failure. A chest x-ray is useful for assessing heart size and the presence or absence of pulmonary congestion or pneumonia. Laboratory testing includes the following: urinalysis, complete blood count, electrolytes, BUN (Note: as discussed elsewhere in this chapter, creatinine clearance is a more specific indicator of kidney disease in the older adult than is serum creatinine), serum albumin, liver function studies, T4, and TSH.

If, after these tests are performed, a high index of suspicion remains for the diagnosis of heart failure, an echocardiogram can furnish information about the etiology and extent. Echocardiography provides assessment of valvular structures as well as data related to chamber size and function. Systolic dysfunction may be differentiated from diastolic dysfunction through echocardiography. An ejection fraction (EF) of less than 35–40% is diagnostic of systolic dysfunction, while an EF greater than 35–40% is indicative of diastolic dysfunction.[23]

With a diagnosis of systolic dysfunction, a referral should be made to nuclear imaging or coronary angiography. This is done to identify the contribution of myocardial ischemia and to undertake appropriate corrective interventions.[26]

Once the diagnosis of heart failure has been made, functional ability needs to be determined. Classification of heart failure, according to the New York Heart Association (NYHA) Functional Classification (Table 3–11), can be helpful regarding prognosis and treatment.[26]

Interventions

Chronic heart failure may be treated by the nurse practitioner in the outpatient setting, while new onset heart failure usually requires physician referral or hospitalization. Identification of the causative factors for heart failure, as well as the type or classi-

Table 3–11   New York Heart Association Functional Classification of Heart Failure

I.	No limitation of physical activity. Asymptomatic with ordinary activities.
II.	Slight limitation in physical activity. Ordinary activities produce symptoms.
III.	Marked limitation in activity. Less than ordinary activities produce symptoms.
IV.	Severe limitation. Symptoms are present at rest.

Symptoms include fatigue, dyspnea, palpitations, or angina[26]

fication of the failure, is central to treatment. Once this identification is made, treatment can be initiated and directed toward the goals of improving quality of life through the relief of symptoms, reducing or reversing progression, and decreasing the morbidity and mortality associated with heart failure.[26]

Clear guidelines have been developed for the treatment of heart failure[23,29,30] and are specific for the treatment of systolic dysfunction; the treatment of diastolic dysfunction is less clear. In general, the treatment of heart failure is aimed at maximizing cardiac output through the manipulation of heart rate and stroke volume. A low-sodium diet, diuretics, and ACE inhibitors are the mainstays of treatment. Dietary sodium restriction and diuretic therapy decrease preload, while ACE inhibitors reduce preload, afterload, and systemic vascular resistance. The combination of these interventions has the potential to decrease pulmonary congestion and reduce myocardial workload and oxygen demand. Other pharmacological agents utilized in the treatment of heart failure include:

- Nitrates to reduce preload
- Hydralazine to provide afterload reduction
- Digoxin to increase myocardial contractility
- Beta blockers to reduce heart rate and myocardial oxygen requirements
- Calcium channel blockers may be used cautiously in the treatment of older persons with diastolic dysfunction; they should not

be used to treat heart failure due to systolic dysfunction.

- Specific recommendations, based on type of dysfunction, can be found in Table 3–12.

Diuretics should be prescribed for older clients with signs and symptoms of fluid overload. Mild overload is managed with thiazide diuretics, while loop diuretics should be utilized for those with more severe volume overload. Because older persons are particularly sensitive to volume depletion and are at risk for dehydration and prerenal azotemia when diuretic therapy is utilized, the minimum effective dose should be prescribed.[31]

It is important to note that an ACE inhibitor may be used as the only pharmacological agent in those who do not have signs of volume overload. If monotherapy is not effective, a diuretic should be added. With contraindications or a history of intolerance to ACE inhibitors, a combination of isosorbide dinitrate and hydralazine may be used.[31]

The use of digoxin in the treatment of heart failure in older adults should be reserved for systolic dysfunction and supraventricular tachycardias, or lack of response to the combination of an ACE inhibitor and a diuretic. Digoxin should not be used to treat diastolic dysfunction, as it may increase ventricular stiffness and filling pressure and worsen the heart failure.[31]

Table 3–12 Treatment of Heart Failure in the Older Adult[32]

Systolic Dysfunction EF < 35–40%	Diastolic Dysfunction EF > 35–40%
Low-sodium diet, diuretic, ACE inhibitors	Low-sodium diet, diuretic, ACE inhibitors
If still symptomatic, add digoxin	If symptoms persist, add one of the following:
If symptoms persist, add isosorbide dinitrate & hydralazine	a beta blocker isosorbide dinitrate & hydralazine or a calcium channel blocker
If symptoms persist, add a beta blocker	

Until recently, the use of beta blockers in the treatment of heart failure was considered investigational.[30,31] These agents were cautiously recommended for use in clients with a history of MI or in those who continued to be symptomatic despite treatment with diuretics and ACE inhibitors.[30] Current research indicates that beta blockers may play a larger role in the future treatment of heart failure. The FDA has approved the nonselective beta blocker/alpha 1 blocker, carvedilol, for treatment of NYHA Class II or III heart failure. Recently, the randomized portion of the Cardiac Insufficiency Bisoprolol Study II was prematurely discontinued when it became apparent to the investigators that Bisoprolol significantly reduced mortality in patients with NYHA Class III or IV heart failure.[32] Because of the potential risks associated with the use of beta blockers in heart failure, especially in the older adult, the nurse practitioner is advised to consult a physician before prescribing these agents.

Although not FDA approved for the treatment of heart failure, angiotensin II receptor antagonists are being evaluated for use in heart failure. Some clinicians are recommending that older adults who cannot tolerate an ACE inhibitor should be treated with this class of drugs.[33]

Recent interest in the use of spironolactone, in combination with diuretics and ACE inhibitors, has emerged for the treatment of NYHA Class III or IV heart failure. The Randomized Aldactone Evaluation Study (RALES) was concluded early after analysis of the data indicated that spironolactone significantly reduced the mortality associated with severe heart failure.[34]

Pharmacological therapy is always appropriate for the treatment of heart failure, even in those persons who are asymptomatic.[23,29,30] Lifestyle modifications must also be implemented for anyone with a diagnosis of heart failure. In addition to dietary sodium restriction, regular exercise should be encouraged. Walking or cycling may improve functional capacity and decrease symptoms with NYHA Class I–III heart failure. Alcohol use should be eliminated or limited. Excess fluid intake should be discouraged and fluid restrictions may be recommended for those with hyponatremia.[23]

While this chapter has focused on the treatment of heart failure, it is important to remember that treatment of heart failure must also include treatment/correction of contributing etiologies. Coexisting coronary artery disease, valvular heart disease, hypertension, as well as pulmonary, thyroid, and renal disease can induce or worsen heart failure symptoms, as can anemia or infection. In order to treat heart failure appropriately, it is imperative that the practitioner identify the existence of these comorbidities and implement treatment strategies.

Education

In order to decrease the morbidity and mortality associated with heart failure, it is crucial for patients and families to understand the condition and the significance of compliance with both pharmacological therapy and lifestyle modifications. The importance of medication use and the rationale for long-term therapy must be stressed. Patients must be taught to take their medications correctly and to identify side effects. Understanding and adherence may be enhanced by providing printed instructions for medication use. In addition to education related to medication use, the following lifestyle modifications should be emphasized:

- Sodium restriction: a 2–3 g sodium diet is usually recommended to prevent volume overload. This can be achieved by eliminating salt use at the table and by avoiding foods that are high in sodium. Older clients often do not realize that canned and processed foods contain large amounts of sodium. Because reading food labels may be difficult for the older adult, instruct to avoid such foods. In order to make food palatable, the use of spices and herbs may be suggested.

- Fluid intake: the use of excessive fluid intake should be discouraged; unless hyponatremia exists, implementation of fluid restrictions is unnecessary.

- Alcohol use: ideally, alcohol use should be eliminated. For persons who resist this, no more than 1 oz. of ethanol per day should be consumed. This is equivalent to one

mixed drink, 12 oz. of beer, or one 5 oz. glass of wine.

- Weight loss: obesity places an extra workload on the heart and, if appropriate, calorie restrictions should be implemented to facilitate weight loss.

- Smoking cessation: use of tobacco and tobacco products must be discouraged.

In addition to the above, teach about exercise within identified limits and protocols to stop if symptoms occur. Planning for daily rest periods, particularly prior to scheduled activity, may be helpful in managing fatigue and promoting enjoyment. Older adults who are sexually active should be counseled on modification of sexual practices in order to accommodate for energy limitations.

It is critically important to teach about the signs and symptoms of worsening heart failure. Advise to notify the practitioner if orthopnea, paroxysmal nocturnal dyspnea, decreased exercise tolerance, or increased lower-extremity edema occur. All persons with heart failure should be instructed to weigh themselves daily and maintain a written log of weights. A weight gain of 3–5 pounds should be reported to the practitioner so that diuretic therapy can be adjusted if needed.

Follow-up care must be directed by individual condition. All hospitalized patients should be seen within one week following discharge in order to ensure understanding of and compliance with the plan of care. It would be prudent to monitor older adults every two weeks until symptoms are stable and weight is maintained.

During follow-up visits, the physical examination should be directed toward the identification of signs of unresolved or worsening heart failure. Neck vein distention, presence of an S3, pulmonary crackles, positive hepatojugular reflux, and lower-extremity edema may indicate the need to reevaluate the treatment plan. Presence of these signs may also be indicative of noncompliance with the plan and should be explored.

In addition to the physical examination, question regularly regarding functional ability, appetite, sleep patterns, sexual function, and maintenance of social and family activities. The practitioner should also ask about the presence of or increase in symptoms of heart failure. Daily weights should be reviewed. The importance of influenza and pneumococcal vaccination should be discussed and administration encouraged, assuming no contraindications exist.

Finally, the first follow-up visit may be an appropriate time to discuss the prognosis if this has not been done previously. Wishes regarding cardiopulmonary resuscitation should be ascertained and, if appropriate, family members or other caregivers advised to learn this skill. Advance directives should be completed along with designation of a durable power of attorney for health-care decision making.

If resuscitation is not desired, the practitioner should discuss with the family, at an appropriate time, the actions to take in the event of a sudden death. Family members or caregivers should be cautioned that calling 911 may initiate a series of events that would be in conflict with the patient's wishes.

Anticipated Outcomes

Outcomes of care should be evaluated on each visit. For patients with a diagnosis of heart failure, the anticipated outcomes include compliance with the therapeutic regimen, as evidenced by absence, decrease, or stabilization of symptoms and stable weight.

Referral

Because the diagnosis and prognosis of heart failure can affect not only physiological health but also psychosocial well being, a referral to staff from other disciplines may be helpful. Social workers, home health agencies, or local support groups provide valuable services that may benefit the older adult with heart failure. A dietary consultation may facilitate appropriate food choices.

Physician referral should be made with new onset heart failure and for those who do not respond to the outlined therapeutic regimen. Because of the potential for adverse effects in the older adult, the physician should also be consulted prior to the initiation of beta blocker therapy in the treatment of heart failure.

Those with heart failure and any of the following findings should be referred for hospital management:[23]

- Evidence of acute myocardial ischemia or MI
- Pulmonary edema or severe respiratory distress
- Oxygen saturation less than 90% in the absence of pulmonary disease
- Severe complicating medical illness, such as pneumonia
- Anasarca
- Symptomatic hypotension or syncope
- Heart failure refractory to outpatient management
- Inadequate social support for safe outpatient management

The treatment and management of the older adult with heart failure presents a clinical challenge to the nurse practitioner. Alleviation of symptoms and prevention of disease progression, through appropriate nursing and medical interventions, can decrease morbidity and mortality and improve quality of life for the older adult with heart failure.

Cardiac Dysrhythmias

Definition and Classification

A cardiac dysrhythmia is most simply defined as a disturbance of cardiac rhythm. It can be identified on the electrocardiogram as a variant from normal sinus rhythm (NSR). The ECG criteria for NSR is as follows:

1. Rate:
   - Atrial: 60–100
   - Ventricular: 60–100
2. Rhythm: regular
3. P waves: present, preceeding each QRS complex
4. PR interval: 0.12–0.20 seconds
5. QRS complexes: present, following each P wave. Complexes generally < 0.12 seconds.

Cardiac dysrhythmias may be classified according to the mechanism of causation or by the site of origin. The mechanisms of dysrhythmia development include automaticity, reentry, and conduction disturbances. Because classifying dysrhythmias in this manner requires in-depth knowledge of the physiology of conduction, use of this method is beyond the scope of this chapter. Identification of dysrhythmias by site of origin provides a useful classification system and is the format that is utilized here.

Prevalence and Significance

Dysrhythmias are a frequently occurring phenomenon in the older population.[35] The normal physiological changes occurring in the cardiovascular system with aging, concomitant disease processes, and medical therapy, alone or in combination, predispose the older adult to the development of cardiac dysrhythmias. The significance of these disorders is dependent on a variety of factors and is discussed, in more detail, related to specific dysrhythmias. Because the nurse practitioner is often the older person's initial contact with the healthcare system, it is imperative that he/she be able to identify the patient with a dysrhythmia and intervene appropriately.

In order to avoid redundancy, the pathophysiology, clinical presentation, history, physical examination, differential diagnoses, and diagnostic tests are presented for dysrhythmias in general. Following this, dysrhythmias common in the older population are identified. In order to assist the nurse practitioner in correctly identifying the dysrhythmia, ECG criteria for each are presented. Specific information is given as applicable to each dysrhythmia, while general interventions and suggestions for education are offered at the end of this section.

Pathophysiology of Dysrhythmias

Age-Related Physiological Changes   Histological changes, occurring in the conduction system with advancing age, contribute to the development of dysrhythmias. The amount of collagen and elastin tissue increases. The number of functioning cells in the sinoatrial node decreases and fat deposits collect around the node. Sclerosis and calcification of the cardiac fibrous skeleton affect the atrioventricular (AV) node, AV bundle, and bundle branches. In addition, amyloid infiltration, idiopathic degeneration and fibrosis may contribute to the problem. A decrease in the sensitivity of beta receptors may also contribute to the development of dysrhythmias.[13]

Relevant Disease Processes   While not considered part of normal aging, older adults often have chronic illnesses. Cardiac, pulmonary, and metabolic diseases are frequent in this population and may be manifested by the occurrence of cardiac dysrhythmias.

Both structural heart disease and CAD may contribute to the development of dysrhythmias. Structural disorders include valvular stenosis and insufficiency, as well as ventricular hypertrophy. CAD, with resulting cardiac ischemia, is often associated with a wide range of cardiac rhythm problems. The presenting symptoms of CAD in the older population may be quite different than those in younger people. While chest pain is still the primary complaint in the majority of older adults, atypical presentations frequently occur. Syncope, palpitations, and sudden cardiac death can be the initial symptoms of CAD.[16] The underlying mechanism of these symptoms is likely to be a disturbance of cardiac rhythm.

Certain pulmonary disorders are common in the older adult and may predispose to the development of hypoxia, with resultant dysrhythmias. Age-associated pulmonary changes may contribute to ventilation–perfusion mismatches and decreased arterial oxygenation. Myocardial cells are sensitive to disruptions in oxygen supply and have limited ability to function anaerobically. The cells of the conduction system have a high rate of oxygen consumption and may exhibit increased irritability during hypoxic states.

Endocrine disorders, specifically diabetes mellitus, and thyroid dysfunction also place individuals at risk for the development of a dysrhythmia. Both of these disorders occur with increased frequency in the elderly. Non–insulin-dependent diabetes mellitus and its complications are a frequent problem for the older adult. Complications of diabetes include accelerated atherosclerosis, promoting the development of CAD. Diabetic neuropathy predisposes to reduced pain perception and the phenomenon of silent ischemia. Dysrhythmias are frequent occurrences during ischemic episodes and may contribute to increased mortality. Diseases of the thyroid also occur with increased frequency in the older population. While bradycardia is commonly associated with hypothyroidism, this finding alone is not useful in establishing a diagnosis. Conversely, dysrhythmia development may offer the first clue to the diagnosis of hyperthyroidism. New onset atrial fibrillation may be the presenting symptom of hyperthyroidism in the elderly population.[36]

Other metabolic derangements such as electrolyte imbalance, infection, fever, and anemia also place the older adult at risk for the occurrence of cardiac dysrhythmias. Additionally, anxiety, digestion, exercise, sleep, and ingestion of caffeine or alcohol have all been implicated in the development of rhythm disorders.

Medical Therapy   Because of their medical problems, older individuals often take multiple medications. Many of these medications place them at risk for the development of cardiac dysrhythmias. Antidepressants, bronchodilators, diuretics, and thyroid hormones are just a few of the drugs implicated in rhythm disturbances. Certain antiarrhythmic drugs, prescribed to treat both atrial and ventricular rhythm disturbances, are sometimes proarrhythmic and can result in a worsening of the dysrhythmia or the development of a new dysrhythmia. These medications, if given in the setting of left ventricular dysfunction, may be responsible for the initiation of life-threatening events such as ventricular tachycardia, ventricular fibrillation, and complete heart block.

Clinical Presentation

Cardiac dysrhythmias result in decreased cardiac output and thus clinical signs and symptoms are

consequences of altered cardiac output. These may include fatigue, dizziness, shortness of breath, palpitations, and syncope. Periods of confusion, weakness, or falls may also be reported. Additionally, angina, myocardial infarction, or heart failure may be the presenting symptom, or consequence, of a cardiac rhythm disturbance.

Identification and management of cardiac dysrhythmias in the older adult present a nursing challenge in the primary-care setting. Because the symptoms of a cardiac dysrhythmia may be vague and atypical, a comprehensive history and physical examination must be performed.

History

In eliciting a history of the present illness from the patient, the nurse practitioner should ask about onset and duration of symptoms. Determine the presence of symptoms specific to dysrhythmias such as fatigue, dizziness, shortness of breath, palpitations, and syncope. Ask if there have been recent falls or periods of confusion.

In reviewing the past medical history and family history, it is important to ask about any previous diagnoses of cardiac disease. Specifically, ask about a history of previous dysrhythmias, CAD, valvular heart disease, hypertension, or heart failure. Question the patient about a history of pulmonary disease, anemia, diabetes mellitus, or thyroid disorders. A family history of sudden death, in one or more members, would be important to note.

Conduct a review of systems and determine if the patient has risk factors for dysrhythmia development. Specifically, ask about daily fluid intake and diet, as both dehydration and electrolyte imbalance can predispose to cardiac rhythm disturbances. Question the patient about life stressors and stress-relieving activities. Review medication use and ask about tobacco, alcohol, and caffeine habits.

Physical Examination

Although the presence of a cardiac dysrhythmia may be obvious during the physical examination, absence of a rhythm disturbance does not exclude this as a diagnosis. Often cardiac dysrhythmias present only intermittently. In this case, the physical examination may be normal and an accurate diagnosis may be dependent on the results of diagnostic testing. Components of the physical examination, specific to the identification of a cardiac dysrhythmia, include the following:

Vital signs: to identify signs of decreased cardiac output and low perfusion.

- Check blood pressure to identify presence of hypotension.
- Check pulse to identify rate, rhythm, and pulse amplitude.
- Check respiratory rate to identify tachypnea or other abnormal respiratory pattern.

Head and neck assessment: to identify evidence of dysrhythmia.

Face:

- Inspect for pallor, perioral cyanosis, or evidence of diaphoresis, which may be secondary to hypoxia or decreased cardiac output.

Eyes:

- Inspect palpebral conjunctiva for pallor, which may indicate anemia. Anemia may decrease myocardial oxygen supply, resulting in dysrhythmia development.
- Perform opthalmoscopic exam to identify retinal vascular abnormalities which may be suggestive of generalized atherosclerosis.

Neck:

- Inspect for distended neck veins. Dysrhythmias can result in abnormal atrial or ventricular contraction causing decreased cardiac output. This may result in increased jugular venous pressure.
- Auscultate for carotid bruits which, if present, suggest atherosclerotic disease.
- Examine thyroid for evidence of thyromegaly. Hyperthyroidism is a frequent cause of atrial fibrillation in the older adult.

Skin assessment: to identify signs of decreased perfusion.

- Check temperature, color, and moisture of the skin. Skin may be cool, pale or cyanotic, and moist, indicating low perfusion.

Cardiac assessment: to identify presence or etiologies of a dysrhythmia.

- Auscultate for presence of:
  1. Tachycardia or bradycardia
  2. Irregular rhythm
  3. Murmurs: valvular heart disease may cause dysrhythmias
  4. S3: Heart failure may be the basis of a dysrhythmia
  5. S4: may indicate coronary artery disease or obstruction to ventricular outflow with resultant dysrhythmia development

Pulmonary assessment: to identify presence of pulmonary disease which may result in hypoxia. Auscultate lungs for presence of:

- Crackles
- Wheezing

Abdominal assessment: to identify signs of generalized atherosclerosis.

- Auscultate for bruits over renal arteries and abdominal aorta.

Peripheral vascular assessment: to identify additional signs of generalized atherosclerosis and low perfusion state.

- Inspect lower extremities for color, temperature, presence/absence of pulses, hair distribution, edema.

Mental status assessment: to identify mental status changes that may be related to decreased cerebral perfusion.

Differential Diagnoses

Because symptoms of cardiac dysrhythmias are also associated with other disorders, differential diagnoses must be symptom based and include multisystem consideration. The following is a listing of symptoms frequently reported with cardiac dysrhythmias and suggested differential diagnoses:

- Fatigue: consider anemia, coronary artery disease, heart failure, thyroid disorders, medication side effects

- Dizziness: consider anemia, orthostasis, cerebrovascular insufficiency, medication side effects

- Dyspnea: consider anemia, coronary artery disease, heart failure, pulmonary disorders

- Syncope: consider aortic valve disease, orthostasis, seizure disorder, vasovagal response, hypoglycemia

- Palpitations: usually indicative of cardiac dysrhythmia

Diagnostic Tests

Diagnostic testing for cardiac dysrhythmias must include laboratory tests and a 12-lead ECG. The practitioner should also consider a chest x-ray to identify the presence of cardiomegaly and an echocardiogram to rule out valvular heart disease as the etiology for the rhythm disturbance.

Thyroid function studies, chemistry studies/electrolytes, and a complete blood count should be evaluated to identify possible causative factors for dysrhythmias. Although the ECG may confirm the presence of a dysrhythmia, absence of this finding is not conclusive. Given appropriate symptoms, in the absence of a positive ECG, 24-hour ambulatory monitoring should be initiated. In addition to monitoring the patient over time and during activities of daily living, computer equipment can produce a signal-averaged ECG (SAE) and heart rate variability data from the monitoring tape. The SAE is highly sensitive in detecting abnormalities in ventricular activity and may be helpful in identifying diagnosis, prognosis, and appropriate medical therapy.

Programmed electrical stimulation, as utilized in electrophysiology studies (EPS), is sometimes used as a diagnostic tool for dysrhythmia identification. EPS is indicated in any patient who survives a cardiac arrest, not associated with a myocardial infarction, or in those with syncope of unknown origin.

Atrial Fibrillation

Definition and Classification

Atrial fibrillation (AF) is a disturbance of cardiac rhythm caused by rapid, repetitive firing of multiple ectopic foci in the atria. Atrial rates are extremely rapid and result in quivering, rather than contraction, of the atrial musculature.

For purposes of treatment, AF is classified as acute or chronic. Acute AF is of short duration, usually less than 48 hours, while chronic AF lasts longer than 48 hours and is persistent or sustained. Both acute and chronic AF can be paroxysmal in nature.[36,38]

Prevalence and Significance

Atrial fibrillation is the most common clinically significant dysrhythmia in the general population.[39] Its prevalence increases significantly with aging and is estimated to be 11% in persons over the age of 70 and 17% in those who are 84 and older.[36] Seventy percent of the population with AF are estimated to be between 65 and 85 years of age.[37]

Atrial fibrillation is associated with both increased morbidity and mortality. Lack of atrial systole may reduce cardiac output by as much as 30%. A 4.8-fold increase in the risk of stroke is associated with AF and mortality rates range from 0.2–16%. The highest morbidity and mortality rates are found in older patients.[36]

Pathophysiology

As previously noted, histological changes, associated with normal aging, predispose older adults to the development of dysrhythmias, including atrial fibrillation. Specifically, atrial dilatation, fibrosis of cardiac and sinoatrial node structures, loss of nodal fibers, and accumulation of fatty deposits in the sinoatrial node and surrounding tissues contribute to the development of AF. In addition to the normal changes of aging, other diseases and conditions support the initiation of AF (see Table 3–13a).

Clinical Presentation

As a consequence of decreased cardiac output, patients with atrial fibrillation can present with a variety of symptoms including fatigue, palpitations, dizziness, syncope, angina, and heart failure. The severity of these symptoms is usually heart rate related. In the older adult, a transient ischemic attack (TIA), related to cerebral arterial embolization, may be the presenting symptom of AF.

In evaluating a patient with suspected atrial fibrillation, the previously identified format for the history and physical examination, differential diagnoses, and diagnostic tests should be utilized. The following ECG criteria provides diagnostic evidence of atrial fibrillation.

1. Rate:
   - Atrial: 400–600
   - Ventricular: variable
2. Rhythm: irregularly irregular
3. P waves: not identifiable. Fibrillatory waves are seen on baseline.
4. PR interval: none, since there are no P waves
5. QRS complexes: usually normal. There may be an occasional widened complex due to aberrant ventricular conduction.

Table 3–13a   Predisposing Factors for Atrial Fibrillation[37]

Atrial dilatation
Atrial ischemia
Atrial disease
Alcohol
Hyperthyroidism
Cardiac surgery
Infection
Metabolic abnormalities
Electrolyte imbalance
Medications

Interventions

Chronic AF can be managed by the nurse practitioner in the outpatient setting, while new-onset AF requires physician referral or hospitalization. Interventions are directed toward controlling the ventricular rate in order to maximize cardiac output, preventing arterial embolization, and, when possible, converting the rhythm to NSR.[37]

The treatment of AF is dependent on the clinical status of the patient, causative factors and the type of AF. When the ventricular rate is uncontrolled (> 100/minute), the patient may be hemodynamically unstable. In this situation, transfer to an acute-care setting for immediate cardioversion must be arranged. Because of AV nodal disease and block, older patients often have a slow ventricular response to AF.[36]

Identification of the type of AF is helpful in directing treatment options. Acute, paroxysmal AF may be precipitated by individual habits, stress, or underlying disease. Lifestyle modification and treatment of contributing medical conditions may be all that is needed to resolve an isolated episode of AF.

Other available treatments require physician collaboration and include direct current cardioversion (DCC) and/or pharmacological therapy. In both acute and chronic AF, DCC may be recommended. DCC frequently produces conversion to NSR; however, it appears that these results may be short-lived in the older population.[36] This may be especially true if cardioversion is not followed with initiation of antiarrhythmic drug (AAD) therapy.

Pharmacological treatment of AF in the elderly requires a careful analysis of the risk/benefit ratio. AADs have a high side-effect profile and may actually be proarrhythmic. When a physician prescribes these agents for treatment of AF, the nurse practitioner must carefully monitor the patient for adverse effects (see Table 3–13b for antiarrhythmic drugs and common adverse reactions). Often, in an older adult, the decision will be made to leave the patient in AF and control the ventricular rate with medications. Digoxin, calcium channel blockers, or beta adrenergic blockade are most often utilized for this purpose.[37,40]

Table 3–13b   Antiarrhythmic Drugs[41,43]

Drug/Class	Adverse Effects
Class IA	
Quinidine sulfate	Diarrhea, tinnitus, thrombocytopenia, anemia, fever, rash, heart failure, torsades de pointes, heart block
Procainamide	Lupus erythematosus, thrombocytopenia, neutropenia, fever, rash, heart failure, torsades de pointes, heart block
Disopyramide	Anticholinergic effects, rash, headache, dizziness, muscle pain or weakness, heart failure, torsades de pointes, heart block
Class IB	
Tocainide	Dizziness, nausea, heart failure, blood dyscrasias, pulmonary fibrosis, exacerbation of ventricular dysrhythmia
Mexiletine	Diarrhea, nausea, anticholinergic effects, tremor, gait disturbance, chest pain, heart failure, exacerbation of ventricular dysrhythmia
Class IC	
Flecainide	Nausea, dizziness, headache, tremor, chest pain, heart failure, ventricular dysrhythmias, heart block
Propafenone	Constipation, other adverse effects same as Flecanide
Class II	
Metoprolol	Bradycardia, AV block, hypotension, worsening of heart failure, bronchospasm, dizziness, fatigue, sleep disturbance, increased triglycerides and total and LDL cholesterol, decreased HDL cholesterol. May mask signs and symptoms of hypoglycemia.
Propanolol	Same as Metoprolol
Class III	
Amiodarone	Photosensitivity, blue-tinged skin, liver and pulmonary toxicity, thyroid disorders, corneal deposits, bradycardia, hypotension, heart failure, torsades de pointes, AV block
Sotalol	Fatigue, bronchospasm, bradycardia, hypotension, heart failure, torsades de pointes, AV block
Class IV	
Verapamil	Constipation, ankle edema, dizziness, fatigue, hypotension, bradycardia, AV block, heart failure
Diltiazem	Same as Verapamil

Because of the high risk of stroke, anticoagulation therapy plays a large role in the treatment of AF. If the decision is made to attempt cardioversion to NSR, the patient is usually anticoagulated for three weeks before and after the procedure.[36,40] Chronic AF requires long-term anticoagulation and warfarin therapy should be considered for all older adults with AF. International Normalized

Ratio (INR) should be closely monitored and maintained at the lower end of the recommended range, which is 2.0–3.0. As with all drug therapy, the risk/benefit ratio should be carefully assessed. Patients with uncontrolled hypertension or those with medical conditions that predispose to bleeding are at high risk for intracranial bleeding, secondary to warfarin therapy.[36] Additionally, in the very old and those with a history of falls, the hazards of anticoagulation must be considered.

Newer interventions for AF may be appropriate for older adults who cannot tolerate, or who have failed, drug therapy. Radiofrequency catheter ablation can be utilized to obliterate intra-atrial conduction pathways or the AV node. Destruction of the AV node requires implantation of a permanent pacemaker.[36,37] The corridor procedure is a surgical intervention that isolates a conduction pathway between the sinus and AV nodes, regulating the heartbeat. With both RFA and the corridor procedure, one or both atria continue to fibrillate; therefore these procedures do not eliminate the need for anticoagulation.[36] A second type of surgical management, the maze procedure, involves surgically incising and repairing multiple sites in both atria with the goal of interrupting the arrhythmogenic foci. This procedure has been successful in restoring sinus rhythm; however, implantation of a permanent pacemaker is often required afterwards.[36]

Heart Block

Definition and Classification

Heart block, as its name implies, may be defined as a block or delay in conduction of the electrical impulse from the sinoatrial (SA) node to the ventricles. The delay may occur in the SA node itself, in the atria, or in the AV node. Heart block is usually classified as follows:

- First degree
- Second degree
  Mobitz I (Wenckebach)
  Mobitz II
- Third degree (Complete heart block)

Prevalence and Significance

The incidence of heart block increases with age. The physiological changes associated with aging, and the prevalence of CAD in the older population, predispose to the development of heart block. Medications such as digoxin, beta blockers, or calcium channel blockers, commonly prescribed for older adults, can cause or exacerbate conduction delays.[39]

Clinical Presentation

First-degree heart block is of no hemodynamic significance and is asymptomatic; it is identified only by routine ECG. Higher-grade blocks often produce symptoms such as dizziness and syncope. Following the history and physical examination, the nurse practitioner should perform a 12-lead ECG. The following are criteria that can be utilized to diagnose heart block from the ECG.

First-degree heart block: defined as a conduction delay between the SA and AV nodes and evidenced by a prolonged PR interval.

1. Rate: may be normal or bradycardic
2. Rhythm: regular
3. P waves: present and preceding each QRS complex
4. PR interval: > .20 seconds
5. QRS complexes: usually normal

Second-degree heart block—Mobitz I (Wenckebach): defined as intermittent nonconducted atrial impulses and evidenced by a progressively prolonged PR interval and dropped beats.

1. Rate: may be normal or bradycardic
2. Rhythm: irregular due to nonconducted impulses
3. P waves: occur regularly, but not always followed by QRS complex
4. PR interval: progressively prolonged until an atrial impulse is not conducted. Following the nonconducted impulse, the PR interval returns to a gradually prolonging pattern.
5. QRS complexes: usually normal, but may be prolonged if the block is lower in the conduction system

Second-degree heart block—Mobitz II: defined as intermittent nonconducted atrial impulses with a constant PR interval.

1. Rate: may be normal or bradycardic and is dependent on degree of block and number of nonconducted impulses. Because not all atrial impulses are conducted to the ventricles, the atrial rate is greater than the ventricular rate.
2. Rhythm: may be regular or irregular
3. P waves: occur regularly, but not always followed by QRS complex
4. PR interval: may be within normal limits or prolonged, but remains constant
5. QRS complexes: usually normal, but may be prolonged if the block is low in the conduction system

Third-degree heart block: defined as atrial and ventricular activity that is completely dissociated. Impulses are not conducted from the atria to the ventricles and each chamber beats at its own inherent rate.

1. Rate: atrial rate > ventricular rate
2. Rhythm: both atrial and ventricular rhythms usually regular
3. P waves: occur regularly, but not always followed by QRS complex
4. PR interval: variable
5. QRS complexes: usually normal but may be prolonged if the block is low in the conduction system

Interventions

As is the case with all dysrhythmias, the treatment of heart block is dependent on the clinical status of the patient. First-degree heart block produces no symptoms and requires no treatment. The condition should be periodically reevaluated for evidence of an increase in the level of block. Identification of a new-onset first-degree block should prompt a review of the patient's medications to ascertain if they may be contributing to the heart block.

Patients with second-degree heart block may or may not be symptomatic. Many times Mobitz I is well tolerated by the patient, while the ventricular rate in Mobitz II may be low enough to produce symptoms. Patients complaining of symptoms such as dizziness or syncope, associated with second-degree heart block, require hospital admission. Mobitz II may also be a precursor to third-degree block. Third-degree heart block is usually a medical emergency and requires immediate transfer to an acute-care facility for cardiac pacing.

While atropine and isoproterenol are utilized in the short term to increase heart rate, the only treatment option for symptomatic heart block is implantation of a cardiac pacemaker. A dual chamber pacemaker facilitates normal atrial and ventricular synchrony and is an appropriate treatment modality for older adults who do not have AF.[39] For active patients, a pacemaker with a rate-responsive feature allows for heart rate increases to meet the metabolic demands of a variety of activities. A newer feature of dual-chamber pacing allows for mode switching and appears to be a good choice in older adults who have periods of AF. This feature allows the pacemaker to switch automatically to the asynchronous mode and pace only the ventricles when it senses a rapid atrial rhythm.[39]

■ Sick Sinus Syndrome

Definition

Sick sinus syndrome, also known as tachy-brady syndrome, is associated with a wide range of dysrhythmias. Patients commonly exhibit atrial tachycardias, which terminate into a bradyarrhythmia. The bradycardic episodes often include long pauses that are the source of the reported symptoms.

Sick sinus syndrome is a conduction disturbance unique to the elderly population. It is usually associated with degenerative, sclerotic changes of the sinus node. It may also be caused by coronary artery disease.

Clinical Presentation

Because sick sinus syndrome includes a variety of dysrhythmias, it can be difficult to diagnose. Patient complaints may be as nonspecific as fatigue, lightheadedness, irritability, and memory loss. Palpitations and syncopal episodes are the most commonly reported symptoms. Criteria for electrocardiographic diagnosis of sick sinus syndrome is difficult to identify because the syndrome consists of different dysrhythmias. A general guideline is as follows:

1. Rate: dysrhythmia dependent
2. Rhythm: irregular
3. P waves: dependent on the dysrhythmia present
4. PR interval: variable
5. QRS complexes: usually normal

Interventions

Once a diagnosis of sick sinus syndrome is made, the practitioner should review the patient's current medications to determine if they may be contributing to the dysrhythmia. If the problem cannot be corrected by discontinuing medications, pacemaker implantation is indicated. Pacemaker therapy may repress the ectopic atrial foci and prevent atrial tachyarrhythmias.[39] If tachycardia continues, despite pacemaker therapy, antidysrhythmic medications may be required.

■ Ventricular Dysrhythmias

Definition and Classification

The term ventricular dysrhythmia or ventricular arrhythmia (VA) refers to a cardiac rhythm that originates in the ventricles, instead of the sinus node. The consequences to the patient with a ventricular dysrhythmia depend on the classification of the dysrhythmia and the presence or absence of underlying heart disease.

Ventricular dysrhythmias may be classified as simple or complex premature ventricular contractions (PVCs), ventricular tachycardia (VT), or ventricular fibrillation. VT is identified as the appearance of three or more consecutive PVCs and is further classified as nonsustained or sustained[38,39,41] (see Table 3–14). Ventricular fibrillation is a lethal rhythm resulting in death unless initiation of full cardiopulmonary support is successful.

Prevalence and Significance

Ventricular dysrhythmias commonly occur in the older adult and, in the absence of underlying heart disease, are not considered to be significant.[38,39,41] However, the presence of ischemic or nonischemic heart disease increases the likelihood of sudden

Table 3–14   Classification of Ventricular Dysrhythmias[41,42]

Classification	Identifying Characteristics	Physiological Consequences
Simple PVC	• Infrequent • Uniform	• None
Complex PVC	• Paired • Multiform • > 6 per minute	• None in patients without heart disease • In the presence of heart disease, may deteriorate into sustained VT or VF
Nonsustained VT	• Lasts < 30 seconds	• None in patients without heart disease • In the presence of heart disease, may deteriorate into sustained VT or VF
Sustained VT	• Lasts > 30 seconds	• May result in hemodynamic collapse

cardiac death from complex PVCs or nonsus-tained VT.[38]

Pathophysiology

While PVCs may not be significant or require treatment in the older adult, their presence should prompt an investigation of possible causes of the dysrhythmia. PVCs occur in healthy people and may be related to stress, anxiety, or use of caffeine, nicotine, or alcohol. Medications, electrolyte imbalances, hypoxemia, and myocardial ischemia are other common causes of PVCs.

Clinical Presentation

Patients with simple or complex PVCs or nonsus-tained VT may be asymptomatic and the presence of any of these dysrhythmias may be identified only through a 12-lead ECG. Conversely, patients may complain of symptoms such as lightheaded-ness, palpitations, chest pain, or syncope.

The diagnostic workup for a patient suspected of having a dysrhythmia must include a 12-lead ECG. In a ventricular dysrhythmia, the electrical impulse originates outside of the sinus node and is transmit-ted through the conduction system in an aberrant manner. As a result, it is usually recognized on the ECG by the presence of one or more widened, bizarre QRS complexes. The following criteria may be utilized to identify a PVC on the ECG:

1. Rate: determined by the underlying rhythm
2. Rhythm: irregular due to the presence of the premature beat(s)
3. P waves: not usually present with the PVC
4. PR interval: because a P wave is usually not visible with the PVC, PR interval cannot be determined
5. QRS complexes: > .12 seconds. Configuration of the PVC varies depending on the site of ori-gin within the ventricle.

Interventions

The identification of simple PVCs on the ECG usu-ally requires no treatment. Because this dysrhythmia

may be precipitated by individual habits, stress, med-ications, or metabolic derangements, elimination or treatment of these factors may abolish the PVCs. These same interventions may be utilized in the man-agement of complex PVCs and nonsustained VT. This approach, however, should be used only after a complete history and physical, diagnostic testing, and physician consultation has ruled out the exis-tence of heart disease. Because of the life-threatening nature and symptoms of sustained VT, these patients usually present to an emergency room rather than the primary-care practitioner. In a patient with undi-agnosed heart disease, complex PVCs or nonsus-tained VT can deteriorate into sustained VT and/or VF in the office setting. This life-threatening situation requires initiation of cardiopulmonary resuscitation and transport to the closest hospital through the emergency medical system.

When required, pharmacological treatment of a ventricular dysrhythmia should be initiated by a physician and may be monitored by the nurse practitioner. Cardioselective beta blockers are indicated as first-line treatment of VA in the older adult. The use of Class I antiarrhythmic drugs (see Table 3–13b) has not been shown to reduce mor-tality and, because of their proarrhythmic side effects, may actually decrease survival rates.[38,39,41] If these agents are used, it is imperative that they be monitored for effectiveness. This may be accomplished through ambulatory Holter moni-toring or by electrophysiological testing. Older patients with persistent life-threatening VA, not controlled by AAD therapy, are candidates for an automatic implantable cardioverter/defibrillator (AICD). In the very frail older adult, with a refrac-tory VA, it may be inappropriate to initiate this type of life-sustaining treatment.[41]

General Interventions and Education for Dysrhythmic Patients

As previously discussed, the nurse practitioner may initially diagnose a dysrhythmia in the older adult. Identification and treatment of coexisting morbidi-ties or contributing conditions may be sufficient to correct the problem. In both the asymptomatic and symptomatic patient, with an identified dysrhythmia (except AF) and no underlying heart disease, the nurse can offer reassurance and instruct the patient about lifestyle changes that may resolve the problem.[39] These changes would include the elimination of tobacco, alcohol, and caffeine. Stress reduction, through relaxation techniques and increased leisure activities, may also be helpful.

Older adults who receive pharmacological therapy for the treatment of a dysrhythmia must be closely monitored for drug efficacy and for the development of adverse effects from their medications. These patients are often followed by a cardiologist, but may be seen for routine visits by the nurse practitioner. During these visits, the practitioner should question the patient about the presence of symptoms suggestive of recurrent dysrhythmia or medication intolerance. The nurse should explore the patient's understanding of the medical problem and attempt to ascertain compliance with the plan of care. Frequent education and reenforcement of the rationale for treatment may be necessary.

Patients with pacemakers or AICDs may have poor comprehension of the mechanism and reason for implantation. Because of the uniqueness of the nurse–patient relationship, the older adult may feel more comfortable acknowledging this to the nurse practitioner, rather than the physician. The practitioner must be prepared to explain, in a way the patient can understand, how these devices work and answer any questions the patient may have regarding this method of treatment.

The nurse practitioner must educate patients and, when appropriate, their families and caregivers regarding symptoms to be reported to the health-care provider. Dysrhythmia symptoms and consequences, and medications and side effects, should be reviewed. Patients and their families must be counseled on what to report and how to do it. Because of the life-threatening nature of some dysrhythmias, it may be appropriate for selected family members to learn the techniques of cardiopulmonary resuscitation.

The diagnosis of a cardiac dysrhythmia represents a complex pathophysiological condition that can be difficult for nonmedical personnel to comprehend. In the older adult, impaired cognition and hearing deficits are further obstacles to understanding this disease process and its therapeutic options. Low educational levels and use of inappropriate terminology by health-care providers may further compromise comprehension. Additionally, low vision, musculoskeletal disorders, and inadequate financial resources may prevent the older adult from obtaining and taking medications appropriately.

The medical diagnosis and treatment of a cardiac dysrhythmia can also be a frightening and unpleasant experience. The nurse practitioner can assist the older patient in coping with these issues by providing information and by encouraging and supporting patient input into treatment decisions.

The nurse practitioner can play an integral role in the health care of the older adult with a cardiac dysrhythmia. As clinician, educator, and patient advocate, the practitioner can assist the patient in meeting the treatment goals of improving quality of life and, when possible, decreasing the morbidity and mortality associated with a cardiac dysrhythmia.

References

1. US Census Bureau, Population Division, Release PPL-91 December 28,1998.
2. Duncan AK, Vittone MD, Fleming KC, et al. Cardiovascular disease in elderly patients. *Mayo Clini Proc.* 1996; 71:184–196.
3. Aronow WS, Tresch DD. Preface. In: WS Aronow, DD Tresch, eds., *Clinics in Geriatric Medicine,* 1996;12(1). Philadelphia: W.B. Saunders.
4. Cefalu CA, Burris JF. Cardiovascular disease in the elderly. *Compr Ther.* 1996;22(8):509–514.
5. Fernandez-Ortiz A, Fuster V. Pathophysiology of coronary artery disease. In: WS Aronow, DD Tresch, eds. *Coronary Artery Disease in the Elderly.* Philadelphia: W.B. Saunders. In series: *Clinics in Geriatric Medicine.* 1996;12(1):1–15.
6. Duprez DA. Angina in the elderly. *Eur Heart J.* 1996; 17(Suppl G):8–13.
7. Kannel WB. Cardiovascular risk factors in the older adult. *Hosp Pract.* 1996;November 15.
8. The Joint National Committee on Prevention, Detection, Evaluation, and Treatment, of High Blood Pressure & the National High Blood Pressure Education Program Coordinating Committee: The sixth report of the joint national committee on prevention, detection, evaluation, and treatment of high blood pressure. *Arch Intern Med.* 1997;157:2413–2444.

9. Dumas MA. Hypertension in primary care. *Am J Nurse Pract.* 1999;3(2):7–32.

10. Sadowski AV, Redeker NS. The hypertensive elder. *Nurse Pract.* 1996;21(5):99–118.

11. Porth CM. *Pathophysiology: Concepts of Altered Health States.* 4th ed. Philadelphia: J.B. Lippincott; 1994.

12. Messerli FH, Grossman E, Goldbourt U. Are beta blockers efficacious as first-line therapy for hypertension in the elderly? A systematic review. *JAMA.* 1998;279:1903–1907.

13. Lakatta EG. Circulatory function in younger and older humans in health. In: WR Hazzard, JP Blass, WH Ettinger, JB Halter, JG Ouslander, eds. *Principles of Geriatric Medicine and Gerontology.* New York: McGraw-Hill; 1999.

14. Burke L, Porth CM. Alterations in cardiac function. In: CM Porth, ed. *Pathophysiology: Concepts of Altered Health States.* 4th ed. Philadelphia: J.B. Lippincott; 1994.

15. Agency for health care policy and research. Unstable angina: diagnosis and management. *Clinical Practice Guidelines.* Rockville, MD: US Department of Health and Human Services; 1994.

16. Tresh DD, Aronow WS. Clinical manifestations and diagnosis of coronary artery disease. In: WS Aronow, DD Tresch, eds. *Clinics in Geriatric Medicine.* 1996;12(1). Philadelphia: W.B. Saunders.

17. Wei JY. Coronary heart disease. In: WR Hazzard, JP Blass, WH Ettinger, JB Halter, JG Ouslander, eds. *Principles of Geriatric Medicine and Gerontology.* New York: McGraw-Hill; 1999.

18. Hill B, Geraci SA. A diagnostic approach to chest pain based on history and ancillary evaluation. *Nurse Pract.* 1998;23(4):20–45.

19. Olson HG, Aronow WS. Medical management of stable angina and unstable angina in the elderly with coronary artery disease. In: WS Arnow, DD Tresch, eds. *Clinics in Geriatric Medicine.* 1996:12(1). Philadelphia: W.B. Saunders Co.

20. Katzel LI, Goldberg AP. Dyslipoproteinemia. In WR Hazzard, JP Blass, WH Ettinger, JB Halter, JG Ouslander, eds. *Principles of Geriatric Medicine and Gerontology.* New York: McGraw-Hill; 1999.

21. LaRosa JC. Dyslipidemia and coronary artery disease in the elderly. In: WS Aronow, DD Tresch, eds. *Clinics in Geriatric Medicine.* 1996;12(1). Philadelphia: W.B. Saunders.

22. Leaf DA. Lipid disorders: applying new guidelines to your older patients. *Geriatrics.* 1994:49(5):35–41.

23. Agency for health care policy and research. Heart failure: evaluation and care of patients with left-ventricular systolic dysfunction. *Clinical Practice Guidelines.* Rockville, MD: US Department of Health and Human Services; 1994.

24. Miller S. Congestive heart failure; Clinical assessment and pharmacologic management. *Adv Nurse Pract.* 1997; June.

25. Havranek EP, Abrams F, Stevens E, et al. Mortality in elderly patients with heart failure. *Cardiol Rev.* 1999;16(6):40–42.

26. Gross SB. Heart failure: a review of current treatment strategies. *Adv Nurse Pract.* 1999;June.

27. Rich MW. Epidemiology, pathophysiology, and etiology of congestive heart failure in older adults. *J Am Geriatr Soc.* 1997;45:968–974.

28. Rich MW. Heart failure. In: WR Hazzard, JP Blass, WH Ettinger, et al., eds. *Principles of Geriatric Medicine and Gerontology.* New York: McGraw-Hill; 1999.

29. American College of Cardiology and American Heart Association. Guidelines for the evaluation and management of heart failure. *J Am Coll Cardiol.* 1995;26(5):1376–1398.

30. American Geriatrics Society. Clinical practice guidelines: heart failure: evaluation and care of patients with left-ventricular systolic dysfunction. *J Am Geriatr Soc.* 1998;46:525–529.

31. Aronow WS. Treatment of congestive heart failure in older persons. *J Am Geriatr Soc.* 1997;45:1252–1258.

32. CIBIS-II Investigators & Committee. The cardiac insufficiency bisoprolol study II (CIBIS-II): a randomized trial. *Lancet.* 1999;353:9–13.

33. Aronow WS. Commentary in Clinical practice guidelines: heart failure: evaluation and care of patients with left-ventricular systolic dysfunction. *J Am Geriatr Soc.* 1998;46:525–529.

34. Pitt B, Zannad F, Remme WJ. The effect of spironolactone on morbidity and mortality in patients with severe heart failure. Available at: *www.nejm.org/content/pitt/1.asp.* Accessed July 19, 1999.

35. Lok N, Lau C. Prevalence of palpitations, cardiac arrhythmias and their associated risk factors in ambulant elderly. *Int J Cardiol.* 1996;54:231–236.

36. Reardon M, Camm AJ. Atrial fibrillation in the elderly. *Clin Cardiol.* 1996;19:765–775.

37. Mackstaller LL, Alpert JS. Atrial fibrillation: a review of mechanism, etiology, and therapy. *Clin Cardiol.* 1997;20:640–650.

38. Van Gelder IC, Brugemann J, Crijns H. Pharmacological management of arrhythmias in the elderly. *Drugs Aging.* 1997; 11(2):96–110.

39. Crossley GH. Arrhythmias in the elderly. In: WR Hazzard, JP Blass, WH Ettinger, et al., eds. *Principles of Geriatric Medicine and Gerontology.* New York: McGraw-Hill, 1999.

40. Chrzanowski DD. Managing atrial fibrillation to prevent its major complication: ischemic stroke. *Nurse Pract.* 1998;23(5):26–42.

41. Aronow WS. Treatment of ventricular arrhythmias in older adults. *J Am Geriatr Soc.* 1995;43(6):688–695.

42. Youngkin EQ, Sawin KJ, Kissinger JF, et al., eds. *Pharmacotherapeutics: A Primary Care Clinical Guide.* Stamford, CT: Appleton & Lange; 1999.

Respiratory Problems in Older Adults

Mary F. Kelley

Introduction

Many factors affect respiratory health, including environmental and hereditary factors, tobacco use, allergens, exposure to carcinogens, comorbidities, and age-related changes in the respiratory system. This chapter briefly reviews these age-related changes. An overview of diagnostic tests is outlined, as well as a more in-depth look at the primary-care diagnosis and treatment of upper respiratory infections, acute bronchitis, chronic obstructive pulmonary disease, asthma, pneumonia, and tuberculosis.

Age-Related Changes

It is unknown whether many age-related changes are a normal part of aging or a result of illness, the environment, heredity, lifestyle, or some combination. Nevertheless, all people experience some of these changes with aging. How these changes affect health and illness is multifactorial and varies among individuals. The following age-related changes may occur in the respiratory system of an older adult[1]:

- diminished muscle strength in the thorax and diaphragm
- stiffer chest wall
- decreased elastic recoil
- decreased elasticity of the alveoli and reduced surface area, with diminished capacity for gas exchange
- decreased vital capacity
- increased residual volume

- decreased sensitivity of the respiratory centers
- drier mucous membranes, leading to more difficult mucous excretion

None of these changes, per se, cause illness, but they can diminish resiliency and ability to withstand and recover from respiratory problems.

Appropriate Diagnostic Tests in Primary Care

Chest X-Ray The chest x-ray is often the first essential step in a diagnostic workup of respiratory illness. It cannot, however, replace the importance of the history and physical examination. It is the integration of the history and physical and diagnostic tests that confirm a diagnosis and direct treatment. It is important to compare current and past x-rays.

The following respiratory illnesses are covered in this chapter, and the radiographic findings for each are listed below[2,3,4]:

Bronchitis	No specific abnormalities
COPD	Normal in mild cases
	Increased radiolucency of lung fields
	Decreased lung markings
	Flattened hemidiaphragm
	Increased retrosternal airspace
	Hyperinflation
Asthma	Usually normal
	Hyperinflation in exacerbations
Pneumonia	Variable depending on causative agent, status of lungs before pneumonia, and comorbidities
	Lobar consolidation or infiltrate
	Pleural effusion

Tuberculosis Active: nodular densities with or
without cavities usually found in
the apex or posterior segments of
the upper lobes or superior
segments of the lower lobes
Latent: calcified granulomas in the
apex

Computed Tomography and Magnetic Resonance Imaging

Computed tomography (CT scan) and magnetic resonance imaging (MRI) are more sophisticated radiological tests and can also be used to aid in the diagnosis of respiratory illnesses.[5] Logistically, both can be difficult for those who are claustrophobic; anyone with a pacemaker or other implanted metal device cannot undergo an MRI.

The CT scan's high-density resolution allows for the distinguishing of fat, cystic, or solid tissues and the visualization of finer details without superimposed parenchymal structures.[5] The mediastinum, hilar regions, blood vessels, connective tissue, and air spaces can be assessed more accurately with the CT scan. It is a more useful tool in the detection of tumors and pulmonary metastasis as well.

MRI provides images in multiple planes with greater differentiation of soft-tissue structures.[5] It also shows blood vessels without use of contrast dye. MRI is not commonly used by the primary-care practitioner. Although the data obtained is very useful and specific, it has limitations. Many people experience feelings of claustrophobia during an MRI. Sedation or even anesthesia may be necessary in order to complete the scan. Open MRI machines are available in some areas and can ease feelings of claustrophobia. The acquisition of images with an MRI is very slow, thereby causing the possibility of motion artifact. Most MRI tests take 30 to 60 minutes to complete. The cost of an MRI can also be prohibitive for patients with inadequate or no health insurance.

The Mantoux Test

The Mantoux test (tuberculin skin test) is relatively easy to administer and interpret.[6,7,8] The tuberculin skin test involves the intradermal administration of purified protein derivative (PPD) into the skin of the inner fore-

arm. The reaction to this injection is assessed in two to three days to allow for development of any delayed cutaneous hypersensitivity. Erythema may develop, but only the amount of induration at the injection site is used to determine whether a test is positive or negative. Although sensitivity to tuberculin after exposure lasts a lifetime, hypersensitivity diminishes with age. For this reason, anyone over age 55 should receive a two-step test.[7,8] One to two weeks after the first test, a second injection is administered and read.

A properly administered Mantoux test for the older adult requires the patient to make four visits to the office or practice site (two visits for each injection and two visits for each interpretation). This may make compliance difficult and orders for such a test need to be judiciously applied. Those with the highest risk factors should be considered for testing: persons who are HIV positive, have a known exposure, have suspicious chest x-rays, are symptomatic, are IV drug abusers, are immunocompromised, are foreign-born (Asia, Africa, Latin America), have comorbidities (silicosis, diabetes, hematologic malignancies), and some in low-income populations. Health-care providers who work with high-risk individuals and residents of long-term care facilities should be screened periodically (at least annually).[7]

The serum used for a Mantoux test is PPD 5 TU (tuberculin units). A small bore needle is used to intradermally inject 0.5 cc into the skin of the inner forearm.[6] A reaction is considered positive if greater than 5, 10, or 15 mm of induration develops within 48 to 72 hours.[8] A 5 mm reaction is positive in individuals who are at greatest risk for the illness (HIV positive, TB exposure, suspicious x-ray, and IV drug abusers). A 15 mm reaction is considered positive in those with no risk factors and a 10 mm reaction is positive in all others (including residents of long-term care).

Pulmonary Function Tests

Pulmonary function tests (PFTs) provide an objective, measurable assessment of lung function,[9] as well as additional data concerning the diagnosis and treatment of certain lung conditions. PFTs may elucidate clinically undetected disease, characterize the type and severity of disease, and demonstrate the response to therapeutic interventions. For the primary-care practitioner, PFTs performed at a reliable laboratory and interpreted by a pulmonologist can provide baseline data, as well as information later about the degree of progression and response to treatment. Pulmonary function testing is indicated for[9]:

- chronic cough or dyspnea, wheezing, orthopnea
- unexplained crackles or other adventitious breath sounds
- hypoxemia, hypercapnia, polycythemia, abnormal chest x-ray
- assessment of the progression of known disease
- assessment of pulmonary rehabilitation or therapeutic intervention
- assessment of preoperative risk
- decreased exercise tolerance
- illnesses or conditions that have an effect on the respiratory system

Upper Respiratory Infections

Common Cold

Definition and Pathophysiology The term "common cold" is a popular phrase for a group of symptoms including sneezing, congestion, and mild malaise. Rhinoviruses, coronoviruses, or adenoviruses (among others) infect ciliated epithelial cells of the nasal mucosa and upper respiratory tract.[10] A mild cellular inflammatory response causes increased production of mucous. Symptoms can continue for two to three weeks. Increased incidence of bacterial sinusitis follows a cold. Viruses are thought to be spread by aerosol method and by contaminated hands which then touch susceptible others who inadvertently infect themselves.[11] The incubation period is usually two to three days, but can be as long as seven days.

Clinical Presentation Symptoms can vary in severity and degree of annoyance. They include sneezing, sore throat, rhinorrhea, mild malaise and achiness, nonproductive cough, sinus congestion, or headache.[11] Signs may include nasal mucosa edema and erythema, nasal secretions, low-grade fever or mild erythema in the pharynx.

If signs or symptoms are of a greater severity, that is, fever, productive cough, purulent nasal discharge, pleuritic chest pain, or shortness of breath, then the differential diagnoses should include sinusitis, bronchitis, pneumonia, or other noninfectious respiratory conditions.

History and Physical Examination The history includes symptoms (onset and duration), possible infectious exposures, and any treatments that already have been tried. The physical exam begins with temperature and vital signs. Otoscopic examination of the ears and nasal mucosa, visualization of the oropharynx, palpation of the neck for lymphadenopathy, auscultation of the lungs, and perhaps transillumination of the maxillary sinuses should also be included.

There are no specific laboratory or diagnostic tests that are indicated in the clinical diagnosis of the common cold.

Management Plan Treatment of the common cold is geared toward symptomatic relief.[10] Antihistamines generally have no role in treatment.[12] Decongestants are helpful to relieve rhinorrhea, sinus congestion, and headache.[13] Gargling with warm salt water often soothes a sore throat and can help clear oropharyngeal secretions.[11] An analgesic such as acetaminophen (up to 3 grams in a 24-hour period) used regularly helps to alleviate malaise and muscle aches.[11] Over-the-counter cough syrups or capsules can quiet a cough due to the common cold. See Table 4–1 for medications commonly used with upper respiratory illnesses.

Simple instructions to the patient may help prevent the spread of a cold and prevent future infections. Good nutrition and adequate sleep strengthen the immune system. Frequent and thorough hand washing, particularly during the cold season, hinders the spread of viruses. It may be useful to wash commonly touched surfaces like

Table 4–1   URI Medications

	Category	Indication	Dose	Prescription (Rx) or Over-the-Counter (OTC)
Phenylephrine 0.5% (Afrin 4 hr, Neosynephrine 4 hr)	Nasal decongestant	Cold, sinusitis	2 sprays each nostril q 4 hrs for 3–4 days only	OTC
Oxymetazoline .05% (Afrin 12 hr, Neo-synephrine 12 hr)	Nasal decongestant	Cold, sinusitis	2 sprays each nostril q 12 hrs for 3–4 days only	OTC
Pseudoephedrine (Sudafed)	Nasal decongestant	Cold, sinusitis	30 mg tabs, 1–2 tabs q 4–6 hrs (max 240 mg/24 hrs)	OTC
Chlorpheniramine maleate (Chlor-trimeton)	Antihistamine	Allergy	4 mg q 4–6 hrs	OTC
Brompheniramine maleate (Dimetapp allergy)	Antihistamine	Allergy	4 mg q 4–6 hrs	OTC
Loratadine (Claritin)	Antihistamine	Allergy	10 mg daily	Rx
Fexofenadine (Allegra)	Antihistamine	Allergy	60 mg BID	Rx
Cetritizine (Zyrtec)	Antihistamine	Allergy	5–10 mg daily	Rx
Guaifenesin syrup (Robitussin)	Expectorant	Cough	10 ml q 4 hrs	OTC
Guaifenesin (Humabid LA)	Expectorant	Cough	600–1200 mg BID	Rx
Guaifenesin/dextro-methorphan syrup (Robitussin DM)	Expectorant/ antitussive	Cough	10 ml q 4 hrs	OTC
Guaifenesin/detro-methorphan (Humabid DM)	Expectorant/ antitussive	Cough	600–1200 mg BID	Rx
Benzonatate (Tessalon)	Antitussive	Cough	100 mg TID	Rx
Acetaminophen (Tylenol)	Analgesic, anti-pyretic	Myalgias, headache, fever	650 mg q 4 hrs or 1000 mg q 6 hrs	OTC (do not exceed 3000 mg/24 hr)

telephone handsets, although there is no evidence that viruses responsible for the common cold live well outside of a live host. A follow-up appointment is not needed unless symptoms do not subside within one to two weeks, or they become worse at any point during the illness.

Influenza

Definition and Pathophysiology   Influenza is a seasonal viral respiratory illness occurring during the late fall and winter months in the United States and capable of reaching epidemic proportions.[14] It is similar to the common cold in mode of infection and transmission, being spread by the aerosol method or close contact.[15] Older adults and those with chronic illnesses are most at risk for complications like pneumonia, exacerbation of comorbidities, and death.[14]

Clinical Presentation   Presenting signs and symptoms include exhaustion, chills, sinus congestion, nonproductive cough, headache, myalgias, fever, pharyngitis, and cervical adenopathy.[15,16] Less common, but not unusual, are nausea, vomiting, and dizziness. Symptoms can be so debilitating that they cause a person to be bedbound for several days. Lungs are usually clear to auscultation.

Diagnosis of influenza is usually made if there has been a local outbreak or it is the flu season. If there is an institutional outbreak, the local health department can provide kits for testing for the offending virus. Differential diagnoses include other viral illnesses, severe sinusitis, or pneumonia.

History and Physical Examination   The history and physical are essentially the same as for the common cold. Diagnostic tests are nonspecific, but a mildly elevated white blood cell count may be seen. If the patient is at risk for respiratory complications, or respiratory status worsens during the course of influenza, then a chest x-ray is warranted.

Management Plan   Treatment of influenza is based on symptomatic relief and detection of complications like bacterial pneumonia. Rest, fluids, and analgesia with acetaminophen are the usual treatment.[15] Those too ill to maintain hydration may need to be hospitalized. If symptoms do not resolve within seven days, further medical attention is needed.[15] Three medications can be considered for influenza, if administration can begin within 48 hours of onset.[16] Amantadine (Symmetrel) and rimantadine (Flumadine) are available in pill form or syrup and oseltamivir (Tamiflu) is available as a capsule. The dose for amantadine and rimantadine is 100 mg daily for 10 days in older adults or in those with renal or hepatic impairment, and 100 mg twice a day for 10 days in all other adults. The dose for oseltamivir is 75 mg twice a day for 5

days or 75 mg daily for 5 days in those with renal insufficiency.

Prevention of influenza is the gold standard of treatment. This is accomplished through yearly vaccination or with chemoprophylaxis. The influenza vaccine is made available every year in the fall and should be administered in October or November.[16] All adults over age 65, residents of long-term care facilities, persons who are HIV positive, anyone with chronic illnesses, and health-care workers and others in contact with persons at high risk for influenza should be vaccinated.[16] Even if in a high-risk group, those with anaphylactic hypersensitivity to eggs or known sensitivity to a component of the vaccine should not be vaccinated. A history of Guillain-Barré Syndrome (GBS) requires weighing the risks of influenza.[16] In rare cases, GBS is also a potential adverse side effect to the influenza vaccine in people with no previous history.

Chemoprophylaxis is useful for persons in high-risk groups who cannot be vaccinated.[15,16] Cost, compliance, and potential side effects must be taken into account before undertaking weeks of amantadine or rimantadine therapy. Either of these medications would need to be administered during the peak period of influenza illness in the community (December through March). The doses are the same as those used in treating influenza. Rest, adequate nutrition, and thorough hand washing are preventive measures for influenza, along with limited contact with infected persons. Follow-up is only necessary if symptoms do not resolve within seven days or if symptoms worsen despite treatment.

Sinusitis

Definition and Pathophysiology   Sinusitis is an inflammation or infection of the mucosal lining of the maxillary or frontal sinuses (the ethmoid sinuses are more often involved in children and sphenoid sinus infection is rare).[17,18] The ostia are the openings through which the sinuses drain into the nasal cavity. Many irritants contribute to inflammation of the ostia, thereby blocking drainage. The ostia are located superiorly which causes mucous to drain against gravity. Obstruction can lead to infection. Sinusitis is considered acute if onset was one day to three weeks prior to reporting of symptoms.[18] Sinusitis is generally considered chronic if symptoms have persisted for six weeks to three months.[18] Acute sinusitis is often preceded by an upper-respiratory infection and has a more obvious onset. Chronic sinusitis is subtle, most commonly caused by an aerobic organism, usually of the *Staphylococcus* species, although anaerobes can also be responsible in a small percentage of cases.[18] Chronic sinusitis most often involves more than one bacteria and needs a complex management approach.

Clinical Presentation   Symptoms of sinusitis initially resemble the common cold, but become more specific and occasionally more severe. Symptoms include diminished sense of smell, cough that can be worse at night, purulent nasal discharge (white, yellow, or green), postnasal drip, headache, facial or upper-teeth pain, fatigue, malaise, unpleasant taste, sneezing, or hoarseness.[17] Signs include fever, purulent secretions, pain upon sinus palpation, and edema and erythema of nasal mucosa. Differential diagnoses are the common cold, allergic rhinitis, brain abscess (note any neurological signs), or other disorders causing facial pain or headaches like dental abscess.

History and Physical Examination   The history is the most important initial tool in diagnosing sinusitis. A thorough discussion of the patient's symptoms is most helpful. The physical exam includes temperature and vital signs, otoscopic examination of the ears and nasal mucosa, visualization of the oropharynx, and palpation of the maxillary and frontal sinuses as well as the neck. Auscultation of the lungs is also important, particularly in those who have other respiratory problems. Transillumination of the maxillary sinuses sometimes detects congestion.

Diagnostic Tests   If chronic sinusitis is suspected and the patient has failed a reasonable course of treatment, then a CT scan of the sinuses is warranted.[17,18] Plain x-rays of the sinuses are probably insensitive in adults. Otolaryngologists can perform nasal endoscopy which can reveal nasal polyps or other pathologic or anatomic causes of ostia obstruction.[18] Nasal endoscopy also enables the sampling of exudate for bacteriological identification.

Management Plan   Once the diagnosis of acute or chronic sinusitis is made, an antibiotic must be identified.[13,17,18] First-line choices include amoxicillin 500 mg every eight hours for 10 to 14 days or trimethoprim/sulfamethoxazole (Bactrim) single strength 400 mg/80 mg or double strength 800 mg/160 mg every 12 hours for 10 to 14 days. If these fail, or if a more serious or chronic infection is suspected, then amoxicillin 250–500 mg with clavulanate 125 mg (Augmentin) every 8 hours for 2 to 4 weeks, or clindamycin (Cleocin) 150 mg every 6 hours for 2 to 4 weeks is chosen. If symptoms do not subside in a reasonable period of time, referral to an otolaryngologist is necessary.

Almost as important as antibiotic therapy are adjuvant measures.[19] Oral and topical decongestants, analgesics, and mucolytics may alleviate symptoms of sinusitis (see Table 4–1). Nasal irrigation with a weak saline solution (eight ounces of water, one-quarter teaspoon salt, and a pinch of baking soda) is very effective in maintaining patency of the ostia.[17] An ear bulb syringe is filled with the solution and squeezed into the nasal passage with the patient leaning over a sink. The solution is allowed to flow back out of the nose and the process is repeated bilaterally two or three times; then the nose is gently blown. This can be done two to four times a day.

A nasally inhaled corticosteroid may also decrease sinus mucosal inflammation. The corticosteroid acts locally and systemic absorption is negligible, but it may cause irritation of the nasal mucosa. Many nasal steroids are available, including flonase, vancenase, and rhinocort. Package labeling states how best to prescribe them. Nasal steroids are most effective if used consistently for a period of time rather than intermittently.

Adequate hydration, avoidance of environmental pollutants, and cessation of smoking are essential in the effective management of chronic sinusitis. Follow-up is necessary if symptoms do not subside with treatment, if they return following a period of quiescence, or after a course of antibiotics (depending on history or severity of symptoms).

Bronchitis

Definition and Pathophysiology

Bronchitis or tracheobronchitis is an infection of the tracheobronchial tree. Its hallmark is a productive cough, which must be distinguished from coughs due to bacterial sinusitis and pneumonia. Bronchitis is generally a self-limiting viral illness that may be caused by a number of viruses, as well as bacteria including *Bordetella pertussis*, *Mycoplasma pneumoniae*, and *Chlamydia pneumoniae*.[20,21] Uncomplicated bacterial bronchitis does not respond to antibiotic therapy any better than uncomplicated viral bronchitis. It is in a more complicated picture that antibiotics are warranted (see Management Plan).[20]

Clinical Presentation

Bronchitis usually presents with a productive cough and sputum. In chronic bronchitis, the cough worsens with increasingly purulent sputum and dyspnea. Complaints of fatigue and malaise are common. Signs may include fever and clear breath sounds or rhonchi upon auscultation. Differential diagnoses include sinusitis and pneumonia.[21]

History and Physical Examination

Ask about respiratory risk factors and environmental exposures. Determine volume and color of sputum and exercise tolerance. If unknown, obtain a complete past medical history. The basic physical exam includes temperature and vital signs, palpation of the neck for lymph adenopathy, auscultation of the lungs and heart, and evaluation of peripheral edema.

Diagnostic Tests

With suspected pneumonia, a complicated past medical history, or particularly severe symptoms, a chest x-ray is indicated. If treatment is unsuccessful, CT scan, pulmonary function tests, and consultation/referral with a pulmonologist may be necessary.

Management Plan

In the absence of previous respiratory problems or immunocompromising illnesses, bronchitis should improve in a matter of days with symptomatic intervention.[20,21] Use of albuterol inhalers or albuterol 2 mg tablets three or four times per day often relieves the cough.[21] Provide adequate instruction to ensure accurate use with albuterol inhalers. Although albuterol tablets are simpler to take, they can cause tremor, tachycardia, and irritability in direct proportion to dosage.

In those with respiratory risk factors, such as smoking or environmental exposure, and who at baseline have a frequent productive cough which has progressively worsened since onset of bronchitis, a course of amoxicillin 250–500 mg every 8 hours for 7 to 10 days, or erythromycin 250 mg every 6 hours for 7 to 10 days,[20] is the first line of treatment. If this fails, other choices include a 7–10 day course of levofloxacin (Levaquin) 250–500 mg once daily, amoxicillin 250–500 mg with clavulanate 125 mg (Augmentin) every 8 hours, clarithromycin (Biaxin) 250 mg every 12 hours, or trimethoprim/sulfamethoxazole (Bactrim) 400/80 mg–800/160 mg every 12 hours.

Patients with compromising respiratory conditions (chronic obstructive pulmonary disease or asthma), and who have worsening symptoms (productive sputum, increased dyspnea), must be treated with a quinolone or macrolide such as levofloxacin (Levaquin) 500 mg for 7 to 12 days or azithromycin (Zithromax) 500 mg on day 1 and 250 mg daily on days 2 through 5. Symptom severity indicates the need for hospitalization and intravenous hydration and antibiotics.

Symptomatic relief of cough can be managed with various cough preparations, as listed in Table 4–1.

Tobacco users should be encouraged to quit smoking. In uncomplicated bronchitis follow-up is necessary only if symptoms do not subside in a week to 10 days or if they suddenly become worse. In more complicated bronchitis, follow-up is prudent after the course of antibiotics is completed.

 ## Chronic Obstructive Pulmonary Disease

Definition and Pathophysiology

Chronic obstructive pulmonary diseases (COPD) are characterized by an irreversible obstruction of expiratory airflow. These disorders include emphysema, chronic bronchitis, and asthmatic bronchitis.[22,23,24] Emphysema is permanent destructive change in the alveoli causing the trapping of air and a decrease in gas exchange. Hyperinflation of the lungs occurs with loss of elastic recoil. Chronic bronchitis is a chronic cough which is productive of sputum on most days during at least three months for a minimum of two years.[24] Overactive, hypertrophied mucous-producing glands can progress to expiratory airflow obstruction. Asthmatic bronchitis encompasses components of chronic bronchitis and asthma (described later). In this section, COPD is used to describe chronic bronchitis or emphysema, since most people with COPD have a combination of both conditions.

COPD is often not diagnosed or treated until several infections have occurred or until exercise tolerance is hindered.[25] Due to the large reserves in normal lungs, much destruction can occur before the presentation of any symptoms. Most people with COPD are smokers or have been exposed to pollutants, often work related.[23] Removal of the offending irritant is crucial to treatment of COPD and prevention of further destruction.

Clinical Presentation

Symptoms generally reveal themselves over the course of office visits and include decreased exercise tolerance (dyspnea with normally manageable tasks) and chronic cough (productive or nonproductive).[22] Signs of COPD are increased hemat-ocrit and wheezing, rhonchi, or decreased air movement upon auscultation.

COPD can be complicated by pulmonary hypertension, cor pulmonale, and right or left ventricular failure.[23] Differential diagnoses include asthma, lung or occult malignancy, tuberculosis, pneumonia, or acute bronchitis.

History and Physical Examination

Obtain a smoking and environmental exposure history, as well as a thorough past medical history. Determine the course and duration of the symptoms and any aggravating or relieving factors. Inquire about associated symptoms such as weight loss, peripheral edema, angina, or paroxysmal nocturnal dyspnea.

Since the etiology of COPD is most often smoking, a thorough physical examination is necessary in order to assess smoking morbidity, as well as any cardiac complications. Note the patient's general appearance, skin color, and ease of movement. Obtain weight and vital signs. Percuss and auscultate the lungs, noting the anterior/posterior diameter of the thorax. Palpate and auscultate the heart. Assess for organomegaly, lymphadenopathy, and palpate peripheral pulses noting edema and skin condition.

Diagnostic Tests

These may include chest x-ray, pulmonary function tests, complete blood count, chemistry panel, electrocardiogram, and a Mantoux test if exposure to tuberculosis is suspected or for those who reside where there is close proximity to others.[22] Arterial blood gases are usually done only in an acute setting or by order of a specialist. Pulse oximetry, if available, may be useful.

Management Plan

Cessation of smoking[25,26,27,28] and avoidance of environmental pollutants is essential in the treatment of COPD. A systematic approach and periodic, supportive counseling are the most effective techniques to help patients quit smoking. Patients need to know that it often takes several attempts to quit and to have realistic expectations. Use of nicotine replacement therapy, either with a patch or chewing gum, is necessary for some people. Doses of 150–300 mg per day of the antidepressant bupropion (Wellbutrin or Zyban)[29,30] may be effective in smoking cessation efforts. Regularly scheduled follow-up appointments to discuss progress are also helpful.

Use of inhalants is a standard therapy in the management of COPD. Beta$_2$-agonists, like albuterol (Proventil), are fast-acting bronchodilators and are often more useful in the treatment of asthma than COPD.[22] Inhaled quaternary anticholinergic agents, like ipratropium bromide (atrovent), may be better bronchodilators for some people with COPD.[22,23,24] Either a metered-dose inhaler (MDI) or nebulizer are effective delivery systems for inhaled medication. A spacer can be prescribed for use with a handheld inhaler in order to enhance effective delivery of the medication to the lungs. Many people, particularly older adults, have difficulty coordinating breathing with release of medication from the inhaler device. Careful instruction with return demonstration is valuable at each appointment. Efficacy of the medication is directly related to accuracy in usage of the metered-dose inhaler or nebulizer.[31]

Airway inflammation is less responsive to inhaled or oral steroids in COPD than in asthma. Because COPD may involve both airway obstruction and reactive airway disease, use of steroids needs to be individualized.[25] Referral to a pulmonologist is indicated when current treatment is ineffective or infections are occurring frequently.

Follow-up appointments are needed to assess effectiveness of medications, presence of infection, progress of smoking cessation, and potential comorbidities. Frequency of appointments is determined by health status. Weekly or monthly appointments may be necessary during exacerbations and quarterly appointments during stable periods.

▪ Asthma

Definition and Pathophysiology

Chronic asthma is characterized by inflammation, airway hypersensitivity, and partially reversible airflow obstruction.[32,33] Environmental allergens, cold air, smoke, or other irritants cause mucosal edema, production of mucous, and infiltration into the cells of leukotrienes. Leukotrienes are compounds derived from unsaturated fatty acids and are potent mediators in the inflammatory process.[34,35] They cause bronchoconstriction, increased vascular permeability, and movement of leukocytes into the area of inflammation.

Older adults may have long-standing asthma or late-onset asthma.[33,36] The former is more likely associated with atopic diseases, is often more severe, and may respond better to combination therapy including interventions for COPD. It is important to determine if both asthma and COPD are present, because treatment must be individualized and geared toward the underlying pathophysiology of the particular illness or combination of illnesses.[22]

Clinical Presentation

Presenting symptoms of asthma are likely to include coughing, shortness of breath, chest tightness, and wheezing.[32] Decreased exercise tolerance and worsening of symptoms may occur simultaneously under certain conditions. Symptoms may be worse in cold air, during periods noted for seasonal allergies, and in the presence of cigarette smoke or other respiratory irritants.[37] Signs may include use of accessory muscles, audible wheezing, or dyspnea with speaking or on minimal exertion. Upon auscultation, wheezing or diminished air movement may be evident. Differential diagnoses include COPD, respiratory infection, bronchiectasis, and heart failure.[31]

History and Physical Examination

Ask about smoking and any history of environmental exposure, as well as details of childhood and adult-onset allergies. Are there symptoms of sinusitis or gastroesophageal reflux disease, since these illnesses can mimic and/or exacerbate asthma.[31] A past medical history and thorough review of systems are important because respiratory illnesses can cause or be exacerbated by comorbidities. As with COPD, a complete physical examination is indicated, as previously described.

Diagnostic Tests

These may include chest x-ray, complete blood count, chemistry panel, electrocardiogram, and a Mantoux test if exposure to tuberculosis is suspected or for those who reside where there is close proximity to others.[22] Pulmonary function tests may help determine any possible reversibility of airway obstruction with bronchodilators. If available, pulse oximetry may be helpful.

Management Plan

As with COPD, cessation of smoking and avoidance of environmental irritants are important first steps in the treatment of asthma.[38] For motivated, cognitively intact patients who want some degree of self-control and self-determination in their care, the use of a peak flow meter may be helpful. A peak flow meter is an instrument used to measure peak expiratory flow. The patient seals the mouthpiece with his/her lips, and gives a complete expiration of air from the lungs. The number obtained is the peak flow. This is done several times during a stable period to determine the patient's baseline "best" results. After determination of the patient's baseline, daily peak flow measurements are obtained and the value is placed in zones labeled as green (80–100% of baseline), yellow (50–80% of baseline), and red (below 50% of baseline).[31] An individualized plan is then laid out for the patient depending on what zone he/she is in.

Inhalants are essential in the management of asthma.[31,33,39,40] Beta$_2$ agonists are an important first step, as they dilate the bronchial tubes and allow for the administration of corticosteroids. A metered-dose inhaler (MDI), breath-activated metered-dose inhaler, or nebulizer are effective delivery systems. A spacer can be prescribed for use with a handheld inhaler in order to enhance effective delivery to the lungs. The most common beta$_2$ agonist is albuterol (Proventil, Ventolin), 2 puffs every three to four hours, depending on symptoms or results of peak flow readings. The breath-

activated MDI is pirbuterol acetate (Maxair) and the dose is the same as for albuterol.

A long-acting beta$_2$ agonist is salmeterol (Serevent). It is useful for patients prone to bronchospasm associated with exercise or nocturnal symptoms. The dose is 2 puffs twice a day only. This is not a rescue drug and cannot be used to treat acute symptoms, because its onset of action is 30–60 minutes. Patients need to understand how to use salmeterol and to have available a short acting bronchodilator like albuterol. Ipratropium bromide (Atrovent) is not an effective bronchodilator for asthma, but may be useful as an adjunct in the treatment of patients with both COPD and asthma.[31,40]

Inhaled corticosteroids are an effective therapy for controlling bronchial inflammation.[31,33,38,39,40,41] Oral steroids are used for exacerbations and in some severe cases, low-dose daily steroids are needed. Examples of inhaled corticosteroids are beclomethasone dipropionate (Beclovent, Vanceril), flunisolide (Aerobid), and triamcinolone acetonide (Azmacort). The dose is 2–6 puffs two to four times per day. Four puffs twice a day is a manageable and effective dose. If a total of 16 puffs a day is insufficient, then a high-potency, inhaled corticosteroid such as fluticasone 220 mcg (Flovent) may be necessary at a dosage of 2 puffs two times per day. Patients must thoroughly rinse the mouth after using an inhaled corticosteroid to prevent oral candidiasis.[31] When multiple inhalers are prescribed, it is important to tell the patient in what order to use them. The bronchodilators are used first, followed by inhaled corticosteroids.

Zafirlukast (Accolate) and montelukast (Singulair) are leukotriene receptor antagonists used for the treatment of chronic asthma. They help block bronchoconstriction, mucous production, and airway edema caused by the inflammatory response of leukotrienes.[35,41,42] These agents are not effective in the management of acute asthma attacks or symptoms.[41,42] They should be taken during symptom-free periods. Zafirlukast is prescribed at 20 mg twice a day on an empty stomach and montelukast at 10 mg taken once daily at bedtime. Another agent that has similar benefits as the leukotriene receptor antagonist is the leukotriene synthesis inhibitor called zileuton

(Zyflo). Zileuton is prescribed at 600 mg four times a day.

Oral theophylline is used only as a second-line therapy when inhaled broncholilators are not effective or well tolerated.[40] Drug levels must be monitored, but even at standard therapeutic levels, adverse side effects can occur. Nausea, headaches, and tachycardia are among the more common side effects. Arrhythmias and seizures are less common, but have been reported. Many commonly prescribed medications interact adversely with theophylline, including cimetidine, ciprofloxacin, and phenytoin.[33]

Referral to a pulmonologist is indicated when treatment is ineffective or infections occur frequently. Referral to an allergist may be necessary to determine what other factors are exacerbating the asthmatic symptoms. Follow-up is the same as described in COPD.

Pneumonia

Definition and Pathophysiology

Pneumonia is a lower respiratory tract infection characterized by inflammation of the lung with consolidation and exudate. It can have a bacterial or viral cause, but most commonly results from pneumococcal bacteria *(Streptococcus pneumoniae).*[14,43,44] Causative agents are generally found in the upper respiratory tract, invading the lower respiratory tract and cause infection when resistance is lowered. Pneumococcal pneumonia accounts for 90% of all bacterial pneumonias and is the focus of this section.

Pneumonia is the most common infectious disease leading to death in older adults. Comorbidities, immobility, and older age increase susceptibility to pneumonia and make death more likely.[44,45,46]

Clinical Presentation

Pneumonia may present with a productive cough, fever, and dyspnea, or it may present more insidiously with tachypnea, lethargy, weakness, falls, unexplained change in functional status or behavior, or pleuritic chest pain, or a modest increase in temperature.[46,47] Decreased appetite and dehydration may appear before any of the more obvious signs and symptoms.

Clinical signs found upon auscultation may be decreased breath sounds or crackles over one or more lung fields. Wheezing may also be heard. Clear breath sounds do not rule out pneumonia. Differential diagnoses include bronchitis, tuberculosis, aspiration pneumonia, or any other chronic lung conditions. A lower respiratory tract infection, however, is likely to present with acute symptoms and the patient probably looks quite ill.

History and Physical Examination

Determine the onset of symptoms and any exacerbating or relieving factors. Ask about a cough (productive or nonproductive), fever, chills, dyspnea, malaise, and decreased appetite. Inquire about any falls, changes in behavior, and decreased ability to care for self. Observe for tachypnea, color, diaphoresis, and strength. The physical exam begins with temperature and vital signs including orthostatic blood pressures. Palpate the neck for lymphadenopathy, percuss and auscultate the lungs, listen to the heart, and check for cyanosis and peripheral edema.

Diagnostic Tests

A chest x-ray should be obtained; however, radiographic findings may lag behind the clinical picture especially with dehydration.[48] A complete blood count to determine leukocytosis and an electrolyte panel with blood urea nitrogen and creatinine help to determine dehydration.[47] Pulse oximetry, if available, is useful to ascertain the need for oxygen and hospitalization.[48] If immediate treatment is unsuccessful, then CT scan of the chest and pulmonary function tests, as well as consultation with a pulmonologist, may be necessary.

Management Plan

A decision has to be made immediately concerning hospitalization. This depends on the availability of qualified caregivers. Presence of underlying chronic illnesses (COPD, cardiac, diabetes, renal disease), immunosuppression, or bilateral or multi-lobe infiltrates may mean hospitalization is appropriate.[48] If the patient is markedly dyspneic, tachypneic, hemodynamically unstable (as evidenced by orthostatic hypotension or tachycardia), or hypoxic, then hospitalization is essential.[44,48]

Many antibiotics are available for the treatment of pneumonia. Treatment should last for two weeks and choice of antibiotic is dependent on patient compliance/social support, drug allergy profile, potential interaction with other medications, and cost.[44,46,47]

Second- or third-generation cephalosporins are generally a good choice. Some examples of these are: second generation: cefuroxime (Ceftin) 250–500 mg every 12 hours and cefaclor (Ceclor) 250–500 mg every 8 hours; third generation: cefixime (Suprax) 400 mg daily and ceftriaxone (Rocephin) 1 gm IM daily. Amoxicillin 250–500 mg with clavulanate 125 mg (Augmentin) every 8 hours or trimethoprim/sulfamethoxazole (Bactrim) 400/80 mg–800/160 mg every 12 hours can be used. If the patient has a drug allergy or adverse reaction to any of the above drugs or does not respond, then other choices include: macrolides, such as azithromycin (Zithromax) 500 mg on day one and 250 mg on days two through five; or clarithromycin (Biaxin) 250–500 mg every 12 hours. The quinolones ciprofloxacin (Cipro) can also be used at 250–500 mg every 12 hours, or levofloxacin (Levaquin) 250–500 mg every 24 hours.

The Advisory Committee on Immunization Practices for the U.S. Public Health Service (ACIP) recommends that every person over the age of 65 receive the yearly influenza vaccination (unless allergic to eggs or known hypersensitivity to the vaccine) and the "once in a lifetime" pneumovax which protects against 23 strains of *Streptococcus pneumoniae*.[14] ACIP recommends that if someone over age 65 received the pneumovax greater than five years ago *and* he/she was under 65 when it was first given, or if the vaccination history is not known, then the pneumovax should also be administered.

Adjunctive therapy includes chest percussion, oxygen, bronchodilator inhalers (albuterol inhaler two puffs every four hours), cough preparations

(see Table 4–1), and adequate nutrition and hydration.[44,46] Careful monitoring is important since pneumonia resistant to first-line therapy is common. Family caregivers, nursing facility staff, or the patient must be diligent about reporting response to treatment and resolution or worsening of symptoms.

Follow-up appointments are always warranted in any case of pneumonia. If the infection required hospitalization, or was in the presence of serious comorbidities, then a follow-up chest x-ray helps determine the effectiveness of treatment, as well as the possibility of any underlying chronic or neoplastic condition.

Tuberculosis

Definition and Pathophysiology

Tuberculosis (TB) is a communicable disease caused by *Mycobacterium tuberculosis*, an acid-fast bacillus (AFB).[4,46,48] It is primarily found in the lungs, but can be systemic. Most older adults infected with *M. tuberculosis* were exposed earlier in life, but did not contract an active illness. The AFB were encapsulated in tubercles, lying dormant until compromise of the host's immune system. This is known as latent infection.[4] The reactivation of such an infection, due to immunosuppression or concomitant illness in the presence of older age, is called recrudescence or secondary TB.

M. tuberculosis is transmitted through droplet nuclei in the air.[4,49] People living in crowded dwellings or in close contact with others are considered high risk. Closed ventilation systems found in many such settings often circulate unfiltered air containing higher concentrations of organisms such as *M. tuberculosis*.[3,50] Older adults comprise the largest pool for TB infection in the developed world.[51]

Clinical Presentation

Presenting symptoms of TB may be fatigue, night sweats, weight loss with or without loss of appetite, persistent low-grade fever, persistent cough, hemoptysis, dyspnea, or pleuritic chest discomfort.[3,50]

Many of these symptoms mimic other chronic conditions in older adults, so the index of suspicion needs to be high.[53] Patients may be unaware of prior exposure to TB. Upon auscultation of the lungs, crackles may be heard in the apex lung fields or breath sounds may be clear. Differential diagnoses include pneumonia, occult malignancy, or any other chronic or infectious respiratory condition.

History and Physical Examination

Review all symptoms common to the usual clinical picture, as well as foreign travel or possible TB exposures (i.e., frequent visits to a nursing home). Obtain a past medical history. The physical exam begins with temperature and vital signs. A head-to-toe physical exam is warranted since the presenting symptoms may signify any one of a number of illnesses.

Diagnostic Tests

These include a Mantoux test (see the section on Appropriate Diagnostic Tests in Primary Care earlier in the chapter), chest x-ray, and three sputum cultures for acid-fast bacilli. The results of an AFB smear are ready within one to two days and are highly specific for *Mycobacterium tuberculosis*.[4] Sputum samples for culture and antibiotic susceptibility take three to eight weeks depending on the lab.[4] Regardless, drug therapy should begin based on results of the sputum smear and clinical judgement.[3] It is recommended that all risk groups be screened for TB with the Mantoux test every 6–12 months.

Management Plan

A positive Mantoux test found with no other symptoms requires further work-up, including a chest x-ray and three sputum cultures. Results determine whether or not to treat with preventive therapy (isoniazid (INH) 300 mg daily for 6 months).[3] If exposure to active TB has occurred, it may be wise to treat empirically with preventive therapy. In the presence of a positive Mantoux test, with no radiographic findings and negative sputum cultures, preventive therapy should be given in cases of HIV infection, diabetes, immunosuppressive therapy, poor nutritional states, rapid weight loss, lymphoma or leukemia, and silicosis.

If fibronodular scars are found on chest x-ray, and measure greater than or equal to 2 cm, and the Mantoux test is positive, then treat with INH 300 mg daily and rifampin 600 mg daily for 4 months or INH alone for 12 months.[4] When rifampin is prescribed, vitamin B_6 (pyridoxine 25–50 mg daily) should be given to reduce the incidence of peripheral neuropathy and CNS disturbance.

In cases of active TB in older adults, a four-drug regimen is given, including INH and rifampin for six months, and pyrazinamide and ethambutol for the first two months.[3,4,50,53] Baseline tests are recommended prior to the initiation of antituberculosis therapy and periodically during treatment: hepatic enzymes, bilirubin, serum creatinine, CBC, platelet count, serum uric acid (if pyrazinamide is prescribed), and visual acuity (if ethambutol is prescribed).[3] Conservative follow-up recommendation is to obtain weekly sputum smears for AFB.[53] If they are not negative after three weeks of therapy, then treatment for resistant TB should be considered. Another recommendation is to obtain sputum smears for AFB every two weeks with consideration for treatment of multidrug-resistant TB if smears are not negative within three months.[50]

Drug therapy for multidrug-resistant TB includes the use of at least six agents: INH, rifampin, ethambutol, pyrazinamide, and two of the following agents: ciprofloxacin, ofloxacin, para-aminosalicylic acid or cycloserine, and streptomycin, capreomycin, or kanamycin.[3,50,53]

Consultation with a pulmonologist or infectious disease specialist is prudent for the management of active TB or multidrug-resistant TB. Follow-up needs to be on a regular basis to ensure medication compliance, monitor for adverse drug reactions, and monitor response to therapy.

▇ Summary

Treatment summaries for the respiratory illnesses presented above are given in Table 4–2.

Table 4–2   Treatment Summaries

Illness	Clinical Presentation	History & Physical	Diagnostic Tests	Management
Common cold	Sneezing, sore throat, rhinorrhea, malaise, achiness, headache, nonproductive cough, sinus congestion, low-grade fever	Onset & duration of symptoms; vital signs; examine ears, nose throat, neck, lungs	None	Decongestants, cough medicine, analgesia (see Table 4–1), warm salt water gargle
Influenza	Exhaustion, chills, sinus congestion, cough, headache, myalgias, fever, pharyngitis, cervical lymphadenopathy	Same as for common cold	Consider WBC, CXR	Same as for common cold and if within 48 hrs of onset, amantadine or rimantadine 100 mg daily x10 days or oseltamivir 75 mg BIDx5days
Sinusitis	Same as for common cold and purulent nasal discharge, postnasal drip, facial or upper-teeth pain, pain upon sinus palpation	Same as for common cold and palpation of sinuses	Consider sinus CT scan and nasal endoscopy if treatment fails	**See text for details.** Amoxicillin 500 mg q 8 hrs x10–14 days or trimethoprim/sulfa-methoxazole single or double strength BID x 10–14 days or amox/clavulanate 250–500 mg q 8 hrs x 2–4 weeks or clin-damycin 150 mg q 6 hrs x 2–4 weeks. See Table 4–1
Bronchitis	Productive cough, fatigue, dyspnea, malaise, fever	PMH, volume & color of sputum, exercise tolerance, vital signs, examine neck, lungs heart, lower extremities	Consider CXR	**See text for details.** Amoxicillin 250–500 mg q 8 hrs x 7–10 days or erythromycin 250 mg q 6 hrs x 7–10 days or levofloxacin 250–500 mg q 24 hrs x 7–10 days or clar-ithromycin 250 mg q 12 hrs x 7–10 days
COPD Asthma	Decreased exercise tolerance, chronic cough, wheezing, increased hematocrit	PMH, smoking & environmental exposure history, vital signs, weight, examine neck, lungs, heart, lower extremities	Consider CXR, PFTs, CBC, chemistry panel, ECG, Mantoux test, pulse oximetry	**See text for details.** Ipratropium bromide or albuterol inhaler 2 puffs QID. Consider inhaled corticosteroids. Leukotriene receptor antagonists for asthma

Table 4–2 *(continued)*

Illness	Clinical Presentation	History & Physical	Diagnostic Tests	Management
Pneumonia	Productive cough, fever, dyspnea, tachypnea, lethargy, falls	Symptoms, change in behavior, appearance, vital signs, examine neck, heart, lungs, extremities	Same as for COPD, asthma	**See text for details.** Same as for bronchitis, but for 2 weeks. Or 2 weeks of: cefuroxime 250–500 mg q 12 hrs, cefaclor 250–500 mg q 8 hrs, cefixime 400 mg daily, ceftriaxone 1 gm IM daily

Tuberculosis: see text.

■ References

1. Rossi A, Ganassini A, Tantucci C, et al. Aging and the respiratory system. *Aging.* 1996;8(3):143–161.
2. Dahnert W. *Radiology Review Manual.* 3rd ed. Baltimore, Md: Williams & Wilkins, 1996:337.
3. Moran GJ. Multi drug-resistant TB: diagnosis and treatment. *Emerg Med.* 1995; 27(2):99–100, 103–104,106,109.
4. Leiner S, Mays M. Diagnosing latent and active pulmonary tuberculosis: A review for clinicians. *Nurse Pract.* 1996;21(2):86–107.
5. Novelline RA. *Squire's Fundamentals of Radiology.* 5th ed. Cambidge, Mass.: Harvard University Press; 1997.
6. McConnell EA. Administering intradermal injections. *Nursing.* 1996;26(2):18.
7. Skelskey C, Leshem OA. Tuberculosis surveillance in long-term care. *Am J Nurs.* 1997;97(10):16BBB–16DDD.
8. Fein AM. The tuberculosis skin test. *Emerg Med.* 1996:28(7):89–90.
9. Crapo RO. Pulmonary function testing. *New Engl J Med.* 1994;331(1):25–30.
10. Mossad SB. Treatment of the common cold. *BMJ.* 1998;317(7150):33–36.
11. Patient Education. Managing the common cold. *Nurse Pract.* 1996;21(4):143–144.
12. Schaeffer SM. Decongestants and antihistamines in rhinosinusitis. *Contemp Int Med.* 1997;9(2):62–63.
13. Alloway RR, Dempster J. Continuing education forum: treatment of rhinitis. *J Am Acad Nurse Pract.* 1996;8(3):135–144.
14. Sneller VP. CDC guidelines for influenza, pneumococcal, and tetanus vaccinations. *Symp Coverage, Spec Rep.* 1998;11–20.
15. Kennedy MM. Influenza viral infections: presentation, prevention, and treatment. *Nurse Pract.* 1998;23(9):21–37.
16. Advisory Committee on Immunization Practices. Prevention and control of influenza. *MMWR Morb Mortal Wkly Rep.* 1998;47(RR-6):1–21.
17. Lockey RF. Management of chronic sinusitus. *Hosp Prac.* 1996;31(3):141–151.
18. Clerico DM, Kennedy DW. Chronic sinusitis: diagnostic and treatment advances. *Hosp Med.* 1994; 30(7):15–18.
19. Knutsen JW, Slavin RG. Sinusitis in the aged. Optimal management strategies. *Drugs Aging.* 1995;7(4):310–316.
20. Grossman RF. Acute exacerbations of chronic bronchitis. *Hosp Pract.* 1997;32(10):85–89, 92–94.
21. Leiner S. Acute bronchitis in adults: commonly diagnosed but poorly defined. *Nurse Pract.* 1997;22(1):104–108, 113–117.
22. Alberts WM, Rolfe MW. A step care approach to managing COPD. *Hosp Formulary.* 1994;29:756–767.
23. Ferguson GT, Cherniack RM. Management of chronic obstructive pulmonary disease. *New Engl J Med.* 1993;328(14):1017–1022.
24. Chapman KR, Bowie DM, Golstein RS, et al. Guidelines for the assessment and management of chronic obstructive pulmonary disease. *Can Med Assoc J.* 1992;147(4):420–428.
25. Chapman KR. Therapeutic approaches to chronic obstructive pulmonary disease: an emerging consensus. *Am Acad Med.* 1996;100(suppl 1A):5S–9S.
26. Agency for Health Care Policy and Research. Centers for Disease Control and Prevention: Smoking cessation: information for specialists. *Clin Pract Guide;* 1996.

27. Weavers ME, Ahijevych KL, Sarna L. Smoking cessation interventions in nursing practice. *Nurs Clin N Am.* 1998;33(1):61–74.

28. Gorman M. Helping patients to quit smoking. *Am J Nurs.* 1997;97(3):64–65.

29. McAfee T, France E. Correspondence: sustained-release bupriopion for smoking cessation. *N Engl J Med.* 1998;338(9):619.

30. Hurt RD, Sachs DP, Glover ED, et al. A comparison of sustained-released bupropion and placebo for smoking cessation. *N Engl J Med.* 1997;337(17):1195–1202.

31. Anderson CJ, Bardana EJ. Asthma in the elderly: the importance of patient education. *Comp Ther.* 1996; 22(6):375–383.

32. Davies RJ, Wang J, Abdelaziz MM, et al. New insights into the understanding of asthma. *Chest.* 1997;111(2): 2S–10S.

33. Smyrinios NA. Asthma: a six part strategy for managing older patients. *Geriatrics.* 1997;52(2):36–44.

34. O'Byrne PM. Leukotrienes in the pathogenesis of asthma. *Chest.* 1997;111(2):27S–34S.

35. Spector SL. Leukotriene inhibitors and antagonists in asthma. *Ann Allergy, Asthma, and Immunol.* 1995;75: 463–469.

36. Ariano R, Panzani CR, Augeri G. Late onset asthma clinical and immunological data: importance of allergy. *J Investig Allergy Clin Immunol.* 1998;8(1):35–41.

37. MacDonald P. Asthma in older people. *Nurs Times.* 1997;93(19):42–43.

38. Sherman CB. Late-onset asthma: making the diagnosis, choosing drug therapy. *Geriatrics.* 1995;50(12):24–26, 29–30, 33.

39. Braman SS. Drug treatment of asthma in the elderly. *Drugs.* 1996;51(3):415–423.

40. Barnes PJ. Current therapies for asthma. *Chest.* 1997; 111(2):17S–26S.

41. Smith LJ. Newer asthma therapies. *Ann Int Med.* 1999; 130(6):531–532.

42. New drugs: zafirlukast (Accolate): after 20 years, a new class of asthma drug. *Am J Nurs.* 1997;97(5):54,56.

43. Pello J, Rodriguez R, Jubert P, et al. Severe community-acquired pneumonia in the elderly: epidemiology and prognosis. *Clin Infect Dis.* 1996;23(4):723–728.

44. Norman D, Verghese A, Dorinsky D, et al. Treating respiratory infections in the elderly: current strategies and considerations. *Geriatrics.* 1997;52(Suppl 1):S1–S28.

45. Metlay JP, Schulz R, Li YH, et al. Influence of age on symptoms at presentation in patients with community-acquired pneumonia. *Arch Int Med.* 1997;157(13): 1453–1459.

46. Cassiere HA, Fein AM. Pneumonia in the elderly: an update. *Emerg Med.* 1997;29(7):38, 43–46, 51–52.

47. Yoshikawa TT, Norman DC. Approach to fever and infection in the nursing home. *J Am Geriatr Soc.* 1996; 44(1):74–82.

48. Moroney C, Fitzgerald MA. Pharmacologic update: management of pneumonia in elderly people. *J Am Acad Nurse Pract.* 1996;8(5):237–241.

49. Centers for Disease Control and Prevention. Guidelines for preventing the transmission of mycobacterium tuberculosis in healthcare facilities. *MMWR Morb Mortal Wkly Rep.* 1994;43(RR–13):1–120.

50. Hopkins ML, Schoener L. Tuberculosis and the elderly living in long-term care facilities. *Geriatr Nurs.* 1996; 17(1):27–32.

51. Davies PD. Tuberculosis in the elderly. Epidemiology and optimal management. *Drugs Aging.* 1996;8(6):436–444.

52. Kemp WE, Jones W, Sohur S, et al. Late generalized tuberculosis: unusual features of an often overlooked disease. *South Med J.* 1995;88(12):1221–1225.

53. Roistacher K. TB-emerging resistance concerns. *Hosp Med.* March 1995;42–50.

CHAPTER 5

Genitourinary Problems

Christine Wanich Bradway
Gale Yetman

Introduction

Genitourinary (GU) problems, including urinary incontinence (UI), urinary tract infections (UTIs), and prostate disease, are common in older individuals and are often managed either independently or collaboratively by advanced practice nurses (APNs). This chapter focuses on the evaluation and management of GU problems in community-residing and institutionalized elderly.

Urinary Incontinence

UI is defined as the involuntary loss of urine sufficient to be a problem.[1] More than 17 million adults in the United States suffer from UI,[2] and although it is not a "normal" consequence of aging, older adults are affected more often than younger adults. Eight to 34% of noninstitutionalized elderly,[3,4] 50–60% of those in long-term care,[5,6] and at least 11% of older adults admitted to acute care suffer from UI.[7] In most cases, UI is not life threatening; however, adverse consequences such as UTIs, indwelling catheter use, dermatitis, skin infections, pressure ulcers, decreased functional status, embarrassment, and isolation can have devastating effects on general health and quality of life.[8,9,10,11] APNs in a variety of health-care settings are in ideal positions to identify, evaluate, and provide care for older individuals with UI.

Requirements for Continence

Requirements for continence include intact urinary tract function, cognitive and functional ability to recognize voiding signals and appropriately use a toilet, motivation to maintain continence,

and an environment that facilitates the process. In adults, micturition involves voluntary and reflexive control of the bladder, urethra, detrusor muscle, and urethral sphincter. When bladder volume reaches approximately 400–500 cc, receptors in the bladder wall send a message to the brain, an impulse for initiating a void is sent back to the bladder, the detrusor contracts, and the urethral sphincter relaxes.[12,13] Adults also have the ability to inhibit micturition reflexes (at least for a time) to reach an appropriate place for voiding or until they desire to void. UI occurs as a result of a disruption at any point in the process.

Age-Associated Changes and Risk Factors for UI

Age-associated changes also affect continence. Older men with benign prostatic hyperplasia (BPH) often complain of urinary urgency, hesitancy, dribbling, frequency, and urge or overflow UI. Menopause, estrogen loss, and atrophic vaginitis and urethritis are the most significant changes in older women. Men and women experience age-associated increases in post-void residual (PVR) urine, a delay in the onset of the desire to void (e.g., increased urinary urgency, especially after the bladder sends the "signal" to void), a decreased bladder capacity, and a reversal of voiding patterns from young age (e.g., more voiding at night, and less in the daytime).[14,15,16] In addition to age and menopause, other risk factors include diabetes mellitus (DM), hysterectomy, stroke, and obesity.[17] Moreover, general health conditions frequently affect continence in older adults. For example, visual impairments may alter an individual's ability to recognize an appropriate place for voiding, functional impairments can result in problems such as getting clothes on and off quickly enough to avoid "accidents," and mental status impairments can affect one's ability to recognize or respond to voiding signals appropriately.

Types of Urinary Incontinence

UI can be transient, established, or a combination of each.[7] Transient UI is characterized by the sudden onset of potentially reversible symptoms. Causes of transient UI include delirium, infection, atrophic vaginitis or urethritis, drugs, psychological disorders that affect motivation or function (e.g., depression), excessive urine production, restricted mobility, and constipation or impaction. Transient UI is common in older adults and can go undetected unless health-care providers are attuned to the various etiologies. If, however, the underlying cause is discovered or treated, transient UI can often be prevented or reversed.

Established UI usually has a more protracted onset and may not be discovered until an abrupt change in an older adult's environment or daily routine occurs.[18] Examples of established UI include:

- Stress UI: defined as involuntary urine loss that occurs as a result of urethral hypermobility or an intrinsic sphincter deficiency.[7] Stress UI is common in women and also in men post-prostatectomy. Most often, individuals complain of small amounts of daytime urine loss associated with physical activity or during activities that increase intra-abdominal pressure (e.g., sneezing, coughing).

- Urge UI: defined as involuntary urine loss associated with urinary urgency,[7] most often associated with involuntary contractions of the detrusor muscle (located on the inside of the bladder), and sometimes referred to as detrusor instability (DI). In addition to an immediate desire to void, individuals frequently describe moderate to large amounts of UI associated with urinary frequency, nocturia, and enuresis. When individuals suffer from both stress and urge UI, the incontinence is called *mixed;* this type of UI is quite common in older women.

- Overflow UI: may be caused by an underactive detrusor muscle or outlet obstruction,[7]

and is characterized by frequent, constant, or post-void dribbling; urinary hesitancy; urinary retention; or an uncomfortable sense of fullness in the lower abdomen. Older men with BPH and women with pelvic prolapse (e.g., uterine prolapse, cystocele, rectocele) may present with signs and symptoms of overflow UI.

- Functional UI: caused by nongenitourinary factors such as cognitive or physical impairments that diminish an individual's ability to use the toilet or commode.[19]

Assessment of Urinary Incontinence

APNs play a key role in assessment and management of UI and complement professional nursing care by adding specific physical examination (PE), diagnostic, and treatment components to a basic evaluation[4] (see Table 5–1). Assessment techniques and recommendations for practice that can be adapted to any setting are presented in this chapter.

History   The history can be quite simple or fairly complex depending on the setting, ability of the individual or caregiver to describe the problem, and the APN's comfort level regarding UI. At the very least, APNs should ask all older adults general questions to identify UI or risk factors for its development. Some examples include:

> "Can you tell me about the problems you are having with your bladder?"
>
> "How often do you lose urine when you don't want to?"
>
> "What activities or situations are linked with leakage?"[20]

If UI is identified, more specific questions focused on precipitants of UI (e.g., cold weather, laughing, coughing), lower urinary tract symptoms (e.g., hematuria, nocturia), past evaluations, and past or current management strategies are helpful. The goal of history taking is to achieve a clear picture of the older adult's pattern of UI and how, or if, it affects his/her daily life.

A bladder diary provides additional, objective information about an individual's voiding pattern,

Tables 5–1 Educational Competencies for Continence Care: Master's Preparation for Advanced Practice[4]

In addition to the competencies of a professional nurse, an APN should be able to:

1. Conduct a physical examination that includes:
   a. A general examination if indicated to detect conditions such as edema and other problems that may contribute to UI
   b. An abdominal exam to detect masses and evaluate bowel sounds
   c. A neurological exam
   d. A pelvic exam to evaluate pelvic muscle strength, perineal structure, perineal skin status (estrogenization of vaginal mucosa), signs of pelvic descent
   e. A rectal exam to evaluate presence or absence of reflexes, resting anal sphincter tone, anorectal sensation, sphincter function
   f. Provocative stress testing
   g. With additional education may include urodynamic testing such as uroflowmetry, cystometry, simple cystometry, a filling cystometrogram, or a voiding cystometrogram and may also include videourodynamics and interpretation of urodynamic data

2. Evaluate assessment findings including:
   a. Identifying patients in need of further laboratory tests
   b. Identifying patients in need of medical referral

3. Identify patients who may benefit from behavioral intervention for their UI and prescribe and direct comprehensive continence program (may include prescriptions), may include:
   a. Bladder training
   b. Directing caregivers regarding specifics of a habit-training program, prompted toileting, and other scheduled voiding regimes
   c. Directing caregivers regarding specifics of a prompted toileting program
   d. Teaching patients to perform pelvic muscle exercises. May include the use of vaginal cones, electrical stimulation, and biofeedback
   e. Individualizing a plan that incorporates drug management
   f. Designing and implementing continence programs for patients with neurogenic bladders (clean intermittent cath, self-catheterization)

4. Recommend topical therapy for management of perineal skin breakdown, dermatitis related to UI

5. Evaluate individual patient outcomes on an ongoing basis

6. Develop management program for chronic, long-term UI to include the use of alternative measures and supportive devices

---

episodes of UI, fluid type and amount, bowel habits, and UI severity. Moreover, diaries help engage older adults (or their caregivers) as active participants in assessment and treatment of UI, provide a focus for discussions regarding voiding patterns, and are used as therapeutic aids for behavioral treatments such as bladder retraining.[21] Several examples of diaries are available;[7,22] APNs should choose the type that best fits the setting and population. For example, complex diaries can give providers a significant amount of information, but only if the individual or caregiver has the time and ability to complete the diary. Even a one-day bladder diary can provide important information and identify individuals who need further evaluation.[19]

Comprehensive questioning regarding additional historical events and conditions that can affect continence complement the specific UI history. For example, questions regarding pregnancy, labor, and delivery; menopause; past surgical events; sexual history; smoking history; and bowel habits identify transient causes or risk factors for UI in older women. A sexual history should also be included for older men as well as an inquiry of symptoms associated with BPH and prostate cancer. Because a wide variety of over-the-counter and prescription medications affect continence, a careful drug history is also essential. Functional, environmental, and mental status assessments should also be part of the UI history in older adults as non-GU factors often affect continence.

Examination Important components of a UI examination include abdominal, genital, rectal, and skin examinations.[19] If possible, the APN should observe the patient using toilet facilities to assess mobility, dexterity, obstacles that interfere with toilet use, and quality (e.g., force, presence of urinary hesitancy) of voiding. This is also an ideal time to inquire about and visualize any continence products or devices that the older individual uses for UI management.

After asking the person to void, the abdominal examination should include inspection, assessment of bowel sounds, and general and focused percussion and palpation (e.g., for identification of bladder fullness, tenderness, masses). Inspection of male and female genitalia should include observation of perineal irritation, lesions, or discharge. In older women, atrophic vaginitis as evidenced by perineal inflammation, tenderness, and thin, pale tissues should be identified. Women should also be asked to perform Valsalva's maneuver (unless medically contraindicated) to identify pelvic prolapse or stress UI.[19] A simple test to quantify cough-related urine loss has been described by Miller and colleagues;[23] in an upright position, women hold a brown paper towel lightly against the perineum and cough three times. A one- or two-finger vaginal examination can further identify prolapse, and can also be used to identify an older woman's ability to identify the vaginal muscle, and to assess its strength (e.g., by asking the woman to squeeze around the APN's fingers). A rectal examination is essential for identification of rectal tone, innervation of sacral nerves, muscle strength, constipation, and abnormalities that require further assessment including masses or abnormalities of the prostate gland.

Finally, in addition to the above, evaluation of UI should include a urinalysis (e.g., to identify hematuria, confirm symptomatic UTI, or other abnormalities) and assessment of the older person's PVR urine (e.g., to rule out urinary retention).[5,7] Additional blood tests that identify acute UI etiologies or chronic conditions that affect continence include electrolytes, blood urea nitrogen, creatinine, thyroid function tests, calcium, blood glucose, and urine cytology;[24,25] controversy exists as to the value of some of these tests, thus APNs must make individual decisions and carefully inform

patients and caregivers of the rationale associated with their use.

Because of time limits, or limits in the setting in which the APN practices, some or all of the basic examination or more sophisticated testing (e.g., urodynamic evaluation), may require referral to other members of the health-care team.[26] Continence nurse specialists, gynecologists, urologists, urogynecologists, geriatricians, geriatric nurse practitioners, and physical therapists are examples of health-care providers who frequently have expertise in this area, and can often provide assistance with completion of the basic evaluation. Additional criteria for referral to a specialist include: an abnormal urinalysis or urine culture, palpable abdominal or pelvic mass, PVR > 200 cc, an abnormal prostate examination, abnormal vaginal discharge or bleeding, symptoms suggestive of obstruction, identification of a new, underlying disorder unrelated to UI, and patients who are candidates for surgical therapies or who require complex medication adjustments or prescribing.

Management of Urinary Incontinence

Individuals and health-care providers have three choices regarding treatment of UI: behavioral therapies, medications, or surgery. In addition, a number of older adults or their caregivers use self-care strategies and a variety of products to complement other treatments. All have advantages and disadvantages; individualized care strategies contrived by the older adult, APN, and other members of the team work best.

First, transient causes of UI should be identified and treated. In some instances, treatment of these causes eradicates the UI; for example, management of constipation often alleviates urinary urgency and urge UI. APNs are also in an ideal position to identify nursing strategies for treatment of immobility, drug-induced UI, or nocturia associated with age-associated fluid shifts (e.g., asking older individuals with significant dependent edema to elevate their legs for 15–30 minutes twice daily often decreases episodes of nocturia), and they play an important role in assisting other members of the health-care team in planning appropriate treatment regimes based on the APN's assessment and diagnosis.

Behavioral Therapies Behavioral therapies include pelvic muscle exercises (PMEs), bladder retraining, habit training, and prompted voiding, and are recommended as a first choice for stress, urge, and mixed UI because they effectively reduce UI without adding significant side effects.[7] Approaches such as PMEs, biofeedback, and other nonmedical strategies can achieve significant reductions in stress, urge, and mixed UI in older adults.[27,28]

PMEs strengthen the voluntary periurethral and perivaginal muscles (e.g., the pubococcygeus muscle [PC]),[29,30] relax spasm in the detrusor muscle, and are used to treat stress UI associated with urethral hypermobility,[31,32] urge, and mixed UI (see Table 5–2). For community-dwelling older women, PME can be as effective as pharmacologic therapy for treatment of stress UI.[32] Experts also recommend PMEs post-radical prostatectomy to improve or maintain continence.[33] Biofeedback supplements verbal or manual PME instructions and is particularly effective with older individuals who have difficulty identifying the correct muscle for PME, or as a means of improving extremely weak muscles. Biofeedback typically involves a measurement of pelvic or abdominal tracings that are visible to the patient, thus providing "feedback" about the effectiveness and correct identification of the PC muscle.

Vaginal weights and electrical stimulation (e-stim) have also been used to augment the effects of PMEs. Vaginal weights of the same size and shape but increasing weight are retained in the vagina by contracting the pelvic muscles, thereby allowing women sensory biofeedback to perform a pelvic muscle contraction when they feel the weight slipping out. The literature regarding use of vaginal weights in premenopausal women with stress UI is quite positive;[34] information regarding use and effectiveness in postmenopausal women is encouraging, but preliminary.[35] E-stim involves either a removable vaginal or anal probe, or surface electrodes that deliver stimulation to either the perivaginal/periurethral muscles (for stress UI), the detrusor muscle (if urge UI is being treated), or both (for individuals with mixed UI). Two recent randomized controlled trials of women with stress[36] or stress or urge UI[37] have been reported; however, the use of e-stim in older individuals requires further investigation.

Bladder retraining is used primarily to manage urge UI[7] and typically involves a combination of behavior modification techniques (e.g., learning to inhibit urges to void) and a voluntary voiding schedule.[38] For example, individuals are instructed to begin the program by voiding every 30–60 minutes and use behavior modification and inhibition techniques to gradually increase the intervals between voids. Bladder retraining techniques are most successful if the individual is motivated, can learn the techniques, receives support from an APN or continence specialist during the process, and has urge UI or urinary urgency and frequency.

Table 5–2 Tips for Instructing Patients in Pelvic Muscle Exercises[19]

- Explain the purpose: PMEs or Kegel exercises strengthen the pelvic muscles and can improve stress and urge UI.

- Help patients find the correct muscle by either: verbally explain that they should gently squeeze the rectal or vaginal muscle, or manually assist them to identify the muscle by instructing them to squeeze around your finger during a vaginal or rectal examination.

- Instruct patients not to squeeze the stomach, buttocks, or thigh muscles (because this only increases intra-abdominal pressure), but to concentrate on the pelvic muscle.

- Explain that ideally each exercise should consist of squeezing for 10 seconds and relaxing for 10 seconds. Some patients may need to start with 3 or 5 seconds and then increase as their muscles get stronger.

- Encourage patients to do 50 exercises per day but not more than 25 at once.

- Point out that patients may notice improvement in 2 to 4 weeks, but not immediately.

Age does not affect an individual's ability to participate in a bladder retraining program.[38]

Habit training and prompted-voiding are additional behavioral therapies that can help restore or improve continence in cognitively impaired individuals. These therapies require significant commitment from all members of the health-care team, and, in particular, direct caregivers. Habit training involves arrangement of an individualized elimination schedule in anticipation of episodes of UI; caregivers are instructed to have older adults void at specific times based on information gained from history, PE, and interpretation of bladder diaries.[39,40] Prompted voiding involves prompting and praising incontinent individuals in combination with individualized habit training. A typical prompted voiding regime includes monitoring for episodes of wetness and dryness, prompting and assistance in use of toilet facilities, and praise (positive feedback) when individuals correctly identify wetness or dryness and/or appropriately use toilet facilities.[40,41]

In summary, behavioral techniques have few side effects, can improve control of detrusor and pelvic muscle function, and can be used alone or in combination with other therapies for the treatment of stress, urge, or mixed UI.[7]

Pharmacologic Measures   Pharmacologic therapies offer additional nonsurgical options for the treatment of UI. Several medications have been proven to be beneficial; as with all pharmacologic interventions, individual risk–benefit ratios must be considered prior to recommendation by the APN.

In postmenopausal women, estrogen replacement therapy (ERT) is commonly used for the treatment of stress, urge, and mixed UI. The specific effects of ERT remain unclear, but experts hypothesize that ERT is effective because the genital and urinary tracts share a common embryology and because high concentrations of estrogen receptors are found in the lower urinary tract and urethra.

Despite limitations, varied doses and preparations (e.g., oral, intravaginal cream or ring, estrogen patch),[42,43,44] and controversy as to the type of UI best treated with ERT, a number of studies have shown improvement in urinary symptoms, stress,[44,45,46] urge, and mixed UI[47] for post-

menopausal women who receive some type of ERT. A common regime for women with an intact uterus is 0.625 mg of conjugated estrogen (days 1–25) combined with 5–10 mg of progestin (days 16–25).[48] Intravaginal estrogen cream (0.5–1 g at night) alone or in combination with oral ERT is another option.[48]

Other medications used to treat stress UI in men and women include alpha-sympathomimetic agonists (e.g., pseudoephedrine, ephedrine) and tricyclic antidepressants (e.g., imipramine). These medications improve the symptoms associated with stress UI because stimulation of urethral alpha receptors causes smooth muscle contraction and increases bladder outlet resistance.[49] In normotensive and medically controlled hypertensive adults, alpha-sympathomimetic agonists may be safe;[48] however, a significant number of older individuals have hypertension, and therefore blood pressure should be carefully monitored if alpha-sympathomimetic agonists are considered.

Medications commonly used for treatment of urge UI and urinary frequency include anticholinergic drugs (e.g., propantheline bromide), and antispasmodic agents (e.g., oxybutynin chloride, hyoscyamine sulfate, tolterodine tartrate), because they are thought to act on the detrusor muscle to inhibit DI. Side effects including dry mouth, constipation, blurred vision, increased PVR, and mental status changes may occur; thus, careful dosage initiation and titration are required to minimize untoward effects while achieving therapeutic effects. Imipramine is often used to treat mixed UI as it has both alpha-sympathomimetic and anticholinergic properties.

Nocturia is a particularly bothersome condition; thus many older individuals seek pharmacologic or nonpharmacologic therapies to relieve or reduce nighttime urinary frequency. Although desmopressin diacetate arginine vasopressin (DDAVP) has been used with success in children with enuresis, it has not been studied adequately in an elderly population and serious side effects (e.g., hyponatremia) warrant limited use in this population.[48] APNs can suggest alternative solutions including daytime use of pressure stockings to reduce venous pooling, short-acting diuretics, and limiting fluids before bed to individuals with significant (greater than three times per night) nocturia.

Pharmacologic management of overflow UI using cholinergic agents (e.g., bethanacol chloride) or alpha-adrenergic blockers (e.g., terazosin) can improve detrusor contractility and thus aid in overcoming bladder outlet resistance. Older adults are at increased risk of experiencing significant cholinergic side effects (e.g., abdominal pain, diarrhea, bronchoconstriction) and postural hypotension.[50] Consequently, nonpharmacologic therapies (e.g., clean intermittent catheterization [CIC], Credé maneuvers, instruction in double voiding techniques) are often of greater benefit to older adults who suffer from overflow UI.

In summary, pharmacologic therapies can be effective, but APNs must be cautious and consider reduced dosages for treatment of UI in older individuals.[51] Moreover, before medications are prescribed, APNs should carefully consider, and treat or discontinue, other conditions or medications that may be adversely affecting continence.

Surgery   Surgery is recommended when nonsurgical approaches fail and UI is causing social distress.[1,7] In older men, the most common surgical procedures involve those aimed at treating BPH,[50,52] or those to correct stress, urge, or mixed UI occurring as an untoward effect of prostatectomy (e.g, artificial urinary sphincter, urethral bulking agents).

In older women, stress UI is the type most amenable to surgical intervention. Over 100 operations have been described and an ongoing debate exists as to the "best" procedure and underlying anatomy and pathophysiology of stress UI in women.[53,54] As a result, it is extremely difficult to compare the various procedures, identify their "true" effectiveness,[55,56,57,58] and evaluate long-term results in younger or older women.[57,59]

The most common surgical procedures for treatment of stress UI in women include slings (to provide firm, long-term support of the bladder neck and underlying tissues), colposuspension (to elevate vaginal tissues and restore proper urethral support), colporrhaphy (repair of anterior or posterior pelvic floor prolapse) combined with a sling procedure,[54,60,61] and periurethral or transurethral bulking agents (to decrease the urethral lumen and increase outlet resistance to urine flow).[62] Older women may do as well as younger women who undergo sling procedures,[63] some colposuspension procedures (laparoscopic or abdominal Burch, Raz),[64,65,66] and injections of urethral bulking agents.[55,62,67,68] Frail elderly women who are not sexually active and experience UI as a result of total vaginal vault eversion, may elect colpocleisis (vaginal vault closure) rather than colporrhaphy in combination with a sling procedure because of decreased operative and recovery time and lower overall morbidity.

In summary, surgery is an option for older adults, but most often is considered after other less-invasive strategies have failed. Surgical experiences and decision making regarding this option are highly individualized. Thus, the role of the APN is to recognize when noninvasive strategies are not working, secure an appropriate referral, and encourage and facilitate communication between older individuals, surgeons, and other health professionals at all stages of decision making and recovery.

Self-Care Strategies and Products   Older individuals and their caregivers employ a variety of self-care strategies and use an array of products to manage UI.[69,70,71,72,73] These practices supplement therapies for treatment of stress, urge, mixed, and overflow UI, and are often effective for treatment of functional UI. Some strategies are less than desirable and may contribute to misdiagnosis or prolongation of UI. Thus, it is important that APNs recognize these strategies and provide advice regarding potential benefits or side effects. For example, noncompliance with diuretics and self-restriction of fluids are common strategies,[71,73,74] yet potentially detrimental to the individuals who use them. Additional self-care strategies used by older men and women include frequent voiding,[70,73] wearing special clothing,[73] avoiding public transportation,[71] decreasing lifting or carrying heavy objects,[71] isolation,[71] avoiding sexual intercourse,[71] and locating or staying near a bathroom.[70]

Incontinent individuals use a wide variety of products; some are specifically manufactured to contain or treat UI or factors that contribute to UI (e.g., protective undergarments, plastic bedcovers, external devices for women and men, pessaries), and others are not (e.g., menstruation pads, towels, toilet tissue).[70,73,75,76,77] It is beyond the scope of this chapter to review all available products; it is recommended that APNs who work with incontinent individuals obtain a copy of *The Resource Guide* published by the National Association for Continence.[78] This publication is updated every year and, for a minimal fee, provides an excellent resource regarding almost anything that individuals use or might inquire about. It is extremely important to remember that while products are not a first-line strategy, nor do they "cure" UI, many older individuals use these adjuncts and APNs often get involved in recommendations or evaluation.

Finally, indwelling catheterization may be necessary in some individuals with overflow UI. Sterile or CIC may result in a lower incidence of infection and may be an alternative to a permanent indwelling catheter;[79,80] however, bacteriuria does develop over time.[81] Therefore, ongoing, detailed evaluations of dexterity, mental status, motivation, and correct techniques are essential[50] if intermittent catheterization strategies are employed.

Health Promotion and Prevention

Ideally, health promotion and prevention should be the priority for APNs who care for older individuals in any setting. Controlled studies that document the success of preventive strategies in all age groups are limited. Suggestions for possible preventive strategies include:

- avoidance of cigarette smoking[82,83,84]
- teaching PMEs[84] to symptomatic and asymptomatic younger and older women[85] and to men who undergo prostate surgery
- treatment of symptomatic perimenopausal women with ERT[85]
- counseling regarding healthy bladder and bowel habits and the effects of alcohol and caffeine on the bladder
- instruction in proper lifting techniques to avoid abdominal strain.[85]

Palmer[86] has developed a conceptual model for continence promotion and prevention that suits the needs of older individuals particularly well. In her model, primary prevention strategies include public education regarding prevention of UTIs, constipation, straining, and normal GU function; environmental modifications such as adequate toilet facilities in public buildings; and caregiver education that stresses the importance of maintaining independence and the expectation of continence. Secondary prevention strategies include treatment with behavioral strategies and drugs, tertiary prevention includes knowledgeable use of equipment and supplies, and surgical therapies.

Recommendations for Practice

UI can be effectively evaluated and managed by APNs in a variety of settings.[87,88] Thus, APNs should:

1. Ask older individuals or their caregivers about the presence of UI and evaluate as necessary.[7,85]
2. Incorporate primary prevention strategies and health promotion into routine visits.[85,86]
3. Inquire about self-care strategies and assist individuals in developing a plan that aims to improve, cure, or prevent further UI.[70,89]
4. Consider minimally invasive, nonsurgical therapies first for those with stress, urge, and mixed UI. These include behavioral therapies and judicious use of medications.
5. Refer to specialists if further assessment is necessary, or if appropriate treatments are unavailable.[36,88,90]

APNs play an essential role in prevention, assessment, and treatment of UI in older individuals. A variety of individualized interventions can be initiated in community, long-term care, and tertiary care settings. Moreover, APNs can be instrumental in promoting changes in system-wide attitudes, educational endeavors, and policies regarding care of those with UI. Appropriate specialist referrals complement basic assessment and treatment strategies, and can benefit APNs, individuals with UI, and their caregivers.

Urinary Tract Infections

UTIs are one of the most frequently encountered problems in older adults, and are a significant cause of morbidity and hospitalization in ambulatory and institutionalized populations.[91,92,93] As individuals age, the risk of developing a UTI increases and, in contrast to younger individuals where the prevalence in women greatly outnumbers men, prevalence rates for older women and men are quite similar.[92,94] Although nursing home residents have the highest UTI rate, (e.g., up to 20% of men and 50% of women),[95] frail and healthy older adults in all settings are affected.[96] Thus, APNs play a key role in diagnosis, management, and prevention of new-onset or recurrent UTIs in older individuals.

Definitions

Because of differences in assessment and management, it is important to understand the various definitions and clinical classifications associated with UTI. Significant bacteriuria is defined as at least 100,000 organisms per milliliter of urine, with or without symptoms.[92] Bacteriuria that elicits a host response is considered a UTI. UTIs are further classified as asymptomatic (e.g., without clinical symptoms), symptomatic, uncomplicated (e.g., UTI without structural or functional abnormalities of the urinary tract), or complicated. The prevalence of asymptomatic bacteriuria increases with age; reported prevalence rates for community-dwelling women and men are 20% and 5–10%, respectively.[92] Uncomplicated infections are usually caused by one organism. Complicated UTIs are often polymicrobial; advancing age is the most significant risk factor.[97] Infections are also complicated if they do not resolve after treatment, are associated with bacteremia or sepsis, present atypically or have an atypical clinical course, or occur in conjunction with renal calculi, obstruction, impaired renal function, anatomic abnormalities, or cystic renal disease.[92,98,99] Finally, some experts also differentiate lower (e.g., cystitis) from upper tract infections (e.g., pyelonephritis).[98]

Age-Associated Changes and Risk Factors

Bacteriuria in older individuals is a complex condition and in most cases, multifactorial. Endocrine, immune, and functional changes associated with aging, combined with other risk factors, put older individuals at extremely high risk of developing bacteriuria and asymptomatic and symptomatic UTI. Common predisposing factors for postmenopausal women include pelvic prolapse[97,100] and estrogen deficiency, which may promote increased organism colonization.[99,100] BPH occurs with aging and can predispose older men to UTIs, as a result of obstruction and increased residual urine volumes, decreased prostatic antibacterial factor, and chronic prostatitis.[96,99] Age-associated changes affecting women and men include altered immunity, increased PVR, and an increased prevalence of chronic diseases (e.g., DM).[96,97,99,101] Other common conditions that increase UTI risk include reduced fluid intake, antibiotic use and sexual activity.[100]

Finally, individuals who undergo short- or long-term catheterization are at significantly increased risk of developing bacteriuria, and catheterization accounts for the vast majority of hospital-acquired UTIs.[93] Catheterization increases UTI risk by acting as a foreign body and, in turn, impairing polymorpholeukocyte function, providing direct entry into the bladder, and increasing PVR.[81] Catheterized individuals at greatest risk include those for whom catheters are used inappropriately or for long periods of time, women, and diabetics.[81]

Assessment of UTIs

Diagnosis is based on history and PE findings; however, definitive diagnosis requires microscopic demonstration of significant bacteriuria. "Classic" UTI symptoms include dysuria, flank or suprapubic discomfort, hematuria, urinary frequency and urgency, and foul-smelling or cloudy urine. Older adults are particularly challenging because they frequently present with nonspecific findings attributable to many disorders other than a UTI. For example, older individuals may be afebrile or complain of new-onset or worsening of established

UI, anorexia, confusion, nocturia, or enuresis rather than, or in addition to, more easily recognizable UTI signs and symptoms.

Differential diagnosis is extremely variable and PE findings are often vague. Thus, a fairly comprehensive PE is often required in frail, institutionalized elderly, or in situations in which abnormalities or other risk factors associated with complicated UTI must be discovered. In other situations (e.g., relatively well, community-dwelling elderly), a more focused PE will suffice. Basic components of the PE for all older individuals include vital signs (including temperature and orthostatic blood pressure readings), assessment of costovertebral angle (CVA) tenderness, and abdominal (to identify masses, tenderness, or bladder fullness) and rectal (to estimate prostate size, rectal tone, impaction) examinations. In addition, perineal examination of older women can identify pelvic prolapse, estrogen deficiency, perineal lesions or discharge, and UI. In older men, the genital examination helps rule out infections, masses, or other abnormalities in the differential diagnosis. In some cases, the APN may also want to check PVR urine, or include neurological, skin, functional, or sensory assessments to further differentiate UTIs from other conditions.

Urinalysis and Urine Culture

The majority of young, healthy women with typical UTI symptoms and no evidence of pyelonephritis most often experience an uncomplicated UTI caused by e. coli. In these patients, obtaining a urine culture is probably not necessary and may not be cost effective; experts recommend empiric therapy or use of a urine dipstick or urinalysis alone as sufficient diagnostic tools.[92,102,103] Older individuals (and young men) do not fit the above criteria because of atypical or vague signs and symptoms, differences in causative organisms (e.g., other enterobacteria, enterococci, staphylococci), and a significantly higher incidence of complicated UTI.[92]

Dipstick tests for leukocyte esterase and nitrite are commonly used to screen for pyuria and bacteriuria, respectively when microscopic urinalysis is unavailable; however, they may be less specific than urinalysis and culture and provide little direction regarding appropriate treatment. Urine dipstick tests also have been advocated as a screen for specific conditions where treatment of asymptomatic bacteriuria is appropriate (e.g., pregnant women, older adults undergoing invasive urologic procedures); however, it is probably not effective or appropriate to screen for or treat asymptomatic bacteriuria in most older individuals.[5,96] Thus, if available, midstream or sterile urinalysis and culture are "gold standard" evaluations if UTI is suspected in this population.[92,96]

In older individuals, the diagnosis of UTI is supported by pyuria (5–10 white blood cells/high powered field) and microscopic hematuria on urinalysis, leukocyte esterase and nitrite on urine dipstick or urinalysis, and bacterial colony counts greater than or equal to 10^5 ml of urine on culture. Low-titer bacteremia (colony counts of 10^2–10^4 ml) has been accepted as diagnostic in younger women, but has not been studied in older women or men.[96,103] Although most uncomplicated, non–catheter-related UTIs are caused by e. coli, other pathogens affecting older adults include *Proteus mirabilis, pseudomonas,* and *Klebsiella pneumoniae.*[96,97] Catheter-related infections are often caused by more than one organism; in addition to e. coli, other pathogens found in older individuals with complicated UTIs include other *Proteus* and *Klebsiella* species, *Serratia marcescens, Candida* species, and *Enterococcus* species.[96,97] Thus, in some settings (e.g., well-elderly and community populations) dipstick tests may be useful to screen for the presence of pyuria, leukocytes, or nitrite; urinalysis and culture and sensitivity tests are required when specific etiologies and choices regarding specific therapies are required.

Management of Urinary Tract Infections

Asymptomatic Bacteriuria   The most important group in which to identify and treat asymptomatic bacteriuria are those undergoing traumatic GU examinations (e.g., cystoscopy, transurethral resection of the prostate [TURP]). These individuals are more likely to be exposed to invasive infections as a result of trauma, and should be treated with appropriate antibiotics prior to undergoing the procedure. The duration of therapy has not been well defined;[104] therefore, APNs should provide background information and collaborate with the individual performing the procedure to determine drug choice, dose, and duration.

Treatment of asymptomatic bacteriuria in non-catheterized, institutionalized elderly does not decrease mortality, morbidity, or the severity of chronic UI.[5,104,105] Treatment of asymptomatic bacteriuria in catheterized patients is not likely to prevent symptomatic UTI, and may lead to development of antibiotic-resistant organisms.[81] Therefore, because treatment predisposes older individuals to risks including drug toxicity, development of resistant organisms, and early recurrence,[99] it is imperative that the APN carefully consider characteristics of the individual and setting prior to initiating screening measures, treatment, or prevention of asymptomatic bacteriuria in this population.

Uncomplicated UTI   Expert geriatricians do not recommend abbreviated antibiotic courses for older individuals.[92] The least toxic and most clinically and cost-effective drug should be chosen. Most older women with uncomplicated, lower UTIs can be treated for 7 to 10 days; older men usually require 14 days of therapy.[92,96] Individuals with significant renal impairment require adjusted doses, particularly if antibiotics are used that may further impair elimination (e.g., aminoglycosides).[96]

Complicated UTI   Treatment of complicated UTIs is difficult because of multiple risk factors, a broad array of pathogens, many of which may be resistant to "standard" antibiotics, and an increased incidence of recurrence particularly if underlying causes cannot be corrected.[97,99] Treatment regimes for complicated infections in older individuals with normal renal function are based on culture results and generally involve 7–14 days of parenteral or oral antibiotics.[96,97,99] Narrow-spectrum antimicrobials (e.g., amoxicillin, ampicillin) may be ineffective; however, oral trimethoprim-sulfamethoxazole or floroquinolones (e.g., norfloxacin, ciprofloxacin, ofloxacin, lomefloxacin) are quite effective and often recommended as first-line therapy in complicated UTIs.[97] Individualized regimes must be constructed

that consider renal function or drug interactions that may prohibit use of a specific medication.

Catheter-Associated UTI   Symptomatic catheterized individuals require treatment based on urinalysis and culture results, as UTIs in this population are always complicated and often polymicrobial. Antibiotic therapy can be oral or parenteral, and should be given for as short a period as possible (5–7 days);[92,99] however, older individuals may require 14 days or more of therapy.[92] Some experts suggest the catheter be removed, and if possible, left out during treatment; the risks and benefits of this practice have not been adequately examined.[81,92,99]

Recurrent UTI   Recurrent UTI (greater than three symptomatic infections in one year) in noncatheterized individuals can occur as a result of relapse (the same bacteria recurs shortly after treatment is completed) or reinfection (different bacteria occur after successful treatment).[92] Older adults are at risk for developing relapse UTI if they suffer from comorbid conditions such as renal calculi or abscess, chronic bacterial prostatitis (CBP), pyelonephritis, anatomic abnormalities (e.g., vesicorectal reflux), or urinary diversion (e.g., ileal conduit).[106,107] Treatment is dependent on the underlying cause and organism responsible for relapse. Urinalysis and urine culture should be repeated to differentiate relapse from reinfection. At this point, it is also important that the APN consider urologic referral to further evaluate renal function, diagnose CBP, and determine anatomy and functional capacity of the upper urinary tract prior to initiating a second course of antibiotic therapy. Strategies for management of reinfection are presented in the following section on prevention.

Prevention of Urinary Tract Infections

Asymptomatic Bacteriuria   Two of the most common predisposing factors for development of asymptomatic bacteriuria are age and the presence of multiple, comorbid conditions. Thus, it is not realistic to attempt to prevent asymptomatic bacteriuria in this population. It is more important that

APNs identify and institute appropriate treatment for older individuals with asymptomatic bacteriuria before undergoing traumatic GU examinations.[99]

Bacteriuria in Catheterized Individuals   Because catheterization causes bacteria to develop at a rate of 3–10% per day, most older individuals with long-term catheters (greater than one month) have bacteriuria.[92] Rather than attempting to prevent bacteriuria, the APN should focus efforts on avoidance of long-term catheterization unless absolutely necessary. The Agency for Health Care Policy and Research clinical guideline for UI[7] outlines specific situations in which it is appropriate to consider long-term, indwelling catheterization. These include:

1. urinary retention that cannot be managed by any other means (surgery, medications, intermittent catheterization),
2. UI that exacerbates pressure ulcers, and
3. care of terminally ill individuals where clothing or bed changes would be uncomfortable.

Recurrent, Symptomatic Reinfection in Older Women   As many as 10–15% of women over 60 suffer from recurrent, symptomatic UTIs.[97,100,108] APNs are in an ideal position to provide guidance and initiate pharmacologic, behavioral, or other nonpharmacologic interventions to improve and maintain bladder health.

Low-dose, antimicrobial prophylaxis is often beneficial for younger and older women who experience recurrent reinfection[100,109] and should be considered for older women diagnosed with more than three uncomplicated UTIs per year. If the UTIs seem to be temporarily related to coitus, the APN can suggest patient-initiated, postcoital antibiotic prophylaxis. Recommended antibiotic regimes include one trimethoprim (40 mg)/sulfamethoxazole (200 mg), 250 mg cephalexin, or 50–100 mg nitrofurantoin as needed.[97] The data available regarding the utility of postcoital voiding is limited and older women are rarely included in clinical trials;[110,111] however, the practice has few or no known side effects and is often recommended by clinicians as an adjunct to postcoital antibiotic use.

If the UTIs have no relation to coitus, antibiotic prophylaxis three times per week, or daily with low doses of medications such as trimethoprim/sulfamethoxazole (40–200 mg), nitrofurantoin (50–100 mg), norfloxacin (200 mg), or cephalexin (250 mg) is appropriate.[96,97] Although most clinicians initiate therapy for six months and then discontinue the antibiotics to reassess the patient's condition, many women are likely to return to baseline and require reinitiation of prophylaxis.[100] In summary, antibiotic prophylaxis for older women with more than three episodes of reinfection per year is a reasonable and frequently used preventive strategy. Side effects related to antibiotic use, consistent compliance, antibiotic resistance, or persistent vaginal candidiasis must be considered when suggesting this option.

Estrogen encourages growth of lactobacilli that lower vaginal pH; maintains vaginal, urethral, and trigonal epithelium; and inhibits growth of uropathogens.[97,109] Thus, institution of intravaginal ERT should be considered for UTI prevention in postmenopausal women; this strategy may work best in combination with other preventive measures.[97]

Behavioral and other nonpharmacologic methods for symptomatic UTI prevention are often cited in the literature, but the degree to which these strategies have been objectively examined in any age group, including the elderly, varies. For example, increased fluid intake helps "flush bacteria out of the system"[93] and is often cited as a preventive strategy by nurse authors.[93,95] Nevertheless, suggesting that older individuals drink eight, 8-oz. glasses of fluid per day may conflict with fluid restrictions imposed as a result of other chronic conditions, or be *so* much more than the individual typically drinks that compliance becomes difficult. Patients, caregivers, and the APN need to work together to identify whether fluid intake is low enough to predispose the individual to concentrated urine that irritates the bladder wall and in turn, may be affecting the incidence of recurrent infection. Individualized fluid regimes can then be constructed to optimize bladder health.

One potentially effective measure that has been studied to some extent is the use of cranberry juice for prevention of recurrent UTI. More than 70 years ago, Blatherwick[112] and colleagues[113] noted increased urinary acidity after ingestion of cranberries or their by-products. Acidification of the urine increases bladder emptying,[95] prevents adherence of bacteria to the bladder wall,[93] and thus may be helpful in preventing UTIs. Although the practice of using cranberry products to acidify the urine has been controversial and is not without side effects (e.g., may worsen symptoms for individuals who suffer from an irritable bladder), recent reports suggest that younger and older women with recurrent UTIs may benefit from daily ingestion of relatively small amounts of cranberry concentrate (capsules containing 400 mg of cranberry solids),[114] or cranberry juice (136–300 ml/day).[95]

Poor or incomplete bladder emptying, or lack of good personal hygiene, may contribute to reinfection in older adults.[92] Thus, suggesting double-voiding techniques for older women who have a tendency to retain urine (e.g., diabetics, women with pelvic prolapse) and attention to careful personal hygiene may be useful adjuncts to other pharmacologic and nonpharmacologic measures.

Scientists have hypothesized that women prone to recurrent *e. coli* UTIs are predisposed as a result of an alteration in host resistance after an initial infection, or as a result of a defect in local defenses.[115,116] Thus, investigators are currently engaged in human trials of vaccines aimed at blocking UTI-causing *e. coli*.[115,117] Although controversial and potentially damaging to beneficial intestinal flora,[116] these vaccines may pave the way for other vaccines or strategies to prevent UTIs.

Conclusions

In summary, APNs who work with older women and men evaluate and manage bacteriuria and symptomatic, complicated, and uncomplicated UTIs in a variety of settings. Some older adults present with "classic" symptoms, receive typical therapies, and have no complications or UTI recurrence. Others, however, require more intense evaluation and management, collaboration with other health professionals, and, in some cases, referral for specialized evaluations or treatments.

APNs are also involved in evaluation and guidance regarding implementation of preventive strategies for older women with symptomatic, recurrent reinfections.

Prostate Disease

Prostate disease is a major public health concern for men over the age of 40 years. BPH affects approximately 75% of men over the age of 50 years.[118] Prostate cancer is the most common cancer diagnosed in men in the United 1States and the second most common cause of cancer death.[119] It is estimated that prostate cancer will affect one in every six American men in their lifetimes[120,121] with an estimated cost of direct medical expenses of $1.5 billion per year.[122] Given the size of this population, APNs need to understand the etiologies, differential diagnoses, and therapeutic interventions for diseases of the lower urinary tract. Moreover, to reduce the burden of costs and suffering caused by this major public health issue, early diagnosis and treatment is crucial.

Pathophysiology

The prostate, a walnut-shaped gland, weighs approximately 20 g and is located within the pelvic area, immediately below the bladder, and encircling the urethra at the bladder neck. Its primary function is to secrete fluid that carries sperm. During ejaculation, seminal fluid mixes with sperm in the prostate; when the bladder neck closes, retrograde ejaculation is prevented and semen is propelled forward through the penis.

The prostate has four zones in concentric circles around the urethra: anterior, peripheral, central, and transitional. The anterior fibromuscular zone has no glandular tissue. It is comprised of smooth muscle and accounts for 30% of prostate mass. The peripheral zone is the largest and contains 75% of the glandular tissue. It is the area palpated with digital rectal exam (DRE) and is the site of origin of 75% of prostate cancer tumors. The central zone, with 25% of the glandular tissue, surrounds the ejaculatory ducts and is rarely a site of cancer. The transitional zone, surrounding the upper urethra and comprising 15–39% of the prostate's volume, has a small portion of glandular tissue and is the site of BPH.

Benign Prostatic Hyperplasia

The prostate gland begins growth during fetal development and attains adult size by the end of puberty. A second growth period occurs beginning in the fifth decade. Approximately 50% of men 51–60 years of age have an enlarged prostate, with 90% of men over 80 years showing evidence of BPH.[123]

BPH is one of the most common disease processes affecting the aging male, yet the exact etiology and pathophysiology are unknown.[123] Testicular androgens clearly contribute to the continued growth of BPH,[123] with the only other substantiated risk factors being age and family history.

BPH is a hyperplastic process characterized by increasing numbers of epithelial and smooth muscle cells.[124] As the prostate lobes enlarge, they cause varying degrees of mechanical obstruction, leading to lower urinary tract symptoms of hesitancy, weak stream, frequency, urgency, and nocturia. The resulting bladder changes include thickened detrusor musculature, high-pressure voiding to empty the bladder, and urinary retention.[125]

BPH develops in the transition zone or periurethral region.[126,127] Severity of symptoms is determined by lobe enlargement and the resulting obstruction of the urethra, which affects the preprostatic sphincter.[125]

Assessment and Management of Benign Prostatic Hyperplasia

The evaluation and diagnosis of BPH begins with a voiding history—frequency of urination, nocturia, urinary stream, feeling of incomplete emptying, UTI, and hematuria. The history should also include a review of the neurologic system (Parkinson's disease, stroke, DM), medications (e.g., anticholinergics may impair bladder contractility, alpha-sympathomimetics increase outflow resistance), and previous surgeries. PE includes assessment of CVA tenderness and bladder disten-

tion, as well as the condition of the external urethral meatus, testes, and spermatic cord. A DRE is done to detect prostatic size, prostate or rectal malignancy, and to evaluate sphincter tone. Dipstick urinalysis can rule out UTI or hematuria; additional laboratory studies include a total serum prostatic specific antigen (PSA) for prostatic disease and serum creatinine to determine evidence of renal insufficiency. The American Urological Association (AUA) and American Cancer Society recommend annual DRE and PSA for men older than 50 years of age with a life expectancy of greater than 10 years. Most patients seek treatment for BPH because symptoms affect quality of life. The AUA Symptom Index[124] is a useful baseline questionnaire. A series of seven self-administered questions are each scored from 0–5 points. A score of 0–7 is mild, 8–19 is moderate, and 20–35 is severe. The index is useful in the initial evaluation of symptom severity, and response to therapy over time. Symptom relief is clearly the major goal for patients and clinicians.

Treatment for BPH is based on symptom management and quality of life. The patient should be counseled regarding therapeutic options. Patients with AUA Symptom Index scores of 0–7 are good candidates for lifestyle changes. A decrease in caffeine, alcohol intake, and liquids after 7:00 PM, and medication review (e.g., use of diuretics in the morning) may help control symptoms. The herb saw palmetto has been linked to decreased nocturia and increased urinary flow. It is sold as tea, capsules, tincture, and extract in health-food stores and pharmacies. Lifestyle changes, watchful waiting, periodic evaluation, and reassurance are usually sufficient measures for most men with mild BPH.

For men with severe symptoms and higher scores on the AUA Symptom Index, drug therapy offers clinically significant outcomes with the possibility of fewer side effects than surgery. Alpha-adrenergic blockers decrease bladder resistance to urinary outflow by decreasing contraction of prostatic smooth muscle. Approved alpha-blockers include terazosin hydrochloride, doxazosin mesylate, and tamsulosin hydrochloride. Higher doses of alpha-blocking drugs provide greater improvement in symptoms.[128] Patients should be titrated up to 10 mg of terazosin, 8 mg of doxazosin, and 0.8 mg tamsulosin for optimal results.[128] However, a major side effect of concern for older individuals is a drop in blood pressure, especially with terazosin and doxasin. Consider controlling hypertensive patients and achieving BPH response with a single drug.

Finasteride is a 5-alpha reductase inhibitor, which reduces prostate volume, increases urinary flow rate, and slows progression of BPH.[128,129] A serum half-life of eight hours in older men allows once daily dosing of 5 mg. Adverse effects are related to sexual function and include erectile dysfunction (ED), decreased libido, and decreased ejaculatory volume. Finasteride is recommended for patients with a large prostate (over 20 g); however, because the drug suppresses androgen production over a six-month period, men with BPH may continue to experience urinary symptoms until the drug reaches its full efficacy. Thus, many patients receive maximum benefit from a combination of finasteride and an alpha-adrenergic blocker (e.g., terazosin hydrochloride)

Patients who fail to benefit from drug therapy may require surgery. TURP is the gold standard of treatment to reduce symptoms by improving flow rates and decreasing PVR.[130] TURP is done under anesthesia with an instrument called a resectoscope inserted through the penis and obstructing prostate tissue is removed. The cost, hospital time, and adverse effects (bleeding, UI, sexual dysfunction) make this procedure less than ideal. Other alternatives include transurethral incision of the prostate (TUIP), balloon dilatation of the urethra, intraurethral stents, hyperthermia, thermal therapy, and laser ablation of the prostate.[131]

Current treatment options for BPH range from watchful waiting to medication to surgery. Intervention is based on symptoms along with a balancing of the risks, costs, and benefits of the available choices for treatment.

Prostate Cancer

Cancer of the prostate is the most common cancer in American males and is a disease of older men, rarely occurring in men under age 50.[121,125] Precise etiology of prostate cancer is unknown but its occurrence depends on the presence of testosterone.[121] Disease progression has a variable course. Most malignancies begin in the peripheral zone of the prostate, with approximately 20% in the transition zone and 5–10% in the central zone.[121,132]

Risk factors associated with prostate cancer include age, diet, family history, and ethnic background. Age increases the risk of prostate cancer. Ninety-five percent of prostate cancers are diagnosed in men between 45 and 89 years of age with the median being 72 years. Less than 1 in 10,000 men younger than 39 years develop prostate cancer; 1/103 men aged 49 years to 59 years and 1 in 8 aged 69–79 years are affected.[120] Family history has been linked with a higher risk of developing prostate cancer and at an earlier age.[132] Prostate cancer is also the most common malignant disorder among African American men.[125] Probability of developing prostate cancer among African American men is 9.4%, compared to 8.7% in Caucasian men and a low incidence in Asian males. Intake of saturated fats is linked to increased risk, possibly accounting for the lower incidence of prostate cancer in Japanese males who have less fat in their diets.[121]

In addition to the above major risk factors, potential risks include high exposure to cadmium, a trace mineral in cigarette smoke, and lack of Vitamin D. Northern countries have higher rates of prostate cancer possibly due to decreased exposure to ultraviolet radiation, which is necessary for synthesis of Vitamin D. In laboratory studies, Vitamin D has been shown to slow the growth of prostate cells.[121]

Assessment and Management of Prostate Cancer

Prostate cancer is usually asymptomatic early in the disease because most adenomas arise in the peripheral areas of the gland. If symptoms are present, it usually indicates advanced or metastatic disease. Symptoms may include urinary frequency, obstruction, ED, decreased ejaculation, pelvic lymph node involvement with leg edema, and bone pain.[125]

Due to the asymptomatic nature of the disease, early detection is essential. The primary screening tools are DRE and serum PSA.[133] Screening is recommended yearly for men over 50 years of age with a life expectancy of at least 10 years, and yearly for men over 40 years with a family history of prostate cancer.[122] PSA is a glycoprotein demonstrated to be specific for prostate tissue.[127] Produced by both benign and malignant prostate cells, PSA normally leaks into circulation in small concentrations of less than 4 mg/ml.[134] A PSA of less than 4 mg/ml is within the acceptable range.[124] Increased levels indicate prostatic disease; however, a number of benign conditions and procedures can elevate PSA levels, including prostatitis, BPH, acute urinary retention, cystoscopy, TURP, and prostate biopsy.[135] A rapidly rising PSA has a 55% reliability for detecting a prostate cancer.[133]

DRE is a simple, cost-effective procedure. The practitioner palpates the prostate for asymmetry, induration, and nodules. Benign tissue is soft and feels like the thenar eminence of the thumb. Adenomas are firm nodules that may be indurated and asymmetrical. Other causes of an abnormal DRE include BPH, prostatitis, prostatic calculi, focal infarct, and prior prostate biopsies or TURP.[133]

Referral for prostate biopsy is recommended with an abnormal DRE or elevated PSA. Biopsy is usually performed as an outpatient procedure using transrectal ultrasound. A needle is inserted through the perineum or rectum and into the prostate gland in order to aspirate tissue for analysis. Histologic grading usually follows the Gleason Sum System[136] based on five patterns of prostate cells. A primary grade is assigned to the cancer pattern occupying the largest area of specimen and a secondary grade to the second largest area of specimen.[125,133]

Once the adenocarcinoma is histologically confirmed, the stage or extent of the disease is determined. The most commonly used system is the tumor, nodes, and metastasis (TNM) classification of the Joint Cancer Committee. Treatment of prostate cancer is based on tumor stage, patient age, and health status.

Radical prostatectomy is the most common procedure for patients under 70 years of age with cancer confined to the prostate and no major medical problems. During radical prostatectomy, the entire prostate, prostatic capsule, and seminal vesicles are removed. Preservation of sexual function is dependent on nerve sparing outside of the capsule. Continence depends on preservation of the urethral external sphincter with anastomosis of the bladder neck to the urethral stump.[125,137]

External beam radiation therapy is an alternative to radical prostatectomy and may avoid ED and UI. Radiation doses and targeting are operator dependent and complications include problems in the gastrointestinal (diarrhea, rectal pain, tenesmus) and GU (frequency, dysuria, urethral stricture, and ED) tract.[119]

Other treatments include the implantation of radioactive seeds. New evidence suggests that dietary changes may slow the progression of existing prostate cancer. For example, APNs can recommend that patients reduce fat and increase Vitamin E, selenium, and soy protein.[138] This holistic approach should be encouraged in combination with traditional medicine. Further evaluation of the long-term effects of these procedures is needed.

Advanced disease, when the prostate cancer invades the prostatic capsule and metastasizes, requires hormone ablation therapy to inhibit testosterone. Approximately 95% of testosterone is produced by the testes, making bilateral orchiectomy the most direct choice. Pharmacological approaches for androgen deprivation include estrogen therapy (inhibits testosterone synthesis), leutenizing hormone-releasing hormone (LHRH) agonists (inhibit the release of pituitary gonadotropins), and combined androgen blockade with LHRH agonists plus antiandrogens (block androgens at target site). Androgen deprivation is not a cure, but eases symptoms and can extend life.[132]

Knowledge of prostate disease allows the APN to identify risks, provide screening, and refer patients for early diagnosis and treatment. Moreover, because radical prostatectomy is associated with complications such as ED and UI, APNs are in an ideal position to provide care; educate patients and family members; initiate supportive, pharmacologic, and behavioral treatments; and collaborate with other members of the health-care team to minimize frustration and suffering associated with the diagnosis and treatment of prostate cancer.[33,139]

References

1. Urinary Incontinence Guideline Panel. *Urinary Incontinence in Adults: Clinical Practice Guideline.* Rockville, Md: Agency for Health Care Policy and Research, US Department of Health and Human Services, 1992. AHCPR Pub. No. 92-0038.

2. National Association for Continence [news release]. Release of findings from consumer survey on urinary incontinence. Dissatisfaction with treatment continues to rise. Spartansburg, SC, December 4, 1998.

3. Herzog AR, Fultz NH. Prevalence and incidence of urinary incontinence in community-dwelling populations. *J Am Geriatr Soc.* 1990;38:273–281.

4. Jirovec MM, Wyman JF, Wells TJ. Addressing urinary incontinence with educational continence-care competencies. *Image: J Nurs Scholarship.* 1998;30:375–378.

5. Ouslander JG, Schapira M, Schnelle JF, et al. Does eradicating bacteriuria affect the severity of chronic urinary incontinence in nursing home residents? *Ann Intern Med.* 1995;122:749–754.

6. National Institutes of Health Consensus Development Conference. Urinary incontinence in adults. *J Am Geriatr Soc.* 1990;38:265–272.

7. Fantl A, Newman DK, Colling J, et al. *Urinary Incontinence in Adults: Acute and Chronic Management.* Rockville, Md: Agency for Health Care Policy and Research, US Department of Health and Human Services, 1996. AHCPR Publication No. 96-0682.

8. Panel for the Prediction and Prevention of Pressure Ulcers in Adults. Clinical Practice Guideline Number 3: *Pressure Ulcers in Adults: Prediction and Prevention.* Rockville, Md: Agency for Health Care Policy and Research, US Department of Health and Human Services, 1992. AHCPR Publication No. 92-0047.

9. Sier H, Ouslander J, Orzeck S. Urinary incontinence among geriatric patients in acute care hospitals. *JAMA.* 1987;257:1767–1771.

10. Wyman JF. The psychiatric and emotional impact of female pelvic floor dysfunction. *Curr Opinion Obstet Gynecol.* 1994;6:336–339.

11. Jackson S. The patient with an overactive bladder—symptoms and quality-of-life issues. *Urology.* 1997;50 (suppl 6A):18–22.

12. Gray M, Ramone R, Moore K. The urethral sphincter: an update. *Urol Nurs.* 1995;1(5):40–53.

13. Wanich C, Chapman E. *Long Term Care Patient Management Simulations.* Rowayton, Ct: Medical Age Publishing; 1989.

14. Madersbacher S, Pycha A, Schatzl G, Mian C, Klingler CH, Marberger M. The aging lower urinary tract: A comparative urodynamic study of men and women. *Urology.* 1998;51:206–212.

15. Colling JC, Owen TR, McCreedy MR. Urine volumes and voiding patterns among incontinent nursing home residents. Residents at highest risk for dehydration are often the most difficult to track. *Geriatr Nurs.* 1994; 15:188–192.

16. Kirkland JL, Lye M, Levy DW, Banerjee AK. Patterns of urine flow and electrolyte excretion in healthy elderly people. *BMJ.* 1983;287:1665–1667.

17. Luft J, Vrheas-Nichols AA. Identifying the risk factors for developing incontinence: can we modify individual risk? *Geriatr Nurs.* 1998;19:66–70.

18. Palmer MH. *Urinary Continence: Assessment and Promotion.* Gaithersburg, Md: Aspen Publishers; 1996.

19. Bradway C, Hernly S, the NICHE Faculty. Urinary incontinence in older adults admitted to acute care. *Geriatr Nurs.* 1998;19(2):98–102.

20. Fantl A, Newman DK, Colling J, et al. *Managing acute and chronic urinary incontinence; Clinical Practice Guideline. Quick Reference Guide for Clinicians.* Rockville, Md: Agency for Health Care Policy and Research, US Department of Health and Human Services, 1996. AHCPR Publication No. 96-0686.

21. Siltberg H, Larsson G, Victor A. Frequency/volume chart: the basic tool for investigating urinary symptoms. *Acta Obstet Gynecol Scand.* 1997;76(suppl 166):24–27.

22. National Institute of Diabetes and Digestive and Kidney Diseases. *Your daily bladder diary.* Bethesda, Md: National Kidney and Urologic Diseases Information Clearinghouse, National Institutes of Health; 1997.

23. Miller JM, Ashton-Miller JA, Delancey JOL. Quantification of cough-related urine loss using the paper towel test. *Obstet Gynecol.* 1998;91:705–709.

24. McIntosh LJ, Richardson DA. 30-minute evaluation of incontinence in the older woman. *Geriatrics.* 1994; 49:35–44.

25. Duldulao KE, Diokno AC, Mitchell B. Value of urinary cytology in women presenting with urge incontinence and/or irritative voiding symptoms. *J Urol.* 1997;157: 113–116.

26. Wozniak-Petrofsky J. Urodynamics for the primary care nurse. *Geriatr Nurs.* 1996;17:115–119.

27. Burgio KL, Whitehead WE, Engle BT. Urinary incontinence in the elderly: bladder/sphincter biofeedback and toileting skills training. *Ann Intern Med.* 1985;103:507–515.

28. McDowell BJ, Burgio KL, Dombrowski M, Locher JL, Rodriguez E. An interdisciplinary approach to the assessment and behavioral treatment of urinary incontinence in geriatric outpatients. *J Am Geriatr Soc.* 1993;40:370–374.

29. Dougherty MD, Bishop KR, Abrams RM, Batich CD, Gimotty PA. The effect of exercise on the circumvaginal muscles in postpartum women. *J Nurse Midwifery.* 1989;34(1):8–14.

30. Huisman AB. Aspects on the anatomy of the female urethra with special relation to urinary continence. *Contrib Gynecol Obstet.* 1983;10:1–31.

31. Bo K, Hagen RH, Kvarstein B, Jorgensen J, Larson S. Pelvic floor muscle exercise for the treatment of female stress urinary incontinence: III. Effects of two different degrees of pelvic floor muscle exercises. *Neurol Urodynamics*. 1990;9:489–502.

32. Wells TJ, Brink CA, Diokno AC, Wolfe R, Gillis GL. Pelvic muscle exercise for stress urinary incontinence in elderly women. *J Am Geriatr Soc*. 1991;39: 785–791.

33. Robinson JP. Managing urinary incontinence following radical prostatectomy. *J Wound, Ostomy, and Continence Nurs*. 2000;27(3):138–145.

34. Jonassan A, Larsson B, Bschera H. Testing and training of the pelvic floor muscles after childbirth. *Acta Obstet Gynecol Scand*. 1989;68:301–304.

35. Wilson PD, Borland M. Vaginal cones for the treatment of genuine stress incontinence. *Aust N Z J Obstet Gynecol*. 1990; 30:157–160.

36. Sand PK, Richardson DA, Staskin DR, et al. Pelvic floor electrical stimulation in the treatment of genuine stress incontinence: a multicenter, placebo-controlled trial. *Am J Obstet Gynecol*. 1995;173(1):72–79.

37. Smith JJ. Intravaginal stimulation randomized trial. *J Urol*. 1996;155:127–130.

38. Fantl JA, Wyman JF, McClish DK, et al. Efficacy of bladder training in older women with urinary incontinence. *JAMA*. 1991; 265:609–613.

39. Colling J, Ouslander J, Hadley BJ, Eisch J, Campbell E. The effects of patterned urge response toileting (PURT) on urinary incontinence among nursing home residents. *J Am Geriatr Soc*. 1992;40:135–141.

40. Thompson DL, Smith DA. Continence restoration in the cognitively impaired adult. *Geriatr Nurs*. 1998; 19(2):87–90.

41. Schnelle JF. Treatment of urinary incontinence in nursing home patients by prompted voiding. *J Am Geriatr Soc*. 1990;38:433–459.

42. Faber P, Heidenriech J. Treatment of stress incontinence with estrogen in postmenopausal women. *Urolog Int*. 1977;32(2–3):221-223.

43. Bhatia NN, Bergaman A, Karram MM. Effects of estrogen on urethral function in women with urinary incontinence. *Am J Obstet Gynecol*. 1989;160: 176–181.

44. Makinen JI, Pitanen YA, Salmi TA, Gronroos M, Rinne R, and Paakkari I. Transdermal estrogen for female stress urinary incontinence in postmenopause. *Maturitas*. 1995;22:233–238.

45. Eckerling B, Goldman JA. Conservative treatment of uterovaginal prolapse and stress urinary incontinence. *Int Surg*. 1972;57:221–222.

46. Sartori MGF, Baracat EC, Girao MJBC, Goncalves WJ, Sartori JP, Rodrigues de Lima G. Menopausal genuine stress urinary incontinence treated with conjugated estrogens plus progesterone. *Intl J Obstet Gynecol*. 1995;49:165–169.

47. Samsioe G, Jansson I, Mellstrom D, Svanborg A. Occurrence, nature, and treatment of urinary incontinence in a 70-year-old female population. *Maturitas*. 1985;7:335–342.

48. Goode PS, Burgio KL. Pharmacologic treatment of lower urinary tract dysfunction in geriatric patients. *Am J Med Sci*. 1997;314(4):262–267.

49. Weinberger MW. Conservative treatment of urinary incontinence. *Clin Obstet Gynecol*. 1995;38:175–188.

50. Rousseau P, Fuentevilla-Clifton A. Urinary incontinence in the aged, part 2: management strategies. *Geriatrics*. 1992;47(June):37–48.

51. Tapp AJS, Cardozo LD, Versi E, Cooper D. The treatment of detrusor instability in postmenopausal women with oxybutinin chloride: a double blind placebo controlled study. *Br J Obstet Gynecol*. 1990;97:521–526.

52. Igbal P, Castleden CM. Management of urinary incontinence in the elderly. *Gerontology*. 1997;43: 151–157.

53. DeLancey JOL. The pathophysiology of stress urinary incontinence in women and its implications for surgical treatment. *World J Urol*. 1997;15:268–274.

54. Keane DP, Eckford SD, Abrams P. Surgical treatment and complications of urinary incontinence. *Curr Opinion Obstet Gynecol*. 1992;4:559–564.

55. Duckett JRA. The use of periurethral injectables in the treatment of genuine stress incontinence. *Br J Obstet Gynecol*. 1998;105:390–396.

56. Lam TC, Hadley HR. Surgical procedures for uncomplicated ("routine") female stress urinary incontinence. *Urol Clin N Am*. 1991;18:327–337.

57. Riggs JA, Riggs JC. Update on retropubic incontinence surgery. A comparison of two procedures. *The Fem Patient*. 1997;22:13–24.

58. Zivkovic F, Tamussino K. Effects of vaginal surgery on the lower urinary tract. *Curr Opinion Obstet Gynecol*. 1997;9:329–331.

59. Kelly MJ, Zimmern PE, Leach GE. Complications of bladder neck suspension procedures. *Urol Clin N Am*. 1991;18:339–348.

60. Cross CA, Cespedes D, McGuire EJ. Treatment results using pubovaginal slings in patients with large cystoceles and stress incontinence. *J Urol*. 1997;158:431–434.

61. Raz S, Little NA, Juma S, Sussman EM. Repair of severe anterior vaginal wall prolapse (grade IV cystourethrocele). *J Urol*. 1991;146:988–992.

62. Stanton SL, Monga AK. Incontinence in elderly women: is periurethral collagen an advance? *Br J Obstet Gynecol*. 1997;104:154–157.

63. Carr LK, Walsh PJ, Abraham VE, Webser GD. Favorable outcome of pubovaginal slings for geriatric women with stress incontinence. *J Urol*. 1997;157:125–128.

64. Langer R, Golan A, Arad D, Pansky M, Bukovsky I, Caspi E. Effects of induced menopause on Burch colposuspension for urinary stress incontinence. *J Repro Med*. 1992;37:956–958.

65. Langer R, Golan A, Ron-El R, et al. Colposuspension for urinary stress incontinence in premenopausal and postmenopausal women. *Surg Obstet Gynecol.* 1990;171:13–16.

66. Nitti VW, Bregg KJ, Sussman EM, Raz S. The Raz bladder neck suspension in patients 65 years old and older. *J Urol.* 1993;149:802–807.

67. Griebling TL, Krieder KJ. Efficacy of periurethral collagen injection for stress urinary incontinence in elderly women [abstract]. *J Am Geriatr Soc.* 1998; 46(9):S76.

68. Khular V, Cardozo LD, Abbott D, Anders K. GAX collagen in the treatment of elderly women: a two-year follow-up. *Br J Obstet Gynecol.* 1997;104:96–99.

69. Diokno AC, Brock BM, Brown MB, Herzog AR. Prevalence of urinary incontinence and other urological symptoms in the noninstitutionalized elderly. *J Urol.* 1986;136:1022–1025.

70. Engberg S, McDowell BJ, Burgio KL, Watston JE, Belle S. Self-care behaviors of older women with urinary incontinence. *J Gerontol Nurs.* 1995;21(8):7–14.

71. Norton PA, MacDonald LD, Sedgwick PM, Stanton SL. Distress and delay associated with urinary incontinence, frequency, and urgency in women. *BMJ.* 1998;297: 1187–1189.

72. Sandvik H, Hunskaar S. The epidemiology of pad consumption among community-dwelling incontinent women. *J Aging Health.*1995;7:417–426.

73. Sandvik H, Kveine E, Hunskaar S. Female urinary incontinence—psychosocial impact, self-care, and consultations. *Scand J Caring Sci.* 1993;7:53–56.

74. McKeever MP. An investigation of recognized incontinence within a health authority. *J Adv Nurs.* 1990;15:1197–1207.

75. Vierhout ME, Lose G. Preventive vaginal and intra-urethral devices in the treatment of female urinary stress incontinence. *Curr Opinion Obstet Gynecol.* 1997;9:325–328.

76. Moore KH, Foote A, Siva S, King J, Burton G. The use of bladder neck support prosthesis in combined genuine stress incontinence and detrusor instability. *Aust N Z J Obstet Gynecol.* 1997;37:440–445.

77. Wu V, Farrell SA, Baskett TF, Flowerdew G. A simplified protocol for pessary management. *Obstet Gynecol.* 1997;90:990–994.

78. National Association for Continence. *The Resource Guide.* 10th ed. Spartansburg, SC: author; 2000.

79. Dowd TT, Campbell JM. Urinary incontinence in an acute care setting. *Urol Nurs.* 1995;15:82–85.

80. Terpenning MS, Allada R, Kauffaman CA. Intermittent urethral catheterization in the elderly. *J Am Geriatr Soc.* 1989;37:411–416.

81. Warren JW. Catheter-associated urinary tract infections. *Infect Dis Clin N Am.* 1997;11:609–621.

82. Bump RC, McClish DM. Cigarette smoking and pure genuine stress incontinence of urine: a comparison of risk factors and determinants between smokers and nonsmokers. *Am J Obstet Gynecol.* 1994;170:579–582.

83. Koskimaki J, Hakama M, Huhtala H, Tammela TJ. Association of smoking with lower urinary tract symptoms. *J Urol.* 1998;159:1580–1582.

84. Swaffield J. Avoiding incontinence—health education and preventative care for women. *Nurs: J Clin Pract Educ Manage.* 1986;3(10):6–7.

85. Webb M. Urinary incontinence in younger women. *Nurse Pract Forum.* 1994;5(3):164–169.

86. Palmer MH. A health promotion perspective of urinary continence. *Nur Outlook.* 1994;42(4):163–169.

87. Seim A, Sivertsen B, Bjarne C, Hunskaar S. Treatment of urinary incontinence in women in general practice: observational study. *Br Med J.* 1996;312:1459–1462.

88. Wyman JF. Level 3: comprehensive assessment and management of urinary incontinence by continence nurse specialists. *Nurse Pract Forum.* 1994;5(3): 177–185.

89. Turner SL, Plymat KR. As women age: perspectives on urinary incontinence. *Rehab Nurs.* 1988;13(3): 132–135.

90. Zhao CX. Postmenopausal urinary incontinence. *J Trad Chinese Med.* 1987;7:305–306.

91. Stam WE, Hooton TM. Management of urinary tract infections in adults. *N Engl J Med.* 1993;329: 1328–1334.

92. Yoshikawa TT, Nicolle LE, Norman DC. Management of complicated urinary tract infection in older patients. *J Am Geriatr Soc.* 1996;44:1235–1241.

93. Marchiondo K. A new look at urinary tract infection. *Am J Nurs.* 1998;98(3):34–39.

94. Bacheller CD, Bernstein JM. Urinary tract infections. *Med Clin N Am.* 1997;81:719–730.

95. Jackson B, Hicks LE. Effect of cranberry juice on urinary pH in older adults. *Home Healthcare Nurse.* 1997;15:199–202.

96. Wood CA, Abrutyn E. Urinary tract infection in older adults. *Clin Geriatr Med.* 1998;14:267–283.

97. McCue JD. Complicated, recurrent, and geriatric UTI. *Clin Focus.* 1995;March:11–17.

98. Funstuck R, Smith JW, Tschape H, Stein G. Pathogenic aspects of uncomplicated urinary tract infection: recent advances. *Clin Nephrol.* 1997;47(1):13–18.

99. Nicolle LE. Asymptomatic bacteriuria in the elderly. *Infect Dis N Am.* 1997;11:647–663.

100. Stapleton A, Stamm WE. Prevention of urinary tract infection. *Infect Dis Clin N Am.* 1997;11:719–733.

101. Sobel JD. Pathogenesis of urinary tract infection. *Infect Dis Clin N Am.* 1997;11:531–547.

102. Barry HC, Ebell MH, Hickner J. Evaluation of suspected urinary tract infection in ambulatory women: a cost-utility analysis of office-based strategies. *J Fam Pract.* 1997;44(1):49–59.

103. Cattell WR. Urinary tract infection in women. *J Royal Coll Physicians London.* 1997;31(2):130–133.

104. Melillo KD. Asymptomatic bacteriuria in older adults: when is it necessary to screen and treat? *Nurse Pract.* 1995;20(8):50–66.

105. Nicolle LE, Mayhew JW, Bryan L. Prospective randomized comparison of therapy and no therapy for asymptomatic bacteriuria in institutionalized women. *Am J Med.* 1987;83:27–33.

106. Lipsky BA. Urinary tract infections in men: epidemiology, pathophysiology, diagnosis, and treatment. *Ann Int Med.* 1989;110:138–150.

107. Yoshikawa TT. Chronic urinary tract infections in elderly patients. *Hosp Pract.* 1993;28:103–106, 111, 115–118.

108. Iosif CS, Bekassy Z. Prevalence of genito-urinary symptoms in the late menopause. *Acta Obstet Gynecol Scand.* 1984;63:257–260.

109. Cardozo L, Benness C, Abbott D. Low dose oestrogen prophylaxis for recurrent urinary tract infections in elderly women. *Br J Obstet Gynecol.* 1998;105:403–407.

110. Hooton TM, Scholes D, Hughes JP, et al. A prospective study of risk factors for urinary tract infections in young women. *N Engl J Med.* 1996;335:468–474.

111. Strom BL, Collins M, West SL, et al. Sexual activity, contraceptive use, and other risk factors for symptomatic and asymptomatic bacteriuria: a case-control study. *Ann Int Med.* 1987;107:816–823.

112. Blatherwick NR. The specific role of foods in relation to the composition of the urine. *Arch Int Med.* 1914;14:409–450.

113. Blatherwick NR, Long ML. Studies of urinary acidity. *J Biol Chem.* 1923;57:815–818.

114. Walker EB, Barney DP, Mickelsen JN, Walton RJ, Mickelsen RA. Cranberry concentrate: UTI prophylaxis [letter]. *J Fam Pract.* 1997;45:167–168.

115. Cramer DA. Recurrent urinary tract infection: new theories and an old remedy. *Ann Int Med.* 1998;128:333–334.

116. Service RF. New vaccines may ward off urinary tract infections. *Science.* 1997;276:533.

117. Uehling DT, Hopkins WJ, Balish E, et al. Vaginal mucosa immunization for recurrent urinary tract infection: phase II clinical trial. *J Urol.* 1997;157:2049–2052.

118. Karlowicz KA. *Urologic Nursing Principles and Practice.* Philadelphia: WB Saunders; 1995.

119. Walsh P. The natural history of localized prostate cancer: a guide to therapy. In: Walsh P, Retik A, Vaughn E Jr, Wein A, eds. *Campbell's Urology.* Vol 3. 7th ed. Philadelphia: WB Saunders; 1998;2539–2546.

120. Wingo PA, Tong T, Bolden S. Cancer statistics 1995. *Cancer J Clin.* 1995;45:8–31.

121. Pienta KJ. Etiology, epidemiology, and prevention of carcinoma of the prostate. In: Walsh P, Retik A, Vaughn E Jr, Wein A, eds. *Campbell's Urology.* Vol 3. 7th ed. Philadelphia: WB Saunders; 1998;2489–2496.

122. Frydenberg M, Stricker PD, Kaye KW. Prostate cancer diagnosis and management. *Lancet.* 1997;349:1681.

123. McConnell JD. Epidemiology, etiology, pathophysiology and diagnosis of benign prostatic hyperplasia. In: Walsh P, Retik A, Vaughn E Jr, Wein A, eds. *Campbell's Urology.* Vol. 2. 7th ed. Philadelphia; WB Saunders; 1998:1429–1452.

124. McConnell JD, Barry MJ, Bruskewitz RC, et al. *Clinical Practice Guideline Number 8:* Benign prostatic hyperplasia: Diagnosis and Treatment. Clinical Practice Guideline, Number 8. Rockville, Md: Agency for Health Care Policy and Research, US Department of Health and Human Services, 1994. AHCPR Publication No. 94-0582.

125. Weiss RE, Fair WR. *Management of Prostate Disease.* New York: Professionals Communication; 1997.

126. McNeal JE. Pathology of benign prostatic hyperplasia. *Urol Clin N Am.* 1990;17:477–486.

127. Partin A, Coffey D. The molecular biology, endocrinology and physiology of the prostate and seminal vesicles. In: Walsh P, Retik A, Vaughn E Jr, Wein A, eds. *Campbell's Urology.* Vol 2. 7th ed. Philadelphia: WB Saunders; 1998:1381–1428.

128. Lepor H. Natural history, evaluation and nonsurgical management of benign prostatic hyperplasia. In: Walsh P, Retik A, Vaughn E Jr, Wein A, eds. *Campbell's Urology.* Vol 2. 7th ed. Philadelphia: WB Saunders; 1998:1453–1478.

129. Roehrborn CG. Meta-analysis of randomized clinical trials of finasteride. *Urology.* 1998;51(Suppl 4A):46.

130. McCullough D. Minimally invasive treatment of benign prostatic hyperplasia. In: Walsh P, Retik A, Vaughn E Jr, Wein A, eds. *Campbell's Urology.* Vol. 2. 7th ed. Philadelphia: WB Saunders; 1998: 1479–1510.

131. Improte L, Reilly N. Diagnosing and treating benign prostatic hyperplasia. *Innovation Urol Nurs.* 1995;5:4.

132. Oesterling JE, Moyad MA. *The ABCs of Prostate Cancer: The Book That Could Save Your Life.* New York: Madison Books; 1997.

133. Carter HB, Partin AW. Diagnosis and staging of prostate cancer. In: Walsh P, Retik A, Vaughn E Jr, Wein A, eds. *Campbell's Urology.* Vol. 3. 7th ed. Philadelphia: WB Saunders; 1998:2519–2538.

134. Carter HB, Landis PK, Metter J, Fleisher L, Pearson J. Prostate specific antigen testing of older men. *J Nat Cancer Inst.* 1999;91:1733.

135. Grumet SC, Brunner DW. The identification and screening of men at high risk for developing prostate cancer. *Urol Nurs.* 2000;20(1):15–18, 23–24, 46.

136. Gleason DF. Classification of prostatic carcinomas. *Cancer Chemother Rep.* 1960;50:125–128.

137. Oesterling JE. Retropubic and suprapubic prostatectomy. In: Walsh P, Retik A, Vaughn E Jr, Wein A, eds. *Campbell's Urology.* Vol 2. 7th ed. Philadelphia: WB Saunders; 1998:1529–1542.

138. McClain R, Grey M. Prostate cancer: a primer. *Clin Advisor.* 2000;3(2):37–50.

139. Stanford JL, Feng Z, Hamilton AS, et al. Urinary and sexual function after radical prostatectomy for clinically localized prostate cancer. *JAMA.* 2000;283:354–360.

6

Diabetes Mellitus

Barbara J. Maschak-Carey
Patricia Katheder Bourne
Izzie Brown-Gordon

◼ Diabetes Statistics: Facts and Figures

Diabetes mellitus is a significant health problem in the United States. It affects all age, racial, and ethnic groups, but is particularly prevalent in the older adult population, as well as among African Americans, Asian Americans, Hispanic Americans, Pacific Islanders, and Native Americans (Figure 6–1). The incidence of diabetes is rising, with 16 million people affected in the United States. Health-care costs associated with diabetes are estimated at greater than $100 billion dollars annually. Long-standing diabetes incurs devastating long-term complications such as retinopathy and blindness, nephropathy and renal failure, and neu-

ropathy and amputations. Macrovascular disease is twice as prevalent in diabetes, with 50–65% of patients with diabetes dying from cardiovascular and cerebrovascular disease. The challenge is finding those who are undiagnosed and treating them earlier to prevent the complications. It is estimated that of the 16 million people with diabetes about one half of them are undiagnosed.[1]

Diabetes mellitus is a metabolic disorder, with two major types, type 1 and type 2. The etiology and pathology of type 1 and type 2 differ, but the end result, hyperglycemia, is the same.

Type 1 diabetes accounts for 10% of the diabetic population and results from lack of insulin production by the beta cells of the islets of Langerhans in the

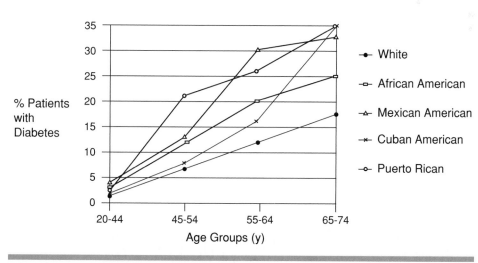

Figure 6–1
Increase in type 2 diabetes prevalance with age in the US population.
Source: Harris. Diabetes Care. 1991;14(Suppl 3):639.

pancreas. The etiology of type 1 diabetes is believed to be autoimmune in nature, with destruction of the beta cells by islet cell antibodies. The absence of insulin production results in hyperglycemia, which leads to an osmotic diuresis (polyuria), dehydration (thirst), ketone production (weight loss), and if untreated with insulin, ketoacidosis. All patients with type 1 diabetes must be treated with insulin injections. Type 1 diabetes has an abrupt onset and the patient is typically symptomatic with the classic polyuria, polydipsia, and polyphagia. Many newly diagnosed patients present in ketoacidosis at diagnosis. Type 1 diabetes was formerly called "juvenile" diabetes because onset occurred in childhood. Type 1 diabetes, however, can present in adults. Many older adults have long-standing type 1 diabetes and must continue treatment with insulin. Monitoring for and treating the long-term complications of diabetes is a major part of care in type 1 diabetes.

Type 2 diabetes is the more common type, and results from several concurrent abnormalities (Figure 6–2). In the simplest terms, glucose metabolism is regulated by several factors. First, carbohydrates are ingested and broken down to monosaccharides. Enzymes called alphaglucosidase in the small intestine are active in this process, resulting in the release of glucose into the blood stream. The elevation of blood glucose stimulates the release of insulin from the beta cells of the pancreas. Insulin is necessary for glucose to cross the cell membranes and enter the cells where it is utilized for energy (glucose transport). Insulin receptors on the cells are required for this action to take place. Glucose that is not utilized is stored in the liver where it is converted to glycogen. Fluctuations in blood glucose affect the conversion of glucose to glycogen and vice versa.

In type 2 diabetes, any or all of these processes may be affected. The earliest dysfunction is the inadequacy or deficiency of insulin receptors in the cells. This results in inefficient insulin action. Prior to the actual occurrence of diabetes, a compensatory response by the pancreas results in a state of hyperinsulinemia, or insulin resistance. Diabetes results when the pancreas fails to keep up with the demand of insulin and hyperglycemia occurs. Figure 6-3 depicts the natural history of the development of type 2 diabetes, showing that pathology begins long before diagnosis. Furthermore, increased hepatic glucose production contributes to hyperglycemia as well.

Type 2 diabetes is insidious in onset and is often asymptomatic. Unfortunately, undetected diabetes

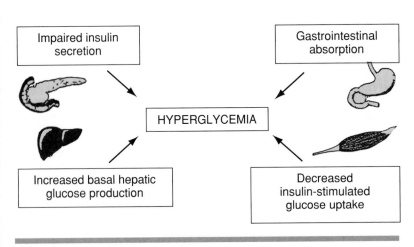

Figure 6–2
Pathogenesis of type 2 diabetes.

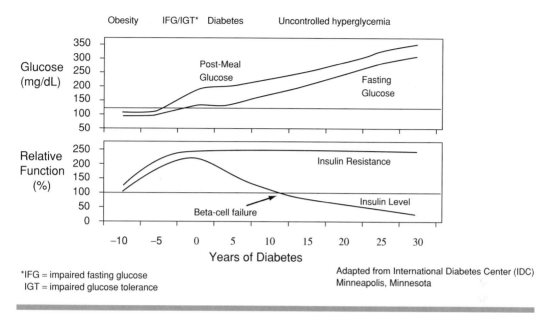

Obesity   IFG/IGT*   Diabetes   Uncontrolled hyperglycemia

Figure 6–3
Depicts the natural history of the development of type 2 diabetes, showing that
pathology begins long before diagnosis.

goes untreated, causing complications before the patient is even aware of the disease. Complication of diabetes can be evident at diagnosis or may be the presenting symptom of disease. In such cases, the diabetes is long-standing. For obvious reasons, all people need to be routinely screened for diabetes.

In the field of diabetes, two recent landmark studies have had the greatest impact on the care and treatment of the patient with diabetes. The Diabetes Control and Complications Trial (DCCT) was completed in 1993, and dramatically demonstrated that intensive control of blood glucose in type 1 patients reduces the risk of long-term complications by as much as 78%.[2] The United Kingdom Prospective Diabetes Study (UKPDS), reported in 1998, had similar results for type 2 diabetes,[3] suggesting that for both types, control of glucose is a major goal of all treatment.

The first purpose of this chapter is to alert the nurse practitioner of the importance of screening for diabetes to promote early treatment and the prevention of complications. Second, the chapter outlines the current standard of care for diabetes from diagnosis within the context of the latest treatment options.

Screening for Diabetes

The American Diabetes Association recommends screening for all persons at risk for the disease. Since the incidence of diabetes increases with age, all those over the age of 45 should be screened every three years. If specific risk factors for diabetes exist, screening should be done annually. Table 6–1 lists major risk factors for diabetes mellitus. Screening should consist of a fasting blood glucose. In 1997, in an effort to enhance early detection, the American Diabetes Association lowered the criteria for diagnosis to a fasting blood glucose of 126 mg/dl. If the blood glucose falls within the equivocal range of 115–126, this is considered "impaired glucose tolerance" and carries a higher risk of

Table 6–1   Major Risk Factors
for Diabetes Mellitus

Family history of diabetes (i.e., parents or siblings
with diabetes)

Obesity (i.e., ≥20% over desired body weight or BMI
≥27 kg/m²)

Race/ethnicity (e.g., African American, Hispanic
American, Native American, Asian American,
Pacific Islander)

Age ≥45 years

Previously identified IFG or IGT

Hypertension (≥140/80 mmHg)

HDL cholesterol level ≤35 mg/dl (0.90 mmol/l)
and/or a triglyceride level ≥250 mg/dl (2.82 mmol/l)

History of GDM or delivery of babies over 9 lb

Source: *Clinical Practice Recommendations. Diabetes Care
Supplement 1*. Alexandria, Va: American Diabetes
Association, 2001.

increases, it is realistic to consider that a new diagnosis of type 2 diabetes in a 60-year-old means sufficient time exists to develop the complications of diabetes related to blood glucose levels.[5]

Treatment of diabetes must be considered in light of patient characteristics at the time of diagnosis. If symptoms of diabetes (polyuria, polydipsia, polyphagia) and a very high blood glucose are present, insulin injections may be necessary. When hyperglycemia has subsided, a trial of oral antidiabetic medications can be attempted. Patients with type 1 diabetes always must be treated with insulin injections for life, but type 2 diabetes can be treated with insulin intermittently and oral agents. It is unlikely that anyone over the age of 50 will present with new type 1 diabetes. If necessary, a blood test called a c-peptide determines the amount of endogenous insulin being produced, thus differentiating between type 1 and symptomatic type 2 diabetes. Type 1 diabetes has minimal or absent insulin production and very low c-peptide. Type 2

developing diabetes in the future. Efforts should be directed at delaying or preventing the onset of type 2 diabetes, such as instituting a program of weight loss and exercise. Table 6–2 lists the diagnostic criteria for the diagnosis of diabetes.[4]

 Treatment

Treatment goals for the patient with diabetes are to decrease/obliterate symptoms, and to maintain as normal a blood glucose as possible without inducing hypoglycemia. This is necessary to decrease the risk of long-term complications from diabetes, which are retinopathy, nephropathy, neuropathy, and macrovascular disease. Avoidance of acute complications such as hypoglycemia/hyperglycemia is also very important.

Consensus does not exist regarding target glucose levels in the older adult. Therefore, the goals should be individualized to reduce the risk of hypoglycemia while considering the long-term effects of elevated glucose level. The life expectancy of a 65-year-old female/male is 19/15 years respectively. At age 75, it is 12/9 years. Therefore, as life span

Table 6–2   Criteria for the Diagnosis
of Diabetes Mellitus

Normoglycemia	IFG or IGT	DM*
FPG <110 mg/dl 2-h PG[†] <200 mg/dl	FPG ≥110 and <126 mg/dl (IFG) 2-h PG[†] ≥140 and <200 mg/dl (IGT)	FPG ≥126 mg/dl 2-h PG[†] ≥200 mg/dl Symptoms of DM and random plasma glucose concentration ≥200 mg/dl

*A diagnosis of diabetes must be confirmed, on a subsequent day, by measurement of FPG, 2-h PG or random plasma glucose (if symptoms are present). The FPG test is greatly preferred because of ease of administration, convenience, acceptability to patients, and lower cost. Fasting is defined as no caloric intake for at least 8 h.
†This test requires the use of a glucose load containing the equivalent of 75 g anhydrous glucose dissolved in water. DM, diabetes mellitus; 2-h PG, postload glucose.
Source: *Clinical Practice Recommendations. Diabetes Care Supplement 1*. Alexandria, Va: American Diabetes Association, 2001.

diabetes most likely has increased c-peptide signifying hyperinsulinemia, which precedes type 2 diabetes. Regardless of the pharmacologic treatment for diabetes, lifestyle modifications are an essential part of treatment.[6,7]

Nutrition

Individuals identified as at risk for diabetes and every newly diagnosed person should be referred to a dietitian for assessment of nutritional needs and individualization of meal plans, with appropriate follow-up visits. Once the patient is stabilized, a nutritional consult should be done every six months to a year. If the patient is experiencing fluctuations in blood glucose, visits should occur more often. Since older adults usually have type 2 diabetes, they have impaired release of insulin and increased insulin resistance. Thus, even a modest weight loss (10–20 pounds) regardless of starting weight can improve glycemic control, decrease lipids, and lower blood pressure.

Several goals for nutrition therapy in diabetes are important. The first is to maintain blood glucose values as close to normal as possible. Ideally, the blood glucose goals are 80–120 before meals, 100–180 after meals, and 100–180 at bedtime. These may need modification in light of complications such as neuropathy and other medical conditions, which may require the avoidance of hypoglycemia.

The second nutritional goal is to achieve and maintain a reasonable weight. Most older adults with type 2 diabetes have impaired insulin secretion and obesity related to insulin resistance. It is important also to achieve and maintain normal cholesterol and triglycerides, as diabetes is a risk factor for heart disease.

The third goal is to emphasize healthy eating habits matched to a treatment and dietary plan for optimal control, without feeling that the diet is too restrictive. Patients on insulin or other medications with hypoglycemia as a side effect, must eat regularly scheduled meals and should not skip meals.[8] The food guide pyramid is the most useful tool in describing the amounts and kind of foods to eat (Figure 6–4).

Carbohydrate Counting

Carbohydrate counting is a method of meal planning that promotes evenly spaced carbohydrate sources throughout the day. The practice of carbohydrate counting often improves meal compliance due to increased decision making and meal flexibility. This empowerment often results in improved metabolic control. The principle of carbohydrate counting is based on two tenets. First, carbohydrate is the main factor affecting postprandial blood glucose and insulin requirements. Second, all carbohydrates convert to glucose within the first two hours after eating. The recommendation to avoid sugar or simple carbohydrate sources in favor of starches and complex carbohydrates is outdated. All carbohydrates increase blood glucose and therefore insulin requirements. Additionally, it is important to follow a low-fat, moderate protein diet if kidney function is normal.

Total carbohydrate requirements for the day depend on gender, level of activity and work, and participation in physical exercise. An active male requires more carbohydrates than a sedentary female. Generally, women require between fourteen and eighteen servings of carbohydrate per day and men require eighteen to twenty-two servings. Level of activity and participation in regular exercise will increase requirements. It is important to know portion sizes of carbohydrate-containing foods. One carbohydrate serving equals 12–15 g of carbohydrate. This equals one serving of bread/starch, one serving of fruit, or one serving of milk. Figure 6–5 shows a sample meal pattern for a day for various caloric levels. Ideally patients should be referred to a dietitian for a customized meal plan. If that is not possible, or until that can happen, a sample meal plan such as in Figure 6–5 can be used.

Careful record keeping aids the dietitian, physician, nurse practitioner, and the patient with designing and implementing an appropriate treatment plan. Care must be taken to record quantity and timing of meals, medication, physical activity, and blood glucose. Label reading, incorporating combination foods, and identifying glycemic patterns associated with particular foods or meals aid in improving glucose control.

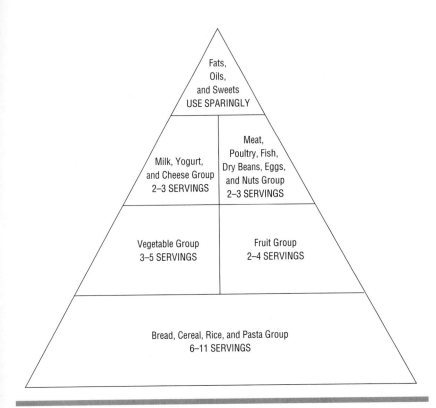

Figure 6–4
The food guide pyramid is the most useful tool in establishing healthy eating habits.

Choose foods to fit type 2 diabetes meal plan:

- Find total daily calorie level on the chart to the right.

- Using the chart, plan menus for the day with serving amounts from each food group.

- Give meals variety by choosing other items from the same food groups.

Calorie Meal Plans (Daily)	1,200	1,500	1,800	2,000	2,500
Starch (servings)	5	7	8	9	11
Fruit (servings)	3	3	4	4	6
Milk (servings)	2	2	3	3	3
Vegetables (servings)	2	2	3	4	5
Meat & meat subtitues (servings)	4	4	6	6	8
Fat (servings)	3	4	4	5	6

Figure 6–5
Meal planning can be achieved with this sample meal plan for various caloric levels.

Exercise

Many health problems associated with diabetes may be improved with exercise, including coronary artery disease, hypertension, hypertriglyceridemia, low HDL cholesterol, hypercholesterolemia, hyperinsulinemia, renal disorders, and obesity and its related co-morbidities. While stress testing for high-risk individuals is recommended for those initiating an aggressive exercise program, almost any individual can begin a walking program or other mild-intensity program with the recommendation of a primary health-care provider.

The benefits of participation in a mild exercise program for the person with type 1 or type 2 diabetes far outweigh the risk of atherosclerosis and heart disease. Hypertension and elevated blood lipid profiles are better controlled with exercise. Regular exercise aids in weight loss and weight maintenance. It can improve quality of life, enhance sleep patterns, modify stress and reduce the depression often associated with chronic disease. Exercise increases lean body mass. Exercisers demonstrate increased insulin sensitivity by virtue of increased insulin efficiency and glucose uptake by the cells. Regular exercise decreases hepatic glucose production and may delay or prevent the onset of type 2 diabetes.

While the benefits of exercise are unquestionable, risk factors differ for type 1 and type 2 diabetes. Patients with type 1 diabetes are much more prone to hypoglycemia during and after a session of exercise, even up to 24 hours after the exercise. Frequent blood glucose monitoring is the best line of defense. Monitoring after appropriate eating; before, during, and after exercising; and throughout the following 24 hours can prevent hypoglycemia. Individuals should be instructed to adjust the therapeutic regimen to allow for safe participation in physical activity and sports.

The American Diabetes Association has set guidelines for participation in safe, exercise. Table 6–3 summarizes these recommendations. Medical clearance is important. A careful history and physical exam should focus on the symptoms and signs of disease affecting the heart and blood vessels, eyes, kidneys, and nervous system. Examination should include careful screening for the presence

Table 6-3   Summary of Exercise Recommendations for Patients With Diabetes

Screening

   Search for vascular and neurological complications, including silent ischemia

   Exercise ECG in patients with known or suspected CAD, >30 years of age with IDDM, with IDDM for >15 years, or >35 years of age with NIDDM

Exercise program

   Type: Aerobic

   Frequency: 3–5 times/week

   Duration: 20–60 min

   Intensity: 50–74% of maximal aerobic capacity

   Energy expenditure: Modulate type, frequency, duration, and intensity to attain an energy expenditure of 700–2,000 calories/week

   Timing: Time participation so that it does not coincide with peak insulin absorption

Avoid complications

   Warm up and cool down

   Careful selection of exercise type and intensity

   Patient education

   Proper footwear

   Avoid exercise in extreme heat or cold

   Inspect feet daily and after exercise

   Avoid exercise when metabolic control is poor

   Maintain adequate hydration

   Monitor blood glucose if taking insulin or oral hypoglycemic agents, and follow guidelines to prevent hypoglycemia

Compliance

   Make exercise enjoyable

   Convenient location

   Positive feedback from involved medical personnel and family

Adapted in part from the American Diabetes Association.

of macrovascular and microvascular complications such as retinopathy, nephropathy, and microalbuminuria, which may be worsened by exercise.

Cardiovascular system evaluation, such as a stress test, should be conducted if a moderate intensity program is to be initiated, if the patient is older than 35 years, if type 2 diabetes has been diagnosed for 10 years, or if type 1 diabetes has been diagnosed for 15 years, if CAD risk factors are present, or if microvascular, peripheral vascular disease or autonomic neuropathy is present.

Evaluation for peripheral arterial disease should be conducted to detect intermittent claudication, cold feet, decreased or absent pulses, and atrophy of subcutaneous tissue. Smoking cessation and participation in a supervised exercise program form the basis of treatment.

Retinopathy screening should be conducted to identify risk of worsening vitreous hemorrhage or retinal detachment. Nephropathy results in a reduced capacity for exercise, which is self-limiting. Peripheral neuropathy limits sensitivity in feet and hands, which can lead to injury, ulceration, and blisters. Consideration of non–weight-bearing activities, such as swimming, bicycling, rowing, and chair exercises, is prudent when peripheral neuropathy is present.

Autonomic neuropathy may limit an individual's capacity to exercise and increase the risk of adverse cardiovascular events due to reduced ability to regulate blood pressure and thermoregulation.

Exercise does not have to be of high intensity to be beneficial in the diabetic population. Approximately 50% of (VO2max) for fifteen to sixty minutes, three to five times a week is sufficient. Exercise should be aerobic and incorporate resistance training. Since glycemic benefits are transient, lasting 24 to 48 hours, exercising every day or every other day is best. Intensity at 50% maximal aerobic activity is enough to decrease glycogen stores within muscle cells, allowing for increased non–insulin-dependent glucose uptake and storage.

Other considerations for patient instruction is the need for comfortable athletic shoes and cotton-polyester socks to keep feet dry and blister free. The insides of shoes should be inspected prior to putting them on, and socks should be examined after exercise for stains and drainage, signs of blisters or sores. The patient should wear some form of identification noting diabetes, and if possible, should exercise with a friend who knows how to recognize and treat hypoglycemia. Blood glucose should be checked before and after exercise and 15 g of carbohydrate should be ingested if the blood glucose is 100 mg/dl or below. Carbo-

hydrate should be carried at all times to treat hypoglycemia if necessary.[9]

Pharmacologic Treatment

Many options now exist for the pharmacologic treatment of diabetes. Selection of a medication depends on patient needs and presentation. Considerations of clinical response and patient safety are important. With more options available, combination therapy is taken into account and different mechanisms of action are becoming the norm. Drug combinations can have a synergistic effect without requiring maximal dosing, thus minimizing side effects. Figure 6–6 outlines the decision tree for initiating oral medication; Table 6–4 lists the drugs available, maximal effective doses, and side effects. The following is a brief discussion of the medications that are currently available.

Sulfonylurea

The oldest of the anti-diabetic drugs, these drugs stimulate the release of insulin from the pancreas. The resulting lowering in blood glucose is desired, but also requires that the patient eat consistent meals on time and on a regular basis. If this is not done, hypoglycemia may result. Sulfonylureas may not be the first choice for older adults, who may eat irregularly and should not be put at risk for a hypoglycemic episode, but are very useful if the patient is symptomatic and needs fast blood glucose lowering. Discussion of prevention, recognition, and treatment of hypoglycemia is essential for any patient placed on a sulfonylurea. Examples are Amaryl (glimepiride), Glucotrol (glipizide), and Micronase (glyburide).

Repaglinide (Prandin)

This class of drugs works by stimulating the release of insulin but is very fast acting and of short duration. For this reason, hypoglycemia is not as high a risk and postprandial hyperglycemia is reduced. Patients need to be instructed to take the medication before each meal and, conversely, not to take the medication if not eating. Patients must carry the medication with them to take before meals.

Match Patient Characteristics to Drug Characteristics

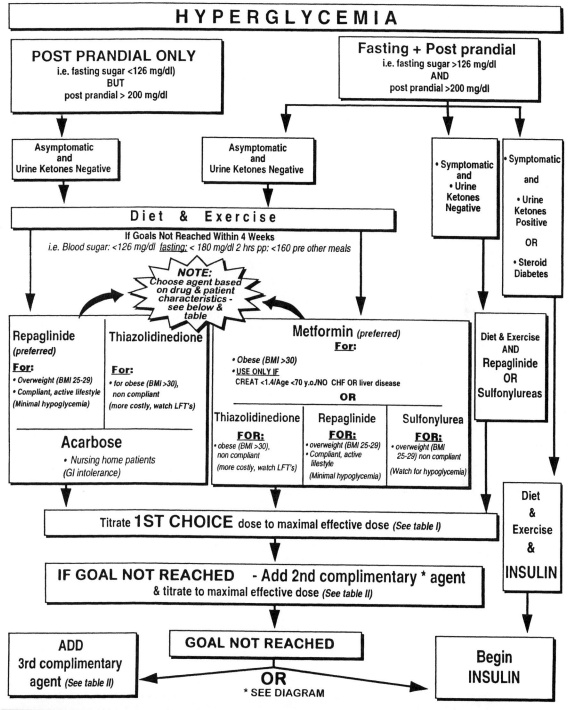

HYPERGLYCEMIA

POST PRANDIAL ONLY
i.e. fasting sugar <126 mg/dl)
BUT
post prandial > 200 mg/dl

Fasting + Post prandial
i.e. fasting sugar >126 mg/dl
AND
post prandial >200 mg/dl

Asymptomatic
and
Urine Ketones Negative

Asymptomatic
and
Urine Ketones Negative

• Symptomatic
and
• Urine
Ketones
Negative

• Symptomatic
and
• Urine Ketones
Positive
OR
• Steroid
Diabetes

Diet & Exercise
If Goals Not Reached Within 4 Weeks
i.e. Blood sugar: <126 mg/dl _fasting_: < 180 mg/dl 2 hrs pp: <160 pre other meals

NOTE: Choose agent based on drug & patient characteristics - see below & table

Repaglinide (preferred)
For:
• Overweight (BMI 25-29)
• Compliant, active lifestyle (Minimal hypoglycemia)

Thiazolidinedione
For:
• for obese (BMI >30), non compliant (more costly, watch LFT's)

Acarbose
• Nursing home patients (GI intolerance)

Metformin (preferred)
For:
• Obese (BMI >30)
• USE ONLY IF CREAT <1.4/Age <70 y.o./NO CHF OR liver disease
OR

Thiazolidinedione
FOR:
• obese (BMI >30), non compliant (more costly, watch LFT's)

Repaglinide
FOR:
• overweight (BMI 25-29)
• Compliant, active lifestyle (Minimal hypoglycemia)

Sulfonylurea
FOR:
• overweight (BMI 25-29) non compliant (Watch for hypoglycemia)

Diet & Exercise
AND
Repaglinide
OR
Sulfonylureas

Titrate **1ST CHOICE** dose to maximal effective dose (See table I)

IF GOAL NOT REACHED - Add 2nd complimentary * agent
& titrate to maximal effective dose (See table II)

Diet & Exercise & INSULIN

ADD 3rd complimentary agent (See table II)

GOAL NOT REACHED
OR
* SEE DIAGRAM

Begin INSULIN

Figure 6–6

Type 2 diabetes mellitus treatment guide.

Source: Schwartz S, Horowitz D. Diabetes Disease Management Program, University of Pennsylvania Health System, 2000. Retrieved from the UPHS intranet: http://uphsnet.med.upenn.edu/dm/diabetes.

Table 6-4 Drug Choices Based on Drug & Patient Characteristics

	Sulfonylurea	Repaglinide	Metformin	TZD	Acarbose
Dosing Frequency	Glimepramide-daily (qd) Glipizide/Glyburide-BID	3x daily with meals	2–3x daily	1x daily	3x daily with meals
Timing of Maximal Effect	Days	Days	Weeks	Months	Months
Efficacy:					
Postprandial	xx	xxx	xx	xx	xxx
FBS	xxx	xx	xxx	xx	x
HgA1	xxx	xxx	xxx	xx	x
Concern/ side effects	hypoglycemia/ wt gain	hypoglycemia/ wt gain	GI upset, lactic acidosis: avoid in patients with CHF, liver disease, acute illness, other acidosis, Cr > 1.4, hospitalized patients and hold 2 days after IV contrast until Creatinine stable	liver toxicity, ? long-term safety	GI side effects Treat hypo with glucose
Hypoglycemic risk when used alone	+	+	None	None	None
Monitor for	hypoglycemia	hypoglycemia	Creatinine & creatinine clearance	LFTs	LFTs
Weight	↑	↑	↓ OR NC	↑ OR NC	NC
Lipids:					
HDL	NC	NC	NC	↑ OR NC	NC
LDL	NC	NC	↓↓	↑↑ (LARGE LDL only)	NC
TG	↓ OR NC	↓ OR NC	↓↓	↓↓	NC
Insulin levels	↑ (less with glim.)	↑	↓	↓	NC
Elderly	Watch for hypoglycemia	Watch for hypoglycemia	AVOID if > 70 years (because ↓ creatinine clearance)	No special risks	No special risks (GI side effects may be beneficial)
Preg risk in pts with polycystic ovary syndrome			+	+	

Other Drug Information					
Primary failure rate	20%	20%	20%	30%	No data
Cost	Xgeneric, XXbrand	XX	XX	XXXX	XX
? ↓ Long-term complications			↓ Age products in vitro	Vit. E attached; ↓ oxidized LDL	

Metformin (Glucophage)

This medication inhibits glucose production by the liver and decreases insulin resistance. Hypoglycemia is not a side effect and metformin contributes to weight loss and lowering of lipid levels which may be a desired effect. Doses should be low initially and titrated over a period of weeks to minimize gastrointestinal side effects (diarrhea). The most serious side effect of metformin, which is rare, is lactic acidosis. For this reason, the drug should not be used in patients with a serum creatinine of 1.4 or greater, who use alcohol, or who are over 70 years of age. The drug should be discontinued 48 hours before or after any contrast dye study. Serum creatinine should be checked before restarting the drug. Because metformin's action takes place primarily in the liver, alcohol consumption should be avoided.

Several new forms of metformin are now available. Glucophage XR is an extended release form of metformin which can be given once a day and have an extended effect. The gastrointestinal side effects are said to be minimized in this form and compliance may be improved with a once-a-day dose. A combination form of metformin and glyburide, Glucovance, is also now available.

Alphaglucosidase Inhibitors (Acarbose, Miglitol)

This category of drugs acts by inhibiting the enzymatic breakdown of carbohydrates in the small intestine. The result is the metabolism of carbohydrates lower in the intestine, allowing slower release into the bloodstream and blunting the rise in glucose postprandially. While this drug is nonsystemic and safe, the side effect of increased flatulence may be unacceptable to patients. For this reason, it is recommended to "start low and go slow," titrating the drug carefully, until a tolerance has been achieved.

Thiazolidendiones (TZDs) pioglitizone (Actos), rosiglitizone (Avandia)

This class of drugs changes the cellular receptor sites to insulin and thereby decreases insulin resistance. These drugs are useful as an adjunct to sulfonylureas, metformin, and insulin and enhance their effects. It may take weeks to months for a response to be seen and sufficient time should be given. Idiopathic liver toxicity is a risk with this class of drugs; therefore, liver function studies must be evaluated prior to therapy, every one to two months the first year, and periodically thereafter. If the patient has abnormal liver function, uses alcohol, or has any other hepatic impairment or risk, these drugs should not be used. If, after the patient has been on the drug, the liver function studies are elevated to three times the normal limit, or if the patient exhibits signs of liver toxicity such as nausea, vomiting, and jaundice, the drug should be discontinued immediately and the patient monitored until the liver function studies return to normal.

Nateglinide (Starlix)

This new drug stimulates the release of insulin from the pancreas in response to blood glucose. The extent of insulin release is glucose dependent and diminishes at low glucose levels, decreasing the risk of hypoglycemia. This drug has a quick onset and peak (one hour) and short duration (six hours). It is taken before meals.

Insulin

Many patients with diabetes are adequately managed with oral medication for many years but may experience a decrease in effect over time. This occurs in about 20% of cases as beta cell function becomes depleted. Since insulin may conjure up fears of injections, many patients need reassurance. Often, when the patient realizes how much better they feel, fear and anxiety are allayed. Assessment of manual dexterity and vision are key to successful implementation of insulin administration. New devices such as pens, syringe magnifiers, and injectors can be very helpful.

Table 6–5 compares the types of insulin. Most patients with type 2 diabetes are started on one injection of long-acting insulin and doses are titrated up from that point. It may be appropriate to take small doses (2–8 units) of long-acting insulin at bedtime with a continuation of oral medications in the daytime. In other cases, oral medications are discontinued and insulin is the sole

Table 6–5   Comparison of Insulins

Type	Source	Color	Approximate Length of Action (Hours)		
			Onset	Peak	End
Rapid-acting					
Lispro	Human	Clear	5 minutes	1	2–4
Short-acting					
Regular	Human, pork	Clear	½–1	2–5	6–16
Intermediate-acting					
NPH	Human, pork	Milky-white when mixed	1–1½	4–12	24+
Lente	Human, pork	Milky-white when mixed	1–2½	6–15	22+
Long-acting					
Ultralente	Human, pork	Milky-white when mixed	4–6	8–30	36+
Mixtures					
NPH 70: R 30	Human	Milky-white when mixed	½	2–12	24
NPH 50: R 50	Human	Milky-white when mixed	½	1–6	14+

Source: Funnell M, Arnold M, Barr P. *Life with Diabetes.* Alexandria, Va: American Diabetes Association; 1998.

treatment. Selection of insulin regimens are based on the patient's eating schedule (Figure 6–7). Insulins that "peak" at the meal times are the most effective. Pre-mixed insulins can often be used in the older population, since older adults may have difficulty mixing two insulins in a syringe. All insulin instruction must be accompanied by additional information on the cause, prevention, and treatment of hypoglycemia.

Monitoring

Blood glucose monitoring is very useful for the evaluation of dietary changes and medication. Goals for blood glucose should be mutually agreed upon, taking into account the medication regimen and any comorbidities that may alter blood glucose. Goals should be set to offer the most protection from the long-term complications of diabetes but ensure

patient safety and the avoidance of hypoglycemia. The frequency of blood glucose monitoring varies with the type of diabetes and its treatment. Those patients with type 1 diabetes must test more frequently, usually before meals and at bedtime. Occasionally, a 3 AM blood glucose test may be requested to rule out nocturnal hyper- or hypoglycemia. Those who are controlled with diet and exercise may only have to test once a day.

It is important to select the blood glucose meter that is most appropriate to the patient's needs and capabilities. Points to consider are manual dexterity, vision, and eye–hand coordination. The patient must be able to obtain an adequate sample size and do the test properly to ensure accuracy. Keeping results in a log book and bringing the log book to office visits helps to evaluate the response to treatment. Blood glucose monitoring technique should be evaluated on a regular basis to ensure accuracy.

Intermediate-Acting
(2 Doses)

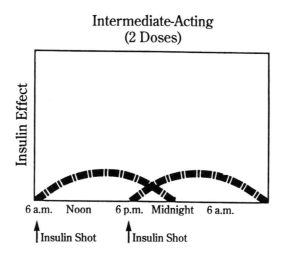

6 a.m.   Noon   6 p.m. Midnight   6 a.m.

↑Insulin Shot   ↑Insulin Shot

Rapid- and Intermediate-Acting

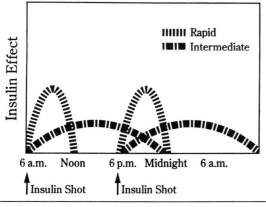

IIIIIII Rapid
I◼I◼ Intermediate

6 a.m.   Noon   6 p.m. Midnight   6 a.m.

↑Insulin Shot   ↑Insulin Shot

Short- and Long-Acting

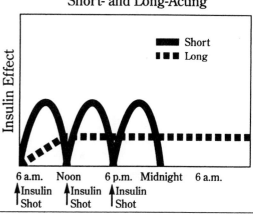

◼◼◼ Short
◼ ◼ ◼ Long

6 a.m.   Noon   6 p.m. Midnight   6 a.m.

↑Insulin   ↑Insulin   ↑Insulin
 Shot   Shot   Shot

Figure 6–7
Insulin programs.
Source: Funnel M, Arnold M, Barr P, *Life with Diabetes,* Alexandria, Va: American Diabetes Association; 1998.

◼ Standards of Care for People with Diabetes

The best care for the patient incorporates a team approach utilizing physicians, nurses, dietitians, pharmacists, physical therapists, podiatrists, and mental health professionals. Other participants also may be required to meet individual needs of the patient.

The goal is to prevent complications using standards of care, based on the DCCT and UKPDS studies, and advanced by the American Diabetes Association. Patients who are medically stable should be seen every three to four months in the office. A laboratory hemoglobin A1C test should be performed every three to four months. This test measures the amount of glycosolated hemoglobin, which reflects the average blood glucose for three months. The goal is 7%. Laboratory blood glucose should be measured each visit pre- or two hours postprandial, if possible.[10] A foot exam, including sensory evaluation, should be done on each visit. Weight and blood pressure should be measured on each visit. The patient should be assessed for hypoglycemic unawareness on each visit; i.e., does the patient know when his/her blood glucose is low and what the symptoms are?

Other laboratory tests should include a urine sample for microalbumin annually, and a lipid profile annually. Urine microalbumin should be less than 30 mg/g. Total cholesterol should be less than 200, HDL 35–45, LDL less than 100 and triglycerides less than 200. An ophthalmology examination should be performed annually, including a dilated eye examination.

It is also important to address additional issues during the course of care. These include smoking cessation and diabetes education with the nurse or dietitian, or in a group, in addition to the usual care of any patient.

Despite the statistics of the incidence of diabetes, there do exist some false beliefs about older adults with diabetes, which can be obstacles to best care practice, as stated in Table 6–6. It is not unusual that in the elderly person, weight loss and anorexia are the presenting features of diabetes.

Other presentations (outside the classic symptoms) may include falls, incontinence, cognitive/behavioral changes, pain intolerance, or even an emergent situation such as hyperglycemic nonketotic syndrome. A description of age-related factors and diseases that can influence diabetes care in the elderly is found in Table 6–7.

Table 6–6   Common Misconceptions About Diabetes in Older Adults

1. The high prevalence of diabetes in older adults is inevitable.
2. Hyperglycemia in the older adult population is usually a benign condition.
3. Reduced life expectancy makes the consequences of chronic hyperglycemia irrelevant.
4. The majority of older adults with type 2 diabetes are obese and need to lose weight.
5. Older patients are less capable of self-monitoring of blood glucose.

Source: Nettles AT. Diabetes in the elderly. In: *A Core Curriculum for Diabetes Education.* 3rd ed. Chicago: American Association of Diabetes Educators; 1998.

Table 6–7   Aging and Disease of the Elderly That Influence Diabetes Care

Ophthalmic
- Decreased acuity
- Slowed light/dark adaptation
- Decreased color perception
- Increased blinding diseases (senile cataracts, macular degeneration)

Cardiovascular
- Conduction defects
- Systolic hypertension
- Decreased cardiac output
- Increased vascular resistance
- Increase in cerebral vascular accidents
- Increase in myocardial infarction
- Peripheral vascular diseases

Gastrointestinal
- Decreased secretion, absorption, motility
- Changes in appetite

Dental
- Tooth loss
- Gum/periodontal disease

Musculoskeletal
- Arthritis, joint diseases
- Decreased muscle mass and strength
- Foot deformities

Neurological
- Slower learning, processing time
- Slower reactions
- Decreased taste, smell, and thirst
- Peripheral and autonomic neuropathies
- Increase in organic brain diseases

Renal
- Decreased glomerular filtration rate (GFR)

Source: Nettles AT. Diabetes in the elderly. In: *A Core Curriculum for Diabetes Education.* 3rd ed. Chicago: American Association of Diabetes Educators; 1998.

The results of the 20-year UKPDS indicate a need for a more vigorous approach to the management of type 2 diabetes. Nevertheless, in this vigorous approach it is also important to realize that the major risk of tight blood glucose control is hypoglycemia. When appropriate, the goals for management include blood pressure below 130/85, and a hemoglobin, HbA_{1c} 7.0 or lower, but avoiding hypoglycemia. Table 6–8 lists the factors that can predispose an older adult with type 2 diabetes to hypoglycemia. In addition to safety issues such as falls and auto accidents, hypoglycemia can cause myocardial infarction and fatal strokes. Therefore, hypoglycemia is of utmost concern. Raising blood glucose goals would be an important consideration in the elderly patient with a history of hypoglycemia.

The health-care professional should assess signs and symptoms on a regular basis as these may change over time. Also, some patients may attribute symptoms of low blood sugar to other reasons such as "normal aging." Some patients may need a snack at bedtime to prevent nighttime hypoglycemia and keep a quick acting source of glu-

Table 6–8   Factors That Predispose Elderly Type 2 Diabetic Patients to Hypoglycemia

- Poor or erratic nutritional intake
- Changes in mental status that impair the perception or response to hypoglycemia
- Increased polypharmacy and noncompliance with medications
- Dependence or isolation that limits receipt of early treatment for hypoglycemia
- Impaired renal or hepatic metabolism
- Presence of comorbid conditions that can mask or lead to misdiagnosis of hypoglycemic symptoms (dementia, delirium, depression, sleep abnormalities, seizures, myocardial infarction, cerebrovascular accident)

Source: Nettles AT. Diabetes in the elderly. In: *A Core Curriculum for Diabetes Education.* 3rd ed. Chicago: American Association of Diabetes Educators; 1998.

Table 6–9   Hyperosmolarity: Predisposing Factors in the Elderly

- Increased renal threshold for glucose
- Replacement of fluid with sweet drinks
- Decreased sense of thirst
- Limited access to fluids
- Drugs, especially diuretic therapy

Source: Nettles AT. Diabetes in the elderly. In: *A Core Curriculum for Diabetes Education.* 3rd ed. Chicago: American Association of Diabetes Educators; 1998.

cose at the bedside. The blood glucose meter is an essential tool for detecting asymptomatic hypoglycemia secondary to autonomic neuropathy. Oral agents that do not cause hypoglycemia should be chosen whenever possible. For patients with a high risk of hypoglycemia, a "check-in" contact with a friend, neighbor, or relative, or use of emergency system devices may be employed. Prevention of hypoglycemia and treatment should be reviewed at every patient visit.

Hyperglycemic Hyperosmolar Nonketotic Syndrome (HHNS) occurs with uncontrolled type 2 diabetes. It is sometimes overlooked or confused with other illnesses, and may sometimes go unrecognized for several weeks in the older patient. The hallmark features include elevated glucose levels, usually over 800 mg/dl, absence of ketones, and profound dehydration—osmolality greater than 350 mOsm/kg. The mortality rate is higher than in diabetic ketoacidosis (DKA) because of severe metabolic changes and further compromise in older patients secondary to other medical comorbidities. The list of situations in Table 6–9 can predispose the older adult to HHNS.

It is important to educate the patient and family about the risks of HHNS. This includes providing sick-day management guidelines, especially regarding fluid intake. For those in hospitals or nursing homes, make fluids accessible and reinforce the importance of getting prompt attention for mental status changes.

Physical Assessment

Physical assessment of the older adult with diabetes should be conducted as with any adult, with emphasis on the assessment, monitoring, and prevention of the long-term complications. Routine visits should occur every three months, unless treatment is being changed and a new monitoring plan is in place.

Weight should be obtained on each visit, as changes in either direction can be a concern. Weight gain worsens diabetes control and increases insulin resistance. Inappropriate weight loss generally means inadequate nutrition or poor diabetes control. Principles of nutrition stated in this chapter should be reinforced at each visit. A 24-hour diary of dietary intake is helpful.

Blood pressure should be measured on each visit. Many people with diabetes have hypertension, which is also associated with micro- and macrovascular complications. In addition, it is necessary to take orthostatic blood pressure measurements annually to rule out the presence of orthostatic hypotension, a sign of autonomic neuropathy. Orthostatic hypotension is also present if the patient is dehydrated, perhaps due to hyperosmolar syndrome or ketoacidosis.

Physical examination of the heart includes rate, rhythm, and extra heart sounds. A routine electrocardiogram (ECG) should be performed annually, to detect silent myocardial infarction or other abnormalities. Stress testing should be performed on persons over the age of 35 who have had diabetes for more than 10 years.

The thyroid should be palpated as thyroid abnormalities are common with diabetes.

The skin should be assessed for any breakdown or changes from normal, particularly in the extremities. Skin discolorations, called necrobiosis, can appear in diabetes, especially on the shin areas of the legs. Common disorders of the hands include carpal tunnel syndrome and Dupuytren's contracture.

Examine the extremities for edema. Pulses should be elicited and sensory evaluation should be done. Testing sensory response with a 10 g filament determines whether the patient has protective sensation. If protective sensation is lost, aggressive foot care instructions and routine visits to a podiatrist are warranted. Careful examination of the feet, especially between the toes, can result in the early detection and treatment of infections.

Monitoring for Complications

Prevention, early detection, and prompt treatment of chronic complications are important to slow progression of the diabetes. While hyperglycemia plays a part in all complications, other risk factors are associated with specific categories of complications. Most importantly, each individual has a personal profile of risk factors and history.

Various conditions add to the development of complications including insulin resistance, tissue ischemia, coagulation defects, autoimmunity, glycosolation of cellular proteins, accumulation of intracellular sorbitol from the conversion of glucose to sorbitol, and genetic predisposition.

The older adult with diabetes has a greater incidence and accelerated development of complications. It is unfortunate that certain complications, such as retinal changes and lower extremity involvement, are often already present upon initial diagnosis.[11] The following areas are of particular concern to the older patient with type 2 diabetes.

Lower Extremity Amputation

Lower extremity amputation is 15 times more common among people with diabetes, especially those who are over 40 years old with diabetes for over 10 years. Fifty percent of these amputations were probably preventable with earlier identification and treatment of the disease. Many patients with one amputation lose the second limb within a few years, often related to the increased weight bearing on the remaining limb, as well as the ongoing progression of the disease.

The pathophysiology leading to amputation involves a series of events involving the loss of protective sensation, along with foot deformity, from sensorimotor neuropathy, coupled with macrovascular diseases leaving poor blood flow to the affected limb secondary to peripheral vascular insufficiency. This places the limb at great risk for bone and tissue infection and amputation. Foot trauma, such as poorly fitting shoes, burns, cuts, and pressure ulcers, along with ischemia and neuropathy, often precede amputation.[12] To protect and ultimately save limbs, it is extremely important to identify the foot at risk, prevent foot ulcers, treat ulcers aggressively, and prevent recurrences.

To elicit relevant information from patients regarding knowledge of foot care and personal foot care practices, the following questions have been found to be useful:[13]

1. How do you care for your toenails?
2. Do you soak your feet?
3. Do you ever walk barefoot, or only in your socks?
4. What kind of shoes do you wear?
5. Do you smoke, or have you ever smoked?

The Lower Extremity Amputation Prevention Program (LEAP) of Health Resources and Services Administration (HRSA) offers a free filament to enable testing the feet for possible nerve damage. Call National Clearinghouse for Primary Care Information at 1-800-400-2742 or visit online at *www.bphc.hrsa.gov/leap* and click on "Free Filament."

The Medicare Shoe Bill provides coverage to diabetic recipients of Medicare for 80% of the cost for extra-depth shoes and three pairs of orthotics per year.[14]

Adapting personal foot care guidelines for older adults may need to include the training of another person in daily foot care procedures. Limitations, such as decreased joint mobility, decreased dexterity, and impaired visual acuity often impede adequate self-care related to the feet.

Hypertension

People with diabetes are twice as likely to have hypertension than those without the disease. In addition, they are two to four times more likely to suffer a stroke or a myocardial infarction. Hypertension also contributes to renal failure. The diagnosis and treatment of hypertension is addressed in more detail in Chapter 3. Suffice it to say that when medication is considered for hypertension in diabetes, the first line drugs of choice are ACE inhibitors, as they also provide protection against microalbuminuria.[1]

Myocardial Infarction and Stroke

Both myocardial infarction and cerebrovascular incidents are more frequent occurrences in the older adult with diabetes. Prevention of stroke revolves around glucose control, control of hypertension and lipids, and treatment for atrial fibrillation. ECGs should be done routinely, along with monitoring for possible congestive heart failure, to ensure timely detection and treatment of cardiac disease.[15]

Vision Loss

Diabetic retinopathy is a profound microvascular complication of both type 1 and type 2 diabetes. After a 20-year diabetes history, almost all people with type 1 and more than 60% of people with type 2 diabetes have some retinopathy. Unfortunately, as high as 20% of type 2 patients already have eye changes upon diagnosis.

Compounding this problem is the fact that many older adults have other eye conditions secondary to the aging process, such as cataracts and glaucoma. The DCCT and the UKPDS studies have shown that glucose control is imperative in slowing the progression of retinopathy. The presence of hypertension, hyperlipidemia, smoking, and age and genetic factors also contribute to the risk.

Diabetic retinopathy is a condition whereby small vessels that supply the retina are damaged. Retinopathy is catagorized as nonproliferative (ranging from mild to very severe) and proliferative. Nonproliferative diabetic retinopathy (NPDR) occurs prior to the development of new vessel formation in the retina, a characteristic of proliferative retinopathy. This condition usually has no symptoms. Changes that may be seen during a dilated pupil exam include microaneurysms, hard exudates, intraretinal hemorrhages, cotton wool spots, venous beading, and intraretinal microvascular abnormalities. If new vessels form, the condition worsens to proliferative diabetic retinopathy (PDR). Those with the most severe form of NPDR have a 45% chance of developing PDR within one year. Even at this point, a patient may not have any notable visual impairment. PDR probably results from a limited blood supply to the retina, resulting in hypoxia. Neovascularization (NVE) involves new vessel growth on the retinal surface. Vessels, which are weak and prone to rupture, may also grow into the vitreous chamber. This is of added concern with hypertension. New vessel growth can also involve the optic disc; this is called neovascularization of the disc (NVD). If more than 25% of the disc is involved, risk is high for large vision loss.[11]

Other ophthalmic concerns include retinal tears and retinal detachment.

Macular edema is of great concern as it is the area of the eye that allows central vision. It results from leakage of fluids and exudate from the macular vessels. The extent of vision loss can be from mild blurriness to legally blind (20/200). Macular edema can occur with nonproliferative and proliferative conditions. Treatment recommendations include achieving optimal glucose control, blood pressure control, and smoking cessation. Close follow-up with an ophthalmologist is warranted.

Prevention includes an initial eye exam with dilated pupils upon diagnosis for type 2 patients, followed by annual eye exams. Fundus photography and flourescein angiography may be performed at these visits. Patients with type 1 diabetes need an eye exam after five years of diagnosis, then annually.

Evaluation of visual loss, along with the patient's ability to adapt to these changes, requires ongoing monitoring. Adaptive education includes referral to appropriate rehabilitation and psychosocial services, for example, the American Foundation for the Blind (1-800-AFBLIND). Various devices and techniques include low-vision services, special lenses, visual aids for insulin injections, and audio blood glucose meters. It is important to assess safety issues, availability of extended family for assistance, and evaluation of patient and family ability to perform activities of daily living, such as foot care and exercise programs.

Patients with active diabetic retinopathy should avoid heavy lifting, bending the head lower than the waist, Valsalva-type maneuvers related to increasing blood pressure, and rapid head movements.

Nephropathy

Albuminuria, hypertension, and progressive renal insufficiency are the clinical hallmarks of diabetic nephropathy. Recent studies demonstrate, however, that early intervention can significantly alter the progression of nephropathy.

Diabetic nephropathy develops from hyperglycemia, hormonal imbalances, and renal hemodynamic changes. Risk factors are multiple and include hypertension, smoking, poor blood glucose control, genetic predisposition, increased protein intake, duration of diabetes, age at diagnosis, and male gender.[16]

At the University of Pennsylvania Diabetes Disease Management Program, a protocol was developed and is now in place for screening and treatment of diabetic nephropathy (Figure 6–8).

Patient education related to nephropathy should include:

1. Awareness of annual screening for microalbumin
2. Avoidance of nephrotoxic contrast media/drugs
3. Prevention of, and signs and symptoms for, urinary tract infection; discussion about prompt treatment to avoid insult to the kidney
4. Low protein diet when necessary
5. Importance of glucose control
6. Control of hypertension, with emphasis on compliance with medication regimen
7. Smoking cessation (if indicated)
8. Sodium restrictions as indicated
9. Exploration of other treatment options, should they be indicated, as with end-stage renal disease (ESRD). These include hemodialysis, peritoneal dialysis, transplant, or no treatment (with result of death usually within seven months)

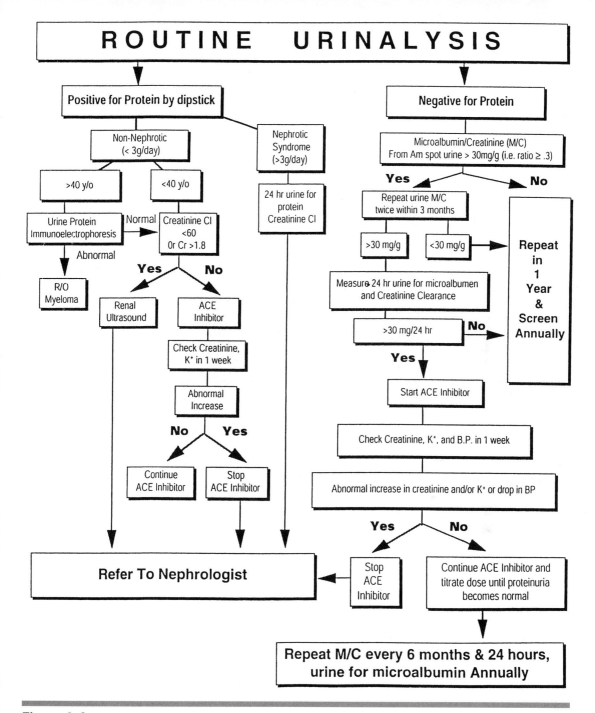

ROUTINE URINALYSIS

Positive for Protein by dipstick

- Non-Nephrotic (< 3g/day)
  - >40 y/o
    - Urine Protein Immunoelectrophoresis
      - Normal → Creatinine Cl <60 Or Cr >1.8
      - Abnormal → R/O Myeloma
  - <40 y/o → Creatinine Cl <60 Or Cr >1.8
    - **Yes** → Renal Ultrasound
    - **No** → ACE Inhibitor
      - Check Creatinine, K+ in 1 week
        - Abnormal Increase
          - **No** → Continue ACE Inhibitor
          - **Yes** → Stop ACE Inhibitor

- Nephrotic Syndrome (>3g/day)
  - 24 hr urine for protein Creatinine Cl

Negative for Protein

- Microalbumin/Creatinine (M/C) From Am spot urine > 30mg/g (i.e. ratio ≥ .3)
  - **Yes** → Repeat urine M/C twice within 3 months
    - >30 mg/g → Measure 24 hr urine for microalbumen and Creatinine Clearance
      - >30 mg/24 hr
        - **No** → Repeat in 1 Year & Screen Annually
        - **Yes** → Start ACE Inhibitor
          - Check Creatinine, K+, and B.P. in 1 week
            - Abnormal increase in creatinine and/or K+ or drop in BP
              - **Yes** → Stop ACE Inhibitor
              - **No** → Continue ACE Inhibitor and titrate dose until proteinuria becomes normal
    - <30 mg/g → Repeat in 1 Year & Screen Annually
  - **No** → Repeat in 1 Year & Screen Annually

Refer To Nephrologist

Repeat M/C every 6 months & 24 hours, urine for microalbumin Annually

---

Figure 6–8

Management of diabetic nephropathy. Complete management also requires tight control of blood sugar and blood pressure & absence of smoking.

Source: Schwartz S, Horowitz D. Diabetes Disease Management Program, University of Pennsylvania Health System, 2000. Retrieved from the UPHS intranet: http://uphsnet.med.upenn.edu/dm/diabetes.

Oral Care

Gum disease, including early inflammation of the gums (gingivitis), sometimes causes elevated blood glucose levels. The infection may go undetected, as it may not be painful or visible. This can extend to peridonitis as the jawbone becomes involved and teeth are lost. This is of special concern in the older adult as it contributes to poor nutritional intake. Those with diabetes are at risk for an accelerated course of gum disease when glucose levels are poorly controlled. Patients should be made aware of symptoms of gingivitis, such as bleeding gums when brushed or flossed; dental pain upon chewing; halitosis or foul taste in mouth; red, swollen, tender gums; pus; or shifting teeth.[17]

For those with dentures or partial plates, a proper fit is very important, along with routine cleaning. With substantial weight loss, dentures may need refitting. Patients should seek dental care every six months, floss, use fluoride toothpaste, use a soft toothbrush, and avoid foods containing concentrated sugars.

Skin Care

The skin is also affected by the metabolic changes accompanying diabetes. Various skin lesions can be present with diabetes; about 30% of people with diabetes have a skin abnormality. Diagnosis may be prompted by an unusual skin change. Appropriate identification of, and treatment for, these conditions are important. Candida infections are likely. When autonomic neuropathy is present, decreased or absent sweat leads to dryness and skin fissures. Diabetic bullae, which are serous blisters, often develop on the toes and soles of the feet. Diabetic dermopathy, which is common in both type 1 and type 2 diabetes, is of unknown etiology.[18]

Principles of good skin care include use of a skin moisturizer with lanolin (except between the toes) and the use of sunscreen with SPF 15. Patients should be made aware that some medications cause increased sensitivity to the sun. Advice regarding adequate hydration and extremity protection, such as gloves and shoes, are important.

Cleansing should include warm, not hot, water and avoidance of skin soaking, friction, and abrasive skin care products. Most importantly, daily self-examination of the skin for changes is critical.

Depression

Depression appears more commonly among people with diabetes and also may be more severe.[19] It often goes unrecognized and therefore untreated. Underdiagnosis is common because symptoms of depression, such as fatigue, can be confused with hyperglycemia. A careful assessment for depression is very useful. Diagnosis and treatment of depression in the older adult are addressed in Chapter 8.

 ## Educational Approaches and the Older Adult

Peyrot and Rubin[20] use the term "patient empowerment" to describe how the health-care professional imparts power to the patient with an appropriate plan of care. Patients have the right to accept or reject the plan and its proposed behavioral changes. This patient-centered view for diabetes treatment supports a strong working partnership between patient and provider(s). In general, patients make changes if they feel the alterations will meet perceived needs. What is acceptable to patients in terms of their unique personal situation and the necessary behavioral changes must be considered. Cultural awareness and the variations within cultures are important.[20]

Another influence on patient ability to manage diabetes is self-efficacy. In other words, does a patient feel confident with regard to what needs to be done? It is important to ask the patient to rate his/her ability (on a scale of 1–10) to manage diabetes on a daily basis. Ask about response to past situations that were perceived to be stressful to determine "coping skills." In general, those who practice positive coping skills have better glucose control. It is important to ascertain beliefs about diabetes. Personal awareness of the disease helps to uncover positive and negative thoughts that affect self care. Helping patients set specific and realistic goals helps improve coping abilities. The patient can identify the one or two changes that are most important and start with these. As reasonable goals are achieved, new ones can be added.

Diabetes does not exist in a vacuum. Patients may have family and friends who are supportive, or sabotaging, regarding self-care choices. The presence of significant others for support generally enables patients to cope with the extra demands imposed by diabetes. Efforts to reach out to other sources of support should be encouraged if needed. These include local chapters of the American Diabetes Association (ADA) and other support groups.

The older adult with diabetes often has other chronic conditions. These actually may be of greater concern to the patient than diabetes and may impede efforts in diabetes self-care management. Principles of adult learning should be applied, and any cognitive and physical challenges considered.[22] The following principles are a guide:

1. Assess what the patient already knows
2. Learn the priorities of the patient
3. Keep the instruction focused to match the patient's goals
4. Encourage rest periods as needed
5. Pace the information provided by observing cues from the patient
6. Provide encouragement and positive feedback
7. Emphasize where control and mastery have been achieved, while being aware of areas that are still difficult for the patient
8. Allow as much time as possible
9. Keep the patient active in the process
10. Review information on a regular basis.[21]

Cognitive and physical limitations must be considered. Table 6–10 provides suggestions for assisting the patient with decreased cognition.

Note cues suggesting hearing impairment such as cupping an ear, leaning closer, looking blank, answering inappropriately (Table 6–11).

Similarly, patients with visual impairment may also show indications of a need for assistance, such as squinting, frowning, withdrawing, and relying on touch (Table 6–12).

Table 6–10   Educational Strategies for Dealing With Decreased Cognition

- Be sensitive to the fact that the patient is encountering new material.
- Address the patient by name and identify yourself.
- Explain your presence.
- Use lay terminology.
- Use signals that aid in memory retrieval (cues) for emphasis, such as verbal analogies, hands-on experience, demonstrations, and models.
- Use short, simple sentences.
- Frequently summarize important points.
- Focus on one topic at a time.
- Sequence the teaching of tasks from simple to complex.
- Supply simple handouts for patients to keep for later use.

Source: Nettles AT. Diabetes in the elderly. In: *A Core Curriculum for Diabetes Education.* 3rd ed. Chicago: American Association of Diabetes Educators; 1998.

Table 6–11   Educational Strategies for Dealing With Hearing Impaired Individuals

- Eliminate visual and auditory distractions.
- Speak toward ear with the best hearing.
- Frequently repeat what you say.
- Write or draw important points.
- Use gestures, objects, and touch whenever possible.
- Enunciate clearly and slowly.
- Use short sentences and do not change topics abruptly.
- Often the hearing impaired use lip reading. To facilite lip reading, be on same level with the patient and try to arrange seating in the room so the lights or windows illuminate your face. Don't cover your mouth or chew gum.
- It is also beneficial to know how to help with a hearing aid.

Source: Nettles AT. Diabetes in the elderly. In: *A Core Curriculum for Diabetes Education.* 3rd ed. Chicago: American Association of Diabetes Educators; 1998.

Table 6–12   Educational Strategies for Dealing With Visually Impaired Individuals

- Try not to move the patient's personal belongings.
- Use bright illumination.
- Allow a longer time to change visual focus.
- Keep the field where you are working narrow.
- Female educators can wear bright lipstick.
- Use more detailed verbal explanations and involve the other senses such as touch.
- Use low-vision aids such as magnifiers.
- When you are using handouts, be sure the paper has no glare or shine. The handouts should have large type, at least 14 point, and be printed in very dark ink on white or pale yellow paper.

For more information, refer to the AADE and the Visually Impaired Persons Specialty Prectice Group, *Recommendations for Producing Education Materials* available on AADE fax, 800-338-3633, documents 9009 and 9070.

Source: Nettles AT. Diabetes in the elderly. In: *A Core Curriculum for Diabetes Education.* 3rd ed. Chicago: American Association of Diabetes Educators; 1998.

Evaluation of patient progress remains ongoing. Have goals been met? What needs to be to learned next? Is there readiness to proceed or need for review? Documentation of outcomes is important. Evidence of patient progress and positive feedback and encouragement maintain motivation and the psychological energy to deal with any chronic condition.[21]

Suggested Patient and Professional Resources

- www.diabetes.org (American Diabetes Association) or 1-800-DIABETES
- www.AADE.org (American Association of Diabetes Educators)
- www.diabetes.com (patient resource)
- Arthritis Foundation Programs (check local listings) provide free video: *PACE* (People with Arthritis Can Exercise)

- Foundation of the American Academy of Ophthalmology: 1-800-222-EYES
- American Foundation of the Blind: 1-800-AFBLIND
- American Printing House for the Blind: 1-800-223-1839
- Diabetes Forecast (patient magazine): 1-800-232-3472
- Diabetes Self Management (patient magazine): 1-800-234-0723

References

1. American Diabetes Association. *Diabetes: The Facts and Figures.* Alexandria, Va: American Diabetes Association; 2000.
2. The DCCT Research Group. The effects of intensive treatment of insulin dependent diabetes on the long-term complications of diabetes. *N Engl J Med.* 1993;329:977–986.
3. American Diabetes Association. Implications of the United Kingdom Prospective Diabetes Study. *Diabetes Care.* 1998;21:2180–2184.
4. American Diabetes Association. Position statement: screening for type 2. *Diabetes Care.* 2000;23(Suppl): 20–23.
5. Van Nostrand JF, Furner SE, eds. Health data on older Americans: national center for health statistics. *Vital Health Stat.* 1998;3:27.
6. American Diabetes Association. *Physician's Guide to Type 1 Diabetes.* Alexandria, Va: American Diabetes Association; 1999.
7. American Diabetes Association. *Physician's Guide to Type 2 Diabetes.* Alexandria, Va; American Diabetes Association; 1999.
8. American Diabetes Association. Nutrition therapy for diabetes. *Diabetes Care.* 2000;23(Suppl):24–26.
9. American Diabetes Association. *The Health Professional's Guide to Diabetes and Exercise.* Alexandria, Va: American Diabetes Association; 1999.
10. Turner RC, Holman RR. Lessons from UK Prospective Diabetes Study. *Diabetes Res Clin Pract.* 1995;28: 151–157.
11. Pfiefer MA. Chronic complications of diabetes: an overview. In: Funnell M, Hunt C, Kulkani K, Rubin R, Yarborough P, eds. *A Core Curriculum for Diabetes Education.* 3rd ed. Chicago: American Association of Diabetes Educators; 1998.
12. Lorber DL. Complications of diabetes: foot problems. *Practical Diabetol.* 1994;13:10–15.
13. Robert SS. Caring for feet. In: *The American Diabetes Association Resource Guide.* Alexandria, Va: American Diabetes Association; 2000:10–12.

14. Helfand A. What you need to know about therapeutic footware. *Practical Diabetol.* 1996;15:4–9.
15. Kiuusisto J, Mykkanen L, Pyorala K, Laakso M. Non-insulin dependent diabetes and its metabolic control are important predictors of stroke in elderly subjects. *Stroke.* 1994;25:1157–1164.
16. American Diabetes Association. Diabetic nephropathy. *Diabetes Care.* 1999;22(Suppl):66–69.
17. American Diabetes Association. Don't gamble with your gums. *Diabetes Adv.* 1999;7:30.
18. Feingold KR, Elias PM. Dermatologic complications: association with diabetes. *Diabetes Spectrum.* 1990;3:282–287.
19. Rubin RR. Psychological disorders. In: Funnell MM, Hunt C, Kulkani K, Rubin R, Yarlborough P, eds. *A Core Curriculum for Diabetes Education.* Chicago: American Association of Diabetes Educators; 1998.
20. Peyrot M, Rubin R. Living with diabetes: the patient-centered perspective. *Diabetes Spectrum.* 1994;7:204–205.
21. Haas LB. Education strategies for geriatric patients. American Association of Diabetes Educators. *Today's Educator*; 2000.
22. Rubin RR. Psychological disorders. In: Funnell MM, Hunt C, Kulkani K, Rubin R, Yarlborough P, eds. *A Core Curriculum for Diabetes Education.* Chicago: American Association of Diabetes Educators; 1998.

CHAPTER 7

Thyroid Disorders

Michelle A. Feil
Valerie T. Cotter

Introduction

Thyroid disorders in older adults often go unrecognized, despite increased prevalence with age. The classical symptoms of thyroid disease, which are pronounced in younger people, typically become blunted and more subtle in older adults. Vague complaints and muted symptoms may be attributed to normal aging or concurrent illness by both the older adult and the clinician. Undetected, and therefore untreated, thyroid disorders lead to potentially serious complications and even death.

Like the rest of the human body, the thyroid gland undergoes certain structural changes with aging. It was once thought that insufficient production of thyroid hormones caused aging, but it is currently assumed that aging brings about changes in the thyroid, thus altering thyroid function. Normally, the thyroid gland increases in nodularity and fibrosis with age; whether thyroid size changes remains controversial. Hormone levels are not significantly altered, and any change in production should be viewed as an abnormal finding.

This chapter provides an overview of thyroid disorders commonly encountered by primary-care nurse practitioners. Special attention is given to the clinical presentation and management strategies specific to older adults. It is critically important to raise the index of suspicion for thyroid disease, and to increase detection and treatment aimed at improved quality of life for older adults with the disease.

Hyperthyroidism

Hyperthyroidism, also referred to as thyrotoxicosis, is a heterogeneous group of disorders characterized by an excess amount of thyroid hormone thyroxine (T4) and/or triiodothyronine (T3). It is more prevalent with advancing age and in women, with the reported prevalence ranging from 0.5–6% in older adults.[1] The clinical diagnosis of thyrotoxicosis is hampered in older adults because of nonspecific and subtle signs and symptoms, or attribution to normal aging.

Typically, hyperthyroidism presents with sweating, palpitations, nervousness, fine tremor, hyperactive reflexes, polydipsia, and increased appetite. Along with some of these signs and symptoms, older adults are more likely to present with tachycardia, fatigue, apathy, anorexia, weight loss, or atrial fibrillation. Older adults tend to present with fewer clinical signs and symptoms than younger adults (Table 7–1)[2].

Screening for Hyperthyroidism

Routine screening of the asymptomatic older adult for hyperthyroidism with thyroid stimulating hor-

Table 7–1 Hyperthyroidism Clinical Presentation

Younger Adults	Older Adults
Classic signs & symptoms:	Nonspecific signs & symptoms:
• Sweating	• Tachycardia
• Palpitations	• Fatigue
• Nervousness	• Apathy
• Fine tremor	• Anorexia
• Hyperactive reflexes	• Weight loss
• Polydipsia	• Atrial fibrillation
• Increased appetite	

mone (TSH) is controversial.[3] Nevertheless, such practice may be important in the differential diagnosis of many acute and chronic conditions and may lead to earlier diagnosis and treatment.

Subclinical hyperthyroidism is defined as a suppressed TSH with normal T4, free T4, free T3, and T3 radioimmune assay (RIA) levels. It occurs in about 3–4% of the population over age 60.[4] Patients generally have few, if any, symptoms. Most older adults do not progress biochemically or clinically toward overt hyperthyroidism.[5] The significance of subclinical hyperthyroidism is unclear, but may possibly carry an associated risk of atrial fibrillation and osteoporosis.[6,7] Although clinical observation and repeated laboratory studies with TSH and thyroid hormone levels appear reasonable, supportive evidence in the literature is limited.

Diagnosis and Evaluation

Because symptoms are usually subtle and may involve many body systems, a thorough review is necessary. Chest pain, dyspnea, palpitations, and edema may indicate cardiac decompensation. Gastrointestinal (GI) symptoms (constipation, diarrhea, appetite changes, or weight loss) and visual changes (photophobia, eye irritation, and diplopia), as well as inquiry about sleep disturbances, sweating or heat intolerance, anterior neck pain, or history of goiter are important.

A complete medication history is essential, including prescribed and over-the-counter drugs. Note any thyroid-replacement drugs and iodide-containing drugs such as Amiodarone hydrochloride and radiocontrast dye. Ascertain from the past medical history or family history any previous thyroid problems. Determine any functional, cognitive, and emotional changes. Gradual or sudden decline in activities of daily living (ADLs), instrumental activities of daily living (IADLs), or cognitive or emotional functioning may be indicative of hyperthyroidism.

The American Thyroid Association[8] recommends a thorough physical examination during the initial evaluation. Observe general appearance, paying attention to affect, nervousness, and apathy. Check blood pressure, pulse rate and regularity, respirations, temperature, weight, and height. Inspect and palpate the skin, observing for pretibial myxedema of the shins or soft and slightly sweaty skin. Inspect the hair for reduced texture and the nails for redness or tenderness. Examine the eyes, noting proptosis, diminished blinking, exopthalmos, and ophthalmopathy, and test visual acuity. Palpate the thyroid gland for enlargement or nodularity, and auscultate for bruits. Goiter is much less common in older adults and its absence does not exclude a diagnosis of hyperthyroidism. Inspect, palpate, and auscultate the heart for rate, regularity, murmurs, and cardiac enlargement. Palpate, percuss, and auscultate the lungs for fluid consolidation associated with heart failure. Complete a focused neurological examination, noting brisk deep tendon reflexes, fine tremor, and proximal muscle weakness. Evaluate for dementia, depression, and delirium; mental status changes, such as restlessness, agitation, withdrawal, or decreased interest in pleasurable activities are highly suggestive of hyperthyroidism.

Laboratory and Diagnostic Workup

To establish the diagnosis of hyperthyroidism, the TSH level should be measured (it will be lower than normal or undetectable in hyperthyroidism), as well as a free thyroxine (T4) and triiodothyronine resin uptake (T3RU) (both levels are elevated in hyperthyroidism) (Table 7–2). When the free thyroxine level is elevated and the TSH is not suppressed in a clinically hyperthyroid patient, consider hyperthyroidism secondary to a TSH-producing pituitary tumor. The TSH level is the most sensitive and specific test for hyperthyroidism, as well as the single best screening test. Thyroid antithyroglobulin and antimicrosomal antibody titers, two autoantibody tests, are elevated in Graves' disease.

The radioactive iodine uptake (RAIU) test differentiates Graves' disease or toxic multinodular goiter from other causes such as thyroiditis. Radioactive iodine tracer is taken up in greater amounts in hyperfunctioning areas of the thyroid gland. A nodule showing increased tracer uptake is referred to as "hot." Likewise, a hypofunctioning nodule that does not take up the tracer is

Table 7–2   Laboratory Values of Thyroid Conditions

	TSH	T4	T3	Thyroid Antibodies	
Hyperthyroidism	↓	↑	↑		
Subclinical hyperthyroidism	↓	Normal	Normal	+	−
Graves' disease (and other autoimmune processes)	↓	↑	↑		+
Hypothyroidism	↑	↓	↓		
Subclinical hypothyroidism	↑	Normal	Normal	+	−
Hashimoto's thyroiditis (and other autoimmune processes)	↑	↓	↓		+

referred to as "cold." RAIU values are elevated in Graves' and toxic multinodular goiter, but not in thyroiditis.

Differential Diagnosis

Graves' disease is the most common cause of hyperthyroidism in younger and older adults. It is an autoimmune disorder resulting from production of immunoglobulin (IgG), which activates the TSH receptor, stimulating thyroid hormone synthesis and gland growth. It is difficult to diagnose in older adults and often presents with cardiac manifestations, weight loss, and a normal-sized thyroid gland. The TSH is always suppressed and the thyroid scan shows diffuse isotope uptake. The T4, T3 RU, free T4 index, free T4, T3 RIA, and free T3 are usually elevated, although some individuals may have elevations of T3 RIA or free T3 (T3 toxicosis) only.

A toxic adenoma, or "hot" nodule is associated with elevations in the T4 and/or T3 RIA levels with a suppressed TSH. The thyroid scan demonstrates a functioning nodule with the extranodular thyroid tissue suppressed. Laboratory findings in toxic multinodular goiter are the same as those associated with a "hot" nodule, but the thyroid gland is enlarged and composed of multiple nodules. In both cases, the RAIU test is usually elevated, but may be in the normal range.

Subacute thyroiditis, iodine-induced hyperthyroidism, and factitious thyroxine-induced hyperthyroidism all have elevated T4 and T3 RIA levels and a low radioiodine uptake with poor thyroid gland imaging on thyroid scan.

Subacute thyroiditis is thought to be of viral origin and usually follows an upper respiratory infection. On exam, the thyroid gland is usually painful. The inflamed gland releases stored thyroid hormone leading to hyperthyroidism. The early hyperthyroid phase leads to a hypothyroid phase over a two- to-three month period before normalizing.

Iodine-induced hyperthyroidism occurs most often in older adults with nontoxic nodular goiter. The minimum daily requirement for iodine intake is 100–200 mcg. The typical American diet far exceeds this amount due to the iodination of salt, milk, and bread. Iodide-containing drugs such as Amiodarone and radiocontrast dye can also cause already high iodine levels to reach excessive levels, causing hyperthyroidism.

Factitious thyroxine-induced hyperthyroidism is self-explanatory. Excess intake of exogenous synthetic thyroxine mimics the hyperthyroidism caused by increased endogenous production of the hormone.

Management

Goals of therapy are to normalize the circulating thyroid hormones quickly and prevent recurrence. Severity of clinical signs and symptoms and underlying medical conditions usually dictate whether thyroid gland ablation or antithyroid drugs are selected. Consider physician consultation and/or collaboration, depending upon acuity.

Beta-adrenergic blocking agents, such as atenolol (Tenormin) 50 mg daily or timolol (Blocadren) 10 mg BID, are prescribed to decrease adrenergic symptoms like tachycardia, restlessness, and tremor, and then gradually discontinued as soon as a euthyroid state is achieved.

Thyroid tissue ablation by oral radioactive iodine is generally safe and is the treatment of choice in older adults. Pretreatment with antithyroid drugs, such as propylthiouracil (PTU) or methimazole (Tapazole), is advisable in older adults or cardiac patients with Graves' disease to reduce T4 released during thyroid ablation. Adverse drug reactions associated with antithyroid drug treatment include minor skin rashes and, in rare instances, agranulocytosis and hepatitis.

Hypothyroidism frequently occurs within the first 6 to 12 months following radioactive iodine therapy, but may occur at any time.[8] To identify hypothyroidism, patients should be seen at frequent intervals, approximately every 2 to 3 months, after receiving radioactive iodine.

Antithyroid drugs may also be useful as a primary form of treatment. It usually takes 4–6 weeks for methimazole (10–20 mg daily) and 6–12 weeks for propylthiouracil (75–100 mg three times daily) to cause a euthyroid state. Recurrence of hyperthyroidism with antithyroid drugs is higher if no other treatment is utilized. Mild disease and small goiters are mostly likely to respond to antithyroid drugs.

Thyroidectomy is infrequently recommended for Graves' disease. It is usually appropriate only for individuals with very large goiters, allergies to antithyroid drugs, or unwillingness to receive treatment with radioactive iodine.[8]

▪ Hypothyroidism

In hypothyroidism, the thyroid gland fails to secrete adequate amounts of thyroid hormone. The disease affects many individuals between the ages of 30 to 60. Women are 10 times more likely than men to develop hypothyroidism in their lifetime.[9] Eleven million people in the United States are diagnosed each year, with an increased prevalence among older adults. Ten percent of women over the age of 65 suffer from the disease[10] compared to 2% of men aged 60 and older. Among those 70 and above, 15% have hypothyroidism.[3] The prevalence has been found to be as high as 27% of older adults in acute-care settings such as hospitals and in-patient rehabilitation centers.[11]

The classic clinical presentation of hypothyroidism includes dry skin, brittle hair, and alopecia; fluid retention and weight gain (usually 7–10 pounds, no more than 20); facial puffiness; pallor; cold intolerance; headache; malaise; myalgias; fatigue or lethargy; confusion and decreased concentration; insomnia; goiter; difficulty breathing or swallowing; constipation; anorexia; delayed deep tendon reflexes (relaxation phase); and manifestations of a decreased basal metabolic rate.[9,12,13,14] In contrast to this classic presentation, older adults experience an insidious onset and subtle signs and symptoms, often mistakenly attributed to heart failure, depression, dementia, anorexia, and gastrointestinal disorders. Most patients over 70 commonly report only two clinical signs, fatigue and weakness[12] (Table 7–3).

Screening for Hypothyroidism

Screening asymptomatic older adults for hypothyroidism is generally not recommended. Periodic screening in older women, however, may be more cost effective and produce a favorable return for the effort, especially in women over the age of 50.[1,15]

Subclinical hypothyroidism is defined as an elevated TSH level in the presence of a normal-serum free T4 level. It may be associated with nonspecific symptoms of thyroid hormone deficiency. Prevalence increases with age and is higher in women. Although controversial, strong arguments favor screening for

Table 7–3   Hypothyroidism Clinical Presentation

Younger Adults	Older Adults
Classic signs & symptoms:	Classic signs & symptoms are subtle and insidious in onset, often mistakenly attributed to:
• Dry skin	
• Brittle hair and alopecia	• Heart failure
• Fluid retention	• Depression
• Weight gain (usually 7–10 lbs, no more than 20)	• Dementia
• Facial puffiness, pallor	• Anorexia
• Cold intolerance	• Gastrointestinal disorders
• Headache	
• Myalgias	**Most patients report only two clinical symptoms:**
• Fatigue or lethargy	• Fatigue
• Decreased concentration	• Weakness
• Insomnia	
• Goiter	
• Difficulty breathing or swallowing	
• Constipation	
• Anorexia	
• Delayed deep tendon reflexes (relaxation phase)	

subclinical hypothyroidism.[1] Progression to overt hypothyroidism, usually associated with positive thyroid autoantibody titers, occurs in up to one-fourth of all patients with subclinical hypothyroidism; thus, early screening and treatment could prevent hypothyroidism. Furthermore, hypercholesterolemia induced by mild thyroid failure and a significant risk factor for coronary artery disease (CAD) could be reduced. Of significance to the patient is the alleviation of symptoms of thyroid deficiency that decrease quality of life, as well as consume diagnostic and therapeutic resources.[15]

Overt hypothyroidism is associated with increased levels of low-density lipoprotein (LDL) cho-

lesterol and lipoprotein-a, and decreased high-density lipoprotein (HDL) cholesterol, thus increasing the risk of premature atherosclerosis.[16,17] It is unclear whether subclinical hypothyroidism is a risk factor for cardiovascular disease.[18] A recent population-based cross-sectional study in the Netherlands, however, found subclinical hypothyroidism was associated with a greater prevalence of aortic atherosclerosis and myocardial infarction.[19]

The National Cholesterol Education Program recommends screening for subclinical hypothyroidism every five years for women starting at the age of 35.[15] According to the American College of Physicians and U.S. Preventative Services Task Force, women aged 45–65 and men aged 35–65 should also be screened periodically. Cost of the TSH assay and importance of the symptoms to the patient need to be considered whenever screening is undertaken. Treatment of subclinical hypothyroidism must be individualized; however, most patients with positive thyroid autoantibodies should receive levothyroxine.[20]

Diagnosis and Evaluation

Because age modifies the clinical presentation of hypothyroidism, and symptoms are subtle and affect many systems, a comprehensive history is important. A query about the following clinical symptoms is essential: fatigue and weakness, mental slowness, drowsiness, chilliness, dry skin, constipation, hearing loss, hoarseness, ataxia, or hair loss.[8,12] Fatigue, weakness, and hearing loss are especially common; typically the mean number of clinical signs and symptoms is half that of younger adults.[12]

A complete medication history must also be obtained. Amiodarone is a common cause of iodine-induced hypothyroidism and may be transient or persistent. Patients with antithyroid antibodies who are given Amiodarone are at an increased risk of developing hypothyroidism due to unmasking of underlying autoimmune thyroiditis.[21] Lithium can also cause hypothyroidism and is more common in a patient with thyroid antibodies.[22]

Past medical and family history should be directed toward any previous thyroid problems. Thyroid gland ablation with radioactive iodine therapy, head or neck irradiation, thyroidectomy, and a familial history of chronic autoimmune thyroiditis all predispose to hypothyroidism. In women, inquire specifically about a history of postpartum thyroiditis, a transient form of autoimmune thyroiditis lasting three to four months and occurring within the first eight months after giving birth. Thirty percent of women with this disorder go on to develop permanent hypothyroidism later in life. Repeated bouts with later pregnancies increase this risk, a condition that is often familial. The present cohort of older women may have been misdiagnosed with postpartum depression rather than classic hypothyroidism.[23] Other autoimmune disorders such as diabetes mellitus, rheumatoid arthritis, adrenal insufficiency, pernicious anemia, and hypoparathyroidism also increase the risk of hypothyroidism.

Inquire about gradual or sudden changes in function, cognition, or depressive symptoms, which may be the only clinical manifestations of hypothyroidism in older adults. The mental slowing associated with hypothyroidism is commonly mistaken for normal aging or evidence of dementia in the elderly. A thorough dementia workup should always include screening for hypothyroidism. In some cases even severe cognitive dysfunction can be reversed with thyroid hormone replacement.[14]

On physical examination, obtain blood pressure, pulse rate and rhythm, respiration, temperature, height, and weight. Inspect the skin for yellowing or dryness. In advanced cases of myxedema, observe for periorbital swelling and puffiness of the jowls, hands, and feet. Examine the hair for coarseness or loss. Palpate the thyroid gland for enlargement or nodularity and auscultate for bruits; goiter is less common in older adults.

Examine the heart for rate, regularity, murmurs, and enlargement; atrial fibrillation may be present with hypothyroidism.[24,25] Hypothyroidism is generally severe if cardiac manifestations occur.[26] Bradycardia may result from overall slowing of the metabolic rate. Assess the lungs for consolidation from heart failure.

Complete a focused neuromuscular examination. Delayed relaxation of deep tendon reflexes, decreased muscle strength, and ataxia occur more often in younger adults. Evaluate mental function for signs of dementia, depression, or delirium.

Laboratory and Diagnostic Workup

Based on guidelines from the American Association of Clinical Endocrinologists, the TSH assay should always be used to establish the diagnosis of hypothyroidism.[20] In primary hypothyroidism, the TSH will be elevated > 10 mIU/L, and the T4 and free T4 decreased. Hypothyroidism resulting from hypothalamic pituitary disorders shows a normal or subnormal TSH and a subnormal free T4 (Table 7–2).

Thyroid antibodies, such as antithyroid peroxidase (anti TPO), antimicrosomal, and antithyroglobulin (anti Tg), are positive in 95% of patients with autoimmune thyroiditis; high titers suggest the diagnosis (Table 7–2).[20] Thyroid antibody tests are used to diagnose Hashimoto's disease or Graves' disease and should always be checked in cases of goiter and in subclinical hypothyroidism. A positive result indicates high risk for progression to overt disease.

RAIU and thyroid scan should never be used in the workup of hypothyroidism, as uptake is usually normal.[27] Such tests may be indicated if a nodule or other structural abnormality is palpable.

A CBC to detect anemia, frequently associated with hypothyroidism, should be done. Microcytic, hypochromic, or macrocytic anemias need to be evaluated for their underlying etiology.[28]

Obtain a lipid profile with specific attention to elevated levels of serum total and LDL cholesterol and decreased serum HDL cholesterol. Hypercholesterolemia is reversible with thyroid hormone replacement therapy. Hypothyroid patients with TSH values greater than 40 mU/L exhibit the greatest reduction in total and LDL cholesterol as a result of treatment.[29]

Creatinine kinase, normally metabolized by the kidneys, can be elevated up to 20 times the level found with a myocardial infarction, because of mild hypothyroid myopathy and decreased renal clearance. This elevation can occur rapidly, but is reversible.[30]

An electrocardiogram (ECG) may be indicated in markedly hypothyroid patients. Bradycardia, diffuse flattened or inverted T waves, prolongation of the QT interval, and generalized low voltage of all the complexes may be seen.[28]

Differential Diagnosis

Most cases of hypothyroidism are due to primary thyroid gland failure from Hashimoto's thyroiditis, an autoimmune disorder involving T lymphocyte activation by thyroid cells, secretion of thyroid autoantibodies, and subsequent thyroid gland destruction.[22] The TSH is always elevated. The presence of anti Tg or antimicrosomal antibodies confirms the diagnosis.[22] The T4, T3 RU, free T4 index, free T4, T3 RIA, and free T3 are decreased. Thyroid imaging is unnecessary and can be very misleading; radioiodine uptake characteristically is normal or elevated in goitrous autoimmune thyroiditis and low in subacute thyroiditis. The pattern of uptake on thyroid scan may be similar to Graves' disease, multinodular goiter, or a hyperfunctioning or hypofunctioning nodule.[22]

Central hypothyroidism caused by hypothalamic or pituitary disease is rare. The TSH level is low, inappropriately normal, or insufficiently elevated in the presence of low levels of T4, T3 RU, free T4 index, free T4, T3 RIA, and free T3.

Iatrogenic hypothyroidism develops from ablative therapy with radioactive iodide or surgery for hyperthyroidism, iodine-containing or antithyroid medications, and head or neck irradiation. About half of all patients who receive radioactive iodine treatment for sporadic nontoxic goiter develop hypothyroidism (26% subclinical hypothyroidism and 22% overt hypothyroidism), usually within two years of treatment. The presence of antithyroid antibodies and smaller thyroid size are correlated with a higher risk of hypothyroidism.[31] Of patients who are treated with antithyroid drugs (e.g., PTU or Tapazole), or have a partial thyroidectomy, only 5–25% develop hypothyroidism. Less commonly, hypothyroidism may be iatrogenic from lithium and amiodarone.[32] Because low dose irradiation to the neck was common practice in the mid-1950s and 1960s for enlarged tonsils and adenoids, enlarged thymus, and skin infections such as acne, older patients are at special risk for hypothyroidism.[33]

Worldwide, dietary iodide deficiency is the main cause of hypothyroidism, especially in developing countries where there is no iodination of salt, milk, and bread, as in the United States.

Management

The goal of therapy is to restore the thyrotropin concentration to a normal level and the body to a euthyroid state. Thyroxine, in the form of levothyroxine sodium (Synthroid, Levoxyl, Levothroid), is the most commonly prescribed treatment for hypothyroidism. Other thyroid preparations, such as desiccated thyroid or combinations of T3 and T4, should be avoided. Maintenance should be with the same brand of drug throughout treatment, because levothyroxine products are not always bioequivalent.[20] A study comparing two brand-name drugs (Synthroid and Levoxyl) with two generic levothyroxine preparations found them to be bioequivalent within FDA regulations.[34] Although not statistically significant, slight differences existed between Synthroid and the other preparations in the levels of thyrotropin and total T3 achieved. The implications are important because of the potential cost savings of prescribing generic brands over name brands. In the United States, 15 million prescriptions for levothyroxine are filled annually.

In older adult patients or those with comorbid disease, the adage "start low and go slow" holds true. The usual starting dose of levothyroxine is 12.5 to 25 mcg with an average daily maintenance dose of 50–100 mcg. Levothyroxine is titrated slowly at 12.5 to 25 mcg increments until the TSH is normalized and the patient's clinical status improves.[32] The serum TSH level should be measured in six to eight weeks after initiating therapy and after each dosage adjustment. The TSH is most important, but a T4 and T3 RU or free T4 may be included.

Older adults are at risk for exacerbation or unveiling of undiagnosed CAD; special precautions are thus warranted in starting them on the lowest dose possible and titrating upward slowly. Hypothyroidism often masks the symptoms of CAD by decreasing oxygen demands on the heart with an overall decreased metabolism. Older patients with hypothyroidism and undiagnosed

CAD therefore may have never experienced angina, yet could be at high risk for acute myocardial infarction or fatal cardiac arrhythmias with aggressive thyroid hormone repletion.[14] If angina is present, full thyroxine replacement therapy is not usually tolerated. The hypothyroid patient in need of cardiac surgery may safely undergo balloon angioplasty, after which full thyroxine dosage may be achieved.[9]

Treatment of hypothyroidism must be individualized. Once the TSH is normalized, follow-up visits in six months and annually are recommended. During follow-up visits, an interim history and physical examination should be performed in conjunction with appropriate laboratory tests.

The use of levothyroxine replacement therapy in euthyroid individuals may improve fatigue and depression[13] and impaired cognitive functioning.[35] More research concerning this therapy is needed. At present, it is not recommended to treat for subclinical hypothyroidism until the TSH is consistently between 5–10 mU/L and symptoms are present.[32] When treatment of subclinical hypothyroidism is deemed appropriate, levothyroxine replacement usually ranges from 25–50 mcg a day in order to maintain a normal TSH.

Thyroxine has numerous interactions with other medications. Patients must not self-medicate, especially with over-the-counter drugs. The sympathomimetic agents in many cold preparations, such as pseudoephedrine, increase the cardiovascular effects of thyroxine-induced angina or arrhythmias. Anti-inflammatory drugs may compete for plasma binding sites. The effect of oral anticoagulants may be increased, and drugs like Coumadin should have dosages decreased. Blood glucose concentrations may be increased, requiring diabetics to increase insulin dosages. The effect of digitalis is reduced with an increased likelihood of toxicity.[9]

Ferrous sulfate, cimetidine, sucralfate, aluminum hydroxide antacids, or cholestyramine will decrease absorption of levothyroxine.[8] Fiber can also interfere with absorption. Levothyroxine should be taken four to six hours apart from any of these preparations and on an empty stomach. Phenytoin, anticonvulsants, and rifampin accelerate the clearance of thyroxine

from the body, increasing dosage requirements. Levothyroxine taken at bedtime may cause insomnia from an increase in metabolism; generally, the drug is better tolerated if taken in the morning.[9]

With a half-life of seven days, thyroxine treatment brings symptomatic relief of hypothyroidism within two to three weeks. Edema and facial puffiness resolve quickly, while improvements in skin and hair texture may take up to six months.[9]

Elevated cholesterol levels may return to normal after several months of treatment with thyroxine. Symptoms of obstructive sleep apnea may diminish in about four months. Electrolyte abnormalities should be corrected almost immediately (e.g., hyponatremia, SIADH, elevated creatinine and creatinine kinase, and carotenemia).

Patient education about the importance of taking medication daily for life is critical; missed doses cannot be made up. Follow-up is essential. Early in treatment, patients need to alternate periods of rest with gradual increases in exercise. A low-fat, low-cholesterol, high-fiber diet should be encouraged to manage weight loss, improve lipid profile, and prevent constipation. If there are psychomotor symptoms, patients must be cautioned against driving or operating machinery. Patients need to be familiar with the signs and symptoms of hypo- and hyperthyroidism in order to monitor for medication side effects or the need for change in dosage requirements of thyroxine replacement. The aging process may continually alter thyroxine requirements over time.

Patients deserve as much detailed information as desired concerning the disease. Because of possible hereditary links, families must be educated about signs and symptoms and be prepared to seek treatment as necessary. Fatigue and depression can persist after treatment, but the dose of hormone replacement should never be increased without consultation with a health-care provider.[28]

Nodular Thyroid Disease

Palpable thyroid nodules occur in an estimated 4–7% of the population; as much as 30–60% of the population has them based on autopsy findings. Only 4–5% of these nodules are found to be malignant. Thyroid nodules occur eight times more often in women than men, and increase after the age of 45. Palpable nodules are twice as likely to be malignant in men than in women. Older adults are at greater risk for an aggressive form of thyroid cancer, anaplastic carcinoma, which is quite rare in the overall population (2–4% of thyroid cancers); it can lead to death within a matter of months.[36,37,38]

The older adult presenting with a thyroid nodule may or may not have signs of thyroid hormone imbalance. Occasionally, signs of hyperthyroidism exist with an autonomously hyperfunctioning adenoma. Benign multinodular goiter in older adults can present with or without hypothyroidism.

Screening for Thyroid Nodules

Thyroid nodules may be detected during a routine physical exam, though a great number of nodules are found by coincidence during imaging of the head and neck or mediastinum for reasons unrelated to the thyroid. These nodules are referred to as incidentalomas and are generally less than 1.5 cm in diameter and nonpalpable.

Diagnosis and Evaluation

A thyroid nodule raises the index of suspicion for malignancy, especially in the presence of a hard, fixed nodule; vocal cord paralysis; history of irradiation to the neck; age (very old or very young); sex (male); rapid growth; sudden change in size of the thyroid nodule; compression symptoms of neighboring structures; recurrent cystic nodules; and certain environmental factors.[38] Always ask the older patient about any history of head and neck irradiation. The incidence of thyroid cancer in individuals who received head or neck irradiation is 50%.

Inquire about possible environmental exposures that increase the risk for thyroid cancer. While uncommon in the United States, disasters such as nuclear accidents in Belarus and the Ukraine, or conditions of endemic iodine deficiency, such as in the Himalayas, Alps, and Middle-Eastern countries, contribute to nodules and other thyroid problems.

The presence of a hard, fixed thyroid nodule, vocal cord paralysis, and the presence of lymph node metastases almost always mean thyroid cancer. A rapidly enlarging mass in an elderly individual is highly suggestive of anaplastic carcinoma. Explore the patient's subjective description of the nodule/s in detail to screen for these high-risk characteristics.

Laboratory and Diagnostic Workup

Serum TSH should be obtained with the presence of thyroid nodules. Hyperthyroidism in the presence of a thyroid nodule is most likely an autonomously hyperfunctioning adenoma, while hypothyroidism with a nodular thyroid suggests Hashimoto's thyroiditis. An abnormal thyroid function test does not exclude cancer, but it may decrease the index of suspicion.

Controversy exists over the use of RAIU and other thyroid scans in the evaluation of nodules. Less than 5% of nodules are labeled as "hot," 10% are labeled "warm" (uptake similar to surrounding tissue), and the remaining 85% are "cold." The finding of a "hot" nodule can be reassuring, as less than 5% of these are malignant. At the same time, however, only 5–15% of "cold" nodules are malignant, so using "hot" versus "cold" can lead to false positives. Thyroid scans help distinguish between a solitary nodule and a multinodular goiter; however, it is not the test of choice for differential diagnosis.[36,38]

Ultrasonography (US) provides detailed information on the size and structure of thyroid nodules, but not function or histopathology. US is useful in differentiating solitary versus multiple nodules. It also shows whether a nodule is cystic or solid. Nodules over 1–1.5 cm are considered significant enough to biopsy. Malignant nodules are usually solitary, solid, and found in the upper half of the thyroid. They often have poorly defined boundaries and may contain fine punctuate areas of calcification. If a malignant nodule is growing, US may show increased blood flow; however, avascular, necrotic areas can also be located within a tumor.[39]

A recent innovation in color Doppler ultrasonography, the power Doppler (PD), reportedly increases sensitivity to 100% and specificity to 98.1%, compared to 91% and 86.2% respectively for color Doppler ultrasound. Better characterization of thyroid nodules aids in more appropriate selection of patients for fine needle aspiration biopsy (FNAB).[40]

Ultrasound-guided FNAB may be the single most cost effective, sensitive, and accurate test for evaluating thyroid nodules. It is the recommended first step in evaluation of any patient with a palpable thyroid nodule. The results of FNAB can be classified as clearly malignant, suspect, benign, or indeterminate. If the results are not satisfactory, the test can be repeated in four to six months.[38]

A computed tomography (CT) scan is useful in the evaluation of the extent of disease and the proximity to, or involvement of, the trachea with diffuse enlarged or substernal goiters. Otherwise, the routine use of CT scanning in evaluating thyroid nodules or masses is not recommended.

Magnetic resonance imaging (MRI) is also quite limited in the evaluation of thyroid nodules or masses. It is very expensive and simply identifies the presence of a nodule or nodules. Many incidentalomas are discovered during MRIs of the cervical spine.

Differential Diagnosis

Most thyroid nodules are benign based on FNAB. The nodules may be part of a benign multinodular goiter, which may or may not be related to thyroiditis and hypothyroidism. Nodules can be solid or cystic. Risk factors for thyroid cancer, such as a history of radiation to the head and neck, suggest that nodules could eventually become malignant.

Solitary thyroid nodules may be autonomously hyperfunctioning "hot" nodules associated with subsequent symptoms of hyperthyroidism. On thyroid scan, the tracer is almost exclusively taken up by the hyperfunctioning nodule in relation to the surrounding tissue. Less than 5% of these nodules develop into cancer. If there are multiple "hot" nodules, the diagnosis is toxic multinodular goiter.

In at least one documented case,[41] a solitary, painless thyroid nodule turned out to be subacute

thyroiditis. Although this is clearly atypical, it must be considered in the differential diagnosis of thyroid nodules.

In solitary, solid, "cold," or hypofunctioning nodules, the greatest concern is for malignancy. Papillary carcinoma is the most common form of thyroid cancer, accounting for up to 78% of cases. The second and third most common forms are follicular cell carcinoma, 13% of cases, followed by Hürthle cell carcinoma (a variant of follicular cancer), which accounts for 3% of cancerous nodules. Papillary carcinoma has the best prognosis, as it is usually noninvasive and slow to progress. Follicular cell cancers are more aggressive and angioinvasive, and may present with metastases to the bones and lungs while bypassing local nodes. Still, the prognosis for follicular cell carcinoma is better than for medullary and anaplastic thyroid cancer.

Medullary and anaplastic carcinoma are the most aggressive forms of thyroid cancer. Medullary carcinoma, which originates in parafollicular cells, accounts for 4% of all thyroid cancers. Three-fourths of patients diagnosed with medullary thyroid cancer have the "sporadic" form of the disease. The remaining 25% have a hereditary form that may be part of the multiple endocrine neoplasia type 2 (MEN-2) syndromes. The remaining 2% of thyroid cancers are anaplastic carcinomas. Older adults are most at risk for this type of thyroid cancer, which presents with a rapidly expanding thyroid mass, severe compression symptoms, hoarseness, and occasionally respiratory distress. In some cases, an incidental thyroid mass may have been present for years before recent rapid expansion. Despite aggressive therapies, the outcome in anaplastic thyroid cancer is universally fatal, usually within six to nine months from diagnosis.[36,38]

Management

Any patient presenting with a thyroid nodule should be referred immediately to an endocrinologist. Nevertheless, it is important for nurse practitioners to know the standards of care for thyroid nodules in order to assure appropriate care and adequate counseling concerning treatment and prognosis.

Management of benign thyroid nodules and benign multinodular goiter is subject to some debate. For incidentalomas and other nodules found to be less than 1.5 cm in diameter, observation alone is recommended. Nodules greater than 1.5 cm in diameter should undergo FNAB.

Fine needle aspiration of benign cystic nodules is often performed. The procedure is rarely therapeutic, however, because a cyst must be fully aspirated to relieve compressive symptoms. Relief is short-lived, as the cystic fluid reaccumulates rapidly. Percutaneous injection of a sclerosing agent, such as tetracycline or ethanol, has also been used to shrink cystic nodules. This is an extremely dangerous procedure unless a diagnosis of benign disease has been confirmed by FNAB.[42]

Suppression with supplemental thyroxine is the current standard of care for benign nodular thyroid disease, both cystic and solid. A trial of 6–12 months of suppressive therapy is recommended with nodule size assessments every 6 months. The National Institutes of Health (NIH) guidelines recommend overt thyroid suppression with maintenance of TSH serum concentrations within the low-normal range. The benefits of this therapy are greater for multinodular disease than for solitary benign nodules.[37]

The main indications for surgery in thyroid nodules are fear of malignancy, compression symptoms, and cosmetic reasons. Total thyroidectomy for benign nodular disease[43] may seem a bit extreme, but it can be justified in cases where other factors place patients at high risk for thyroid cancer, or where compressive symptoms are severe. The long-term recurrence is relatively high when abnormal thyroid tissue and nodules are left behind. The main risks associated with total thyroidectomy are recurrent laryngeal nerve injury and permanent hypoparathyroidism.

Subtotal thyroidectomy or lobectomy is indicated in most cases of papillary and follicular carcinoma. The clinical incidence of recurrence in the contralateral lobe is less than 5%. Disagreement exists as to whether radioactive iodine ablation of

the remaining thyroid tissue is warranted. Some argue for long-term suppression with thyroxine. Total thyroidectomy is recommended if there is any evidence of microscopic disease in the remaining lobe. Promising work is currently under way to investigate a minimally invasive video-assisted (MIVA) approach to resecting nodules up to 3 cm in diameter that border on intact thyroid lobes.[44]

The recommended treatment for medullary cancer is total thyroidectomy with central compartment neck dissection, as these central nodes have a high incidence of microscopic metastatic invasion. The lateral nodes should be dissected if there is clinical evidence of metastases. Patients may need ablation and/or suppression if any thyroid tissue is left behind.

The current treatment approach for anaplastic thyroid disease is chemotherapy and radiation. Total surgical resection is almost impossible unless the tumor is quite small and intrathyroidal. Even with resection, the local recurrence is extremely high. Most patients die within six to nine months, regardless of treatment, from massive local disease or distant metastases to the lung causing pulmonary problems.[36,38]

◼ Conclusion

Thyroid disorders are more common with advancing age and can lead to potentially serious complications and decreased quality of life for older adults. It is important to recognize the clinical presentation of thyroid disorders in the differential of many acute and chronic conditions. Evidence to screen for hypothyroidism and hyperthyroidism is limited and controversial. Primary-care nurse practitioners have a responsibility to evaluate and manage thyroid disorders by applying strategies specific to older adults.

References

1. Helfand M, Redfern CC. Screening for thyroid disease: an update. *Ann of Int Med.* 1998;129(2):144–158.
2. Trivalle C, Doucet J, Chassagne P, et al. Differences in the signs and symptoms of hyperthyroidism in older and younger patients. *J Am Geriatr Soc.* 1996;44:50–53.

3. U.S. Public Health Service. *Clinicians Handbook of Preventive Services: Put Prevention into Practice.* Washington, DC: U.S. Government Printing Office; 1998.

4. Lazarus JH. Hyperthyroidism. *Lancet.* 1997;349: 339–343.

5. Wallace K, Hofmann MT. Thyroid dysfunction: how to manage overt and subclinical disease in older patients. *Geriatrics.* 1998;53(4):32–41.

6. Sawin CT, Geller A, Wolf P, et al. Low serum thyrotropin concentrations as a risk factor for atrial fibrillation in older persons. *N Engl J Med.* 1994;331(19):1249–1252.

7. Faber J, Galloe AM. Changes in bone mass during prolonged subclinical hyperthyroidism due to L-thyroxine treatment. *European J Endocrin.* 1994;130:350–356.

8. Singer PA, Cooper DS, Levy EG, et al. Treatment guidelines for patients with hyperthyroidism and hypothyroidism. *JAMA.* 1995;273(10):808–812.

9. White J, Jordan S. The endocrine system: hypothyroidism. *Nurs Times.* 1998;94:50–53.

10. Trotto NE. Hypothyroidism, hyperthyroidism, hyperparathyroidism. *Patient Care.* 1999;33:186–188, 191, 195–200.

11. Christian A, Berlow A, Ravishankar T, Root B. Hypothyroidism: its incidence and prevalence in adults older than 55 years of age in an acute rehabilitation unit. *Arch Phys Med Rehabil.* 1999;80:468–469.

12. Doucet J, Trivalle CH, Chassagne PH, et al. Does age play a role in clinical presentation of hypothyroidism? *J Am Geriatr Soc.* 1994;42:984–986.

13. Dzurec LC. Experiences of fatigue and depression before and after low-dose 1-thyroxine supplementation in essentially euthyroid individuals. *Res Nurs Health.* 1997;20:389–398.

14. Mazzaferri EL. Decision making in medicine. Recognizing the faces of hypothyroidism. *Hosp Pract.* 1999;34:93–96, 101–105, 109–110.

15. Danese MD, Powe NR, Sawin CT, Ladenson PW. Screening for mild thyroid failure at the periodic health examination: a decision and cost-effectiveness analysis. *JAMA.* 1996; 276(4):285–292.

16. Becerra A, Bellido D, Luengo A, Piedrola G, De Luis DA. Lipoprotein(a) and other lipoproteins in hypothyroid patients before and after thyroid replacement therapy. *Clin Nutr.* 1999;18:319–322.

17. Klein I, Ojamaa K. The cardiovascular system in hypothyroidism. In: LE Braverman, RD Utiger, eds. *Werner and Ingbar's the Thyroid: A Fundamental and Clinical Text.* 7th ed. Philadelphia, Pa: Lippincott-Raven, 1996;799–804.

18. Lindeman RD, Schade DS, LaRue A, et al. Subclinical hypothyroidism in a biethnic, urban community. *J Am Geriatri Soc.* 1999;47(6):703–709.

19. Hak AE, Pols HAP, Visser TJ, Drexhage HA, Hofman A, Witteman JCM. Subclinical hypothyroidism is an independent risk factor for atherosclerosis and myocardial infarction in elderly women: the Rotterdam study. *Ann Int Med.* 2000;132:270–278.

20. American Association of Clinical Endocrinologists. Clinical practice guidelines for evaluation and treatment of hyperthyroidism and hypothyroidism. 1996. Available at: www.aace.com/clinguideindex.htm. Accessed February 28, 2001.

21. Harjai KJ, Licata AA. Effects of amiodarone on thyroid function. *Ann Int Med.* 1997;126(1): 63–73.

22. Dayan CM, Daniels GH. Chronic autoimmune thyroiditis. *N Engl J Med.* 1996;335(2):99–107.

23. Gregerman RI. Thyroid disorders. In: LR Barker, JR Burton, PD Zieve, eds. *Principles of Ambulatory Medicine.* Baltimore, Md: Williams & Wilkins; 1999; 1066–1095.

24. Krahn AD, Klein GJ, Kerr CR, et al. How useful is thyroid function testing in patients with recent-onset atrial fibrillation? The Canadian Registry of Atrial Fibrillation Investigators. *Arch Int Med.* 1998;157: 2221–2224.

25. Wong PSC, Hee FLL, Lip GY. Atrial fibrillation and the thyroid. *Heart.* 1997;78(6):623–624.

26. Tielens ET, Pillay M, Storm C, Berghout A. Cardiac function at rest in hypothyroidism evaluated by equilibrium radionuclide angiography. *Clin Endocrinol.* 1999;50:497–502.

27. Braverman LE, Dworkin HJ, MacIndoe JH II. Thyroid disease: when to screen, when to treat. *Patient Care.* 1997;31:18–20, 29, 34.

28. Heitman B, Irizarry A. Hypothyroidism: common complaints, perplexing diagnosis. *Nurse Pract.* 1995; 20(3):54–60.

29. Diekman T, Lansberg PJ, Kastelein JP, Wiersinga WM. Prevalence and correction of hypothyroidism in a large cohort of patients referred for dyslipidemia. *Arch Int Med.* 1995;155(14):1490–1495.

30. Kreisman SH, Hennessey JV. Consistent reversible elevations of serum creatinine levels in severe hypothyroidism. *Arch Int Med.* 1999;159:79–82.

31. Le Moli R, Wesche MF, Tiel-Van Buul MM, Wiersinga WM. Determinants of long term outcome of radioiodine therapy of sporadic non-toxic goitre. *Clin Endocrinol.* 1999;50:783–789.

32. Adlin V. Subclinical hypothyroidism: deciding when to treat. *Am Fam Phys.* 1998;57:776–780.

33. Maxon HR, Thomas SR, Saenger EL. Ionizing radiation and the induction of clinically significant disease in the human thyroid gland. *Am J Med.* 1977;63:967–978.

34. Dong BJ, Hauck WW, Gambertoglio JG, et al. Bio-equivalence of generic and brand-name levothyroxine products in the treatment of hypothyroidism. *JAMA.* 1997;277:1205–1213.

35. Prinz PN, Scanlan JM, Vitaliano PP, et al. Thyroid hormones: positive relationships with cognition in healthy, euthyroid older men. *J Gerontol Ser A, Biol Sci Med Sci.* 1999;54: M111–M116.

36. Castro MR, Gharib H. Thyroid nodules and cancer: when to wait and watch, when to refer. *Postgrad Med.* 2000;107(1):113–116, 119–120, 123–124.

37. Csako G, Byrd D, Wesley RA, et al. Assessing the effects of thyroid suppression on benign solitary thyroid nodules: a model for using quantitative research synthesis. *Medicine.* 2000;79:9–26.

38. Shaha AR. Controversies in the management of thyroid nodule. *The Laryngoscope.* 2000;110:183–193.

39. Barraclough BM, Barraclough BH. Ultrasound of the thyroid and parathyroid glands. *World J Surg.* 2000; 24:158–165.

40. Cerbone G, Spiezia S, Colao A, et al. Power Doppler improves the diagnostic accuracy of color Doppler ultrasonography in cold thyroid nodules: follow-up results. *Horm Res.* 1999;52:19–24.

41. Bianda T, Schmid C. De Quervain's subacute thyroiditis presenting as a painless solitary nodule. *Postgrad Med. J.* 1998;74 (876):602–603.

42. McHenry CR, Slusarczyk SJ, Khiyama A. Recommendations for management of cystic thyroid disease. *Surgery.* 1999;126:1167–1172.

43. Liu Q, Djuricin G, Prinz RA. Total thyroidectomy for benign thyroid disease. *Surgery.* 1998;123:2–7.

44. Miccoli P, Berti P, Conte M, Bendinelli C, Marcocci C. Minimally invasive surgery for thyroid small nodules: preliminary report. *J Endocrinol Invest.* 1999;22: 849–851.

8

Delirium and Depression

Lenore H. Kurlowicz

Introduction

Delirium and depression are prevalent mental problems in older adults that contribute to poor health outcomes and more frequent institutionalization.[1,2,3] Despite this evidence, the detection of these disorders is poor, resulting in unnecessary morbidity and mortality in this population. A substantial number of older adults encountered by advanced practice nurses have delirium and/or depression. Advanced practice nurses remain at the front line in early recognition of delirium and depression and facilitation of older adults' access to mental health care. This chapter summarizes the literature as it relates to delirium and depression in older adults with emphasis on risk factors, age-related assessment considerations, atypical symptomatology, clinical decision making, and interventions. Standardized protocols on delirium and depression for use by advanced practice nurses in a variety of practice settings also are presented.

Delirium

Delirium, also known as acute confusion, is a highly prevalent and serious health problem for acutely ill older adults.[4] Delirium is defined as a transient and etiologically nonspecific organic mental syndrome characterized by a reduced ability to focus, sustain, or shift attention; disturbance of consciousness or cognition (such as memory loss, disorientation, or language disturbance); or the development of perceptual disturbance.[5] Perceptual disturbances often are accompanied by delusional (paranoid) thoughts further contributing to behavioral and emotional manifestations.[6] The onset of delirium is always acute or subacute, developing over a short period of time (usually hours to days), tending to fluctuate over the course

of the day, and often worsening at night.[5] Prior to onset, a prodromal phase with symptoms including anxiety, restlessness, insomnia, and disturbing dreams may be evident. The clinical course of delirium is variable. The possibilities are full recovery with early detection and intervention, or progression to stupor or coma, seizures, and death. Recovery is the most common outcome and in most cases completely resolves within one to four weeks.[5] Following recovery, some patients are amnestic for the entire episode, while others may have islands of memory.[7]

Significance

Delirium is associated with loss of function, falls, and other complications. Patients with delirium are at increased risk for longer lengths of hospital stay, more likely to be institutionalized post-hospital, and require more nursing and home health-care services.[8] Agitated behaviors frequently associated with delirium also can lead to use of physical and chemical restraints, further compounding the risk of functional loss and serious complications.[9] Cost of delirium has been assessed at $4 billion a year.[10] General medical conditions, substance intoxication, and substance withdrawal are common causal factors.[10] The frequent misdiagnosis of delirium, often as depression or dementia, and subsequent failure to recognize the etiology of delirium, results in high morbidity and mortality.[11] Because of its clinical impact and potential reversibility, efforts for primary prevention, early recognition, and prompt treatment of delirium are essential. Failure to diagnose delirium, or the misdiagnosis as depression or dementia, and the subsequent failure to recognize the etiology of delirium, compounds the poor prognosis and outcomes associated with delirium.

Epidemiology and Risk Factors

Delirium occurs in approximately 10% of all hospitalized patients.[4] Older patients are especially susceptible to this disorder, with delirium rates ranging from 22–38% in older hospitalized patients.[12] Little is known about delirium in long-term care or community settings. Recently, however, a 40.5% prevalence of delirium in an older long-term care population was reported.[13] Delirium rates increase significantly as the number of underlying risk factors accumulates (Table 8–1). The marked variability in the epidemiology of delirium results from the differences in study populations, diagnostic criteria, case finding, and research techniques.[2,14,15] Studies employing standardized definitions of delirium that are criteria based by the Diagnostic and Statistical Manual of Mental Disorders[5,16,17] report prevalence (delirium on admission) rates from 11% to 33% among older hospitalized patients, while incidence (delirium developed during hospital stay) rates vary from 3% to 42%.[2,18] Older patients, in particular those with a preexisting dementia, may be discharged from the hospital while still delirious.[8,19,20]

Any condition that compromises brain function can cause delirium. Table 8–2 lists the common causes of delirium in hospitalized elders. Patients who are older, sicker, and cognitively impaired are

Table 8–1   Risk Factors for Delirium

Advanced age (especially >80 years)

Dementia

Severe illness

Comorbidity of illness

Alcoholism

Depression

Sensory impairment

Dehydration

Polypharmacy (>4 medications daily)

Symptomatic infection

Previous episodes of delirium

Table 8–2   Common Causes of Delirium in Older Hospitalized Patients[27]

Medication

Pain

Dehydration

Electrolyte and metabolic disturbances

Infection

most vulnerable to delirium during hospitalization.[21] Anticholinergic medications, which block cholinergic transmitters in the brain, are thought to be the primary drug-related causes of delirium.[18,22] Fourteen of the 25 drugs most commonly prescribed for the elderly, including furosemide (Lasix), lanoxin (Digoxin), theophylline, and nifedipine (Adalat and Procardia), have detectable anticholinergic effects.[22] Alcohol withdrawal or sedative-hypnotic drug withdrawal also may underlie delirium. Over-the-counter (OTC) "home remedies" may increase an older adult's risk for delirium because many have anticholinergic effects (NSAIDS, nasal sprays, cold and flu medicines).[23]

Infections, especially pyelonephritis and pneumonia, commonly cause delirium in older adults, even in the absence of sepsis.[24] Fluid and electrolyte disturbances and major organ system failure often induce delirium,[24] as does anesthesia given for surgery or trauma. For example, a 61% incidence of delirium has been reported among older patients undergoing surgery for hip fracture.[25] Hospitalization is stressful and can contribute to the development of delirium. When several potential etiologies exist, the delirium rate is very high.

Delirium research increasingly has focused on the identification of risk factors or predictors to target high-risk patients in medical and surgical settings. Numerous equations predicting the occurrence of delirium have been developed. A recent model by Inouye and Charpentier[26] consists of variables that are easily identifiable, measurable, and controllable by nurses. This model relies on the interaction of predisposing host baseline factors (vision impairment, severe illness, preexisting cognitive impairment, and dehydration) present on hospital admission with hospital and treatment-related precipitating factors (use of physical restraints, malnutrition, use of bladder catheter, more than three medications added, and any iatrogenic event). Inouye and Charpentier's model is the most clinically useful in identifying and quantifying risk for delirium, while providing direction for minimizing such risk. The model is particularly useful because it allows for adjustment based on a patient's risk for delirium depending on changes in status over the course of hospitalization. Because the model was developed and tested on a hospitalized older population, it may not be applicable in other settings where predictability may be altered.

Clinical Presentation

Three clinical subtypes of delirium have been described: hyperactive, hypoactive, and mixed. Hyperactive patients show increased psychomotor activity, such as rapid speech, irritability, and restlessness. Providers recognize and seek treatment for the hyperactive-hyperalert variant of delirium more readily than the other subtypes, as the resultant behaviors often disrupt or interfere with diagnostic activities, medical therapies, and nursing care.[27] Hypoactive patients present with lethargy, slowed speech, decreased alertness, and apathy. Patients with hypoactive delirium are not disruptive to others and are often overlooked or misdiagnosed as being depressed. Patients with mixed delirium shift between hyperactive and hypoactive states. Thus, it may be assumed that delirium has improved, whereas it actually may have worsened.[27,28] Knowledge of these clinical subtypes may facilitate identification of the underlying etiologic agent(s).[27] For example, the hyperactive subtype may be related to hypoxia or a rapid weaning of corticosteroids;[13,27] the hypoactive variant may result from a drug or metabolic impairment (altered hepatic or renal function). One study of delirium subtypes found that 52% were mixed, 19% were hypoactive, and 15% were hyperactive; 14% were neither (patients classified as "neither" did not demonstrate a cluster of hyperactive or hypoactive symptoms).[29,30]

Diagnostic Evaluation

History   The history is extremely helpful in establishing a diagnosis of delirium and its cause. Family members and nursing staff should be questioned regarding baseline mental function and any recent mental status changes.

> When did the confusion begin?
>
> Does the condition change over a 24-hour period?
>
> Have sleep patterns changed?
>
> Have problems in thinking occurred?
>
> Is there a history of mental illness or similar thought disturbance?
>
> Has there been a sudden decline in physical function or a new onset of falls?

Interviews with knowledgeable family or caregivers is key when attempting to detect delirium with chronic dementing illness.

Since delirium has an organic etiology, the current history is essential for identifying acute organic illness. New onset urinary incontinence often occurs with delirium. Obtaining the patient's past medical history, medications, social habits, and review of systems is critical to the identification of possible causes of delirium.

Physical Examination   The hallmark of delirium is an abnormal mental status examination. Mental status screening tests are helpful in identifying cognitive deficits and should be performed routinely in older patients.[31] Several instruments for routine, standardized, and systematic assessment of changes in cognitive status or detection of delirium have been described and reviewed in the literature.[32]

The Mini-Mental State Examination (MMSE) is most favored as a helpful screening test for assessing cognition.[33,34] The range of scores on the MMSE is 0–30, with a score of 23 or less indicative of cognitive disturbance.[35] For those with low scores, consideration should be given to advanced age, lower education level, fatigue, and characteristics of the testing environment.[36] If drawing is difficult, the Short Portable Mental Status Questionnaire (SPMSQ) is appropriate.[37]

Further investigation of mental status helps to confirm suspected delirium. The letter-recognition test highlights attention problems.[38] After instructing the patient to raise his or her hand only when the letter "A" is heard, the examiner then begins saying letters from the alphabet randomly. Delirious patients have inconsistent responses.

Two instruments specific for detecting delirium based on observation of behavior rather than formal testing have been developed. Both instruments are suitable for use at the bedside and can aid the nurse in identifying patients who are likely to suffer from delirium.

The NEECHAM Confusion Scale[39] allows rapid evaluation for acute confusion at the bedside using a structured database derived during routine nursing assessments and interactions with patients. Testing can be repeated at frequent intervals to monitor changes in mental status because the scale is comprised of items that have no learning effect. Additional advantages of the NEECHAM scale are its capacity to detect delirium in its early stages and its sensitivity to both the hyperactive and hypoactive forms of delirium.[39] Nine components of information processing, performance, and vital function items are evaluated in this scale, allowing detection not only of changes in mental status, but also changes and different patterns of physiologic and behavioral manifestations over short time periods. The range of scores is 0–30. The following cut-off scores for clinical practice are suggested: 0–19 = moderate to severe delirium; 20–24 = mild or early development of delirium; 25–26 = no delirium, but high risk for acute confusion; and more than 24 = no delirium.

The Confusion Assessment Method (CAM) diagnostic algorithm[40] (Figure 8–1) is also an easy-to-use, standardized method for quick, accurate screening of delirium. The CAM, based on criteria from the Diagnostic and Statistical Manual of Mental Disorders (DSM-III-R),[17] captures information about the cardinal elements of delirium (i.e., acute onset and fluctuating course, altered level of consciousness, disorganized thinking, inattention), based on specific observations relevant to each of these elements. Patients are identified as positive for delirium using the CAM if 3 out of 4 features are present.

A comprehensive physical examination usually uncovers the likely causes of delirium. Careful examination of the chest and abdomen, as well as hypo- and hyperthermia, may reveal infectious etiologies. Tachycardia may be a sign of infection, alcohol withdrawal, or heart failure. Other signs of heart failure include a third heart sound, basilar rales, and dependent edema. Suprapubic and rectal examination may reveal urinary retention and fecal impaction. A neurological examination might uncover the focal deficits of cerebrovascular injury. Signs of meningitis, subdural hemorrhage, and normal-pressure hydrocephalus may also be found. Tremor and restlessness suggest alcohol withdrawal. Asterixis and myoclonus are suggestive of a metabolic encephalopathy, such as that associated with liver failure.[38]

Diagnostic Tests   The choice of diagnostic tests is based on the history and physical findings.[34,41] Baseline laboratory studies include a complete blood count, urinalysis, and determination of electrolyte, calcium, blood urea nitrogen, creatinine, glucose, albumin, liver enzyme levels, and thyroid function tests. Electrocardiography and chest radiographs also are indicated.

Thyroid function tests, determination of vitamin B_{12} and folic acid levels, and screening for syphilis are warranted in selected patients with chronic mental status changes. To detect toxic ingestions, it is helpful to obtain drug and heavy metal screens and determine drug levels. When central nervous system trauma or vascular injury are suspected, computed tomographic (CT) scanning or magnetic resonance imaging (MRI) are beneficial. Signs of infection call for appropriate culture, and lumbar puncture is indicated if meningitis is a diagnostic consideration. If cardiopulmonary disease is a possibility, determination of cardioenzymes and arterial blood gases should be performed. Debate continues about the nature of the relationships between sensory impairment, the environment, and delirium. Some argue that the relationship between sensory impairment and delirium is causal, while others maintain that it is coincidental. Extremes in environmental characteristics are common with delirium, but it is

Feature 1. Acute onset and fluctuating course
This feature is usually obtained from a family member or nurse and is shown by positive responses to the following questions: Is there evidence of an acute change in mental status from the patient's baseline? Did the (abnormal) behavior fluctuate during the day; that is, tend to come and go, or increase and decrease in intensity?

Feature 2. Inattention
This feature is shown by a positive response to the following question: Did the patient have difficulty focusing attention; for example, being easily distractible or having difficulty keeping track of what was being said?

Feature 3. Disorganized thinking
This feature is shown by a positive response to the following question: Was the patient's thinking disorganized or incoherent, such as rambling or irrelevant conversation, unclear or illogical flow of ideas, or unpredictable switching from subject to subject?

Feature 4. Altered level of consciousness
This feature is shown by any answer other than "alert" to the following question: Overall, how would you rate this patient's level of consciousness? (alert [normal], vigilant [hyperalert], lethargic [drowsy, easily aroused], stupor [difficult to arouse], or coma [unarousable]

Figure 8–1
The Confusion Assessment Method (CAM): diagnostic algorithm. The diagnosis of delirium by the CAM requires the presence of features 1 and 2 and either 3 or 4.

unknown whether or not environmental factors are related to the genesis of delirium.[42]

When it is difficult to differentiate delirium from an acute psychotic state, electroencephalography is helpful. The electroencephalogram reveals diffuse slowing in most cases of delirium, fast activity in cases of delirium related to drug withdrawal, and normal patterns in patients with acute functional psychosis.[18]

Differential Diagnosis

The clinical history, physical examination, and laboratory studies usually differentiate delirium from other causes of confusion. The chronic confusion of dementia occurs gradually, persists greater than one month, and is usually irreversible. Although both dementia and delirium cause cognitive impairment, most demented patients are alert and able to maintain attention in the early stages. Sudden cognitive or functional deterioration of a patient with dementia suggests a superimposed delirium.[38] Depression with apathy, slowed speech, and mood disturbance may mimic hypoactive delirium. Acute functional psychosis also can resemble delirium. Functional psychosis usually has its onset at an earlier age and most older patients with functional psychosis have a history of psychiatric illness. In patients with functional psychosis, hallucinations tend to be auditory and delusions are more elaborate than those associated with delirium. Consultation with a psychiatrist or a neurologist may be necessary in difficult cases.[38]

Table 8–3   Prevention of Delirium
in Older Adults[38]

Community support systems

Immunizations

Early treatment of medical illness

Rapid diagnosis and treatment of medical illness

Elimination of deliriogenic medications

Pain control

Early detection

Identifying risk factors

Rapid treatment of underlying organic cause(s)

Prevention

Preventing delirium in older patients requires addressing the components of sound geriatric care[38] (Table 8–3). Community support systems, such as home health care and geriatric daycare, can assist family and friends in the care of frail older persons. Immunizations for influenza and pneumococcal pneumonia may prevent a serious illness leading to delirium. Frequent evaluations for early treatment of medical illness may prevent hospitalizations that contribute to delirium. If hospitalization is required, efforts can be made to ensure rapid diagnosis and treatment. Medications known to precipitate or worsen delirium, especially anticholinergics, sedative-hypnotics, and narcotics, should be used sparingly. Stressful situations should be addressed, such as the control of pain and avoidance of critical care settings.[38] Family and community support must be enlisted to detect delirium in early stages. Prevention of delirium rests on the recognition of risk factors and the rapid treatment of the underlying organic cause.

Prognosis

The prognosis of older hospitalized patients with delirium is worse than the prognosis of those without delirium.[12,14,43] Delirious patients are sicker and have longer periods of hospitalization.[12,43] Hospital mortality rates are high, rang-

ing from 6–35%.[43,44] After hospitalization, delirious patients show more cognitive impairment and have greater rates of institutionalization.[10,45] Mortality rates after hospitalizations are also high: 14–26% at six months, [22,46] 39% at two years,[12] and 66% at four years.[47]

Management

Effective management of delirium requires prompt treatment of the underlying cause and creation of a maximum supportive environment.[4] Immediate medical treatment is necessary because further deterioration may occur rapidly. Medications thought to be deliriogenic should be discontinued or reduced to a minimum. Adequate nutrition and hydration are essential, since many delirious patients present in a malnourished state with a low serum albumin level. When oral feeding is not tolerated, enteral tube feeding or hyperalimentation may be necessary. Treatment of the underlying pathology typically results in rapid improvement of delirium.[48]

The importance of a supportive environment should be emphasized in the care of the delirious patient. Presence of family members, friends, or those who have a familiar and calming influence on the patient provide needed reassurance, relieve anxiety, prevent disorientation, and enhance connections to the immediate environment.[38] Having a relative present on admission to the hospital is generally helpful. Familiar items from home, such as photographs, a favorite pillow, or piece of clothing may be comforting. Sensory losses that contribute to misperceptions can be minimized with eyeglasses and hearing aids. A night-light and minimal noise can provide a soothing environment for sleep. Sleep should not be interrupted unless absolutely necessary. Consolidation of nighttime treatments, rescheduling of medications, as well as other unit-wide noise reduction strategies can help create an environment conducive to sleep.[49,50] In order to maximize visualization of the delirious patient and to monitor frequently for changes in behavior, placement in a room with a window near the nurses' station is useful.

Specific interventions, such as techniques to reinforce orientation and increase continuity of care, decrease the incidence of delirium after hip fracture.[51] Having someone remain with the patient on a one-to-one basis allows constant supervision to prevent injury and provides respite for family members during periods of increased psychomotor agitation.[49] Creative strategies to enhance protection of medical therapies (e.g., roll bandages over IV sites or an abdominal binder over abdominal dressings or tubes) should be employed, thus avoiding the use of physical restraints altogether or using for very brief periods only.[11]

Planning effective communication strategies provides patients with the information needed to maintain control and remain connected to the immediate environment. Communication aimed at reorienting the patient to surroundings (e.g., large, easily visible clock and calendar, a board with names of care team members, the daily schedule, and integration of orienting cues into the daily routine) is key. Cognitive enhancement strategies (e.g., discussion of current events, discussion of specific interests, structured reminiscence, and word games) should be incorporated into the plan of care and initiated several times a day.[40] Efforts must be taken to maintain a sense of independence and control with the uncertainties of hospitalization.[27]

Care must be taken to avoid the complications of immobility. Skin breakdown can be minimized by frequently turning the patient, ambulating at regular intervals when permitted, providing appropriate bedding, and by maintaining a dry skin surface. Bowel and bladder problems, especially constipation, diarrhea, and urinary incontinence, warrant prompt attention. Pulmonary care often is necessary to avoid atelectasis and pneumonia. Early ambulation, strengthening exercises, active and passive range of motion, and minimal use of immobilizing equipment (bladder catheters or physical restraints) help to preserve function.[50] Physical therapy should be utilized routinely.[52]

Pharmacologic Intervention

Pharmacologic agents may be useful when behaviors associated with psychotic thinking and perceptual disturbances (e.g., hallucinations) pose a safety risk for the patient and others, if the delirium interferes with needed medical therapies, or in those cases in which behavioral interventions fail.[27] Medication should not be a substitute for detection, correction, or elimination of the underlying cause or causes of delirium. In addition, medication should be used with caution because older delirious patients are especially sensitive to the anticholinergic side effects of antipsychotic drugs, which may worsen the delirium. Drugs should be given in low doses over the shortest possible time period.

Typically, low-dose, high-potency neuroleptics like haloperidol have been used as a first-line therapy in the treatment of delirium.[53] Although these drugs in general have a tolerable side effect profile and can be administered parenterally, they are frequently associated with extrapyramidal symptoms (EPS) such as dystonic reactions, akathisia, and tardive dyskinesia. EPS is more common in older and severely medically ill patients, who are more likely to develop delirium especially in the hospital setting. Newer antipsychotics, such as olanzapine and risperidone, with a lower incidence of EPS, may be better tolerated than typical antipsychotics in older patients, and may be useful alternatives to haloperidol in the treatment of delirium.[53,54] Neuroleptic Malignant Syndrome (NMS), a more serious side effect of antipsychotic therapy, can occur with high-potency, as well as with novel, antipsychotics.[55] Benzodiazepines such as lorazepam are recommended for the treatment of delirium associated with alcohol-withdrawal. In cases of non-alcohol-withdrawal delirium, benzodiazepines have the potential to worsen delirium and should be used with caution.

Aftercare

An important focus for care after resolution of the acute confusion is to provide an opportunity to discuss the experience and its meaning. Understanding the bizarre and bewildering experience of delirium can be therapeutic.[56] Delirium represents a stressful life event and psychiatric care can facilitate its resolution. Sensitive retrospective exploration may help the patient to understand the temporary loss of control within the context of physical disease. Schofeld found that many older patients were willing to describe their experiences, especially those that had elaborate illusions and/or hallucinations.[56] Increasing the older patient's understanding and acceptance of the condition could lead to a more optimistic view of the future and, in turn, a more rapid recovery. At the time of any future hospitalization, patients should be instructed to inform health-care providers of their prior episode of delirium and suspected etiology. Comprehensive discharge planning, including referrals to home-care services, such as psychiatric nursing home-care services, and physical and occupational therapy, should be initiated for this high-risk group of older adults.

Conclusion

Historically, delirium has been considered a benign condition accompanying acute illness in older patients and receiving little attention by health-care providers. Delirium, however, is a serious health problem associated with significant negative consequences. Because of its clinical impact and potential reversibility, prompt treatment is essential. Nurses are most often at the front line in the early identification of patients most at risk for delirium, as well as early detection of symptoms. Routine and systematic assessment for confusion is key in order to prevent and effectively treat delirium and reduce its negative consequences (Figure 8–2).

Depression

The NIH Consensus Statement on the Diagnosis and Treatment of Depression in Late Life noted that depression in older adults is a major public health problem.[57] Central to its importance is the suffering experienced by those whose depression remains unrecognized, the burden experienced by families and institutions who provide care to older adults, and the increased health-care needs and costs associated with depressed older adults. Depression afflicts a considerable portion of the

---

A. Assess patient's risk for delirium:
    1. Older adults (especially 80 & older)
    2. Preexisting chronic confusion (i.e., dementia or other brain disease/injury)
    3. Severe illness or high medical comorbidity (≥ 2 chronic health conditions)
    4. Vision/hearing impairment
    5. Polypharmacy (≥ 4 medications)
    6. Chronic alcohol and/or drug use
    7. Dehydration
    8. History of acute confusion

B. Assess for key features of delirium using the Confusion Assessment Method (CAM) (Figure 8–1).

C. Assess for evidence of other features of delirium as evidenced by the *acute* onset of any of the following symptoms that are a *change* from the patient's baseline mental status:
    1. Increasing lethargy
    2. Appears frightened or suspicious of others
    3. Illusions, hallucinations (may be manifested by climbing out of bed, pulling at tubes, refusing treatments, calling out for family)
    4. Disorientation (mostly time)
    5. Nighttime agitation
    6. New onset of memory problems

Figure 8–2
Nursing guide for assessment and management of acute confusion/delirium.[49]

D. Interview consistent caregivers and family (when possible) to determine patient's baseline mental functioning and behavior.

E. Assess organic etiologic factors contributing to acute confusion:
1. Lab profile, especially blood chemistries (BUN/creatinine, CBC, glucose, ammonia, liver enzymes, albumin), drug levels, urinalysis, pulse oximetry, and ABG
2. ECG, chest x-ray, CAT scan (if applicable)
3. Medication record (especially those with CNS/anti-cholinergic side effects; e.g., narcotics, sedative-hypnotics, steroids, antihistamines, H_2 receptor blockers, or antispasmodics)
4. Vital signs (especially elevated temperature)
5. Assess pain control
6. Assess for alcohol and/or drug withdrawal

NOTE: Explore all possible etiologic factors since multiple causal agents are usually involved in the origin of delirium.

F. Review medication records daily; discontinue and minimize use of nonessential medication, especially those with CNS/anti-cholinergic effects; substitute alternatives less likely to cause delirium. In particular, explore whether there was a recent (within the previous 72 hours) change (especially addition of new drugs) in medication regimen.

G. Monitor vital signs, oxygenation, and I & O q shift and as needed. Implement other target-specific nursing interventions to correct the underlying problem(s) as warranted by the medical evaluation and based on the individual needs of the patient (e.g., hydration, antibiotic therapy, blood transfusion, pain regimen change).

H. Ensure adequate pain control.

I. Eliminate urinary and other catheters/tubes as soon as possible.

J. Increase and maintain close observation of patient (observation room, unit staff or family member to stay with patient—including nighttime—private duty staff, companions) until patient's confusion resolves.

K. Avoid/minimize use of restraints/medical immobilization (may increase a patient's risk for delirium).

L. Decrease stimulation, but avoid sensory deprivation (private room if possible; maintain consistency/continuity of care; decrease room clutter and noise level).

M. Provide frequent verbal orientation on an ongoing, consistent basis. Enhance orientation through the use of aids such as a clock, calendar, and familiar objects from home, such as eyeglasses, hearing aid, and nightlight.

N. Normalize sleep pattern; reorganize care, especially at night, to provide increased amounts of uninterrupted sleep; i.e., consolidate treatments, medications, vital signs.

O. Consult physical and occupational therapy.

P. Consider consultation by psychiatry and/or neurology for psychosis, severe agitation, complex interplay of etiologic factors (for diagnostic evaluation and medication regimen), or if symptoms worsen or do not resolve within 48 hours.

Q. Clarify use and dosage of existing ordered neuroleptic psychotropic medications. Neuroleptic agents such as haloperidol (Haldol) should only be used for target symptoms such as hallucinations, paranoid thoughts, and severe agitation. These agents should be used with caution in older adults. Benzodiazepines are usually the drug of choice for alcohol withdrawal but have the potential to worsen delirium in non–alcohol-withdrawal cases.

R. Assess and document mental function and behavior every shift until acute confusion is resolved.

S. Provide emotional support, especially reassurance, for patients.

T. Reassess daily for delirium and prior to discharge using the CAM.

U. Debrief patient/family after delirium resolves.

Figure 8–2 (Continued)

older population, but the coexistence of many physical, social, and economic problems frequently impedes timely recognition and treatment, with subsequent unnecessary morbidity and mortality.[58]

Depression Defined

Everybody gets the "blues" now and then. Transient depressed mood or being "down in the dumps" is a part of life, especially in response to the loss of a loved one, hospitalization, separation from one's family, or other stressful life events.[59] When depressed mood persists with loss of enjoyment or pleasure after visiting with family or friends or after performing an activity that was previously enjoyable, or when general daily functioning and well-being are limited, a more serious depression may exist requiring clinical attention, regardless of the situation or circumstances.[60]

In the broadest sense, depression is defined as a syndrome comprised of a constellation of affective, cognitive, and somatic or physiological manifestations.[57] Depression may range in severity from mild symptoms to more severe forms, both of which can persist over longer periods of time with negative consequences for the elderly patient. Suicidal ideation, psychotic features, especially delusional thinking, and excessive somatic concerns frequently accompany more severe depression.[57,61]

The 4th edition of the Diagnostic and Statistical Manual of Mental Disorders (DSM-IV)[62] currently lists specific criteria that are necessary for a diagnosis of a Major Depressive Disorder (MDD), the most serious form of depression, and that are frequently used as the standard by which older adults' depressive symptoms are counted in clinical settings (Table 8–4).[62] Five symptoms from a list of nine (affective, cognitive, and somatic) must be present nearly every day during the same two-week period and must represent a change from previous functioning.

Ambiguous and Atypical Symptomatology

Older adults may manifest additional atypical symptoms of depression that are not included in the DSM criteria for depression. In particular,

Table 8–4   Key Diagnostic Criteria for Major Depressive Disorder[62]

1. Depressed mood indicated either by subjective account or observation by others
2. Markedly diminished interest or pleasure in almost all activities
3. Significant weight loss or weight gain or decrease or increase in appetite
4. Insomnia or hypersomnia
5. Psychomotor agitation or retardation
6. Fatigue or loss of energy
7. Feelings of worthlessness or inappropriate guilt
8. Diminished ability to think or concentrate
9. Recurrent thoughts of death or suicide

A major depressive disorder is defined as a minimum of five symptoms present nearly every day during the same two-week period and representing a change from previous functioning; at least one of the symptoms is either #1 or #2.

older adults may more readily report somatic or physical symptoms than depressed mood.[63] The somatic or physical symptoms of depression are often difficult to distinguish from somatic or physical symptoms associated with acute or chronic physical illnesses, especially in the hospitalized elderly patient, or the somatic symptoms that are part of common aging processes.[64] For example, disturbed sleep may be associated with a chronic lung disease, heart failure, or changes in sleeping patterns or habits. Diminished energy or an increased lethargy may be caused by an acute metabolic disturbance or drug response. Somatic symptoms may indicate a more serious depression when they are severe or persist, despite treatment of the underlying medical illness or discontinuance of a depressogenic medication.[64] Several experts also have suggested that the presence of affective and cognitive symptoms may be more useful in detecting a serious depression in the presence of multiple somatic complaints in medically ill older adults.[65,66] Furthermore, symptoms of anxiety also frequently coexist in as many as 90% of depressed older adults; dementia-like symptoms also may be exhibited.[61] Moreover, depression may be expressed nonverbally through repetitive verbalizations (e.g., calling out for help) or agitated vocalizations (e.g., screaming, yelling, or shouting), irritability, demandingness, repetitive questions, expressions of unrealistic fears (e.g., fear of abandonment, being left alone), repetitive statements that something bad will happen, and repetitive health-related concerns or complaints.[67] Nurses should remain alert to these nonverbal cues of depression in persons with coexisting dementia in whom the somatic/vegetative symptoms of depression (e.g., psychomotor retardation, weight loss, insomnia, fatigue, decreased libido) may be attributable simultaneously to the dementing illness.

Minor Depression

Although major depression appears to be less common among older than younger cohorts, there is increasing evidence of a high prevalence of less severe depressive symptoms that do not meet the duration criteria or show the number of symptoms necessary for major depression, but that are states of clinical significance and for which treatment may be warranted.[68] Such depressive symptomatology has been variously referred to in the literature as "minor depression," "subsyndromal depression," "subdysthymic depression," "subclinical depression," and "elevated depressive symptoms" and "mild depression." Minor depression is two to four times as common as major depression in older adults and is associated with increased risk of subsequent major depression and greater use of health services, as well as having a negative impact on physical and social functioning and quality of life.[68,69,70]

Course, Etiology, and Risk Factors

Depression in late life can occur for the first time late in life, or it can be part of a long-standing affective or mood disorder. Some studies of hospitalized elders have shown that elevated depressive

symptoms, even in the absence of a discrete depressive disorder, may be a continuation or exacerbation of a preexisting psychological condition and not an "expected" reaction to acute physical illness or hospitalization.[71] Older depressed hospitalized medically ill patients were also more likely to have had a previous depression or other psychiatric illness, including alcohol abuse.[72] As in younger people, the course of depression in older adults is characterized by exacerbations, remissions, and chronicity.[57]

Despite major advances, the etiology of depression occurring at any age is not fully understood, although biological and psychosocial etiologies for late-life depression have been proposed. These play an important and interactive role. Genetic factors or heredity are less likely to be associated with depression in older adults, especially for those who are experiencing depression for the first time in late life. Heredity seems to play a more major role when elders have suffered with depression throughout life. Additional biological causes proposed for late-life depression include neurotransmitter or "chemical messenger" imbalance and dysregulation of endocrine function.[73] A final pathway to late-onset depression, suggested by CT and MRI studies, may involve structural, neuroanatomic factors. Enlarged lateral ventricles, cortical atrophy, increased white-matter hyperintensities, decreased caudate size, and vascular lesions in the caudate nucleus appear to be especially prominent in late-onset depression associated with vascular risk factors.[74] Possible psychosocial etiologies for depression in older adults include cognitive distortions, stressful life events, especially loss, chronic stress, and low self-efficacy expectations.[73,75]

While age alone is not a risk factor for depression, age-related social and demographic risk factors for depression in late life include being female, unmarried (particularly widowed), stressful life events, and the absence of a supportive social network.[57] In older adults, there is additional emphasis on the cooccurrence of specific physical conditions such as stroke, cancer, dementia, arthritis, hip fracture surgery, myocardial infarction, chronic obstructive pulmonary disorder (COPD), and Parkinson's disease. Medical co-morbidity is the hallmark of depression in older adults and this factor represents a major difference from depression in younger cohorts.[58] Those older adults with functional disabilities, especially those with new functional loss, also are at risk. The more severe the medical illness and associated functional disability, the greater the likelihood of depression in older adults.[60] Specific subgroups of older adults who are at greater risk for depression include the chronically physically ill, institutionalized elders, the recently bereaved, and older family members caring for chronically ill relatives.[57]

Prevalence

Depression in late life is common. Nearly 5 million of the 31 million Americans aged 65 and older suffer from depression.[58] Prevalence studies report significant rates of combined major and minor depression in various populations of older adults: community dwelling (13%), medical outpatients (24%), acute care (30%), and nursing homes (43%).[73] Certain populations have higher levels of depressive symptoms, particularly those with more severe or chronic disabling conditions, such as those elders in acute and long-term care settings. Depression also frequently coexists with dementia, specifically Alzheimer's disease, with prevalence rates ranging from 10%–40%.[76,77] Cognitive impairment may be a secondary symptom of depression, or depression may be secondary to dementia.[73]

Consequences of Depression in Late Life

Research has shown that untreated depression is associated with serious negative consequences for older adults, especially for frail elders, such as those recovering from a severe medical illness or those in nursing homes. Consequences of depression include amplification of pain and disability, delayed recovery from medical illness or surgery, worsening of medical symptoms, risk of physical illness, increased health-care utilization, alcoholism, cognitive impairment, worsening social impairment, protein-calorie subnutrition, and increased rates of suicide and nonsuicide mortality.[76] The recent "amplification" hypothesis states that de-pression can "turn up the volume" on several aspects of physical, psychosocial, and behavioral functioning in elderly patients, ultimately accelerating the course of medical illness.[60] For older nursing-home residents, depression is also associated with poor adjustment to the nursing home, resistance to daily care, treatment refusal, inability to participate in activities, and further social isolation.[79] Major depression can also contribute to both cognitive impairment and functional disability in older adults with Alzheimer's disease.[77] Comorbid depression in dementia, through its influence on motivation, motor responsivity, and cognition, is a major source of excess disability in this population.

Suicide   Mortality rates by suicide are higher among older persons with depression than among their nondepressed counterparts and cannot be accounted for by sociodemographic factors or preexisting illness.[80] Older adults commit suicide at disproportionate rates that appear to be increasing, and they are more successful at completing suicide than any other age group.[80] Although older adults make up only 12% of the population, they account for 21% of suicides.[81] White males over 80 are at greatest risk and are six times more likely to commit suicide than the rest of the population.[80] Suicide among older adults is associated with diagnosable psychopathology, most often major depression, in approximately 90% of the cases.[80] Depression can also influence decision-making capacity and may be the cause of indirect life-threatening behavior such as refusal of food, medications, or other treatments in elderly patients.[81] Studies also have shown that more than half of those over age 65 visited a physician within one week of death, 75% within one month, and 90% within three months.[60,82,83] Most of the patients were suffering from their first episode of major depression, which was only moderately severe, yet the depressive symptoms went unrecognized and untreated.

Treatment Efficacy for Depression

Depression is the most treatable of the mental disorders in late life.[73] If recognized, the treatment response for depression is good in 60–80% of the cases and approximately 80% of elders can remain relapse free with medication maintenance for 6 to 18 months.[57] Recurrence is a serious problem with up to 40% experiencing depression chronically, especially following acute illness and hospitalization.[84] A "wait and see approach" with regard to treatment is not recommended. Continuation and maintenance treatment is necessary to prevent early relapses or recurrences.[60] Even in those patients with depression who have a co-morbid medical illness or a dementia, treatment response is good. In patients with dementia, treatment of depression also improves cognitive performance, mood, and physical and social functioning, as well as family well being.[76] Thus, appropriate and timely treatment of depression can help older adults get well and stay well.[58]

Barriers to Recognition and Treatment

Depression in older adults is highly underrecognized, misdiagnosed, and subsequently undertreated. It is estimated that as many as 90% of older adults who are considered to need mental health care, particularly those in institutions, receive no services for primary psychiatric disorders, including depression.[83] Barriers to care for older adults with depression exist at many levels. In particular, some older adults refuse to seek help because of perceived stigma of mental illness. Others may simply accept their feelings of profound sadness without realizing they are clinically depressed. Recognition of depression also is frequently obscured by the various atypical manifestations of depression in older adults or because both patients and providers believe that depression is a "natural" part of the aging process or is an understandable and logical reaction to medical illness, hospitalization, relocation to a nursing home, or other stressful life events. Thus, patients and providers frequently use age as an explanation of depression or substitute understanding or rationalization of the depression for timely recognition and appropriate treatment, with subsequent negative consequences for the elderly patient. The frequently heard statement by patients and providers, "Wouldn't you feel depressed if you were in this situation?" reflects these beliefs.

Assessment of Depression

Figure 8–3 depicts a protocol assessment and intervention of depression in older adults. Early recognition of depression is enhanced through the use of methods that are routine, standardized, and systematic, employing both a depression screening tool and individualized depression assessment or interview.[86]

Depression Screening Tool   Assessment of depression in older patients can be facilitated by the use of tools such as the Geriatric Depression Scale (GDS) (Figure 8–4).[87] The GDS is a 30-item screen by self-report that is frequently used in a variety of clinical settings. This GDS has been validated and used extensively with older adults including those who are medically ill, mild to moderately cognitively impaired, and/or institutionalized. It has a brief yes/no response format and takes approximately 10 minutes to complete. When patients cannot complete the GDS by hand, the scale can be administered by the clinician without changes in its psychometric properties. Validity and reliability are supported in clinical practice and research. In addition, the GDS contains few somatic items that may potentially confound symptoms caused by a medical illness. A GDS score of 11 or greater is considered significant for a more serious depression.[87] The GDS is not a substitute for an individualized assessment or a diagnostic interview by a mental health professional, but is a useful screening tool in a variety of clinical settings, especially when baseline measurements can be compared to subsequent scores.

Individualized Assessment and Interview Central to the individualized depression assessment or interview is assessment of the full range of symptoms (nine) for major depression as delineated by the DSM-IV.[62] A challenge in clinical settings is not to overlook or disregard atypical depressive symptoms while also looking beyond such complaints to assess the full spectrum of symptoms. Older patients should be asked directly and specifically about suicidal ideation, that is, thoughts that life is not worth living or contemplation of or attempted suicide. The number of symptoms, type, duration, frequency, and patterns

Part I.   Depression Screening Tool: Geriatric Depression Scale (GDS) (Figure 8–4)

Part II. Individualized Assessment Component

A. Depressive symptoms (depressed mood, anhedonia, appetite/sleep changes, fatigue/loss of energy, diminished concentration, psychomotor slowing/agitation, worthlessness/guilt, suicidal thoughts/hopelessness); number of symptoms, duration (esp. 2 weeks or >); frequency, patterns, clustering; type: affective, cognitive, somatic; change from normal mood, behavior, functioning

B. Psychosis (i.e., delusional/paranoid thoughts, hallucinations)

C. Personal and/or family history of depression, suicide

D. Previous coping style, history of substance abuse (esp. alcohol)

E. Anniversary dates

F. Changes in physical health status, relationships, roles

G. Recent losses or crises (death of relative, friend, pet; retirement; move to another residence, nursing home, different facility within nursing home complex; possessions)

H. Depressogenic medications (e.g., narcotics, sedatives/hypnotics, benzodiazepines, steroids, anti-hypertensives, alcohol, antipsychotics, immunosuppressives, beta-blockers, H_2 antagonists)

I. Related systemic and metabolic processes (e.g., infection, anemia, hypothyroidism, hypnatremia, hypercalcemia, CHF, renal failure)

Part III. Clinical Decision Making/Interventions

A. For severe depression (GDS score ≥ 11, 5 to 9 depressive symptoms, plus other positive responses on individualized assessment component [esp. suicidal thoughts, psychosis, coexisting substance abuse and/or dementia]), refer for a geriatric psychiatry evaluation. Treatment options: hospitalization, medication, psychotherapy (individual, group, family), and/or ECT. For suicidal thoughts, psychosis, coexisting substance abuse and/or dementia, referral for a geriatric psychiatry evaluation always should be made.

B. For less severe depression that does not meet all of above criteria, but that persists and interferes with day-to-day functioning and/or recovery from illness, refer to mental health services (for counseling/psychotherapy [individual, group, family] esp. for issues identified in individualized assessment component, and to enhance sense of mastery/personal control/self-efficacy, as well as further evaluation).

C. Consider for all levels: safety precautions for suicide risk; remove/control etiologic agents; monitor nutrition, elimination, sleep/rest patterns, physical comfort; support system enhancement (identify confidant, peer, and/or health-related support groups); structured and regular activity/exercise (PT, OT, RT); identify strengths; engage in pleasurable activities, relaxation therapies; provide spiritual guidance; offer bibliotherapy; assist with problem solving, listening empathetically, supportively, encourage expression of feelings/pleasant reminiscences; instill hope; support adaptive coping; educate about depression and treatment.

Figure 8–3
Nursing assessment guide for depression in older adults.

Choose the best answer for how you felt the past week:

1. Are you basically satisfied with your life?	Yes	No*
2. Have you dropped many of your activities and interests?	Yes*	No
3. Do you feel that your life is empty?	Yes*	No
4. Do you often get bored?	Yes*	No
5. Are you hopeful about the future?	Yes	No*
6. Are you bothered by thoughts you can't get out of our head?	Yes*	No
7. Are you in good spirits most of the time?	Yes	No*
8. Are you afraid that something bad is going to happen to you?	Yes*	No
9. Do you feel happy most of the time?	Yes	No*
10. Do you often feel helpless?	Yes*	No
11. Do you often get restless and fidgety?	Yes*	No
12. Do you prefer to stay at home rather than going out and doing new things?	Yes*	No
13. Do you frequently worry about the future?	Yes*	No
14. Do you feel you have more problems with memory than most?	Yes*	No
15. Do you think it is wonderful to be alive now?	Yes	No*
16. Do you often feel downhearted and blue?	Yes*	No
17. Do you feel pretty worthless the way you are now?	Yes*	No
18. Do you worry a lot about the past?	Yes*	No
19. Do you find life very exciting?	Yes	No*
20. Is it hard for you to get started on new projects?	Yes*	No
21. Do you feel full of energy?	Yes	No*
22. Do you feel that your situation is hopeless?	Yes	No
23. Do you think that most people are better off than you are?	Yes*	No
24. Do you frequently get upset over little things?	Yes*	No
25. Do you frequently feel like crying?	Yes*	No
26. Do you have trouble concentrating?	Yes*	No
27. Do you enjoy getting up in the morning?	Yes	No*
28. Do you prefer to avoid social gatherings?	Yes*	No
29. Is it easy for you to make decisions?	Yes	No*
30. Is your mind as clear as it used to be?	Yes	No*

Note: Each answer indicated by an asterisk counts 1 point. Scores between 15 and 22 suggest mild depression; scores above 22 suggest severe despression. The 15-item short form includes questions 1–4, 7–10, 12, 14, 15, 17, and 21–23. On the short form, scores between 5 and 9 suggest depression; scores above 9 generally indicate depression.

Figure 8–4
The Geriatric Depression Scale.[87]

of depressive symptoms, as well as a change from the patient's normal mood or functioning should be noted. The presence of concurrent medical conditions, including dementia, does not preclude a comprehensive assessment for a diagnosis of depression. Additional components of the individualized depression assessment would include:

- evidence of psychotic thinking, especially delusional thoughts
- anniversary dates of previous losses or nodal/stressful events
- previous coping style, specifically alcohol or other substance abuse
- relationship changes
- physical health changes
- a personal or family history of depression, suicide, and/or other psychiatric illness
- a general loss and crisis inventory

Older adults, with and without cognitive impairment, should be asked directly about conventional depressive symptoms. Subsequent questioning of the family, caregiver, or other individuals who observe and interact with the elder on a consistent basis and have direct knowledge of the elder's behavior, both in and out of institutions, is then recommended to obtain further information about verbal and nonverbal expressions of depression.

Table 8–5   Common Illnesses Associated with Depression in Older Adults

Hypothyroidism

Congestive heart failure

GI malignancy (esp. pancreatic)

Degenerative arthritis

Stroke

Alzheimer's dementia

Parkinson's disease

Anemia

Vitamin deficiencies

Hematologic and other systemic malignancies

Table 8–6   Common Drugs Associated with Depression in Older Adults

Alcohol

Antihypertensives

Anti-Parkinson drugs

Antipsychotics

Benzodiazepines

Beta-blockers

H-2 antagonists

Immunosuppressives

Opiate analgesics

Sedative/hypnotics

Steroids

Differentiation of Medical or Iatrogenic Etiologies of Depression   Once depressive symptoms are recognized, medical and drug-related etiologies should be explored. Tables 8–5 and 8–6 list common physical illnesses and pharmacological agents associated with depressive symptoms in older adults. In medically ill older adults with multiple medical diagnoses and medications, assessment may be more difficult.[88] Efforts should be directed toward treatment, correction, or stabilization of associated metabolic or systemic conditions and, when medically feasible, depressogenic medications should be eliminated, minimized, or substituted.

Clinical Decision Making and Treatment

The majority of depressed older adults are diagnosed and treated within primary-care practice settings. Referral to a geriatric psychiatrist should be made if symptoms indicate a major depression, suicidal thoughts, psychosis, coexisting dementia, or substance abuse are present, and scores on a depression screening tool (e.g., ≥ 11 on the GDS) are above the established cut-off for depression. Cases of less severe depressive symptoms without suicidal thoughts, psychosis, dementia, or substance abuse, but scores above the cut-off for depression, should be referred to available psychosocial services (i.e., psychiatric liaison nurses, geropsychiatric advanced practice nurses, social workers, psychologists) for psychotherapy and/or other psychosocial therapies, and for evaluation of response to medication.

The two major categories of treatment for depression in older adults are biological therapies (e.g., pharmacotherapy and electroconvulsive therapy) and psychosocial therapies (e.g., cognitive-behavioral, interpersonal, and brief psychodynamic) in both individual and group formats.[57] Marital and family therapy also may be beneficial in treating depressed elders. The type and severity of depressive symptoms influence the approach to treatment. In general, more severe depression, especially with suicidal thoughts or psychosis, requires intensive psychiatric treatment including hospitalization, medication with an antidepressant or antipsychotic drug, electroconvulsive therapy, or intensive psychosocial support.[73] Less severe depression without suicidal thoughts or psychosis may require treatment with psychotherapy or medication, often on an outpatient basis.

The specific goals of treatment are to decrease and resolve depressive symptoms, restore psychosocial function, prevent recurrence, relieve excess disability, and ease adaptation to irreversible losses. A goal of treatment also may include acceptance of medical therapies that might otherwise be refused because of hopelessness or pessimistic feelings.

Pharmacologic Intervention

Table 8–7 lists antidepressants (in the United States market) having particular relevance for older adults. In general, the agents listed are considered equally effective, although differences in tolerability may exist. Specific tricyclic antidepressants (TCAs) such as amitriptyline (Elavil), imipramine (Tofranil), or doxepin (Sinequan) are considered unsuitable in older adults because of significant side effects. The greatest problem with depression in older adults is undertreatment, in particular underdosing. Unfortunately, treatment is often withheld in the very old and the very sick.

Table 8–7   Antidepressants of Relevance to Older Adults

Tricyclics	
Nortriptyline	(Pamelor)
Desipramine	(Norpramin)
SSRIs	
Fluoxetine	(Prozac)
Sertraline	(Zoloft)
Paroxetine	(Paxil)
Fluvoxamine	(Luvox)*
Citalopram	(Celexa)
MAOIs	
Phenelzine	(Nardil)
Tranylcypromine	(Parnate)
Others	
Bupropion	(Wellbutrin)
Nefazodone	(Serzone)
Trazodone	(Desyrel)
Venlafaxine	(Effexor)
Mirtazepine	(Remeron)

*Marketed in the United States for treatment of obsessive-compulsive disorder

Tricyclic Antidepressants (TCAs)   TCAs have been used for decades, are effective in a variety of depressive conditions (including melancholia), have generally predictable kinetics, and require once-a-day dosing. Limitations of the TCAs include orthostasis (although it is rare with nortriptyline), persistent anticholinergic effects (constipation, dry mouth, urinary retention, cognitive impairment, delirium), tachycardia, sedation, and conduction defects. An ECG is required prior to and during TCA therapy. When initiating TCA therapy, "start low, go slow, but don't stop too soon."

Selective Serotonin Reuptake Inhibitors (SSRIs)
SSRIs generally are as effective as tertiary TCAs in medically well, depressed patients. Fewer data are

available on the efficacy of SSRIs in older, frail, hospitalized, medically ill patients, and further work is needed regarding effectiveness in more severely depressed patients. Many clinicians prefer the newer SSRIs because tolerability allows more adequate dosing and may be a major factor in medication compliance. Limitations include insomnia, fatigue, nausea, anorexia, restlessness, headache, sexual dysfunction, and variable drug interactions. Fluvoxamine, although used as an antidepressant in Europe since 1983, is marketed in the United States for the treatment of obsessive-compulsive disorder (OCD). Unlike the other SSRIs, this drug contributes to drowsiness and may best be given at bedtime. In addition, dose adjustments (generally a decrease) in the usual doses of certain drugs taken concurrently may be required, due to inhibition of cytochrome P450 by fluvoxamine.

Monoamine Oxidase Inhibitors (MAOIs)

Although effective and reasonably safe in young-old depressed patients (in their 60s), MAOIs often are underutilized in older adults. Benefits of MAOIs include few anticholinergic side effects and no effects on cardiac conduction. Limitations include food and drug interactions (fatalities when used with meperidine), hypo- and hypertension, weight loss or gain, and insomnia or somnolence.

Others   Buproprion has fewer side effects than the TCAs, but seizures may occur at high doses. Multiple (BID or TID) dosing is required. Since the risk of seizures is fairly low, the drug should not be eliminated entirely from consideration. Nefazodone and Trazododone have distinctive sedative effects that may be both useful and problematic. Subtle or more obvious cognitive toxicity with these drugs, and orthostatic hypotension with trazodone, limit their value for more severe geriatric depressions. Venlafaxine's relative freedom from anticholinergic effects is an advantage over TCAs for some patients. Some data suggest efficacy of venlafaxine in more severe depression or in treatment-refractory patients. Nausea is the most common side effect, leading to premature termination of therapy, and hypertensive effects must be monitored. Multiple (BID or TID) dosing

also is recommended. Mirtazapine has an attractive pharmacological profile and has been shown to have fewer anticholinergic side effects than the TCAs, as well as little effect on sexual function. Increase in appetite is frequent and may be advantageous when used with depressed patients with anorexia and weight loss.

Individualized Nursing Interventions for Depression

Psychosocial and behavioral nursing interventions for depressed elderly patients, based on individualized needs, can be incorporated into the plan of care in any practice setting.

Safety   Provision of safety precautions for patients with suicidal thinking is a priority. Institutional policies combining continuous surveillance of the patient and environmental safety measures are critical. In acute medical settings, patients may require transfer to the psychiatric service when suicidal risk is high and staffing is not adequate to provide continuous observation. In outpatient settings, continuous surveillance should be provided while emergency psychiatric evaluation and disposition are obtained. Suicidal patients also should not leave the setting unattended until the psychiatric evaluation is completed.

Psychosocial and Behavioral Interventions   Additional nursing interventions for depression include monitoring and promotion of nutrition, elimination, sleep/rest patterns, and physical comfort. Provision of adequate pain control is recommended specifically for depressed medically ill elderly patients.[89] Relaxation strategies should be offered to relieve anxiety and as an adjunct to pain management. Nursing interventions should also focus on enhancement of physical function through structured and regular activity and exercise, referrals to physical, occupational, and recreational therapies, and the development of a daily activity schedule; enhancement of social support by identifying, mobilizing, or designating a support person such as family, a confidant, friends, volunteers and other hospital resources, church members, support groups, patient or peer visitors, and particularly by accessing appropriate clergy for spiritual support; and maximization of autonomy, personal control, self-efficacy, and decision making about clinical care, daily schedules, and personal routines.[90] The use of a graded task assignment where a larger goal or task is subdivided into several small steps can be helpful in enhancing function, assuring successful experiences, and building confidence in performance of various activities.[89] Participation in regular, predictable, pleasant activities or events such as watching TV, grooming, wearing certain clothes, completing a task, or thinking pleasant thoughts can also result in more positive mood changes for depressed elderly patients.[91] A pleasant-events inventory can reveal pleasurable activities for incorporation into an elderly patient's daily schedule in a variety of settings.[91] Encouragement of pleasurable reminiscence also enhances self-esteem and alleviates depressed mood in many elderly patients.[92] Nursing interventions to encourage reminiscence include asking about their past or linking historical events with the patient's life experiences. The use of photographs, old magazines, scrapbooks, and other objects frequently stimulate discussion. Nurses provide emotional support to depressed elders by empathic, supportive listening, encouraging expression of feelings in a focused manner on issues such as grief and/or role transition, facilitating adaptive coping strategies, identifying and reinforcing strengths and capabilities, maintaining privacy and respect, and instilling hope. Emotional support is easily provided during routine contacts with the patient (e.g., while talking and during treatments or procedures).[88] Helping older patients problem solve as well as offering practical assistance with social and economic concerns (e.g., family conflict, housing, transportation, medical insurance, Social Security income, payment of medical debts), also are recommended for depressed hospitalized older patients.[90]

Monitoring and Followup   Once treatment for depression is initiated, older patients should be monitored closely for therapeutic response and potential side effects of medication. Dose adjustment of antidepressant medication may be warranted, as well as regular clinician contact in the early treatment phase. Although, in general, it is necessary to start antidepressant medication at low doses, it is also necessary to ensure that elders with persistent depressive symptoms receive adequate treatment.[93] Information should be provided to the patient regarding the depressive illness in order to increase awareness of the treatability of symptoms. Adherence to the prescribed treatment regimen should be stressed to prevent recurrence or relapse. Primary caretakers should be included in the medical plans and any education. Emotional support and respite information should be provided as needed. Psychiatric/mental health home-care services should be considered in high-risk older adults.

Conclusion

Contrary to popular belief, depression is not a natural feature of aging. Without depression, older adults have an impressive ability to cope and adapt to the stressful life events commonly encountered in late life and to establish meaningful lives for themselves. Depression often is reversible with prompt and appropriate treatment. Early recognition is central and can be enhanced by the use of a standardized protocol of assessment, early identification, and subsequent intervention and treatment. Nurses can enhance the quality of life for elderly patients and demonstrate to society that depression is the most treatable mental problem in late life. As Blazer stated, "When there is depression, hope remains!"[63]

▮ References

1. Holmes J. Psychiatric illness and length of stay in elderly patients with hip fractures. *Int J Geriatr Psych*. 1996;11:607–611.
2. Pompei P, Foreman M, Rudberg MA, et al. Delirium in hospitalized older persons: outcomes and predictors. *J Am Geriatr Soc*. 1994;42:809–815.
3. Saravay SM, Lavin M. Psychiatric comorbidity and length of stay in the general hospital. *Psychosomatics*. 1994;35:233–252.
4. Lipowski ZJ. Delirium in the elderly patient. *N Engl J Med*. 1989;320:587–592.
5. American Psychiatric Association (APA). *Diagnostic and Statistical Manual of Mental Disorders*. 4th ed. Washington, DC: author; 1994.

6. Stinnett JL, Freimuth LM, Silber SA. Postoperative delirium. In: DR Goldman, FH Brown, DM Guarnieri, eds. *Perioperative medicine*. 2nd ed. New York: McGraw-Hill; 1994:699–704.

7. Wise MG. Delirium. In: RE Hales, SC Yudolfsky, eds. *Textbook of Neuropsychiatry*. Washington, DC: American Psychiatric Press; 1988:89–105.

8. Fick D, Foreman MD. Consequences of not recognizing delirium superimposed on dementia in hospitalized elderly patients. *J Gerontol Nurs*. 2000;26:30–40.

9. Sullivan-Marx EM. Delirium and physical restraint in hospitalized elderly. *IMAGE: J Nurs Scholarship*. 1994;26:295–300.

10. Inouye SK, Schlesinger MJ, Lydon TJ. Delirium: a symptom of how hospital care is failing older persons and a window to improve quality of hospital care. *Am J Med*. 1999;106:565–573.

11. Sullivan-Marx EM, Foreman MD. Delirium. In: *Encyclopedia of Aging*. New York: Springer Publishing; in press.

12. Francis J, Kapoor WN. Delirium in hospitalized elderly. *J Gen Int Med*. 1990;5:651–679.

13. Culp K, Tripp-Reimer T, Wadle K, Wakefield B, Akins J, Mobily P, Kundradt M. Screening for confusion in elderly long-term care residents. *J Neurosci Nurs*. 1996;29(2): 86–100.

14. Levkoff SE, Cleary P, Liptzin B, et al. Epidemiology of delirium: an overview of research issues and findings. *Int Psychogeriatr*. 1991;3:149–167.

15. Rummans TA, Evans JM, Krahn LE, et al. Delirium in elderly patients: evaluation and management. *Mayo Clin Proc*. 1995;70:989–998.

16. American Psychiatric Association (APA). Diagnostic and statistical manual of mental disorders. 3rd ed. Washington, DC: author; 1990.

17. American Psychiatric Association (APA). Diagnostic and statistical manual of mental disorders. 3rd ed., revised. Washington, DC: author; 1987.

18. Francis J. Delirium in older patients. *J Am Geriatr Soc*. 1992;40:829–838.

19. Furstenberg AL, Mezey MD. Mental impairment of elderly hospitalized hip fracture patients. *Compr Gerontol*. 1987;1:80–85.

20. Rogers MP, Liang MH, Daltroy LH, et al. Delirium after elective orthopedic surgery: risk factors and natural history. *Int J Psych Med*. 1989;19:109–121.

21. Foreman MD. Acute confusion in the elderly. In: J Fitzpatrick, J Stevenson, eds. *Annual Review of Nursing Research*. New York: Springer Publishing; 1993.

22. Tune L, Carr S, Hoag E, Cooper T. Anti-cholinergic effects of drugs commonly prescribed for the elderly: potential means for assessing risk of delirium. *Am J Psych*. 1992;149:1393–1394.

23. Foreman MD, Zane D. Nursing strategies for acute confusion in elders. *Am J Nurs*. 1996;96:44–52.

24. Rockwood K. The occurrence and duration of symptoms in elderly patients with delirium. *J Gerontol*. 1993;48:M162–M168.

25. Gustafson Y, Brannstrom B, Berggren D, et al. Acute confusion in elderly patients treated for femoral neck fracture. *J Am Geriatr Soc*. 1988;36:525–530.

26. Inouye SK, Charpentier PA. Predicting factors for delirium in hospitalized elderly persons. *JAMA*. 1996;275:852–857.

27. Milisen K, Foreman MD, Godderis J, Abraham IL, Broos LO. Delirium in hospitalized elderly—nursing assessment and management. *Nurs Clin N Am*. 1998; 33:417–439.

28. Blass JP, Nolan KA, Black R, et al. Delirium: phenomenology and diagnosis. A neurobiologic view. *Int Psychogeriatr*. 1991;3:121–133.

29. Liptzin B, Levkoff SE. An empirical study of delirium subtypes. *Br J Psych*. 1992;161:843–845.

30. Francis J, Martin D, Kapoor WN. A prospective study of delirium in hospitalized elderly. *JAMA*. 1997;263: 1097–1001.

31. Foreman MD, Fletcher K, Mion LC, Simon L. Assessing cognitive function. *Geriatr Nurs*. 1996;17: 228–233.

32. Smith MJ, Breibert WS, Platt MN. A critique of instruments and methods to detect delirium, diagnose, and rate delirium. *J Pain Symptom Man*. 1995;10:35–77.

33. Folstein MF, Folstein SE, McHugh PR. "Mini-Mental State": a practical method for grading the cognitive state of patients for the clinician. *J Psych Res*. 1975; 12:189–198.

34. O'Brien JG. Evaluation of acute confusion. *Primary Care*. 1989;16:349–360.

35. Tombaugh TN, McIntyre NJ. The Mini-Mental State Examination: a comprehensive review. *J Am Geriatr Soc*. 1992;40:922–935.

36. Crum RM, Anthony JC, Bassett SS, Folstein MF. Population-based norms for the Mini-Mental Status Examination by age and educational level. *JAMA*. 1993;269:2386–2391.

37. Pfeiffer E. A short portable mental status questionnaire for the assessment of organic brain deficit in elderly patients. *J Am Geriatr Soc*. 1975;23:403–411.

38. Bross MH, Tatum NO. Delirium in the elderly patient. *Am Fam Phys*. 1994;50:1325–1332.

39. Neelon VJ, Champagne MT, Carlson JR, et al. The NEECHAM Confusion Scale: construction, validation and clinical testing. *Nurs Res*. 1996;45:324–330.

40. Inouye SK, vanDyck CH, Alessi CA, Balkin S, Siegel AP, Horwitz RI. Clarifying confusion: the Confusion Assessment Method—a new method for detection of delirium. *Ann Intern Med*. 1990;113:941–948.

41. Johnson JC. Delirium in the elderly. *Emerg Clin N Am*. 1990;8:255–265.

42. Foreman MD, Zane D. Nursing strategies for confusion in elders. *Am J Nurs*. 1996;96:44–52.

43. Francis J, Martin D, Kapoor WN. A prospective study of delirium in hospitalized elderly. *JAMA*. 1990;263:1097–1101.

44. Rockwood K. Acute confusion in elderly patients with delirium. *J Am Geriatr Soc*. 1989;37:150–154.

45. Levkoff SE, Safran C, Cleary PD, et al. Identification of factors associated with the diagnosis of delirium in elderly hospitalized patients. *J Am Geriatr Soc*. 1988;36:1099–1104.

46. Levkoff SE, Evans DA, Liptzin B, et al. Delirium: the occurrence and persistence of symptoms among elderly hospitalized patients. *Arch Intern Med*. 1992;152:334–340.

47. Koponen HJ, Riekkinen PJ. A prospective study of delirium in elderly patients admitted to a psychiatric hospital. *Psychol Med*. 1993;23:103–109.

48. Rockwood K. Acute confusion in elderly medical patients. *J Am Geriatr Soc*. 1989;37:150–154.

49. Kane AM, Kurlowicz LH. Enhancing nursing management of acute confusional states postoperatively in older patients. *MED/SURG Nursing*. 1994;3:1–44.

50. Inouye SK, Bogardus ST, Charpentier PA, Leo-Summers L, Acampora D, Holford TR, Cooney LM. A multicomponent intervention to prevent delirium in hospitalized older patients. *N Engl J Med*. 1999;340:669–676.

51. Williams MA, Campbell EB, Raynor WJ, Mlynarczyk SM, Ward SE. Reducing acute confusional states in elderly persons with hip fractures. *Res Nurs Health*. 1985;8:329–337.

52. Wanich CK, Sullivan-Marx EM, Gottlieb GL, Johnson JC. Functional status outcomes of a nursing intervention in hospitalized elderly. *IMAGE: J Nurs Scholarship*. 1992;24:201–207.

53. Sipahimalani A, Masand PS. Use of risperidone in delirium: case reports. *Ann Clin Psych*. 1997;9:105–107.

54. Sipahimalani A, Masand P. Olanzapine in the treatment of delirium. *Psychosomatic*. 1998;39:421–429.

55. Hasan S, Buckley P. Novel antipsychotics and Neuroleptic Malignant Syndrome: a review and critique. *Am J Psych*. 1998;155:1113–1116.

56. Schofeld I. A small exploratory study of the reaction of older people to an episode of delirium. *J Adv Nurs*. 1997;25:942–952.

57. NIH Consensus Development Panel. Diagnosis and treatment of depression in late life. *JAMA*. 1992;268:1018–1024.

58. Lebowitz BD. Diagnosis and treatment of depression in late life: an overview of the NIH consensus statement. *J Am Geriatr Soc*. 1996;4(Suppl. I):S3–S6.

59. Kurlowicz LH. Social factors and depression in late life. *Arch Psych Nurs*. 1993;7:30–36.

60. Katz IR, Streim J, Parmalee P. Prevention of depression, recurrences, and complications in late life. *Prev Med*. 1994;23:743–750.

61. Blazer DG, Hughes DC, George LK. The epidemiology of depression in an elderly community population. *Gerontologist*. 1987;27:281–287.

62. American Psychiatric Association. *Diagnostic and Statistical Manual of Mental Disorders*. 4th ed. Washington, DC: author; 1994.

63. Blazer DG. Depression in the elderly. *N Engl J Med*. 1989;320:164–166.

64. Kurlowicz LH. Depression in hospitalized medically ill elders: evolution of the concept. *Arch Psych Nurs*. 1994;8:124–126.

65. Cavanaugh S, Clark DC, Gibbons RD. Diagnosing depression in hospitalized medically ill. *Psychosomatics*. 1983;24:809–815.

66. Schein RL, Koenig HG. CES–D assessment of geriatric depression in medically ill patients. *Gerontol Abstracts*. 1994;31:237.

67. Cohen-Mansfield J, Werner P, Marx MS. Screaming in nursing home residents. *J Am Geriatr Soc*. 1990;38:785–792.

68. Koenig HG, Blazer DG. Minor depression in late life. *Am J Geriatr Psych*. 1996;4(Supp I):S14–S21.

69. Broadhead WE, Blazer DG, George LK, Tse CK. Depression, disability days, and days lost from work in a prospective epidemiologic survey. *JAMA*. 1990;264:2524–2528.

70. Wells KB, Stewart A, Hays RD, et al. The functioning and well being of depressed patients results from the medical outcome study. *JAMA*. 1989;262:914–919.

71. Mossey JM. Subsyndromal depression in hospitalized elderly: a typical reaction to being sick and hospitalized or a manifestation of pre-existing illness. *Gerontol Abstracts*. 1994;34:237.

72. Koenig HG, Meador KG, Cohen HJ, Blazer DG. Depression in elderly patients with medical illness. *Arch Intern Med*. 1988;148:1929–1936.

73. Blazer DG. *Depression in Late Life*. 2nd ed. St. Louis, MO. Mosby; 1993.

74. Krishnan KR, Gadd KM. The pathophysiologic basis for late life depression. *Am J Geriatr Psych*. 1996;4 (Supp. I):S22–33.

75. Holahan CK, Holahan CJ. Self-efficacy, social support, and depression in aging: a longitudinal analysis. *J Gerontol*. 1987;42:65–68.

76. Teri L, Wagner A. Alzheimer's disease and depression. *J Consulting Clin Psychol*. 1992;60:379–391.

77. Pearson JL, Teri L, Reifler BV. Functional status and cognitive impairment in Alzheimer's patients with and without depression. *J Am Geriatr Soc*. 1989;34;1117–1121.

78. Katz IR. On the inseparability of mental and physical health in aged persons: lessons from depression and medical comorbidity. *Am J Geriatr Psych*. 1996;4:1–16.

79. Parmalee PA, Katz IR, Lawton MP. Depression and mortality among institutionalized elderly. *J Gerontol*. 1992;47:P3–P10.

80. Conwell Y. Suicide in the elderly. In: Schneider LS, Reynolds BD, Lebowitz BD, Friedhoff AJ, eds. *Diagnosis and Treatment of Depression in Late Life: Results of the NIH Consensus Development Conference.* Washington, DC: American Psychiatric Press; 1994.

81. Conwell Y, Caine ED, Olsen K. Suicide and cancer in late life. *Hosp Commun Psych.* 1990;41:1334–1338.

82. Barraclough BM, Bunch J, Nelson B. A hundred cases of suicide: clinical aspects. *Br J Psych.* 1974;125:355–373.

83. Miller M. Geriatric suicide: the Arizona study. *Gerontologist.* 1978;18:488–495.

84. Koenig HG, George L, Peterson B, Pieper C, Fowler N, Sanfelippo T. Course of depression and predictors of recovery in medically ill hospitalized elderly: a preliminary report. *Gerontol Abstracts.* 1996;34:36.

85. Burns BJ, Taub CA. Mental health services in general medical care and in nursing homes. In: Fogel BS, Furino A, Gottlieb G, eds. *Mental Health Policy for Older Americans: Protecting Minds at Risk.* Washington, DC: American Psychiatric Press; 1990.

86. Keane SM, Sells S. Recognizing depression in the elderly. *J Gerontol Nurs.* 1990;16:21–25.

87. Yesavage JA, Brink TL, Rose TL, et al. Development and validation of a geriatric depression screening scale: a preliminary report. *J Psych Res.* 1983;17:37–49.

88. Dreyfus JK. Depression assessment and interventions with medically ill frail elderly. *J Gerontol Nurs.* 1988;14:27–36.

89. Parmalee PA, Katz IR, Lawton MP. The relation of pain to depression among institutionalized aged. *J Gerontol.* 1991;46:15–21.

90. Koenig HG. Depressive disorders in older medical inpatients. *Am Fam Pract.* 1991;44:1243–1250.

91. Teri L, Logsdon RG. Identifying pleasant activities for Alzheimer's disease patients—AD. *Gerontologist.* 1991;31:124–127.

92. Osborn C. Reminiscence: when the past meets present. *J Gerontol Nurs.* 1989;15:6–12.

93. American Association of Geriatric Psychiatry. Position statement: psychotherapeutic medication in nursing homes. *J Am Geriatr Soc.* 1992;40:946–949.

CHAPTER 9

Dizziness and Stroke

Kathleen A. Hill-O'Neill
Marianne Shaughnessy

Introduction

Changes in the structure and function of the nervous system occur with normal aging, and can result in changes in mobility, balance, coordination, sensation, comprehension, cognitive performance, or behaviors. These changes generally reflect a slowing of neurologic responses as fewer neurons are available to provide sensory and motor messages to and from the central nervous system. Remaining neurons may function at reduced capacity due to myelin sheath degeneration and a decrease in available neurotransmitters. Patients may be reluctant to share the history of the development of such symptoms, attributing them to "old age" or a previously diagnosed illness. However, changes in function should never be assumed to be due to normal aging without a full neurologic evaluation of the presenting complaint. Readers are encouraged to consult a physical assessment textbook as needed for review of the nuances of the history and physical examination for neurological complaints.

This chapter focuses on one of the most common neurologic complaints in older adults—dizziness—and one of the most common causes of neurologic disability—stroke. Prompt diagnosis and management of dizziness, and early identification and treatment of stroke can effectively prevent disability and improve function and quality of life.

Dizziness

Overview/Prevalence

Dizziness is reported by about 30% of people aged over 65 years and is the most common presenting complaint in office practice among patients aged over 75 years.[1] Dizziness is a difficult diagnosis in older adults as it has many potential causes and patients often find it difficult to articulate the nature of the symptoms.[1] In older adults, dizziness is often linked to cardiovascular or neurological diseases, medications, or multisensory dysfunction and psychiatric problems such as anxiety and depression.[2,3]

Dizziness is a nonspecific symptom and in a substantial proportion of cases, diagnosis must be based on clinical examination, as a definitive cause may not be confirmed by means of laboratory or other diagnostic investigation.[2]

Age-Related Changes

A variety of anatomic and physiologic changes associated with aging contribute to the susceptibility of older persons to dizziness.[4] Sensory receptors are reduced in the semicircular canals, the saccule, utricle, proprioceptive nerves, and retina. Interneuronal connections (synapses) also diminish with age. In addition, the microenvironment surrounding nerve cells is often impaired because of vascular disease.[5]

Types of Dizziness

Dizziness is categorized into four major types:

1. vertigo
2. pre-syncope (lightheadedness)
3. disequilibrium (imbalance)
4. ill-defined, which is dizziness that does not fit into any other category (Table 9–1).

Benign Positional Vertigo (BPV)   BPV accounts for 40–50% of all dizziness complaints. BPV may occur as a normal part of aging caused by degeneration and deposit of debris on the cupula of the posterior semicircular canals (cupulolithiasis). When the

Table 9–1　Types of Dizziness and Their Causes

Vertigo	• BPV (deposit of debris in semicircular canals) • Vertebrobasilar insufficiency • Acute labyrinthitis/vestibular neuronitis • Meniere's disease
Pre-syncopal (etiology contributes to decreased cerebral perfusion)	• Postural hypotension • Cardiovascular disease • Vasovagal response (causes pooling of blood in the lower extremities) • Medication
Disequilibrium	• Cerebellar diseases • Lesions involving the frontal lobes and basal ganglia • Peripheral neuropathy often associated with a systemic metabolic disorder such as renal failure or diabetes mellitus • Cervical arthritis due to compression of peripheral nerves and spinal cord
Ill-defined/other	• Anxiety • Psychological conditions

patient moves from the sitting to head-hanging position, the posterior canal moves from an inferior to superior position, and because of gravity the debris moves, causing vertigo, a sense of spinning, and nystagmus (Figure 9–1).[6]

Vertebrobasilar Insufficiency (VBI)　Older patients over the age of 50 who complain of vertigo or dizziness often have ischemic brain diseases such as VBI.[7] Vertigo due to VBI usually presents with an abrupt onset, lasting several minutes, and is associated with nausea or vomiting.[8] Whether the vertigo originates from ischemia of the labyrinth, brain stem, or both structures is not always clear since the blood supply to the labyrinth, VIII cranial nerve, and vestibular nuclei originate from the same source, the basilar vertebral circulation.[8] Vertigo due to VBI is

usually diagnosed from accompanying neurological symptoms such as visual disturbance, transient loss of consciousness, and sensory disturbance in upper limbs.[7] VBI episodes may be precipitated by postural hypotension, Stokes-Adams attacks, or mechanical compression from cervical spondylosis.[8]

Infection　Vestibular neuronitis may develop several days or weeks following a viral illness and may cause symptoms of vertigo with associated

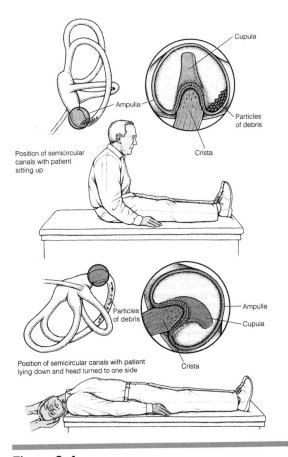

Figure 9–1
Pathophysiology of benign paroxysmal positional vertigo.
Reprinted from Beers MH, Berkow R. *The Merck Manual of Geriatrics.* 3rd ed. Whitehouse Station, NJ: Merck Research Laboratories; 2000.

nausea and/or vomiting. Labyrinthitis (the labyrinth consists of the vestibule, cochlea, and semicircular canals) or a middle ear infection causing fluid to accumulate in the middle ear may also cause vertigo.

Meniere's Disease
The cause of Meniere's disease is unknown. Bacterial, viral, and syphilitic labyrinthitis all can lead to typical symptoms of Meniere's syndrome.[8] Typically, the patient develops a sensation of fullness and pressure along with decreased hearing and tinnitus in one ear. Vertigo rapidly follows, reaching a maximum intensity within minutes, and then slowly subsides over the next several hours. The patient is usually left with a sense of unsteadiness and dizziness for days after the acute vertiginous attack.[8]

Pre-syncope (Light-Headedness)
Pre-syncope, also described as a sense of fainting or light-headedness, is frequently caused by orthostatic hypotension. With a sudden change from a supine to an upright position, a series of venous valves play an important role in slowing the inevitable venous pooling that occurs secondary to gravity.[9] In this capacity, the valves maintain adequate right ventricular filling pressures and prevent an abrupt decrease in preload that can trigger mechanoreceptor and baroreceptor reflexes.[9]

Because of changes that occur with aging, including altered sensitivity of baroreflex and cardiopulmonary reflex, the elderly are more prone to pre-syncopal or syncopal episodes.[9] From the brain's "point of view," light-headedness and its endpoint, syncope, arise in one of three ways:

1. a drop in cerebral blood flow depriving the brain of enough glucose and oxygen to support consciousness
2. oxygen deprivation (hypoxemia)
3. hypoglycemia[10]

Arrhythmia due to underlying heart disease may contribute to decreased cardiac output and pre-syncopal episodes. The elderly are also more susceptible to the side effects of medications such as antihypertensives, diuretics, antidepressants, and sedatives, which may cause orthostatic hypotension.

Disequilibrium
Unsteadiness when walking is often due to disequilibrium. To maintain postural stability when standing and walking, the brain must rapidly process signals from the visual, vestibular, and somatosensory systems.[11] Because balance depends on multiple sensory inputs, it can deteriorate when any of these systems fails individually or collectively. The combined loss of sensory signals from several systems has been proposed as a common cause of imbalance (so-called multisensory dizziness and imbalance).[11]

The three common causes of disequilibrium are vestibular loss, proprioceptive and somatosensory loss, and motor and cerebellar lesions (Figure 9–2). Symptoms include persistent unsteadiness, which may be incapacitating. The imbalance is worse in the dark when the patient is unable to use

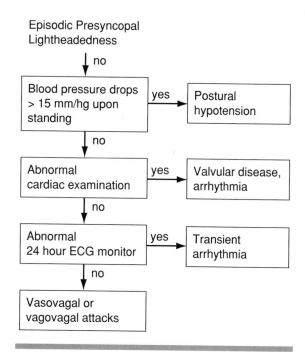

Figure 9–2
Logic for differentiating the common causes of episodic pre-syncope/light-headedness.
Source: Baloh RW. Dizziness in older people. *J Am Geriatr Soc.* 1992;40:713–721.

vision to compensate for the loss. Oscillopsia (a visual sensation that fixed objects are moving back and forth) is a common accompanying symptom.[8] Ototoxic drug exposure is the most common cause of bilateral vestibulopathy, particularly in older patients with renal dysfunction.

Ill-Defined   In ill-defined dizziness the complaint is a vague description of dizziness not fitting into the other categories. The patient may have panic/anxiety disorder or depression.

Clinical Presentation

When taking a history, it is important to remember that dizziness may represent many different abnormal sensations. The initial task of the examining clinician is to determine what the patient means by dizziness.[8] Patients should be encouraged to describe the sensation and how it interferes with their routine activities and determine the type before proceeding with exhaustive diagnostic studies.[8] Dizziness is often self-limited. When it does persist, a direct history and physical examination can establish a presumptive cause in most patients. Vestibular function testing and psychiatric evaluations are the most useful supplemental measures.

History

A thorough history is critical. However, it is important to ask open-ended questions and allow the patient to define and describe the symptoms.

- What does being "dizzy" mean?
- What was patient doing just prior to onset of symptoms?
- What relieves the symptoms if anything?
- What makes dizziness worse?
- Have changes in hearing or other otological symptoms occurred?
- Has the patient had associated diaphoresis, chest pain, shortness of breath, or blood in the stools?
- Have there been recent upper respiratory infections or sinus problems?

Table 9–2   Medications Contributing to Dizziness

| Aminoglycosides |
| Antiarrhythmics |
| Antihistamines |
| Antihypertensives |
| Antipsychotics |
| Calcium channel blockers |
| Diuretics |
| Over-the-counter cold medicines |
| Salicylates |
| Sedatives |

- What medications are being taken, and when are they taken, including over-the-counter products? Review new medications and their side effects (look for inappropriate combinations or timing, i.e., diuretics at bedtime) (Table 9–2).
- Look for a pattern of presenting symptoms while developing a differential diagnosis (Table 9–3).
- Assess for history or presence of anxiety or depression. (Patient may make vague comments such as "I am dizzy all the time," but unable to be specific. May say yes or no to every question about symptoms).

Physical Exam

- Temperature, apical pulse, respirations (irregular heart rate may indicate arrhythmia, fever, and/or other symptoms of upper respiratory infection).
- BP in lying, sitting, and standing positions (looking for orthostatic changes of presyncope).
- HEENT auditory acuity and Rinne test (new hearing loss would lead to consideration of Meniere's disease, acoustic neuroma, or vestibular neuronitis).

Table 9–3   Presenting Symptoms in Common Types of Dizziness

Positional vertigo (40–50% of all dizziness complaints)	• Sudden onset • Turning the head causes severe symptoms • Illusion of motion or rotational sensation on change of position lasting several minutes • May describe rocking, spinning, or tilting
Pre-syncopal	• Periodic reoccurrence • Feeling of impending fainting episode • Palpitations • Perspiration
Disequilibrium	• Most prominent when standing • Unsteady and sense of falling • Numbness or weakness • Oscillopsia
Ill-defined	• Complains of general nonspecific symptoms • Vague symptoms not fitting other categories

The triad of gradually worsening unilateral hearing loss plus tinnitus plus loss of corneal reflex could be indicative of acoustic neuroma (incidence is rare but should be considered if appropriate presenting symptoms).

Table 9–4   Nystagmus in Benign Positional Vertigo

Left ear affected and in the down position	Clinician looks at patient and sees clockwise nystagmus
Right ear affected and in the down position	Clinician looks at patient and sees counterclockwise nystagmus

2. The clinician firmly holds the patient's head and moves the patient quickly from a sitting position into a supine position with the head turned about 30 degrees laterally and about 30 degrees below the level of the exam table.
3. Within a few seconds the burst of nystagmus may occur and the clinician must be observant.
4. The patient is assisted back to a sitting position and the procedure is repeated turning the patient to the opposite side.
5. The clinician observes the patient's eyes for 5–15 seconds after each head-hanging manuever to see whether nystagmus has been induced. It is recommended that the

■ Cardiac, pulmonary, and neurological assessment including deep tendon reflexes (if findings include a new arrhythmia or bruit cardiology, referral may be indicated).
■ Stool for occult blood if positive history.
■ Assessment for positional nystagmus (involuntary fine rhythmic oscillation of the eyes) (Table 9–4). A positive Hallpike would indicate BPV.

This can be done by doing the head-hanging Hallpike's test (Figure 9–3).

1. The patient is positioned so that the head will extend beyond the end of the table when the patient is supine.

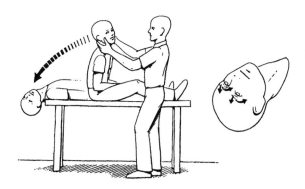

Figure 9–3
Hallpike's maneuver.
Adapted from Froehling D, Silverstein M, Mohr D, Beatty C. Does this patient have a serious form of vertigo? *JAMA.* 1994;271(5).

position change be completed in about two seconds or nystagmus may not be induced.[12] Explaining the procedure prior to beginning the maneuver is important, as well as reminding the patient to keep his/her eyes open even if vertigo develops.

- Romberg test (positive finding indicative of vestibular lesion or cerebellar lesion).
- Gait (the broad-based ataxic gait is common in patients with disequilibrium).

Diagnostic Data (Order Based on History and Physical Findings)

- Fasting blood sugar (to rule out hypoglycemia, a potential cause of pre-syncope)
- Chemistry panel (to rule out electrolyte abnormality)
- Complete blood count (CBC) (to rule out anemia, a potential cause of pre-syncope)
- Electrocardiogram (ECG) or 24-Holter monitor (to rule out arrhythmia, a potential cause of pre-syncope)
- Computed tomography (CT) or magnetic resonance imaging (MRI) if appropriate by history and physical (if slurred speech, visual disturbances, or vertical nystagmus or other cranial nerve abnormality is present, rule out acoustic neuroma, cerebellar CVA, or other cerebrovascular occlusion).

Among various methods used for diagnosing VBI, vertebral artery angiography is reported to be the most reliable. On the other hand, MRI, which is minimally invasive, gives information on blood vessels of the vertebrobasilar system as well as on ischemic changes in the brain.[7]

Assessment/Plan

Vertigo   Usually the diagnosis of BPV can be made based solely on the history and physical exam. BPV is the most common cause of vertigo. When Hallpike's maneuver is positive, the Epley

maneuver should be done (Figure 9–4).[13] Most patients achieve a complete cure with this maneuver. The purpose of this maneuver is to move the loose particles out of the posterior semicircular canal and back into the utricle. The procedure can be repeated until the patient no longer exhibits signs of nystagmus. It is best to advise the patient not to lie flat for several days to prevent the particles from moving back into the semicircular canals.

Exercise may be beneficial to patients with chronic vestibular diseases due to BPV, Meniere's disease, or ototoxicity (Table 9–5).

Pre-Syncope (Light-Headedness)   A drop in blood pressure on standing, though not in line with criteria for orthostatic changes, may contribute to pre-syncopal episodes as blood pressure may fall after prolonged standing. Hypovolemia needs to be corrected when identified, as well as adjusting any medications that may be contributing to reduced fluid volume. Patients need to be taught to change position slowly, that is, waiting two to three minutes before moving when going from lying to sitting to standing. Education about risks of venous pooling and measures to prevent and correct this condition should be reviewed. Additional cardiac workup may be necessary based on physical exam findings (see Figure 9–2).

Disequilibrium (Figure 9–5). Neuroimaging may be necessary based on findings. Home assessment for safety by an occupational therapist may be beneficial. Patients may need a physical therapy program to recommend exercises to strengthen deconditioned muscles or to recommend assistive walking devices for safety.

Referral

Consider neurology, cardiology, or otolaryngology referral if:

- Persistent symptoms of more than two months with no progress
- Episodes are persistent and disabling
- New neurological or cardiological abnormalities are detected

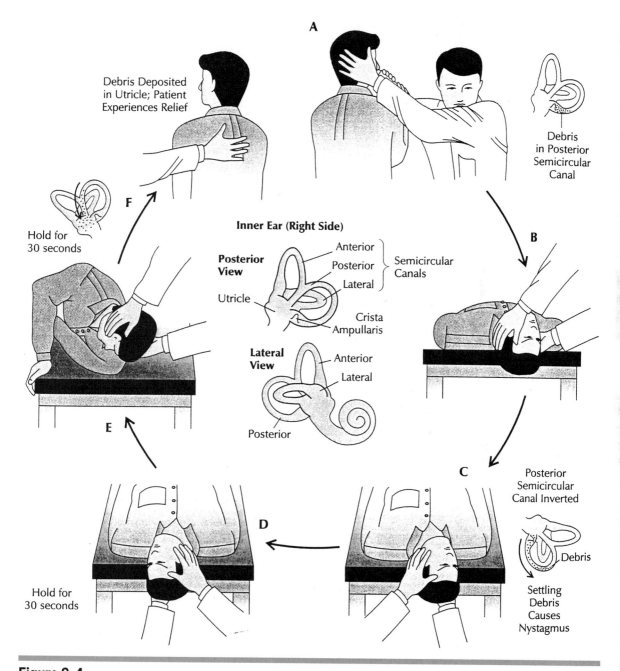

A

Debris in Posterior Semicircular Canal

Debris Deposited in Utricle; Patient Experiences Relief

F

Hold for 30 seconds

Inner Ear (Right Side)

Posterior View

Anterior
Posterior } Semicircular Canals
Lateral

Utricle

Crista Ampullaris

Lateral View

Anterior
Lateral

Posterior

B

E

C

Posterior Semicircular Canal Inverted

Debris

Settling Debris Causes Nystagmus

D

Hold for 30 seconds

Figure 9–4
Epley maneuver.
Source: Baloh R, Baringer JR. Dizzy patients: the varieties of vertigo. *Hosp Pract.* 1998; June:55–77.

Table 9–5   Summary of Treatments for Vertigo

Diagnosis	Duration of Symptoms	Diagnosis/Treatment
Benign positional vertigo	Usually resolved over several weeks. May last several months. Some patients have reoccurrence lasting several years.	Epley maneuver. Anti-vertigo medications if needed to relieve symptoms, i.e., meclizine prn (should only be used for severe episodes and 3–14 days duration). Vestibular rehabilitation may be beneficial which would include maneuvering techniques (works by allowing the brain to adapt by enhancing neural connections in the inner ear).
Vertebrobasilar insufficiency	May have a history of vertigo. Current symptoms are sudden and unprovoked lasting 5–10 minutes. May be associated with nausea, slurring speech, and/or visual disturbances. May be seen in patients with past medical history of atherosclerosis or cerebrovascular disease.	Neurology consult should be considered. MRI brain scan to rule out stroke may be considered. MRI angiography may be considered. ASA or alternative anticoagulation therapy may be prescribed if indicated. Ongoing management of associated risk factors, i.e., lifestyle modifications, hypertension control, etc.
Vestibular neuronitis/ labyrinthitis	Symptoms may last approximately 2–3 weeks. Usually occurs a few days or weeks after a viral infection. Most likely due to inflammation of the vestibular nerve. If hearing (auditory acuity) is affected symptoms are more likely due to labyrinthitis; if hearing is not affected, symptoms are likely due to neuronitis.	Tapered steroids may be considered. Vestibular sedatives may be helpful during the acute phase. Inner ear damage may improve within a few weeks or months but recovery may be slower with symptoms of floating or imbalance lasting several years. Consult ENT if symptoms are not improved within 2–4 weeks.
Meniere's disease	Symptoms may be mild or severe including ringing in the ears or hearing loss caused by fluid buildup in the inner ear. Symptoms may last up to an hour or more.	Treatment is aimed at reducing the accumulation of fluid and may include steroids or diuretics. Surgery may be considered. ENT consult should be considered if symptoms worsen, i.e., more frequent attacks or hearing loss progresses.

Consider psychiatry referral if unable to treat or improve symptoms of anxiety or depression.

In conclusion, many types of dizziness are treatable with improvement in symptoms and often resolve completely. Incurable conditions such as dizziness due to stroke or permanent impairment may be addressed with the goal of maintaining a safe environment and promoting independence with assistive devices when appropriate. Exercise and other therapies under the guidance of a therapist or clinician for vestibular rehabilitation may also be beneficial.

Stroke

Introduction

Stroke is the third leading cause of death and the leading cause of disability in the United States. Approximately 750,000 people suffer strokes each year,[14] and of that number, one-third expire from the stroke itself or other cardiovascular sequelae.[15] An estimated 4.4 million stroke survivors are alive today. The focus of this section of the chapter is on the early identification, management, follow-up, and patient education for stroke survivors and

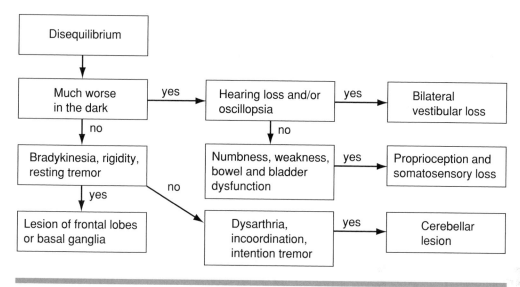

Figure 9–5
Logic for differentiating the common causes of disequilibrium.
Source: Baloh RW. Dizziness in older people. *J Am Geriatr Soc.* 1992;40:713–721.

their families through the acute, rehabilitation, and chronic phases of stroke.

Stroke is also known as "brain attack"—a term chosen to emphasize the need for emergency treatment, just as in a "heart attack." A stroke is indeed a medical emergency created by the interruption of blood flow to some area of the brain. This interruption can occur as the result of an occlusion (thrombus or embolus) or a hemorrhage.

Pathophysiology

Ischemic Stroke   Ischemic strokes, the result of an occlusion, are categorized according to type (thrombotic, embolic, or hemodynamic) and location (hemispheric or lacunar).

Thrombotic Stroke   This occurs in vessels when a thrombus forms on an atherosclerotic plaque, occluding the flow of oxygenated blood distal to the occlusion site.

Embolic Stroke   This occurs when a clot forms elsewhere (usually the result of valvular disorders,

cardiac thrombus, dysrrhythmias, or atherosclerotic plaque in the carotid arteries) and travels to the brain, occluding blood flow. Hypercoagulable states may also play a role in thrombotic or embolic infarction. Infarction (or neuronal death) occurs when these occlusions are uncompensated by collateral flow. Hemodynamic strokes are characterized by lack of flow to the brain tissue due to circulatory failure or occlusion in an artery proximal to the brain.

Between the infarcted area and normally perfused brain tissue is an area of moderately reduced blood flow known as the penumbra. Many of the current treatments for stroke are targeted at rescuing cells in the penumbra. When cerebral blood flow is reduced, synaptic transmission may fail, but cells still have potential for recovery. When cerebral blood flow falls below a certain pressure, a biochemical cascade begins: failure of the sodium-potassium pump results in a rapid loss of potassium from the neurons, subsequent depolarization opens calcium channels, and an extracellular buildup of excitatory amino acids floods calcium into the neuronal cytoplasm, resulting in cell death.[16]

Ischemic strokes are further classified according to location in one of two areas: hemispheric and lacunar. Hemispheric strokes generally occur in the anterior, middle, or posterior artery circulation and result in unilateral deficits. The most common site of occurrence is the middle cerebral artery (MCA) and results in contralateral hemiparesis with or without sensory loss. Lacunar infarcts occur in the deep penetrating arteries where they branch at 90-degree angles from the main intracerebral arteries and are generally also unilateral. The most common sites of occurrence are the basal ganglia, internal capsule, thalamus, or pons. Depending on the site of occlusion, a variety of presentations are possible. Table 9–6 summarizes these likely presentations depending on the location of the infarct.[17]

A transient ischemic attack (TIA) occurs in instances when a small, temporary occlusion is dissolved by endogenous thrombolytics or dislodged and moved to distal, smaller vessels by cerebral blood pressure. Symptoms are felt for a brief period of time (usually minutes) and resolve spontaneously as the affected brain cells are reperfused. By definition, symptoms of a TIA resolve within 24 hours.[18] A TIA generally heralds the oncoming event of a larger, more disabling stroke; patients reporting a TIA are 10 times more likely to experience a major stroke than those without the warning sign.[15]

Hemorrhagic Strokes   Hemorrhagic strokes account for approximately 20% of all strokes and occur when a blood vessel supplying the brain ruptures. The two primary types are intracerebral hemorrhage (ICH), when rupture occurs within the brain, and subarachnoid hemorrhage (SAH), when the ruptured vessel is around the brain itself. Both result in direct damage to brain tissue. Causes of hemorrhagic stroke include hypertension; arteriovenous malformation; use of cocaine, amphetamines, or alcohol; anticoagulation therapy; amyloid angiopathy; or brain tumor. TIAs are generally not associated with hemorrhagic infarctions.

Risk Factors

According to the American Heart Association,[15] the primary risk factors for stroke are:

- Advanced age: the chance of a stroke doubles each decade after age 55.
- Gender: overall, men have about a 19% greater chance of stroke than women.
- Family history: chance of stroke is greater for those with a family history of stroke.
- Prior stroke or TIA: raises the risk for stroke tenfold.
- Hypertension: primary risk factor for stroke. The decrease in stroke deaths is attributed to identification and treatment of hypertension.
- Smoking: significant modifiable risk factor for stroke. Nicotine and carbon dioxide are known to damage the cardiovascular system.
- Diabetes mellitus: independent risk factor for stroke and is strongly correlated with high blood pressure and hyperlipidemia.
- Heart disease: those with heart disease have twice the risk of stroke as those with normal heart function. Atrial fibrillation is a major risk factor in embolus formation.
- Atherosclerosis: buildup of plaque in the carotid arteries can be the source of emboli or occlude flow sufficiently to cause a hemodynamic event.
- Geography: strokes are more common in the southeast United States ("stroke belt").
- Excessive alcohol intake or other drug abuse: intravenous drug use carries a high risk for cerebral embolism, and cocaine and amphetamines are associated with increased risk of hemorrhagic stroke.
- Socioeconomic factors: lower socioeconomic and educational levels are associated with higher risk of stroke.

Clinical Presentation

Patients with suspected stroke generally present with one or more of the following symptoms:

- Abrupt onset of hemiparesis (one-sided weakness) or monoparesis (one-limb weakness)
- Abrupt onset of hemisensory loss

Table 9–6 Common Patterns of Stroke Deficit
by Anatomic Location[17]

Anterior Circulation	
Left Middle and Anterior Cerebral Artery	**Right Middle and Anterior Cerebral Artery**
Aphasia	Neglect of left visual space
Poor reading, writing, calculating	Difficulty drawing and copying
Right visual field deficit	Left visual field deficit
Poor conjugate gaze to right	Poor conjugate gaze to left
Right hemiparesis	Left hemiparesis
Right hemisensory loss	Left hemisensory loss
	Left sensory neglect

Posterior Circulation	
Right Visual Field Deficit	**Left Visual Field Deficit**
Difficulty reading with preserved writing	Left neglect
Difficulty naming objects	Left limb sensory loss
Right limb numbness	

Vertebrobasilar

Vertigo, nausea, vomiting
Diplopia
Ataxia of limbs or gait
Weakness or numbness of all four limbs
Crossed motor or sensory findings
Bilateral blindness or dim vision
Nystagmus or disconjugate gaze
Amnesia
Headache in the occiput, mastoid, or neck

Small Vessel Lacunar

Pure motor stroke (pons, internal capsule)
  • Hemiparesis of the face, arm, and leg
  • Normal sensation
  • Normal higher cortical function and vision

Pure sensory stroke (thalamus)
  • Hemisensory loss or numbness
  • No weakness or incoordination
  • Normal higher cortical function and vision

Sensory-motor stroke (thalamocapsular)
  • Hemisensory loss or numbness
  • Hemiparesis ipsilateral to hemisensory symptoms
  • Normal higher cortical function and vision

Ataxic hemiparesis (pons, internal capsule, midbrain)
  • Ataxia and incoordination of limbs
  • Hemiparesis ipsilateral to ataxia
  • Normal higher cortical function and vision

- Severe headache (usually described as the "worst headache ever experienced")
- Difficulty swallowing
- Difficulty speaking or understanding spoken language
- Sudden loss of vision in one or both eyes, loss of vision in half the visual field, double vision, or horizontal visual field cut (amaurosis fugax)
- Clumsiness or loss of balance, vertigo
- Weakness in all four extremities

Patients may report prior experience with similar symptoms that resolved spontaneously (prior TIA). Physical signs identifiable on physical exam may include:

- Hemiparesis or sensory changes of the face, arm, or leg
- Decreased visual acuity or field cut, diplopia
- Slurred or unintelligible speech, swallowing dysfunction
- Ataxia, balance, or coordination problems
- Acute confusional state
- Elevated blood pressure

Differential Diagnosis

All of the following alternative diagnoses may be suspected when a patient with stroke symptoms presents for evaluation: temporal arteritis, vertebral disk disease, brain tumor, central nervous system (CNS) or meningeal infection. Diagnostic probabilities can be further refined with the history of onset of symptoms, physical examination, and diagnostic studies.

History

Clinicians should attempt to ascertain immediately the type, time since onset, and progression of symptoms, since eligibility for thrombolytic treatment is limited to the first three hours following symptom onset. A complete history of present illness should be obtained. If the patient is unable to provide this information, a caregiver or family member should be questioned, if available. Additional relevant information includes history of trauma or seizures, recent infection, illicit drug use, or other medical problems and medications. Any of the above-mentioned signs or symptoms should alert the clinician to suspect a stroke in evolution.

Physical Examination

Physical examination should include repeated measurement of vital signs and examination of the head and neck for signs of trauma or meningeal inflammation. Positive Brudzinski's or Kernig's signs may suggest the possibility of subarachnoid hemorrhage. A cardiovascular exam should be done to determine evidence of a dysrrhythmia. All peripheral pulses should be palpated and the carotids auscultated for bruits. Finally, a complete neurological exam, including motor, sensory, cranial nerve function, deep tendon reflexes, and mental status should be completed and documented. Focal positive neurologic findings are generally found. Baseline findings should be carefully noted to detect any changes over the subsequent hours and days. If stroke is suspected, clinicians should notify 911 or initiate emergency transport to the nearest appropriately equipped medical facility. If possible, intravenous access should be obtained prior to transport. Supplemental oxygen via mask or nasal prongs is recommended only if patients are in respiratory distress. Recent animal studies have demonstrated that blind adminstration of oxygen may contribute to the formation of free radicals that can contribute to neuronal cell death.[19]

Diagnostic Data

Initial evaluation should include an ECG, cardiac monitoring, pulse oximetry, chest x-ray, CBC, platelet count, prothrombin time, partial thromboplastin time, serum electrolytes, and glucose level. If indicated, serum cardiac markers, arterial blood gases, serum alcohol, toxicology, and pregnancy test may also be helpful. A cranial CT scan (without contrast) should be obtained as quickly as possible, as all subsequent therapeutic decisions depend on the results.[20] CT does not usually show definitive changes of cerebral infarction for 24–48 hours, but often reveals a hemorrhage.

MRI shows better contrast resolution of all parenchymal structures, as well as evidence of ischemic stroke sooner than CT. It offers early delineation of the ischemic penumbra. Also, MRI scanning is superior for detecting posterior circulation strokes, small infarctions, early signs of brain edema, and vascular malformations. MRI is not generally as available, however, and it takes significant time to complete. The patient may have difficulty remaining still during the procedure and monitoring of the patient's neurologic status is difficult. Magnetic resonance angiography (performed during the MRI procedure) is useful for demonstrating large vessel occlusions. Arteriography definitively demonstrates stenoses and occlusions of both large and small vessels, and detects arterial abnormalities. Carotid duplex is a useful, noninvasive technique for identifying internal carotid artery stenosis and is most effective at identifying stenosis > 60%. Echocardiogram may be useful for identification of a cardiac thrombus. Elucidating the specific mechanism of the CVA assists in determining the management plan.[20]

Management

Acute Phase   Patients with a hemorrhagic stroke (ICH, SAH), confirmed with imaging and evolving clinical presentation, should have a neurosurgical consultation immediately. Any compromise of respiration or circulation must be addressed very quickly. Blood pressure elevations should be reduced if the stroke is hemorrhagic. If not, elevations of systemic arterial pressure should not be treated immediately unless:

1. Systolic pressure exceeds 220 mmHg, or diastolic pressure exceeds 115 mmHg on repeated measurements 30 to 60 minutes apart,
2. Cardiac ischemia, failure, or arterial dissection has been identified, or
3. Thrombolytic therapy is used.

If blood pressure needs to be reduced, lower it gradually in 10–15% decrements while observing the patient for clinical change.[20, 21]

Patients with an ischemic stroke should evaluated by a specialized stroke team for evaluation or thrombolytic administration, if criteria are met, within three hours of symptom onset. If seizures occur, anticonvulsant therapy should be initiated. Anticoagulation should not be employed routinely during the acute phase of stroke, but can be considered in the case of a cardioembolic source, or a documented large vessel stenosis. If use of heparin is selected, it should be administered without a bolus, and with close monitoring of the partial thromboplastin time (PTT), aiming for levels approximately 1.5–2.0 times control.[20]

A phenomenon of concern in the management of ischemic strokes is hemorrhagic transformation, or bleeding into the infarcted tissue associated with reperfusion of the affected area. Hemorrhagic transformation is spontaneous, may be microscopic or catastrophic, and has a peak occurrence during the first week after stroke, most often very early in the post-stroke course. It is particularly associated with large embolic strokes. Neurological consultation should be sought in the use of anticoagulant therapy if suspicion for hemorrhagic transformation is high.[22]

Several large clinical trials are under way to define the benefits of alternative neuroprotective agents that may be started safely started on the scene or in the ambulance. The goal is to prolong the time that brain tissue can withstand ischemia prior to thrombolysis treatment.[19]

Rehabilitation Phase   Rehabilitation begins immediately following stabilization of the medical condition. Multiple studies have shown that early mobilization is key to minimizing disability. The choice of rehabilitation setting depends on the severity of brain injury and the patient's endurance level. Studies indicate that specialized stroke units utilizing an interdisciplinary team approach are associated with better functional outcomes following rehabilitation.[23,24] Threshold criteria for admission to a rehabilitation program include:

1. medically stable
2. one or more persistent disabilities
3. capacity to learn
4. sufficient endurance to participate actively in therapy

Patients who are too debilitated to participate in an acute rehabilitation program immediately following the stroke may qualify for subacute rehabilitation prior to transfer to home or into an acute rehabilitation program.

As patients enter the rehabilitation phase following stroke, a multidisciplinary team of professionals is needed to assess clinical status and set realistic goals toward returning stroke survivors to optimal levels of function. Nurses and physicians usually establish the stroke survivor's overall level of neurological disability and clinical status. Physical and occupational therapists complete assessments of upper and lower extremity function and ability to translate motor movement to purposeful activity. Speech and language pathologists specialize in the assessment and treatment of speech, swallowing, and cognitive function. Psychologists and psychiatrists assist with assessment and treatment of cognitive and emotional problems related to stroke. Together, all professionals work to establish baseline data regarding functional levels. Finally, the patient and his/her family contribute to care planning with information regarding the patient's prior functional patterns and desired goals for rehabilitation. During the course of rehabilitation following stroke, all members of the team should communicate regularly regarding the patient's daily progress. The first 12 weeks following stroke is generally the period when the most rapid progress may be expected. Use of standardized validated instruments establishes baseline data for later comparison as the patient progresses through rehabilitation and throughout recovery. Table 9–7 provides a list of standardized measurement instruments recommended for monitoring the progress of stroke patients.[25]

Management Issues/Stroke Sequelae

Depending on the location and extent of damage to brain tissue following stroke, a number of sequelae may follow that should be monitored and addressed by the rehabilitation team.

Mobility Impairment   This includes hemiparesis, ataxia, spasticity, apraxia, and coordination disorders. Hemiparesis is muscular weakness on one side of the body and is the most common consequence of stroke. It may occur in varying degrees in the arm, leg, face, or trunk. Other mobility problems may be

Table 9–7 Recommended Standardized Assessment Instruments for Stroke Survivors[25]

Stroke deficit scales (measures neurologic deficit)
  NIH Stroke Scale
  Canadian Neurological Scale

Measures of disability in basic activities of daily living
  Barthel Index
  Functional Independence Measure

Measures of disability in instrumental activities of daily living
  PGC Instrumental Activities of Daily Living
  Frenchay Activities Index

Mental status screening tests
  Mini-Mental State Exam
  Neurobehavioral Cognitive Status Examination

Motor function
  Fugl-Meyer Scale
  Motor Assessment Scale
  Motricity Index

Balance assessment
  Berg Balance Scale

Mobility assessment
  Rivermead Mobility Index

Speech and language assessment
  Boston Diagnostic Aphasia Examination
  Porch Index of Communicative Ability
  Western Aphasia Battery

Depression scales
  Beck Depression Inventory
  Center for Epidemiologic Studies—Depression
  Geriatric Depression Scale
  Hamilton Depression Scale

Quality of life measures
  Medical Outcomes Study (MOS) 36-Item
    Short-Form Health Survey
  Sickness Impact Profile
  Stroke Impact Scale
  Stroke Specific Quality of Life

attributed to abnormal synergistic organization of movements (ataxia), abnormal muscle tone (spasticity), impaired regulation of force control, or delayed muscle responses. Appropriate range of motion and strengthening exercises should be initiated as soon as possible under the direction of a physical therapist. Patients with severe spasticity may also benefit from muscle relaxants, stretching, or splinting. Botulinum toxin, injected in small amounts to paralyze muscle tissue and therefore reduce spasticity may be an alternative for some patients, but its effectiveness has not been demonstrated in clinical trials. Apraxia is the inability to perform purposeful, learned movements unexplained by deficits in strength, coordination, sensation, or comprehension, and results in difficulties with all tasks and activities. Interventions focus on restoration of performance of habitual or novel movements. Balance and coordination problems may also be present if cerebellar or motor integrative areas are affected.

Sensory Impairment   This includes dysesthesia, hyperesthesia, and visual impairment. Dysesthesia is defined as numbness, tingling, or lack of tactile sensation. Hyperesthesia is a syndrome characterized by excessive reaction to sensory stimuli. Maintaining patient safety is a primary issue when dealing with sensory loss, whether tactile or visual. Patients with sensory loss may not be aware of noxious stimuli and are at risk for injury. Compensatory strategies are the focus of treatment in teaching patients to shift to intact abilities, such as the use of visual scanning, increased use of nonaffected extremities, and regular inspection of body areas with decreased sensation.

Nutrition and Elimination   This includes dysphagia, diarrhea, constipation, and urinary incontinence. Swallowing disorders can quickly lead to dehydration in stroke survivors. Daily weights and intake/output may be helpful in identifying suspected problems. A speech-language pathologist should be consulted to evaluate swallowing function, and a modified barium swallow performed to assess for penetration of liquids. Thickening agents may be required for safe swallowing, along with recommendations regarding special diet and positions for feeding. In cases of severe swallowing dysfunction, a feeding tube may be required.

Fecal incontinence occurs in a substantial proportion of stroke survivors, but clears within two weeks in the majority of cases. Diarrhea may be due to medications, tube feedings, infection, or impaction. Constipation is more common in stroke survivors and may be due to immobility, dehydra-

tion, inadequate food intake, neurogenic bowel, lack of transfer ability, cognitive deficits, depression, or anxiety. Stool softeners and judicious use of laxatives may be helpful to prevent impaction.

Urinary function should be monitored in all elderly patients, and urinary incontinence should be worked up according to standard guidelines. Urinary tract infections may be related to immobility or catheter use. If the incontinence is functional, patients may be regularly assisted to the toilet or shown how to safely maneuver to a bedside commode or bathroom.

Sleep Disturbances   Many elderly patients, and stroke survivors in particular, suffer from disturbances in sleep patterns, especially when in unfamiliar environments. Sleep problems could be due to pain, muscle spasms, inability to move in bed, urinary frequency, depression, or anxiety. Patients often report fatigue secondary to a rigorous therapy schedule. Rest periods during the day may be helpful, but only if the patient does not sleep for too long. Zolpidem (Ambien) or zaleplon (Sonata), two nonbenzodiazepine hypnotics, cause relatively little residual sleepiness and may be helpful in reestablishing a regular sleep pattern. These should be used for a short term (7–10 days) only when necessary. Generally, hypnotics should be avoided because of hypersomnolence.

Cognitive/Perceptual Deficits   Common cognitive deficits following stroke include attention, orientation, short-term memory, problem solving, and visual spatial construction, and are generally related to the area of brain affected. Neglect, or hemi-inattention, refers to lack of awareness of a specific part of the body or external environment. Sensory stimuli in the affected half of the environment are ignored or evoke muted responses. Neglect usually resolves spontaneously, but can significantly hinder rehabilitation efforts. Treatment for cognitive and perceptual deficits emphasizes retraining, substitution of intact abilities, and compensatory approaches.

Communication Disorders   These include aphasia and dysarthria. Aphasia is the loss of ability to communicate orally, through signs or in writing, as well as lost ability to use language appropriately.

Dysarthria is a motor disorder that results in difficulty with motor speech. These disorders commonly coexist. Either disorder may result in high levels of frustration for patient and caregivers alike. Goals of treatment for both are to remediate the ability to speak, comprehend, read, and write, and to assist the patient in developing strategies that circumvent language problems. Speech-language pathologists can provide evaluation, recommendations, and exercises for speech-impaired patients.

Management of Comorbid Illnesses   Clinicians must be mindful of managing comorbid chronic medical illnesses, as these may limit the patient's participation in rehabilitative therapies. Commonly seen illnesses in the stroke survivor are: hypertension, ischemic heart disease, congestive heart failure, chronic pulmonary disease, and diabetes mellitus. Goals of treatment are to limit the impact of these illnesses on rehabilitation through regular monitoring and adjustment of medications as needed. Symptoms suggesting an acute illness (myocardial infarction, pulmonary embolus, etc.) should be evaluated promptly and transfer to an acute facility considered.

Prevention of Secondary Complications   Prevention of complications during the rehabilitation and chronic phases following stroke is critical to minimize disability and optimize outcomes, and requires an interdisciplinary approach. Many secondary complications of stroke are those associated with immobility. Pressure ulcers should be avoided with frequent turning, meticulous skin care, and good nutrition. Nutritional states can be jeopardized by swallowing disorders and should be monitored with regular attention to electrolyte, serum protein, albumin, and prealbumin levels. Swallowing dysfunction is a serious risk factor for aspiration pneumonia, and immobility places patients at risk for venous thrombosis and contractures. The risk for contractures may be worsened by increased muscle tone or spasticity. Early mobilization, frequent range of motion exercises, and low molecular weight heparins may be used unless contraindicated. Muscle weakness and coordination problems may lead to falls. Careful examination of deficit patterns (both physical and cognitive) and proper instruction in use of adaptive equipment is critical to fall risk assessment. Appropriate precautions should be implemented as for any person at high risk for falling.

Shoulder injury and shoulder pain syndromes are common following stroke. This may be due to arthritis, peripheral vascular disease, muscle spasms, or soft tissue or joint injury in the paretic limb. Pain syndromes may be related to reflex sympathetic dystrophy or thalamic pain syndrome. Proper positioning and support of paretic limbs is important and vigorous range of motion exercises should be avoided.

Prevention of Recurrent Stroke   Stroke recurrence is highest during the first 30 days after the initial event, with 30% of recurrences occurring within this time frame. Therefore, it is imperative that clinicians consider prevention of recurrence. Identification of the specific ischemic stroke mechanism guides decision making with regard to prevention therapy. For patients with atrial fibrillation or embolic stroke from a suspected cardiac source, warfarin (Coumadin) is dose-adjusted to an International Normalized Ratio (INR) in 2.0–3.0 range, and recommended as a lifelong therapy. In the case of a left-ventricular thrombus, or recent myocardial infarction, warfarin is indicated for a six-month course.[26] For patients with moderate to severe (> 50%) carotid artery stenosis with significant risk factors, the treatment of choice is carotid endarterectomy. For patients who do not have atrial fibrillation or moderate to severe carotid stenosis, treatment with a daily dose of aspirin (50–325 mg) is of demonstrated benefit. Other anti-platelet agents, such as clopidogrel (Plavix), extended release dipyridamole with aspirin (Aggrenox), and ticlopidine (Ticlid) also appear effective at reducing risk for second ischemic stroke. One study, however, suggested the use of ticlodipine with aspirin following coronary angioplasty and stenting to be complicated by the onset of thrombotic thrombocytopenic purpura in 1 of every 4,184 patients and fatal in > 20% of those affected. Therefore, ticlodipine should be used judiciously, and patients monitored carefully for untoward hemotologic effects.[26] A full assessment of additional modifiable risk factors should be conducted and addressed.

Confusional States   Alterations in mental status, or acute confusion, is quite common in the hospitalized elderly, and stroke patients are at increased risk for this secondary complication. Medication regimens should be evaluated, and any potential sources of infection investigated. A general workup for alteration in mental status may be found in Chapter 8.

Depression   This is very common in stroke survivors and may occur up to several years following the event. Symptoms of depression may be mild or signs of a major depressive disorder may be noted. Patients should be routinely monitored for both affective and vegetative symptoms and treated accordingly.

Chronic Phase

Patients are generally transitioned from acute rehabilitation into community/home settings within several weeks following stroke. Most functional gains continue for up to six months as neural reorganization occurs. Language functions may improve for up to one year following stroke. Both functional and language gains slow following the subacute period, but may still continue up to several years following stroke events.

Long-term follow-up primary care of stroke survivors should include regular visits every three to six months and as needed. Ongoing assessment of physical, functional, cognitive, and emotional states is imperative. Standardized assessments listed in Table 9–7 may be helpful to clinicians treating stroke survivors in the primary-care setting. Patients should be routinely monitored for appearance of each of the stroke sequelae addressed in the previous section. Although such problems are most common during the rehabilitation phase, they can appear at any time following stroke, particularly depression.

Of particular importance to stroke survivors are issues surrounding resumption of previous work, family, and social roles. Patients should be queried regarding the impact of the stroke on social activities, role adaptation, and quality of life. Several assessment tools (noted in Table 9–7) may be helpful in this regard.

Prevention of future cardiovascular events is of primary importance to stroke survivors. Preventive measures should be targeted to modifiable risk factors: elevated blood pressure, smoking, obesity, impaired glucose tolerance, physical inactivity, elevated total low-density lipoproteins (LDL) and elevated plasma homocysteine levels. Every effort should be made to limit these stroke risk factors using lifestyle modification and pharmcologic therapy as needed. Table 9–8 presents a guide to risk reduction for patients with prior stroke. Specific recommendations regarding antiplatelet therapy appear in the preceding section of the chapter. Additionally, clinicians should consider the use of HMG-CoA reductase inhibitors (statin drugs) for lowering LDL levels, as recent studies in post-myocardial infarction patients have shown effectiveness in preventing stroke.[27]

A recent finding from the Heart Outcomes Prevention Evaluation (HOPE) study indicates that the ACE-inhibitor ramipril (Altace) significantly reduces the rate of death, myocardial infarction, and stroke in patients at high risk for cardiovascular events.[28] The specific mechanism of action is not well understood, nor is it known if other ACE-inhibitors are as effective in reducing stroke risk. Clinicians are encouraged to consult guidelines derived from this and future studies for updates on treatment recommendations.

Finally, the role of aerobic and strength-training exercises in the chronic phase of stroke recovery is currently under investigation and shows promise for improving gait, motor strength, and balance, as well as cardiovascular fitness. Regular exercise has been demonstrated to reduce cardiovascular risk factors and improve mood and socialization in well older adult populations, and studies are under way to investigate the potential benefits of a supervised exercise program. In the interim, clinicians should encourage patients to remain active, including as much ambulatory activity in their daily routines as is safely possible.

Conclusion

Care of stroke survivors requires early assessment and quick action during the acute phase, and careful

Table 9–8   Guide to Risk Factor Reduction for Patients with Ischemic Cerebrovascular Disease[26]

Risk Factor	Goal	Recommendations
Hypertension	SBP <140 and DBP <90 SBP <135 and DBP <85	Lifestyle modification and antihypertensive medications
Smoking	Cessation	Strongly encourage patient and family to stop smoking. Provide nicotine replacement counseling and formal programs.
Diabetes mellitus	Glucose <126 mg/dl	Diet, oral hypoglycemics, insulin
Lipids	LDL, 100 mg/dl HDL >35mg/dl TC <200 mg/dl TG <200 mg/dl	Start AHA Step II diet: ≤30% fat, <7% saturated fat, <200 mg/dl cholesterol, and emphasize weight management and exercise. If target goal not achieved with these measures, add drug therapy (statin) if LDL >130 mg/dl, and consider drug therapy if LDL 100–130 mg/dl.
Alcohol	Moderate consumption ≤2 drinks/day)	Strongly encourage patient and family to stop excessive drinking or provide formal alcohol cessation program.
Physical activity	30–60 minutes of activity at least 3–4 times per week	Moderate exercise (e.g., brisk walking, jogging, cycling, or other aerobic activity) Medically supervised programs for high-risk patients (e.g., cardiac disease) and adaptive programs depending on neurologic deficits
Weight	≤120% IBW for height	Diet and exercise

monitoring and vigilance during the rehabilitation and chronic phases. Changes in function may be so insidious as to go unnoticed by the stroke survivor or family, and risk for secondary complications may remain high. A multidisciplinary, comprehensive approach to the care of stroke survivors has been demonstrated to be the most effective means for helping them to attain and maintain optimal recovery and health.

References

1. Colledge NR, Barr-Hamilton RM, Lewis SJ, Sellar RJ, Wilson JA. Evaluation of investigations to diagnose the cause of dizziness in elderly people: a community based controlled study. *BMJ.* 1996;313:788–792.

2. Yardley L, Owen N, Nazareth I, Luxton L. Prevalence and presentation of dizziness in a general practice community sample of working age people. *Br J Gen Pract.* 1998;48:1131–1135.

3. Boult C, Murphy J, Sloane P, Mor V, Drone C. The relation of dizziness to functional decline. *J Am Geriatr Soc.* 1991;39:858–861.

4. Sloan PD. Evaluation and management of dizziness in the older patient. *Clin Geriatr Med.* 1996;12(4):785–801.

5. Sloan PD. Clinical research and geriatric dizziness: the blind men and the elephant. *J Am Geriatr Soc.* 1999; 47:113–114.

6. Beers MH, Berkow R. *The Merck Manual of Geriatrics.* 3rd ed. Whitehouse Station, NJ: Merck Research Laboratories; 2000:187.

7. Miura M, Naito Y, Naito E, Funabiki K, Honjo I. Usefulness of magnetic resonance imaging and diagnosing vertebro-basilar insufficiency. *Acta Otolaryngol.* 1997;528:91–93.

8. Baloh RW. Dizziness in older people. *J Am Geriatr Soc.* 1992;40:713–721.
9. Lurie KG, Benditt D. Syncope and the autonomic nervous system. *J Cardiovasc Electrophysiol.* 1996; 7(8):760–776.
10. Grimm RJ. Dizziness. *Nurse Pract For.* 1996;7(4): 160–166.
11. Kerber KA, Enretto JA, Jacobsen KM, Baloh RW. Disequilibrium in older people. *Neurology.* 1998;51: 574–580.
12. Froehling D, Silverstein M, Mohr D, Beatty C. Does this patient have a serious form of vertigo? *JAMA.* 1994;271(5):385–388.
13. Baloh R, Baringer JR. Dizzy patients: the varieties of vertigo. *Hosp Prac.* 1998;June:55–77.
14. Williams GR, Jiang JG, Matchar DB, et al. Incidence and occurrence of total (first ever and recurrent) stroke. *Stroke.* 1999;30:2523–2528.
15. American Heart Association. Heart and Stroke A-Z Guide. Available at: http://www.americanheart.org/ Heart_and_stroke_A_Z_Guide/. Accessed March 13, 2001.
16. Pulsinelli W. Pathophysiology of acute ischaemic stroke. *Lancet.* 1992;339:533–536.
17. Dashe JF. Acute stroke evaluation and treatment. *Clin Adv Nurse Pract.* 2000;3:43.
18. Miller RM, Woo D. Stroke: current concepts of care. *Geriatr Nurs.* 1999;20:66–69.
19. DeKeyser J, Sulter G, Langediijk M, et al. Management of acute ischaemic stroke. *Acta Clinica Belgica.* 1999; 54:302–305.

20. National Stroke Association. *Stroke, the first hours: guidelines for acute treatment.* NSA consensus statement. Stroke Clinical Updates Special Edition, 2000. Available at:http://www.stroke.org/admin/pdf/out/firsthours.pdf. Accessed March 13, 2001.
21. Stewart DG. Stroke rehabilitation 1. Epidemiological aspects and acute management. *Arch Phys Med Rehabil.* 1999;80:S4–7.
22. Toni D, Fiorelli M, Bastianello S, et al. Hemorrhagic transformation of brain infarct. *Neurology.* 1996;46: 341–345.
23. Langhorne P, Williams BO, Gilchrist W, et al. Do stroke units save lives? *Lancet.* 1993;342:279–283.
24. Indredavik B, Bakke F, Solberg R, Rokseth R, Haaheim LL, Holme I. Benefit of a stroke unit: a randomized controlled trial. *Stroke.* 1991;22:755–759.
25. Agency for Health Care Policy and Research. *Clinical Practice Guideline Number 16: Post-Stroke Rehabilitation.* Rockville Md: U.S. Department of Health and Human Services; 1995. AHCPR publication 95-0662.
26. Wolf PA, Clagett P, Easton JD, et al. Preventing ischemic stroke in patients with prior stroke and transient ischemic attack. *Stroke.* 1999;30:1991–1994.
27. Plehn JF, Davis BR, Sacks FM, et al. Reduction of stroke incidence after myocardial infarction with pravastatin: the Cholesterol and Recurrent Events (CARE) Study. *Circulation.* 1999;95:216–233.
28. Heart Outcomes Prevention Evaluation Study Investigators. Effects of an angiotensin-converting-enzyme inhibitor, ramipril, on cardiovascular events in high-risk patients. *N Engl J Med.* 2000;342:145–153.

10

Dementia

Valerie T. Cotter

Introduction

Dementia is a clinical syndrome characterized by multiple cognitive deficits, severe enough to interfere with daily functioning in an alert individual. The 4th edition of the *Diagnostic and Statistical Manual of Mental Disorders* (DSM-IV) currently specifies criteria for the diagnosis of dementia and these are listed in Table 10–1.[1] Memory impairment (lessened ability to learn new information or to recall previously learned information) and deficits in one or more cognitive domains (aphasia, apraxia, agnosia, and executive function) must be present.

Advanced age is the major risk factor for dementia. The prevalence of dementia ranges from about 1% in individuals 60 years of age and 30–50% in individuals over the age of 85.[2] Prevalence varies by clinical setting with dementia present in about 10% of community-residing older adults over 65 years of age and close to 50% of older adults in nursing homes.[2,3] Other risk factors include history of head trauma, family history of dementia, and lower education.

Dementia is a general term that does not specify the etiology or underlying pathology. It is estimated that more than 55 illnesses are potential causes of dementia. Identification of dementia and determination of underlying cause(s) are essential to prevent further mental and functional decline and to avoid morbidity from unrecognized conditions and inappropriate drug use. Early diagnosis allows patients and family members the time to prepare for future medical, financial, legal, and ethical challenges. Initiating pharmacologic interventions earlier in the course of dementia can provide clinically meaningful improvements in cognition, mood, and function.

The advanced practice nurse (APN) is in a critical role to identify dementia and to work with the patient and family throughout the course of the disease. A biopsychosocial approach aimed at improving the function and quality of life of patients and caregivers should be the focus of care.

This chapter describes the evaluation and diagnosis, clinical features and course, behavioral symptoms, caregiver correlates, and pharmacologic and nonpharmacologic interventions of the most prevalent types of dementia.

Table 10–1 Diagnostic Criteria for Dementia

Multiple cognitive deficits involving both:
1. Memory impairment and
2. One or more of the following cognitive disturbances:
   - aphasia (language disturbance)
   - apraxia (inability to carry out motor activities despite intact motor function)
   - agnosia (failure to recognize or identify objects despite intact sensory function)
   - executive functioning (planning, organizing, sequencing, abstracting)

The cognitive deficits must cause significant impairment in social or occupational functioning and not occur only during the course of a delirium.

Differentiating Normal Aging from Dementia

Cognitive changes, such as a general slowing in the speed of thought processing and slight declines in memory and in the ability to manage multiple tasks simultaneously, are considered part of the normal aging process. Age-associated memory impairment (AAMI), labeled nearly two decades ago by Crook and colleagues,[4] describes progressive memory impairment considered to be a normal age-related change. The DSM-IV currently designates this as "age-related cognitive decline."[1]

More recently, mild cognitive impairment (MCI), a transitional phase between normal cognition and dementia, has been identified. A diagnosis of MCI is made if the patient meets the following criteria:

1. Memory complaint
2. Normal activities of daily living
3. Normal general cognitive function
4. Abnormal memory for age (1.5 SD below age and education-matched cutoff scores)
5. Not demented[5]

Patients with MCI appear to be at an increased risk of developing Alzheimer's disease (AD) at the rate of 10–12% per year, compared to rates of 1–3% in controls.[6] Early recognition of individuals with MCI generally targets those for whom pharmacological interventions would be beneficial in delaying progression to AD and shortening time in the severe stages of AD. The Alzheimer's Disease Cooperative Study, a National Institute on Aging consortium of Alzheimer's disease research groups, is currently involved in a multi-center trial investigating several drugs that may alter the progression of patients with MCI to AD.

Differential Diagnosis of Dementia

The differential diagnosis of dementia includes ruling out a broad range of neurologic, psychiatric, and other possible medical causes. The most common causes of dementia are Alzheimer's disease (AD) (60–80%), frontotemporal dementia (FTD) (10%), dementia with Lewy bodies (DLB) (10%), and vascular dementia (VaD) (5%). Late-life depression is often a prodromal or early sign of dementia, predominantly AD,[7] and can also be mistaken for dementia. Fully reversible causes of dementia, such as neurosyphilis, B_{12} deficiency, hypothyroidism, and drug toxicity are identified in less than 10% of individuals with cognitive decline.[8]

Pathology and Clinical Features

Alzheimer's Disease (AD)

AD is the most common cause of dementia in late life. Insidious onset of progressive loss of recent memory is present in the earliest stages, followed by disorders of language, praxis, and visual perception. Disease progression is gradual and the duration from onset to death averages from 8 to 10 years.[9] The characteristic pathologic changes in AD are B amyloid plaques, tau protein neurofibrillary tangles, neuronal loss, and hippocampal degeneration, yet the etiology of these changes is unknown. Loss of the neurotransmitter acetylcholine in the forebrain and cortical cholinergic neurons is instrumental in the pathogenesis of AD.

The two most widely accepted sets of criteria for the clinical diagnosis of AD are the DSM-IV[1] and the National Institute of Neurological and Communicative Disorders and Stroke-Alzheimer's Disease and Related Disorders Association (NINCDS-ADRDA).[10] The NINCDS clinical criteria for the diagnosis of probable, possible, and definite AD are outlined in Table 10–2. The clinical diagnosis of probable AD is made if a typical insidious onset of dementia with progression is present and if no other diseases could account for the cognitive deficits. The clinical diagnosis of possible rather than probable AD is used when one of two conditions exist:

1. The presentation or course of the dementia is somewhat inconsistent with that of AD, but best fits with AD.
2. Other illnesses are present that contribute to, but do not entirely explain, the dementia.

A diagnosis of definite AD requires pathologic evidence from an autopsy.

AD can be staged into mild, moderate, severe, profound, and terminal categories. This is the most commonly used staging system to categorize the severity of dementia. Many other staging systems are published in the literature and a few are discussed later in this chapter.

In the mild stage of AD, patients experience moderate memory loss interfering with daily func-

Table 10–2   Criteria for Clinical Diagnosis of Alzheimer's Disease[10]

1. The criteria for the clinical diagnosis of probable Alzheimer's disease include:

   - Dementia established by clinical examination and documented by the Mini-Mental Test, Blessed Dementia Scale, or some similar examination, and confirmed by neuropsychological tests
   - Deficits in two or more areas of cognition
   - Progressive worsening of memory and other cognitive functions
   - No disturbance of consciousness
   - Onset between ages 40 and 90, most often after age 65
   - Absence of systemic disorders or other brain diseases that in and of themselves could account for the progressive deficits in memory and cognition

2. The diagnosis of probable Alzheimer's disease is supported by:

   - Progressive deterioration of specific cognitive functions such as language (aphasia), motor skills (apraxia), and perception (agnosia)
   - Impaired ADLs and altered patterns of behavior
   - Family history of similar disorders, particularly if confirmed neuropathologically
   - Laboratory results of:

     normal lumbar puncture as evaluated by standard techniques

     normal pattern or nonspecific changes in EEG, such as increased slow-wave activity, and

     evidence of cerebral atrophy on CT with progression documented by serial observation

3. Other clinical features consistent with the diagnosis of probable Alzheimer's disease, after exclusion of causes of dementia other than Alzheimer's disease, include:

   - Plateaus in the course of progression of the illness
   - Associated symptoms of depression; insomnia; incontinence; delusions; illusions; hallucinations; catastrophic verbal, emotional, or physical outbursts; sexual disorders; and weight loss
   - Other neurologic abnormalities in some patients, especially with more advanced disease and including motor signs such as increased muscle tone, myoclonus, or gait disorder
   - Seizures in advanced disease
   - CT normal for age

4. Features that make the diagnosis of probable Alzheimer's disease uncertain or unlikely include:

   - Sudden, apoplectic onset
   - Focal neurologic findings such as hemiparesis, sensory loss, visual field deficits, and incoordination early in the course of the illness
   - Seizures or gait disturbances at the onset or very early in the course of the illness

5. Clinical diagnosis of possible Alzheimer's disease:

   - May be made on the basis of the dementia syndrome, in the absence of other neurologic, psychiatric, or systemic disorders sufficient to cause dementia, and in the presence of variations in the onset, in the presentation, or in the clinical course
   - May be made in the presence of a second systemic or brain disorder sufficient to produce dementia, which is not considered to be *the* cause of the dementia
   - Should be used in research studies when a single, gradually progressive severe cognitive deficit is identified in the absence of other identifiable cause

6. Criteria for diagnosis of definite Alzheimer's disease are:

   - The clinical criteria for probable Alzheimer's disease
   - Histopathologic evidence obtained from a biopsy or autopsy

7. Classification of Alzheimer's disease for research purposes should specify features that may differentiate subtypes of the disorder, such as:

   - Familial occurrence
   - Onset before age of 65
   - Presence of trisomy-21
   - Coexistence of other relevant conditions such as Parkinson's disease

tioning (e.g., misplacing items, repeating questions, difficulty managing medications or finances, decreased performance in housekeeping). The ability to perform basic activities of daily living (ADLs) is preserved (bathing, dressing, grooming, and using the bathroom). Language dysfunction is manifested by word-finding problems. Some disorientation to time and place occurs. The mildly impaired individual usually appears normal and is able to carry on a social conversation with others.

In the moderate stage, long-term memory is affected and new information is rapidly lost. Patients are no longer independent in activities outside of the home and need reminders or supervision to carry out ADLs. Judgment and problem solving are usually impaired. Behavioral symptoms may occur, including hallucinations, aggression, sleep alterations, and wandering. The exact origins of these behaviors are unknown, but they are thought to be related to psychological factors, neurochemical changes occurring in the brain, and the environment. All behavior has meaning and, therefore, has a cause.[11]

As the disease progresses to the severe stage, few fragments of memory remain. Ability to speak is markedly impaired and patients rely completely on others for personal care. Despite cognitive deterioration, incontinence, and other functional problems, evidence suggests the person retains awareness of self and ability to respond emotionally.[12,13]

Between the severe and terminal stages a period of profound dementia is likely. The profound stage occurs between Functional Assessment Staging (FAST)[14] stage 6 and 7 and is characterized by more frequent incontinence, less verbal output, and loss of ambulation.

The terminal stage is marked by further cognitive and functional deterioration, including urinary and fecal incontinence, unintelligible speech, inability to walk or sit up without assistance, and loss of ability to smile or hold up the head independently. Complications frequently associated with end-stage AD are aspiration pneumonia, urinary tract infection, septicemia, stage 3–4 pressure ulcers, recurrent fevers, and significant weight loss.

Frontotemporal Dementia (FTD)

FTD affects primarily the frontal or temporal cortex. Two histologic types exist: prominent microvacuolar change without specific histologic features (FTD) or severe astrocytic gliosis with or without ballooned cells and inclusion bodies (Pick type). Onset typically occurs early in the fifth or sixth decade of life with gradual progression. Incidence appears familial in origin with mutations on chromosome 17.

Three clinical syndromes occur in FTD: frontal dementia (FD), primary progressive aphasia (PPA), and semantic dementia (SD).[15] FD is a disorder of profound alteration in personality and behavior, characterized by inertia and social disinhibition, but with relative preservation of memory function. PPA and SD are progressive language disorders that occur in the absence of impairment in other cognitive domains. In PPA, expressive language is impaired and characterized by nonfluent speech, with at least one of the following: agrammatism (omission or incorrect use of grammatical terms), phonemic paraphasias (sound-based errors, e.g., "gat" for "cat"), and anomia (inability to find the correct word). SD is characterized by the loss of word meaning, an inability to recognize familiar faces and objects, or both of these impairments.

Dementia with Lewy Bodies (DLB)

Although this neurodegenerative dementia has features of AD and the dementia associated with Parkinson's disease, it is a distinct entity. The pathologic hallmarks are the presence of Lewy bodies (intracytoplasmic inclusions) in the cortex, amygdala, and hippocampus, with atrophy in the substantia nigra and nucleus ceruleus. Clinical criteria for the diagnosis include progressive cognitive decline with prominent or persistent memory impairment and at least one of the following:

1. Fluctuating cognition with variations in attention and alertness

2. Recurrent visual hallucinations that are well formed and detailed

3. Spontaneous motor features of parkinsonism.[16]

In the early stages, short-term memory impairment may be mild and substantial fluctuations in cognition and behavior may occur rapidly or slowly, fluctuate from hour to hour, or be present at times and not present at other times. Daytime sleepiness with transient confusion on waking is common. Repeated falls, syncopal attacks without focal neurologic signs and symptoms, and transient losses of consciousness may support a diagnosis of DLB. Patients are often sensitive to neuroleptic medications and these should be avoided if DLB is suspected.

Vascular Dementia (VaD)

VaD refers to a broad range of cognitive dysfunctions associated with cerebrovascular disease. The symptoms are highly variable because they depend on the location, size, number, and severity of the cerebrovascular lesions. Onset may be acute or subacute, and rather than a course of gradually progressive decline as in AD, cognitive impairment with VaD may fluctuate and even improve. Risk factors for VaD include hypertension, coronary disease, diabetes, hyperlipidemia, smoking, increased age, and history of stroke. Vascular pathology affecting large cortical vessels or small deep white matter and subcortical vessels is often evident on neuroimaging; however, these changes do not exclude the possibility that AD, rather than stroke, may be responsible for dementia. In addition, the presence of cerebral infarctions or other vascular lesions does not necessarily indicate that the lesions are responsible for the dementia.

The most common type of VaD is multi-infarct dementia (MID). It has an abrupt onset, stepwise deterioration and a fluctuating course. Focal neurologic signs are usually present on exam. Autopsy studies of patients with the clinical diagnosis of MID suggest that in most cases the patients have both cerebrovascular disease and AD. This "mixed dementia" is more common than "pure" VaD. Cerebral infarctions accelerate cognitive decline in AD patients.

One guide for diagnosis is the National Institute of Neurological Disorders and Stroke-Association Internationale pour la Recherche et l'Enseignement en Neurosciences (NINDS-AIREN) criteria for classifying VaD.[17] This mandates deficits in memory and two other cognitive domains. The onset of dementia must occur either within three months after the stroke, abruptly or in a fluctuating, stepwise progression. The clinical diagnosis of probable VaD is made if the history of cognitive dysfunction coincides with neurologic deficits, evidence of cerebrovascular disease, and presence of lesions on imaging. When the course is variable, evidence on imaging is absent, or the timing of cognitive dysfunction to cerebrovascular insult does not match, a diagnosis of possible VaD is given. A diagnosis of definite VaD is made when there is pathologic evidence of cerebrovascular disease, without neurofibrillary tangles and neuritic plaques, and a prior diagnosis of probable VaD.

Identifying Signs of Dementia

Patients often lack insight and awareness about functional and cognitive declines; therefore, the APN must interview both the patient and a knowledgeable informant. Informants are usually the adult child, spouse, partner, or close friend. The history should focus on the functional, cognitive, mood, and behavioral symptoms, as listed in Table 10–3.[18] A review of the chronology, duration, and progression of symptoms, and their effects on the patient and the caregiver, are essential.

Functional declines, such as difficulty with medications, finances, driving, organizing and cooking meals, and decreased performance in housekeeping chores and shopping, occur early in dementia. In most types of dementia, especially AD, ADL skills are preserved until the moderate stage of disease.

Prominent signs of dysfunction are present in one or more cognitive domains in dementia: decline in memory (e.g., asking the same question repeatedly, difficulty retaining new information), language (e.g., difficulty with word finding or understanding conversation), constructional praxis (e.g., getting lost in familiar places), executive function (e.g., difficulty planning, organizing, and

Table 10–3 Symptoms That May Indicate Dementia[18]

Does the person have increased difficulty with any of the activities listed below?

- *Learning and retaining new information.* Is more repetitive; has trouble remembering recent conversations, events, appointments; frequently misplaces objects.

- *Handling complex tasks.* Has trouble following a complex train of thought or performing tasks that require many steps such as balancing a checkbook or cooking a meal.

- *Reasoning ability.* Is unable to respond with a resonable plan to problems at work or home, such as knowing what to do if the bathroom is flooded; shows uncharacteristic disregard for rules of social conduct.

- *Spatial ability and orientation.* Has trouble driving, organizing objects around the house, finding his or her way around familiar places.

- *Language.* Has increasing difficulty with finding the words to express what he or she wants to say and with following conversations.

- *Behavior.* Appears more passive and less responsive; is more irritable than usual; is more suspicious than usual; misinterprets visual or auditory stimuli.

In addition to failure to arrive at the right time for appointments, the clinician can look for difficulty discussing current events in an area of interest, and changes in behavior or dress. It also may be helpful to follow up on areas of concern by asking the patient or family members relevant questions.

executing activities), orientation (e.g., difficulty with time, not recognizing familiar places), and judgment (e.g., inappropriate problem solving or decision making). Elicit a careful description of the initial symptoms of dementia to differentiate its etiology: insidious memory loss in AD, behavioral or language changes in FTD, visual hallucinations in DLB, and symptoms of focal neurologic deficits in VaD.

Personality changes (e.g., social withdrawal, apathy, irritability) and mood changes (complaints of diminished ability to think, sense of hopelessness or helplessness, changes in sleep or appetite, behavioral slowing, or agitation) may be signs of dementia, depression, or both syndromes. Depression often coexists with dementia in approximately 20% of individuals with AD[19] and is associated with increased functional impairments and reduced enjoyment in activities.[20] Hopelessness, helplessness, and subsyndromal distress are more common symptoms than depressed mood in older adults.[21] APNs should evaluate individuals for depression in the initial workup of dementia and be attentive for signs of depression throughout its course. Failure to identify and treat depression or related psychological distress has a tremendous impact on the well being and quality of life of both the patient and caregiver.

Dramatic character changes, disordered social behavior, disinhibition, and impulsivity are prominent early behavioral symptoms in FTD. Visual hallucinations, typically recurrent and detailed, and less frequently, auditory hallucinations, occur early and often in DLB.[14] Behavioral symptoms such as hallucinations or verbal or physical aggressiveness are not common in the early stages of AD, but occur frequently in the moderate and severe stages of the disease.

Other Relevant History

Ask about relevant past medical history: neurological disorders, including Parkinson's disease, history of head trauma, or stroke; psychiatric disorders, such as depression, schizophrenia, or alcohol or substance abuse; and other acute or chronic medical conditions, such as infection, hypertension, delirium, or diabetes, that may cause or contribute to cognitive impairment.

Prescription drugs, over-the-counter drugs, and alcohol should be reviewed as possible contributors to cognitive impairment. A wide range of drugs has been associated with cognitive impairment, including anticholinergics, sedative-hypnotics, and beta-blockers.

A family history of dementia in a first-degree relative is a relative risk factor for dementia. In AD, having an affected family member increases an individual's risk about fourfold.[22]

Physical Examination

The physical examination is aimed at identifying neurologic or other medical abnormalities that could cause or contribute to dementia. The examination is usually normal in early AD. Focal neurologic signs may suggest VaD or some other neurologic disorder. Extrapyramidal motor signs, such as rigidity, bradykinesia, stooped posture, and a slow, shuffling gait, are common findings in DLB.[14] Primitive reflexes may be present in early FTD.[13]

Laboratory Evaluation

Laboratory evaluation should include electrolyte, blood chemistry, liver function, complete blood count, thyrotropin, vitamin B_{12}, and when appropriate, a screen for neurosyphilis. Additional laboratory tests are based on individual presentation, other medical comorbidity, and findings from the history and physical examination.

Brain Imaging Studies

Anatomic imaging with either a noncontrast computed tomography (CT) or magnetic resonance imaging (MRI) study of the head rules out conditions such as subdural hematoma, brain tumor, or stroke. Brain atrophy greater than expected for age in the frontal or anterior temporal lobes supports a diagnosis of FTD or AD when reported in the temporal lobes. Functional imaging with positron emission tomography (PET) or single photon emission computed tomography (SPECT) shows a promising role in the diagnosis, but is controversial and currently utilized only in research settings.

Genetic Testing

Genetic testing can be useful in narrowing a differential diagnosis and confirming a diagnosis suggested by clinical assessment. In dementia, however, it is controversial and involves ethical issues. Tests for mutations on chromosomes 1, 14, and 21 can be considered if the family history suggests early-onset AD. Mutations on chromosome 17 in FTD and chromosome 21 in some rare types

of VD have been identified. The presence of one or two copies of the apolipoprotein E (APOE) e4 allele on chromosome 19 has been associated with increased risk of late-onset AD. APOE genotyping is not accurate enough to predict future risk of AD and should not be used as a diagnostic test.

Cognitive Function Assessment

Mental Status Tests   The complete mental status assessment involves level of consciousness, attention, language, memory, constructional praxis, executive function, and judgment. Many short screening instruments exist to assist in the diagnosis and staging of dementia. Brief standardized cognitive tests are useful to screen for early signs of dementia and to provide a baseline measure of cognitive function against which to compare future assessments. Cognitive testing provides a measure of progression, response to treatment, and functional capacity to carry out daily activities. Detailed testing, performed by a neuropsychologist, is helpful in differentiating complex presentations of cognitive dysfunction or if the diagnosis is unclear. Most patients, however, do not require referral for cognitive testing.

The Mini-Mental State Examination (MMSE)[23] is the most widely used of all brief cognitive screening and longitudinal follow-up tests, regardless of clinical setting. It is a 30-item scale that measures orientation, language, concentration, constructional praxis, and memory (Table 10–4). A score of ≤ 24 indicates cognitive impairment. The MMSE is affected by education; patients with higher education may show normal cognitive scores in the presence of actual cognitive impairment, and conversely, patients with lower education may have low MMSE scores and no functional or cognitive decline.

Functional Assessment   Structured assessments of functional performance ought to be utilized in addition to standardized short mental status tests to identify individuals with cognitive impairment, confirm a diagnosis of dementia, and over the course of the disease, provide measures against which to compare future assessments. Such assess-

Table 10–4   The Mini-Mental State Examination

Maximum Score	Orientation
5	What is the (year) (season) (date) (day) (month)?
5	Where are we (state) (county) (town) (hospital) (floor)?

	Registration
3	Name three objects: one second to say each. Then ask the patient to repeat all three after you have said them. Give one point for each correct answer. Repeat them until he or she learns all three. Count trials and record number.

	Attention and Calculation
5	Begin with 100 and count backward by 7 (stop after five answers). Alternatively, spell "world" backward.

	Recall
3	Ask for three objects repeated above.

	Language
2	Show a pencil and a watch and ask the patient to name them.
1	Repeat the following: "No ifs, ands, or buts."
3	A three-stage command: "Take a paper in your right hand, fold it in half, and put it on the floor."
1	Read and obey the following: (show written item) CLOSE YOUR EYES
1	Write a sentence.
1	Copy a design (complex polygon).
30	Total score possible

Source: "Mini-Mental State." A Practical Method for Grading the Cognitive State of Patients for the Clinician. *Journal of Psychiatric Research,* 12(3):189–198, 1975, 1998 Mini Mental LLC.

ments also serve as objective measures of progression and to a lesser extent, response to treatment.

The Dementia Severity Rating Scale (DSRS) is a useful instrument to assess the cognitive-based ability to function in the home environment.[24] This informant-based, 11-item scale has high reliability and correlates with assessment of overall severity and cognitive function in AD. The DSRS assesses the major functional and cognitive domains affected in AD including memory, orientation, judgment, community affairs, home activities, personal care, speech/language, recognition, feeding, incontinence, and mobility/walking (Table 10–5). Scores increase with disease severity; less than 4 in normal cognition; 7–10 in mild cognitive impairment; 11–21 in mild-stage AD; 22–32 in moderate-stage AD; and 33–47 in severe-stage AD. The 11-item DSRS is useful in the longitudinal

Table 10–5   Dementia Severity Rating Scale

Memory

0 Normal.

1 Occasional "benign" forgetfulness of no consequence.

2 Mild consistent forgetfulness with partial recollection of events.

3 Moderate memory loss, more marked for recent events and severe enough to interfere with everyday activities.

4 Severe memory loss; only well-learned material retained with newly learned material rapidly lost.

5 Usually unable to remember basic facts such as the day of the week, month, and/or year, when last meal was eaten, or the name of the next meal.

6 Unable to test due to speech and language difficulty and/or ability to follow instructions.

7 Makes no attempt to communicate and is no longer aware of surroundings.

Orientation

0 Normal.

1 Some difficulty with time relationships, but not severe enough to interfere with everyday activities.

2 Frequently disoriented in time and sometimes disoriented to new places.

3 Almost always disoriented in time and usually disoriented to place.

4 Unable to answer questions related to time of day or name of present location.

5 Is unaware of questioner and makes no attempt to respond.

Table 10–5 *(continued)*

Judgment

0 Normal.

1 Only doubtful impairment in problem-solving ability.

2 Moderate difficulty in handling complex problems, but social judgment usually maintained.

3 Severe impairment in handling problems, social judgment usually impaired.

4 Unable to exercise judgment in either problem solving or social situations.

Social Interactions/Community Affairs

0 No alteration in ability to participate in community affairs.

1 Only mild impairment, of no practical consequence, but clearly different from previous years. Still able to work (if applicable), but performance not up to previous standards.

2 Unable to function independently in community activities, although still able to participate to some extent and, to casual inspection, may appear normal. Unable to hold a job or, if still working, requires constant supervision.

3 No pretense of independent function outside of home. Unable to hold a job but still participates in home activities with friends. Casual acquaintances are aware of a problem.

4 No longer participates in any meaningful way in home-based social activities involving people other than the primary caregiver.

Home Activities/Responsibilities

0 Normal.

1 Some impairment in activities such as money management and house maintenance, but no effect on the ability to shop, cook, or clean. Still watches TV and reads newspaper with interest and understanding.

2 Unable to perform activities related to money management (bill paying, etc.) or complex household tasks (maintenance). Some difficulty with shopping, cooking, and/or cleaning. Losing interest in the newspaper and TV.

3 No longer able to shop, cook, or clean without considerable help and supervision. No longer able to read the newspaper or watch TV with understanding.

4 No longer engages in any home-based activities.

Personal Care

0 Normal.

1 Needs occasional prompting but washes and dresses independently.

2 Requires assistance with dressing, hygiene, and personal upkeep.

3 Totally dependent for help. Does not initiate personal care activities.

Speech/Language

0 Normal.

1 Occasional difficulty with word finding, but able to carry on conversations.

2 Unable to think of some words, may occasionally make inappropriate word substitutions.

3 No longer spontaneously initiates conversation but can usually answer questions using sentences.

4 Answers questions, but responses are often unintelligible or inappropriate. Able to follow simple instructions.

5 Speech usually unintelligible or irrelevant. Unable to answer questions or follow verbal instructions.

6 No response, vegetative.

Recognition

0 Normal.

1 Occasionally fails to recognize more distant acquaintances or casual friends.

2 Always recognizes family and close friends but usually not more distant acquaintances.

3 Alert, occasionally fails to recognize family and/or close friends.

4 Only occasionally recognizes spouse or caregiver.

5 No recognition or awareness of the presence of others.

Feeding

0 Normal.

1 May require help cutting food and/or have limitations as to the type of food, but otherwise, able to eat independently.

2 Generally able to eat independently but may require some assistance.

3 Needs to be fed. May have difficulty swallowing or requires feeding tube. *(continues)*

Table 10–5   Dementia Severity Rating Scale *(continued)*

Incontinence

0   Normal.

1   Rare incontinence. Bladder incontinence (generally less than one accident per month).

2   Occasional bladder incontinence (an average of two or more times a month).

3   Frequent bladder incontinence despite assistance (more than once per week).

4   Total incontinence.

Mobility/Walking

0   Normal.

1   May occasionally have some difficulty driving or taking public transportation, but fully independent for walking without supervision.

2   Able to walk outside without supervision for short distances, but unable to drive or take public transportation.

3   Able to walk within the home without supervision, but cannot go outside unaccompanied.

4   Requires supervision within the home, but able to walk without assistance (may use cane or walker).

5   Generally confined to a bed or chair. May be able to walk a few steps with help.

6   Essentially bedridden. Unable to sit or stand.

---

assessment of AD, but the abbreviated 5-item scale (Table 10–6) is all that is needed for screening purposes. A screening score of greater than 4 suggests clinically meaningful cognitive impairment. The DSRS can be mailed to the informant to expedite the interview process or completed during the visit.

The Global Deterioration Scale (GDS),[25] for the clinical staging of AD, describes seven distinct stages, from normal (stage 1) to severe AD (stage 7). It has been expanded into the FAST system[12] (Table 10–7). Stages 1 through 5 of the FAST correspond to stages 1 through 5 of the GDS. Stages 6 and 7 of the GDS have been subdivided into 5 and 6 subcategories in the FAST. The distinct advan-

Table 10–6   Functional Assessment

(To be completed by knowledgeable informant)

Person completing form _____

Relationship to patient _____

In each section, please circle the *one number* that most closely applies to the patient. This is a general form, so no one category may be exactly right—please circle the answer that seems closest at this time.

Please circle only one number per section.

Memory

0   Normal memory.

1   Occasionally forgets things that s/he was told recently. Does not cause many problems.

2   Mild consistent forgetfulness. Remembers recent events but often forgets parts.

3   Moderate memory loss. Worse for recent events. May not remember something you just told him/her. Causes problems with everyday activities.

4   Substantial memory loss. Quickly forgets recent or newly learned things. Can only remember things that s/he has known for a long time.

Speech and Language

0   Normal ability to talk and understand others.

1   Sometimes cannot find a word, but able to carry on conversations.

2   Often forgets words. May use the wrong word in its place. Some trouble expressing thoughts and giving answers.

3   Usually answers questions using sentences but rarely starts a conversation.

Date and Time

0   Normal awareness of the time and which day of the week it is.

1   Some confusion about what time it is or what day of the week it is, but the problem is not severe enough to interfere with everyday activities.

2   Frequently confused about the date and/or time.

Ability to Make Decisions

0   Normal. As able to make decisions as before.

1   Only some difficulty making decisions that arise in day-to-day life.

2   Moderate difficulty. Gets confused when things get complicated or plans change.

Table 10–6   (continued)

Ability to Get From Place to Place

0 Normal, able to get around on his/her own. (May have physical problems that require a cane or walker.)

1 Sometimes gets confused when driving or taking public transportation, especially in new places. Able to walk places alone.

2 Cannot drive or take public transportation alone, even in familiar distances. Might get lost if walking too far from home.

Source: Clark CM, Arnold SE, Karlawish JHT, Horowitz D. Functional Assessment. From Dementia Disease Management Program, University of Pennsylvania Health System, 1999. Retrieved April 26, 2001 from the UPHS Intranet; http://uphsnet.med.upenn.edu/dm/dementia.

tage of the FAST system is its ability to assess functional change in the very severe, end-stage, immobile patient with AD.[12] Stage 7 or beyond, according to the FAST scale, is currently utilized to determine Medicare eligibility for hospice services for dementia.

Behavioral Symptoms and Mood Assessment

The assessment of behavioral symptoms and mood is important because these often have serious consequences for the patient and caregiver. Depression leads to higher levels of functional impairment and decreased enjoyment in activities with AD.[19] Caregivers also experience higher levels of depression, burden, and distress[26,27] as behavioral symptoms increase. This distress is associated with greater nursing home placement.[28] With even mod-

Table 10–7   Functional Assessment Staging (FAST)

(Check highest consecutive level of disability.)

1. No difficulty either subjectively or objectively.

2. Complains of forgetting location of objects. Subjective work difficulties.

3. Decreased job functioning evident to coworkers. Difficulty in traveling to new locations. Decreased organizational capacity.

4. Decreased ability to perform complex task (e.g., planning dinner for guests, handling personal finances, such as forgetting to pay bills, difficulty marketing, etc.).

5. Requires assistance in choosing proper clothing to wear for the day, season, or occasion (e.g. patient may wear the same clothing repeatedly, unless supervised).

6. A) Improperly putting on clothes without assistance or cueing (e.g., may put street clothes on over night clothes, or put shoes on wrong feet, or have difficulty buttoning clothing) (occasionally or more frequently over the past weeks).

   B) Unable to bathe properly (e.g., difficulty adjusting bath-water temperature) (occasionally or more frequently over the past weeks).

   C) Inability to handle mechanics of toileting (e.g., forget to flush the toilet, does not wipe properly or properly dispose of toilet tissue) (occasionally or more frequently over the past weeks).

   D) Urinary incontinence (occasionally or more frequently over the past weeks).

   E) Fecal incontinence (occasionally or more frequently over the past weeks).

7. A) Ability to speak limited to approximately a half a dozen intelligible different words or fewer, in the course of an average day or in the course of an intensive interview.

   B) Speech ability is limited to the use of a single intelligible word in an average day or in the course of an intensive interview (the person may repeat the word over and over).

   C) Ambulatory ability is lost (cannot walk without personal assistance).

   D) Cannot sit up without assistance (e.g., the individual will fall over if there are not lateral rests [arms] on the chair).

   E) Loss of ability to smile.

   F) Loss of ability to hold up head independently.

Source: Reisberg B. Functional assessment staging (FAST). *Psychopharmacol Bull.* 1988;24:653–659.

Specific Behavior: _____

Client's Name: _____ Room # _____

Date	Exact time	What happened?	Where?	Who else was present?	What could be happening internally (*inside* client) to precipitate behavior?	What could be happening externally (*outside* client) to precipitate behavior?	What interventions help (could help) client?

Figure 10–1
The Behavior Log; a useful assessment tool.[32]

est reductions in behavioral and mood symptoms, substantial improvements in functioning and quality of life are possible.

Behavioral and mood symptoms are common at particular stages in degenerative dementia. Depression and anxiety are more prevalent in the early stages of the disease; behavioral symptoms of verbal or physical agitation, delusions, hallucinations, sleep disturbance, anger, aggressiveness, and emotional lability are more common in the moderate and severe stages. The frequency and severity of behavioral symptoms increase with dementia progression and peak in occurrence before FAST stage 7.[29] Major depression is relatively rare in AD, although minor subsyndromal depression is much more frequent (up to 50% of patients at some point in the illness). Physical aggression is associated with depression in more severe dementia.[30] Assessment can be difficult because of overlap of symptoms of depression and dementia: apathy, social withdrawal, decreased concentration, decreased appetite, agitation, and insomnia are present in both. Assessment of mood and behavior is an important part of the initial evaluation with any cognitive impairment, as well as the periodic assessment with dementia. For comprehensive assessment of depression, see chapter 8.

The environment affects behavior in dementia and must be carefully evaluated when determining patient needs. Environmental design, routines, family interaction, and activities are all critical determinants of behavior. The Progressively Lowered Stress Threshold (PLST) model, a conceptual framework used in long-term care, can be applied in other settings as well. The PLST model uses the following six triggers to identify potential causes of behavioral symptoms:

1. Fatigue in the patient

2. Change of environment, routine, or caregiver

3. Affective responses to perception of loss

4. Responses to overwhelming or misleading stimuli

5. Excessive demand

6. Delirium[31]

The Behavior Log (BL) is a useful assessment tool for the clinical evaluation of behavior.[32] It facilitates observation and documentation of specific behaviors so that pattern(s) and meaning can be understood. The BL is structured to focus on one symptom at a time, noting frequency, location, time of day, associated factors, and caregiver interventions (Figure 10–1).

The Revised Memory and Behavior Problems Checklist (RMBPC)[33] is a 24-item caregiver report of observable behaviors with dementia. The caregiver rates the frequency of memory-related behaviors, depressive behaviors, and noncognitive behaviors, as well as reactions to each behavior. Caregiver reaction ratings are highly correlated with caregiver depression and burden. This is one of the few instruments to measure both patient behavior and caregiver reactions.

Management

The need to focus interventions not only on the patient, but also the caregivers, is increasingly recognized. Skill is required to design the best approaches for effective, humanistic care to enhance function and quality of life. Treatment usually involves appropriate behavioral interventions based on an understanding of the patient's cognitive and emotional state, environmental modifications, medication, and support and education of the caregiver. Pharmacologic treatments for dementia are aimed at improving memory and other cognitive and behavioral symptoms and slowing the progression of disease. Thus far, clinical trials have investigated various drugs for use with AD, to improve symptoms and delay progression, but not in other types of dementia.

Improvement of Cognitive Symptoms and Delay of Progression

Drugs that enhance acetylcholine function, such as the acetylcholinesterase (AchE) inhibitors (e.g., tetrahydroaminoacridine, donepezil, rivastigmine), are approved for the symptomatic treatment of mild to moderately severe AD. Tetrahydroaminoacridine (Tacrine), the first AchE inhibitor, is rarely used because of its significant cholinergic adverse effects (diarrhea, nausea, vomiting) and hepatotoxicity. Donepezil (Aricept), released in 1997, is safer and requires less frequent dosing. It appears to improve global cognitive function at the 5 mg dose, and the 10 mg dose shows somewhat greater improvement.[34] Donepezil is started at 5 mg per day, taken in the morning, to avoid nightmares, and then increased to 10 mg if clinical benefits are not evident. Rivastigmine (Exelon) is started at 1.5 mg twice daily, and then increased to 6–12 mg per day. Thus far, no clinical trials have been conducted directly comparing the safety and efficacy of any of the AchE inhibitors. Treatment can be continued indefinitely with these drugs, although evidence is insufficient to recommend it in the later stages of disease.

Gingko biloba is a widely publicized dietary supplement to improve memory and to relieve anxiety and depression. Several trials have suggested modest beneficial effects in dementia; however, a more recent rigorous trial has failed to demonstrate any clinically meaningful benefit of gingko in older adults with mild to moderate dementia or AAMI.[35]

Alpha-tocopherol (vitamin E), an antioxidant, delays functional deterioration and slows the progression of AD. One large study of AD patients compared alpha-tocopherol (2000 IU daily), seliginine (10 mg daily), alone or in combination with placebo, and the time to institutional placement, loss of the ability to perform ADLs, severe dementia, or death.[36] Significant differences were found in outcomes in the alpha-tocopherol (670 days), selegiline (655 days), and combined group (581 days), as compared to the placebo group (440 days). Unlike selegiline, alpha-tocopherol is generally safe and well tolerated and therefore can be administered to most patients. As long as slowing the disease is a goal, alpha-tocopherol 1000 IU twice daily is recommended in dementia.

Estrogen may improve cholinergic neuron function and cerebral blood flow and decrease production of B amyloid plaques in the central nervous system. It is ineffective for cognitive symptoms or slowing the decline of AD,[37] although clinical trials are under way to evaluate its role in the prevention of AD. Anti-inflammatory drugs may reduce the production of complements, acute phase reactants, and cytokines found in B amyloid plaques. No data supports the use of anti-inflammatory drugs to treat symptoms or slow decline in AD. The role of anti-inflammatory drugs in the prevention of AD is also under investigation.

Behavioral and Mood Symptoms

Three principles guide the treatment of symptoms related to behavior and mood:

1. Something can be done for individuals with dementia.
2. Factors that cause excess disability with dementia must be identified in order to improve function and quality of life.
3. Behaviors represent understandable feelings and/or the expression of needs, even if these cannot be verbally articulated.[38]

Medications are central to the management of psychosis, aggression, and depression, but are generally not helpful with wandering[39] or disruptive vocalizations.[40] Atypical antipsychotics (e.g., Risperidone, Olanzapine, Quetiapine) are indicated for psychotic thinking and hallucinations which are distressing to the patient or lead to aggressive behavior toward others. Start with a very low dose and titrate up to the lowest effective dose. These drugs should be reduced and eliminated when psychotic behaviors are no longer a problem.

No strong evidence favors one drug class over another to treat depressive or agitated behaviors. Behavioral symptoms and underlying etiology(s) and other medical comorbidities need to be carefully considered before deciding on a possibly beneficial course of drug treatment.

Selective serotonergic reuptake inhibitors (SSRIs), trazodone, and anticonvulsants are useful to treat depressive symptoms (irritable mood, withdrawal, verbal hostility). Trazodone (Desyrel) 25–100 mg twice daily is preferred when a more rapidly acting antidepressant is indicated. Valproic acid (Depakote) 125–1500 mg daily in divided doses or carbemazepine (Tegretol) 200–600 mg daily in divided doses are useful with significant agitation, impulsivity, disinhibition, and emotional lability. With the anticonvulsants, carefully monitor for hepatotoxicity, blood dyscrasias, and bleeding disorders. A comprehensive review of antidepressant drug therapy is found in chapter 8.

For event-related agitation, medication may be given on a one-time basis or as needed. Trazodone 25–100 mg every four hours, lorazepam (Ativan) 0.25–1.0 mg every four hours, or oxazepam (Serax) 10–20 mg every four hours, are recommended.

Nonpharmacologic Interventions

Support and education of the caregiver is essential to any set of therapeutic interventions. Caregivers play a significant role in the day-to-day experiences of the patient and the caregiver–patient relationship is important in terms of mood and function in both. Varying levels of distress, depression, and anxiety in the caregiver have a considerable impact on the patient, and vice versa.[27]

A randomized controlled trial of 206 spouse-caregivers of AD patients living at home demonstrated that an intensive program of counseling and support enables caregivers to withstand the difficulties of caregiving and to avoid or defer institutionalization.[28] The program consisted of three components:

1. Two individual and four family counseling sessions over a four–month period, emphasizing problem solving and management of troublesome patient behavior, providing emotional support, and promoting communication among family members.
2. A required weekly support group.
3. Continuous availability of counselors to help caregivers deal with crises and disease progression.

Patients in the experimental group remained at home an average of 329 days longer than those not in the program, in large part because caregivers learned to manage and to decrease the severity of patient behaviors.

With an individualized approach, a structured environment promoting comfort and ongoing involvement, and skillful communication techniques, patient behavior can be understood and modified in a compassionate manner. A supportive environment emphasizes the need for meaningful social interactions that allow persons with dementia to achieve a greater measure of self-fulfillment, as overall functional capacity declines.[41]

A dementia daycare program located in the community or within a nursing home is an excellent environment to support people with dementia through ongoing activity and socialization. Such programs also support the caregiver by providing respite. Patients should attend two to three times weekly to establish a routine and gain maximum benefit. It is often difficult for patient and caregiver to adjust to separation from each other in the initial few weeks. Caregivers need to know the goals of the program and to expect rejection by the patient in the beginning. Within a month, most patients adjust to the program and look forward to attending. Local area agencies on aging and the Alzheimer's Association (www.alz.org or 1–800–272–3900) can assist in locating programs.

Alzheimer disease special care units (SCUs) are widely available in long-term care settings across the United States. SCUs are extremely diverse but are not standardized other than to meet any regulations imposed federally or through the states for nursing homes or assisted living facilities. Often, the units are smaller in size, environmentally designed to promote function and freedom of movement, and provide staff trained in dementia-focused interventions. Evidence for the slowing of functional decline in SCUs for nursing home residents with dementia is negligible, although less easily measured benefits to quality of life may occur.[42]

With all behavioral interventions, communication needs to validate and respect the patients' sense of reality.[43] Consider a variety of approaches, as one single approach rarely produces the desired improvement. A range of behavioral interventions has been shown effective with a variety of behavioral symptoms:

- Wandering as agenda behavior. The term describes how the person uses verbal and nonverbal actions to fulfill unmet social, emotional, and physical needs. Provide visual cues, barriers, meaningful activities, and social interaction to minimize anxiety. Wandering in a safe environment should not be prevented.[39,44] A Safe Return identification bracelet or necklace, developed by the Alzheimer's Association, lists a nationwide, toll-free telephone number, monitored 24 hours a day, and should be worn at all times.

- Disruptive vocalization (excessively loud or repetitive verbal utterances): Provide for mobility, pain relief, and activities, such as music, massage, rocking chairs, stuffed animals, and so on, to create a calm, home-like environment.[40] Control length of activities and socialization to avoid fatigue.

- Dressing problems (dependency-induced dressing routines): Use a series of simple one-step instructions and nonverbal cues to guide the patient,[45] encouraging the patient to do as much as possible.

- Resistance to care. This term describes any patient behavior that prevents or interferes with the caregiver performing or assisting with the patient's ADLs. Proceed in a calm and gentle manner, be flexible, and set realistic goals. Specific interventions include:

1. For elimination needs, use pull-on pants, promote privacy, respond to nonverbal cues indicating need, and create a comfortable atmosphere.

2. For bathing, consider personal preferences for times and routines, use bath products that are pleasant and relaxing, or that elicit positive memories, and provide verbal reassurance.

3. For dressing and grooming, provide simple, comfortable clothing and eliminate choices and unnecessary garments.[46,47]

Conclusion

Dementia is a common clinical syndrome in older adults. The associated cognitive, functional, mood, and behavioral changes not only affect the patient, but also the caregiver. Throughout the course of the disease, the APN is in a unique position to diagnose dementia and to work with family and professional caregivers. Treatment involves individualized behavioral interventions, environmental modifications, medication, and support and education of the caregiver.

References

1. American Psychiatric Association. *Diagnostic Criteria from DSM-IV.* Washington, DC: American Psychiatric Association; 1994.

2. Evans DA, Funkenstein HH, Albert MS, et al. Prevalence of Alzheimer's disease in a community population of older persons: higher than previously reported. *JAMA.* 1989;262:2551–2556.

3. Evans DA. Estimated prevalence of Alzheimer's disease in the United States. *Milbank Q.* 1990;68(2):267–289.

4. Crook T, Bartus RT, Ferris S, et al. Age-associated memory impairment: proposed diagnostic criteria and measures of clinical change-report of a National Institute of Mental Health Working Group. *Dev Neuropsychol.* 1986;2:261–276.

5. Petersen RC, Smith GE, Ivnik RJ, et al. Apolipoprotein E status as a predictor of the development of Alzheimer's disease in memory-impaired individuals. *JAMA.* 1995; 273:1274–1278.

6. Petersen RC, Smith GE, Waring SC, Ivnik RJ, Tangalos EG, Kokmen E. Mild cognitive impairment: clinical characterization and outcome. *Arch Neurol.* 1999;56: 303–308.

7. Devanand DP, Sano M, Tang MX, et al. Depressed mood and the incidence of Alzheimer's disease in the elderly living in the community. *Arch Gen Psych.* 1996; 53:175–182.

8. Weytingh MD, Bossuyt PMM, vanCrevel H. Reversible dementia: more than 10% or less than 1%? A quantitative review. *J Neurol.* 1995;242:446–471.

9. Small GW, Rabins PV, Barry PP, et al. Diagnosis and treatment of Alzheimer disease and related disorders: consensus statement of the American Association for Geriatric Psychiatry, the Alzheimer's Association, and the American Geriatrics Society. *JAMA.* 1997;278: 1363–1371.

10. McKhann G, Drachman D, Folstein M, Katzman R, Price D, Stadlan EM. Clinical diagnosis of Alzheimer's disease: report of the NINCDS-ADRDA work group. *Neurology.* 1984;34:939–944.

11. Hall GR, Buckwalter KC. Progressively lowered stress threshold: a conceptual model for care of adults with Alzheimer's disease. *Arch Psych Nurs.* 1987;1(6): 399–406.

12. Tappen RM, Williams C, Fishman S, Touhy T. Persistence of self in advanced Alzheimer's disease. *Image: J Nurs Scholarship.* 1999;31(2):121–125.

13. Tappen RM, Williams C. Attribution of emotion in advanced Alzheimer's disease: family and caregiver perspectives. *Am J Alzheimer's Dis.* 1998; Sept/Oct: 257–264.

14. Auer S, Reisberg B. The GDS/FAST staging system. *Int Psychogeriatr.* 1997;9(1):167–171.

15. Neary D, Snowden JS, Gustafson MD, et al. Frontotemporal lobar degeneration: a consensus on clinical diagnostic criteria. *Neurology.* 1998;51: 1546–1554.

16. McKeith IG, Galasko D, Koaska K, et al. Consensus guidelines for the clinical and pathologic diagnosis of dementia with Lewy bodies (DLB): report of the consortium on DLB international workshop. *Neurology.* 1996;47:1113–1124.

17. Roman GC, Tatemichi TK, Erkinjuntti T, et al. Vascular dementia: diagnostic criteria for research studies. Report of the NINDS-AIREN International Workshop. *Neurology.* 1993;43:250–260.

18. US Department of Health and Human Services. *Guide Number 19: Early Identification of Alzheimer's Disease and Related Dementias. Quick Reference Guide for Clinicians.* Rockville, Md: Agency for Health Care Research and Quality, 1996. AHCPR Publication 97–0703.

19. Rovner B, Broadhead J, Spencer M. Depression in Alzheimer's disease. *Am J Psych.* 1989;146:350-353.

20. Logsdon RG, Teri L. The pleasant events schedule—AD: psychometric properties and relationship to depression and cognition in Alzheimer's disease patients. *Gerontologist.* 1997;37(1):40–45.

21. Gallo JJ, Anthony JC, Muthen BO. Age differences in the symptoms of depression: a latent trait analysis. *J Gerontol.* 1994;49:P251-265.

22. Silverman JM, Raiford K, Edland S, et al. The consortium to establish a registry for Alzheimer's disease (CERAD): part VI. Family history assessment: a multicenter study of first-degree relatives of Alzheimer's disease probands and nondemented spouse controls. *Neurology.* 1994;44:1253–1259.

23. Folstein MF, Folstein SE, McHugh PR. "Mini-Mental State": a practical method for grading the cognitive state of patients for the clinician. *J Psych Res.* 1975;12:189–198.

24. Clark CM, Ewbank D. Performance of the dementia severity rating scale: a caregiver questionnaire for rating severity in Alzheimer disease. *Alzheimer Dis Rel Disord.* 1996;10(1):31–39.

25. Reisberg B, Ferris SH, deLeon MJ, Crook T. Global Deterioration Scale (GDS). *Psychopharmacol Bull.* 1988;24(4):661–663.

26. Pearson JL, Teri L, Wagner A, Truax P, Logsdon RG. The relationships of problem behaviors in dementia patients to the depression and burden of caregiving spouses. *Am J Alzheimer's Dis Rel Res.* 1993;8(Jan/Feb): 15–22.

27. Schulz R, O'Brien AT, Bookwala J, Fleissner K. Psychiatric and physical morbidity effects of dementia caregiving: prevalence, correlates, and causes. *Gerontologist.* 1995;35(6):771–791.

28. Mittelman MS, Ferris SH, Shulman E, Steinberg G, Levin B. A family intervention to delay nursing home placement of patients with Alzheimer disease. *JAMA.* 1996;276:1725–1731.

29. Reisberg B, Auer SR, Monteiro I, Boksay I, Sclan SG. Behavioral disturbances of dementia: an overview of phenomenology and methodologic concerns. *Int Psychogeriatr.* 1996;8(2):169–182.

30. Lyketsos CG, Steele C, Galik E, et al. Physical aggression in dementia patients and its relationship to depression. *Am J Psych.* 1999;156(1):66–71.

31. Hall GR, Gerdner L, Zwygart-Stauffacher M, Buckwalter K. Principles of nonpharmacological management: caring for people with Alzheimer's disease using a conceptual model. *Psych Ann.* 1995;25(7):432–440.

32. Strumpf NE, Robinson JP, Wagner JS, Evans LK. *Restraint-Free Care: Individualized Approaches for Frail Elders.* New York: Springer Publishing, 1998.

33. Teri L, Truax P, Logsdon RG, Uomoto J, Zarit S, Vitaliano PP. Assessment of behavioral problems in dementia: the Revised Memory and Behavior Problems Checklist. *Psychol Aging.* 1992;7:622–631.

34. Rogers SL, Farlow MR, Doody RS, Mohs R, Friedhoff LT, Donepezil Study Group. A 24-week, double-blind, placebo-controlled trial of donepezil in patients with Alzheimer's disease. *Neurology.* 1998;50:136–145.

35. Van Dongen MCJM, vanRossum E, Kessels AGH, Sielhorst HJG, Knipschild PG. The efficacy of gingko for elderly people with dementia and age-associated memory impairment: new results of a randomized clinical trial. *J Am Geriatr Soc.* 2000;48:1183–1194.

36. Sano M, Ernesto C, Thomas RG, et al. A controlled trial of selegiline, alpha-tocopherol, or both as treatment for Alzheimer's disease. *N Engl J Med.* 1997;336:1216–1222.

37. Mulnard RA, Cotman CW, Kawas C, et al. Estrogen replacement therapy for treatment of mild to moderate Alzheimer's disease: a one-year randomized clinical trial. *JAMA.* 2000;283:1007–1015.

38. U.S. Congress Office of Technology Assessment. *Special Care Units for People with Alzheimer's and Other Dementias.* Washington, DC: U.S. Government Printing Office; 1992;17-21.

39. Coltharp W, Richie MF, Kaas MJ. Wandering. *J Gerontol Nurs.* 1996;22(11):5-10.

40. Sloane PD, Davidson S, Buckwalter K, et al. Management of the patient with disruptive vocalization. *Gerontologist.* 1997;37(5):675–682.

41. Kelley MF. Social interaction among people with dementia. *J Gerontol Nurs.* 1997;23(4):16–20.

42. Phillips CD, Sloane PD, Hawes C, et al. Effects of residence in Alzheimer disease special care units on functional outcomes. *JAMA.* 1997;278: 1340–1344.

43. Fine JI, Rouse-Bane S. Using validation techniques to improve communication with cognitively impaired older adults. *J Gerontol Nurs.* 1995;21(6):39–45.

44. Rader J, Doan J, Schwab M. How to decrease wandering, a form of agenda behavior. *Geriatr Nurs.* 1985;July/August:196–199.

45. Beck C, Heacock P, Mercer SO, Walls RC, Rapp CG, Vogelpohl TS. Improving dressing behavior in cognitively impaired nursing home residents. Paper presented at: World Alzheimer Congress; 2000; July 14, Washington, DC.

46. Sloane PD, Rader J, Barrick AL, et al. Bathing persons with dementia. *Gerontologist.* 1995;35(5):672–678.

47. Potts HW, Richie MF, Kaas MJ. Resistance to care. *J Gerontol Nurs.* 1996;22(11):11–16.

11

Gastrointestinal Problems

William F. Edwards

Gastroesophageal Reflux Disease

Prevalence

Gastroesophageal reflux disease (GERD) is a common problem in the population at large, with heartburn and esophagitis more common after age 50. Although presenting symptoms in the elderly are not markedly different, esophagitis occurs more frequently in the elderly.[1]

Pathophysiology

Several factors are associated with development of GERD:

- decreased tone of the lower esophageal sphincter (LES)

- decreased peristalsis causing poor clearance of refluxed material

- esophageal irritation from refluxed gastric contents

- decreased gastric emptying[2]

The evidence on whether aging itself causes any changes in these factors is unclear, but overall esophageal function seems well preserved.[3]

Healthy individuals can have daily episodes of reflux without symptoms. Others may have occasional heartburn without developing esophagitis. Reflux occurs when the pressure in the stomach is greater than the pressure of the LES. Large meals, tight garments, and outlet (pyloric valve) obstruction can increase pressure in the stomach. The LES pressure is influenced by many factors (Table 11–1) and even a transient decrease in pressure can lead to reflux. When there is decreased LES tone, reflux can occur with recumbency, bending down, and in the presence of a hiatal hernia. These conditions can cause the stomach contents to be located

near the gastroesophageal junction, even in the absence of increased abdominal pressure.[4]

The amount of damage caused by reflux is dependent on the acidity of the refluxed material, the amount of material refluxed, the frequency of episodes, the rate at which the material is cleared from the esophagus, and the degree to which gastric acid is neutralized by saliva. Over time, reflux can cause esophagitis, often with erosion and ulceration. Esophagitis can cause a change in the epithelium of the lower esophagus to columnar epithelium. Known as Barrett's esophagus (Barrett's metaplasia, Barrett's syndrome), this is associated with a significantly greater risk of adenocarcinoma.[4] Older patients with Barrett's esophagus can be significantly less symptomatic than their younger counterparts,[1] leading to undertreatment of the disease and increased risk of cancer.

Clinical Presentation

The most common presenting symptom of reflux disease is heartburn. It is important to get a thorough description of what the patient means by "heartburn," to be sure that it fits the clinical

Table 11–1 Common Causes of Decreased LES Pressure

Caffeine	Medications
Nicotine	Anticholinergics
Alcohol	Estrogen
Peppermint and spearmint	Progesterone
	Theophylline
Chocolate	Calcium channel blockers

definition of pyrosis and to distinguish it from heart disease or other gastrointestinal disorders. Heartburn is often worse with exercise, lying down, or bending over. It usually occurs with eating, particularly large meals. Patients may complain of sour or wet belches.[5]

Dysphagia is another common complaint and is a result of fibrosis and stricture formation from longstanding reflux. Usually these individuals have a history of heartburn for several years, but dysphagia is the presenting symptom in one-third of patients.[4] A careful history often reveals slowly progressive difficulty swallowing solids. Chest pain, which can occur after meals, at rest, or with exercise, is another common presenting symptom. In about one-third of patients with noncardiac chest pain, reflux is the most likely cause.[6]

Individuals with reflux may also present with hoarseness or chronic persistent cough. Patients might also present with wheezing and may have a history of recurrent pneumonia, bronchitis, or chronic asthma.[2]

Diagnosis

All patients suspected of having GERD require a thorough history and physical. The history focuses on obtaining precise descriptions of the symptoms, and attempting to differentiate them from true cardiac disease, respiratory disease from another origin, or some other gastrointestinal disorder. A complete list of medications, including over-the-counter (OTC) products, is an essential part of the history. The physical examination helps to rule out the presence of obvious masses, musculoskeletal chest-wall pain, and occult blood in the stool.

The basic goal of an initial assessment is to determine those patients who can be treated empirically and those who require referral or further diagnostic evaluation. A blood count and chemistry screening can rule out anemia, liver disease, and other abnormalities. Patients complaining of angina or chest pain radiating to other areas should be referred to a cardiologist. Those with evidence of gastrointestinal (GI) bleeding, dysphagia, masses, or unexplained weight loss should be referred to a gastroenterologist.[2]

The advanced practice nurse (APN) working with older adults needs to have a lower threshold for pursuing further evaluation since elderly patients with advanced disease frequently are less symptomatic than younger patients.[1] Those with a history of dysphagia, or a long history of heartburn, alcohol or tobacco abuse, or frequent use of nonsteroidal anti-inflammatory drugs (NSAIDs) are candidates for a barium esophagram or an endoscopy.[2] Endoscopy is usually the preferred option since it offers the opportunity for mucosal biopsy examination for histological changes consistent with esophagitis or for the columnar epithelium indicative of Barrett's esophagus.[5] Other diagnostic procedures, such as acid perfusion, 24-hour pH monitoring, and esophageal manometry are more appropriate for symptoms that do not respond to treatment. The decision to proceed with such testing involves consultation with a gastroenterologist.

Nonpharmacologic Interventions

If the symptoms of GERD are mild and of recent onset, the APN can treat the patient with lifestyle modifications and over-the-counter medications. The goals of interventions include patient education, decreasing the amount and acidity of the refluxate, improving esophageal clearance, and protecting the mucosa.

Education is very important for patients with GERD since it is likely to be a longstanding problem and the first step requires lifestyle modifications. An explanation of pathophysiology can be important in helping patients understand the rationale for interventions. The importance of lifestyle modifications should be emphasized to discourage over-reliance on medications. These behavioral changes should be continued throughout all stages of intervention.

Lifestyle modifications focus on reducing or eliminating factors that increase the risk of reflux. Interventions to decrease intra-abdominal pressure include losing weight if the individual is obese, avoiding large meals, abstaining from food and beverages two to three hours before lying down, and avoiding tight-fitting clothing.[4]

Elevating the head of the bed six inches can be helpful, but is often not tolerated. Using a foam wedge to elevate the head and chest is just as effective and better tolerated.[7]

Dietary changes include limiting acidic and spicy foods and caffeine, which can increase gastric acid secretion as well as directly irritate the esophageal mucosa. Chocolate, excess alcohol, decaffeinated coffee, fatty foods, and mints can decrease lower esophageal sphincter pressure and should also be avoided. Foods high in fat can delay gastric emptying and contribute to increased intra-abdominal pressure.[2]

Smoking increases gastric acid secretion and causes a marked decrease in LES pressure.[6] This provides the clinician with the opportunity to review all other harmful effects of cigarette smoking. Exercise can be helpful with weight reduction, but should be avoided after meals. Some medications, such as NSAIDs (including aspirin and other OTCs), tetracyclines, and quinidine, irritate the mucosa. Other medications, such as theophylline, anticholinergics, calcium channel blockers, diazepam, nitrates, and beta-adrenergic blockers decrease the tone of the lower esophageal sphincter.[8] In some cases, there may be no suitable alternative, but whenever possible these medications should be reduced or eliminated.

Increasing fluids between meals can relieve symptoms by improving esophageal clearance. Gum and lozenges can also be helpful.

Pharmacological Interventions

Antacids after meals and before bedtime can be effective in controlling mild, intermittent symptoms. They work by neutralizing the pH in the esophagus and the stomach and by increasing the LES tone. Although antacids are often considered benign by patients and clinicians alike, it can be well worth the time it takes to make a careful choice. Factors to consider include: patient preference, current bowel function, medical history, and cost. Antacids that are high in sodium should be avoided by patients with hypertension or heart failure. Aluminum and magnesium must be used with caution in renal patients, and calcium preparations are not advisable for persons with a history of kidney stones.[2] Most patients do best with combination products that minimize the adverse effects of any one ingredient.

The over-the-counter H_2 blockers, cimetidine (Tagamet HB), ranitidine (Zantac 75), famotidine (Pepcid AC), and nizatidine (Axid AR) provide another option in the treatment of mild GERD. The APN needs to emphasize that just because medications are available over-the-counter does not mean that they are entirely benign. It can be dangerous to use these products more than two or three times a week, as they may mask more serious disease.[5]

When individuals do not respond to lifestyle modifications and OTC agents, the APN needs to review the history and physical to be certain a cardiac problem is not being overlooked or to determine whether GERD is severe. It is particularly important to remember that heart disease is very common in elderly women and the symptoms described may appear as GI disease rather than the classic symptoms of heart disease seen in a middle-aged male. In the elderly, severity of symptoms may not correspond to severity of the disease.[9] If the older person's symptoms include dysphagia, odynophagia, or GI bleeding, referral to a gastroenterologist for endoscopy is indicated.[10]

If further evaluation indicates that the diagnosis is mild reflux disease, the next step is to add prescription-strength H_2 blockers. It is important to instruct the patient to continue with lifestyle modifications. Antacids may or may not be continued, depending on which H_2 blocker is chosen. Prokinetic agents (bethanechol, metoclopramide, and cisipride) appear to have a very limited role in the treatment of GERD, especially in the elderly, who are much more susceptible to the side effects.[7,10]

When elderly patients with mild symptoms do not respond to the usual doses of H_2 blockers (e.g., Ranitidine 150 mg BID), consultation with a gastroenterologist is appropriate. Esophagoscopy is often needed to determine severity. This is especially important in the elderly to avoid delayed diagnosis of Barrett's esophagus, a precancerous condition that occurs in the absence of severe symptoms.[1,9]

In severe disease, it is more cost effective to switch to a proton pump inhibitor (omeprazole or lansoprazole) than to push the dose of the H_2 blocker.[7] Proton pump inhibitors have been effective even when high doses of H_2 blockers failed to heal esophagitis.[10]

Patients with severe GERD have a high incidence of recurrence within 6–12 months. Maintenance therapy with proton pump inhibitors is more effective than H_2 blockers, even when a prokinetic agent is added to the H_2 antagonist.[7] The doses of the proton pump inhibitors needed to prevent recurrence are often as high as those needed for initial healing. Patients treated with proton pump inhibitors may have an added risk of gastritis (thus increasing their risk for gastric cancer), but this risk seems to be present only in individuals who are infected with *Helicobacter pylori*. Patients requiring long-term treatment with a proton pump inhibitor should therefore be evaluated and treated for *H. pylori*.[10]

Older patients who do not respond to medical therapy, or who are unable to tolerate medical therapy, may be candidates for surgery. This is a complex decision and the role of the APN is to foster patient understanding of the information and advice provided by the gastroenterologist and the surgeon.

Peptic Ulcer Disease

Prevalence

Approximately 500,000 new cases and 4 million recurrences of peptic ulcer occur annually in the United States. Lifetime prevalence for duodenal ulcer (DU) in Western populations is from 6–15%. The precise incidence of gastric ulcer (GU) is not known, although it peaks in the sixth decade, about 10 years after the peak incidence for DU. DU is identified clinically more often than GU; however, autopsy studies show an equal frequency for GUs.[11]

Pathophysiology

Peptic ulcer disease results from an imbalance between aggressive factors (principally pepsin and gastric acid) and protective factors (thick mucosal layer, prostaglandins, and ability to replace cells

rapidly). The use of NSAIDs, hyperacidic states such as Zollinger-Ellison syndrome, and *H. pylori* infection are the most common factors associated with peptic ulcer disease.[12] Infection with *H. pylori* is associated with 95–100% of patients with DU, and 75–85% of those with GU. While the rate of infection with *H. pylori* is about 10% in healthy individuals in the United States, for those over 60 years of age the rate is nearly equal to their age.[11] It is not yet clear whether the risk increases with age or whether these findings represent a greater rate of infection among today's older population when they were younger.

Although infection with *H. pylori* is the most important risk factor for development of peptic ulcer disease, most of those infected do not develop ulcers. In addition to the risk factors noted above, stress, smoking, and genetics also contribute to the pathogenesis of peptic ulcer.[13] Smoking stimulates the aggressive factors and impedes the protective factors, thus making individuals infected with *H. pylori* more likely to develop disease.[14]

Clinical Presentation

The most common presenting symptom of patients with peptic ulcer disease is gnawing epigastric discomfort. This typically occurs an hour or so after meals and may be relieved by food. Patients who complain of an increase in pain immediately after eating are more likely to have a gastric ulcer. Patients with duodenal ulcer may present with back pain, which can delay diagnosis. Symptoms common to both types of ulcers include anorexia, bloating, and change in bowel habits. Chronic blood loss or acute hemorrhage can also occur. Acute hemorrhage is more common in the elderly and in patients who are currently taking NSAIDs.[15] A study from the Netherlands suggests that it is difficult to distinguish patients with peptic ulcer disease from those with dyspepsia on the basis of clinical presentation.[16]

Diagnosis

Diagnosis of peptic ulcer disease is often a two-part process. The first consists of diagnosing the ulcer itself and the second involves determining the presence of *H. pylori* infection. Of course, it is important to rule out cardiac problems, which can present as "indigestion." While history is helpful in raising the possibility of an ulcer, positive identification requires visualization of the stomach and duodenum.[15] Although barium examination with double contrast can identify 90% of DUs, the rate is not as successful with gastric ulcers, and in both cases endoscopy offers advantages. Smaller ulcers can be identified by endoscopy, and it is possible to identify or rule out the ulcer as a cause of active hemorrhage. Endoscopy also makes it possible to obtain a biopsy of the gastric mucosa to detect *H. pylori*. With gastric ulcers, at least six biopsies are obtained from the inner margin of the ulcer to exclude malignancy.[11]

Endoscopy is often not the first step in diagnosis because it is invasive, expensive, and potentially stressful to patients.[12] A reasonable approach is to evaluate those patients who are not taking NSAIDs and who have symptoms of DU with double-contrast barium. Those on NSAIDs or with symptoms that are more consistent with GU might best be evaluated by endoscopy. If there is suspicion of cancer, endoscopy is clearly the best diagnostic choice.

Patients who are diagnosed with uncomplicated duodenal ulcer can reasonably be treated for *H. pylori* without further testing for the organism. Ninety to 100% of individuals with duodenal ulcers are infected with *H. pylori* and this is as accurate as any diagnostic test.[17]

Patients suspected of having GU can be tested for *H. pylori* with endoscopy. Rapid urease testing (also called the *Campylobacter*-like organism [CLO] test) is the least expensive of the tests that require endoscopy and it has high sensitivity and nearly 100% specificity. For those diagnosed with GU by barium examination, the least expensive nonendoscopic method of testing for *H. pylori* is serologic examination for IgG antibodies to *H. pylori*. To test for eradication after treatment, urea breath tests are preferred, since the antibody levels do not drop immediately after the organism is eliminated and the serology tests remain positive for many months.[17]

Controversy exists over how to evaluate patients with uncomplicated dyspepsia with no history of ulcer disease. Based on an analysis of cost-effectiveness, one study suggests nonendoscopic testing to identify *H. pylori* infection followed by eradication therapy for infected patients. However, no comparisons with radiographic examination were made.[18] A European review of research suggests that the fit elderly with dyspepsia should have symptoms promptly investigated. The frail elderly, on the other hand, should be treated empirically.[19] With the availability of noninvasive testing for *H. pylori*, a reasonable approach is testing the frail elderly for the organism. Those who are positive should receive appropriate antibiotic therapy with acid suppression, and those who are negative should be treated with acid suppressors alone.

Clinical Management

Drug Regimens to Eradicate *H. pylori*   Since most peptic ulcers are caused by *H. pylori* infection, clinical management focuses on eradication of the organism. The NIH Consensus Development Panel[20] recommended that all peptic ulcer patients who are infected with *H. pylori* receive antimicrobial therapy. Infected patients with a history of ulcer, and who are on antisecretory therapy, should also be treated with antibiotics. Patients with a history of complicated or refractory ulcer disease should be treated for *H. pylori* even if they are not currently receiving antisecretory therapy.[20]

The principle of minimizing the medication regimen with older patients needs to be modified in the treatment of *H. pylori* infection. For example, if an infected patient is treated symptomatically with only a proton pump inhibitor, the efficacy of subsequent treatment with antimicrobials may be reduced. The use of the proton pump inhibitor by itself might induce the normally spiral shaped *H. pylori* organism to mutate to a spherical shape that is more resistant to antimicrobial therapy.[21] Attempts to limit medications by using a single antibiotic are associated with increased incidence of resistant organisms.[12]

The goal of treatment is eradication rather than clearance, because with eradication reinfection is extremely rare. Clearance refers to the apparent absence of infection by the end of the treatment period. Eradication means that no organisms remain at least four weeks after treatment.[12]

Many therapeutic drug combinations have been used in the effort to eradicate *H. pylori*. The European Study Group concluded that the therapy for *H. pylori* should be well tolerated, conducive to easy compliance, cost-effective, and produce bacterial eradication of at least 80%.[22] The least expensive options are not always the most cost-effective. Inadequate attempts to treat *H. pylori* can make subsequent treatment more difficult. Over the long term, the most expensive therapies are those that do not eradicate the organism.[17]

Since the discovery of *H. pylori* as the cause of most ulcer disease, health-care providers have tried numerous approaches. Single drug therapies do not produce adequate eradication rates. Dual drug therapies have been more successful but have not consistently achieved eradication rates above 80%. The FDA has approved two dual drug therapies. The first is the proton pump inhibitor omeprazole plus clarithromycin. This is associated with eradication rates of 71%. The second regimen with FDA approval is ranitidine bismuth (which itself is a combination of two drugs) and clarithromycin. This approach is associated with eradication rates of 73% and 84% in separate studies. The American College of Gastroenterology recommends the addition of another antibiotic to both of the above regimens.[17]

Therapeutic regimens with three, or even four, drugs have consistently had the highest rates of eradication of *H. pylori*. Most of these regimens last at least two weeks and this, in addition to the number of medications, the cost, and the side effects, can pose problems with compliance. Some of these regimens require that the patient take medication four times daily resulting in over 200 pills over a two-week period. The most effective regimens involve a proton pump inhibitor (omeprazole or lansoprazole), the macrolide antibiotic clarithromycin, and either amoxicillin or metronidazole. This FDA regimen can be completed in 10 days and it requires only twice-daily

dosing (when the second antibiotic is amoxicillin) for a total of 60 pills. Although the initial cost is more expensive, with eradication rates of near 90% or more, this approach is cost effective over the long term.[11] European studies have demonstrated eradication rates of over 90% using this regimen for only 7 days, but U.S. studies have not shown this level of success and the FDA has yet to approve 7-day regimens.[17]

Current research on the control of peptic ulcer disease focuses on two goals. The first is the discovery of an inexpensive, easily tolerated treatment that eradicates *H. pylori*. The second direction of research is the development of a vaccine that will eliminate *H. pylori* infection.[12]

Treating NSAID-Induced Peptic Ulcers and Dyspepsia   Patients with gastroduodenal disease who are taking NSAIDs can be treated effectively with a proton pump inhibitor. One study showed more rapid healing of gastric ulcers in individuals treated with a proton pump inhibitor alone than in those who were also treated with *H. pylori* eradication therapy.[23]

Consultation

Although the advanced practice nurse can manage the care of the patient with peptic ulcer disease, there are several instances when consultation is necessary. The first is when endoscopy is required for diagnosis and in those instances when it is required to assure successful treatment. Consultation might also be appropriate in situations in which the patient's health history and medication tolerance make choice of drug regimen difficult. If an individual is treated for *H. pylori* and symptoms recur, referral to a gastroenterologist is appropriate. Referral is also recommended if a symptomatic patient tests negative for *H. pylori* but does not respond to H_2 blockers.[24]

At times, despite the advances in therapeutic interventions, urgent referral is necessary to stop acute hemorrhage through endoscopic intervention. In some cases, surgery may be required because of obstruction or because of complicated disease.[11]

Follow-Up care

Urea breath testing is the preferred way to determine H. pylori eradication after therapy. This test should be done at least four weeks after therapy is completed to avoid false negatives. Urea breath testing is noninvasive, relatively inexpensive, simple, and specific. Serologic tests measure antibodies that take months to decrease.[12]

Patients who have had bleeding ulcers, or those who required endoscopy to diagnose gastric ulcer, should have an endoscopic examination at the completion of therapy to verify healing and the absence of malignancy. H. pylori is associated with gastric adenocarcinoma and gastric lymphoma, including mucosa-associated lymphoid tissue (MALT) lymphoma.[21]

Patient Education

Since successful treatment of H. pylori requires patient adherence to drug regimens that can be cumbersome and have side effects, educating the patient regarding the role of H. pylori in causing ulcers and the long-term benefits of eradication greatly improve adherence to the prescribed therapy. A 1997 survey of U.S. adults by the Centers for Disease Control reported that 60% believed that ulcers were caused by too much stress. About 17% believed that spicy foods caused ulcers and 27% said that bacterial infection was the cause.[25]

The primary-care provider should recognize that the dosing schedule can be challenging, but if patients maintain it for 10 days, money and time are saved. Side effects are generally tolerable, and numerous options exist for individuals with a history of problems with one of the components.[17] It might further motivate patients to know that H. pylori is considered a carcinogen because of its association with gastric adenocarcinoma and low-grade, B-cell lymphomas of gastric MALT.[21]

Although the role of stress remains controversial, there is no typical "ulcer personality." It is possible that chronic anxiety and psychological stress can exacerbate ulcer symptoms.[11] For this reason, lifestyle issues should be reviewed and techniques for stress management taught. Some patients might benefit from a referral to a nurse specialist for a more in-depth approach to stress management.

Dietary issues are often challenging as well. Patients should be instructed that coffee, with or without caffeine, stimulates gastric acid secretion. Beer and wine also increase gastric acid secretion and should be avoided, at least until the ulcer is healed. Oral calcium may stimulate gastric acid secretion. Milk and cream diets, which used to be the mainstay of therapy, may cause rebound acid secretion. A general rule is to limit foods that exacerbate symptoms. There is no evidence that bland, soft, or low-spice diets promote healing of ulcers.[11]

Smoking is associated with higher rates of peptic ulcer, poorer response to therapy, and a higher rate of mortality. Cessation of smoking can improve physiologic functions of the gastrointestinal system within minutes to hours.[14]

If at all possible, patients should discontinue NSAIDs, at least until the ulcer is healed. For patients who are unable to stop NSAIDs, a proton pump inhibitor should be continued until the ulcer is healed, even after H. pylori is eradicated.[26]

Associated Conditions

Gastritis   Gastritis refers to a group of disorders that cause inflammatory changes in the gastric mucosa. Acute gastritis can occur in response to injury or infection. Alcohol and NSAIDs are the most common causes of injury to the mucosa.[15] The most common infection is H. pylori.[11]

The incidence of chronic gastritis rises to nearly 100% after age 70. The two most common forms are type A, which involves the fundus, or type B, which is often called antral gastritis. Type A can have autoimmune components or can be caused by H. pylori. This is the type of gastritis that is associated with pernicious anemia. Type B gastritis is more common, and in older individuals can affect the fundus as well as the antrum. H. pylori infection is responsible for type B gastritis and eradication of the organism leads to resolution of the histological changes.[11]

Over the course of years, chronic *H. pylori* infection can lead to peptic ulcer disease and chronic atrophic gastritis. Gastric atrophy can progress to adenocarcinoma, and acid-suppressive therapy (both H$_2$ blockers and proton pump inhibitors) can increase the rate of development of gastric atrophy and thus increase the risk of gastric cancer. There is controversy over whether *H. pylori* is an independent risk factor for the development of gastric cancer or whether they both have a common cause, such as low socioeconomic status. The most likely explanation is that multiple factors contribute to the development of gastric cancer, and *H. pylori* is one factor. At this point, *H. pylori* eradication is not recommended in individuals without evidence of peptic ulcer disease or MALT lymphoma.[11]

Upper GI Bleeding   Acute GI bleeding is responsible for 1–2% of all hospital admissions annually in the United States.[27] The risk is increased in the elderly, and the mortality rate for elderly individuals with GI bleeding approaches 10%. Upper GI bleeding is often secondary to esophagitis or peptic ulcer, and symptoms may be subtle.[28]

Compared to younger patients, older patients with upper GI bleeding are less likely to have a history of alcohol consumption and less likely to complain of dyspepsia.[29] Among the elderly, upper GI bleeding is frequently associated with NSAID use. Over 40,000 hospitalizations and over 3,000 deaths a year are associated with NSAID use among the elderly in the United States.[30] One study of adults showed that the use of NSAIDs increased the risk of GI bleeding by a factor of seven.[31]

Since the symptoms of upper GI bleeding can be subtle in the elderly, and the consequences severe, a high index of suspicion is necessary in any at-risk older adult. This includes those with a prior history of ulcers with GI bleeding, and those who are on NSAIDs. Treatment requires prompt action and referral to a gastroenterologist for probable endoscopic examination. In all but the mildest cases, treatment of GI bleeding in the older patient requires hospitalization.

Constipation

Prevalence

Estimates of the prevalence of constipation among older adults vary according to the definition of constipation and the methods used to determine prevalence. From a medical perspective, constipation is often defined as fewer than three bowel movements a week. Individuals complaining of constipation may describe straining, hard stools, or the sensation of incomplete evacuation.[32]

Over half of the elderly who complain of constipation move their bowels at least once daily. In one study, 47% of interview respondents reported constipation but only 17% had two or fewer bowel movements per week.[33] The incidence of constipation varies with setting. A study in England showed prevalence rates varying from 12% in community-dwelling elders, to 41% in hospitalized patients, and over 80% in long-term care residents.[34]

The frequency of bowel movements in healthy older populations is essentially the same as in a younger group. Nevertheless, the use of laxatives is more common in the elderly, even when stools are relatively frequent.[33]

Pathophysiology

Although normal aging apparently does not prolong intestinal transit time nor result in fewer bowel movements, complaints of constipation increase with age.[33] The synergistic effect of multiple contributing factors (Table 11-2) is often responsible for constipation in the elderly. Poor diet, decreased fluid intake, chronic illness, and decreased mobility are relatively common. In addition, many elderly are on medications that contribute to prolonged colonic transit time.

In contrast with healthy elderly individuals, those who have two or fewer bowel movements per week or who strain when defecating have markedly prolonged gut transit times. Studies of colonic motor activity in constipated elderly individuals demonstrate deficits in intrinsic innervation. It is unclear whether this change is the cause of constipation or the result of laxative abuse.[33]

Table 11–2   Common Causes of Constipation

Dietary	Functional
Inadequate caloric intake	Poor bowel habits
Low-fiber diet	Immobility/lack of exercise
Poor fluid intake	Depression
Problems chewing and swallowing	Cognitive impairment

Neuropathies	Drugs
Spinal cord lesions	Anticholinergics
Parkinson's disease	Antidepressants
Stroke	Antiparkinsonian drugs
Multiple sclerosis	Antihistamines
	Antipsychotics
Metabolic Conditions	Muscle relaxants
Diabetes	Narcotics
Hypothyroidism	Diuretics
Electrolyte imbalances	NSAIDs
	Metals
Obstruction	Aluminum
Rectocele or rectal prolapse	Calcium
Neoplasm	Lithium
Barium or bezoars	Iron
Stricture	Bismuth
Prostatic enlargement	Calcium channel blockers
Megacolon	

Internal anal sphincter tone decreases to some extent in some healthy elderly individuals. The external sphincter tone declines more markedly, especially in women. Rectal tone and sensation do not decline with normal aging.[33]

Pathophysiological changes in rectal function noted in older individuals with constipation include rectal dyschezia, pelvic dyssynergia, and increased rectal tone with reduced compliance. Rectal dyschezia can occur as a result of impaired sacral cord function from spinal stenosis. Patients may present with reduced tone and increased compliance, dilatation, and impaired sensation that can reduce awareness of an impaction. Pelvic dyssynergia causes an inability to relax the puborectalis and external anal sphincter muscles during defecation. This is often seen in patients with Parkinson's disease. Increased rectal tone with decreased compliance is usually associated with irritable bowel syndrome.[33]

Clinical Management

History   Successful management of constipation begins with a thorough history. This must include the patient's understanding of constipation and a specific description of all associated symptoms. Many elderly were reared with the idea that daily movements were essential to good health and that failure to move the bowels led to the buildup of dangerous toxins. Patients should keep a bowel log for a two-week period, noting frequency, amount, caliber, color, and consistency of stool, as well as symptoms experienced during defecation. The log should also note whether laxatives were used, whether the patient noticed staining of underwear, and whether digital removal of stool was necessary.

Individuals with a recent change in bowel habits require a thorough evaluation. In patients with recent onset of constipation, the history should focus on excluding underlying causes such as malignancy, adhesions, stricture, or volvulus. The clinician should investigate the possibility of an exacerbation of a known illness. A thorough evaluation of recent changes in diet, medications, level of activity, and emotional state is also warranted. Total caloric intake, fiber content, and fluid intake are the critical elements of a dietary evaluation. The clinician also needs to inquire about problems related to chewing and swallowing. Brief screening tests for cognitive function and depression assist the clinician in detecting non-physiological causes of constipation.

For those with a long-term history of constipation, the focus should be on management. The history should include information about the duration of the problem, fluctuation over time, and exacerbating and relieving factors. The medical history should focus on GI disease (including a history of hemorrhoids or other anorectal disease) and the use of any medications that could affect bowel function. Psychological stressors, anxiety, and depression can have a powerful impact on bowel function.[34] A history of attempted remedies and current strategies can be helpful in avoiding futile interventions.

Physical Examination   If the patient is unknown, a complete physical is needed to rule out systemic causes. The neurological examination is particularly important since constipation is a common complication of many neurological illnesses. For most patients, the focus is on examination of the mouth, abdomen, anorectal area, and assessment for dehydration. The oral examination focuses on adequacy of dentition, and detection of any lesions or tumors.

The abdomen is examined for normal bowel sounds, detection of pain or localized masses (including retained stool), distention, and evidence of prior surgery. The anorectal area is evaluated for sphincter muscle tone, rectal prolapse, presence of stool in the vault, lesions such as hemorrhoids, strictures, fistulas, masses, presence of the anal reflex, and prostatic enlargement.[35]

Diagnostic Testing   Patients with constipation need a complete blood count, fasting blood glucose, chemistry panel, and thyroid-stimulating hormone level to rule out anemia, diabetes, electrolyte imbalances, and hypothyroidism. If the onset of constipation is recent, if there is an acute change in symptoms, or if the patient has pain or has any evidence of rectal bleeding, colonoscopy or sigmoidoscopy and barium enema are essential.[34] In addition to detecting cancer, endoscopy can also reveal the presence of melanosis coli or the absence of haustrations, conditions associated with chronic use of laxatives.[35]

If the patient has seepage of liquid stool or symptoms of impaction with an empty rectal vault, abdominal x-rays can detect a high impaction or other signs of obstruction. Additional diagnostic testing, such as colonic transit studies or anorectal motility studies, are only needed if no response occurs to treatment for constipation. Decisions on these studies should be made in consultation with a gastroenterologist.

Interventions

Patient Education and Goal Setting   Educating the patient and caregivers about normal bowel function can be challenging, but effective in terms of time. Teaching should include the normal range of frequency for bowel movements, the impact of acute and chronic illnesses and their associated medications, as well as the importance of diet, exercise, and other lifestyle issues. The educational approach needs to be tempered by the fact that research supporting many long-held beliefs about the best methods for treating constipation is inconclusive.[33] Treatment is most effective when mutual goals are established. Patient-outcome goals can be stated in terms of frequency and quality of bowel movements and avoidance of adverse symptoms and complications such as fecal impaction.

Nonpharmacological Interventions   Successful treatment of constipation requires an individualized plan that addresses the identified causes, lifestyle issues, and patient preferences. The clinician must balance the patient's desire to get results quickly with the need to make changes slowly in order to have a bowel program that is satisfactory over the long term.

The first step, whenever possible, is the elimination of any medications that could contribute to constipation. In some cases, the medication can be changed to a less-constipating alternative. It is best to start a bowel program with an empty colon. This helps meet the patient's need for rapid results, but may require the use of enemas or even manual disimpaction.

Healthy bowel function requires an adequate intake of fluids and dietary fiber. If there are no health-related reasons for fluid restrictions, 2–3 liters per/day is an appropriate goal. This needs to be done gradually to improve compliance. Water is the ideal fluid—beverages containing caffeine and some fruit juices can cause diuresis.

Dietary fiber should be increased slowly to avoid the unpleasant side effects of bloating and gas pains, and to give the colon a chance to adapt. Although the amount of additional fiber required to improve bowel function varies considerably, the usual range is from 6–30 grams. Supplementing the diet with a mixture made from two parts wheat bran (sometimes given in the form of 100% bran cereal, which is more palatable but less effective than crude bran), two parts applesauce, and one part prune juice is effective and inexpensive. The starting dose is 30 ml daily.

Adequate fluids must accompany the increase in fiber in order to avoid development of a hard, dense, fibrous blockage known as a bezoar. Coarse, uncooked bran can significantly reduce absorption of calcium and iron because of its high phytic acid content.[33] Fiber should not be added to the diet in cases of megacolon or intestinal stricture. In fact, patients with megacolon should be on a fiber-restricted diet and may need to be managed with enemas. Problems are generally few with gradual increases in fiber.

Teaching should emphasize that fiber supplements do not bring overnight results. It is also important to advise a decrease in the consumption of fat and refined foods, as these slow colonic transit time and often take the place of foods higher in fiber.

Maintaining adequate caloric intake is an important component of any program to prevent constipation. This can be particularly difficult for those who live alone and for the frail elderly who are dependent on others for assistance with meal preparation and feeding. Those in institutions require constant vigilance to ensure proper nutrition and healthy bowel function. Care plans should note usual bowel habits and include a protocol for preventing and addressing any problems. Bowel logs noting at least the amount and consistency of each stool are an essential part of such a program.

Regular exercise contributes to healthy bowel function. Encourage walks for 20 minutes daily,

preferably after a meal. For those with limited mobility, stationary exercises can be helpful. Exercises to strengthen the abdominal and pelvic floor muscles can improve defecation. Even bed- or chair-bound patients can benefit from an exercise program.

Work with the patient to establish a routine that promotes normal bowel function. In addition to exercise and maintaining adequate intake of calories, fiber, and fluid, the routine should include taking advantage of the gastrocolic reflex. For most individuals, this is pronounced after breakfast or supper and may be enhanced by a warm drink. It is important to have privacy and adequate time (about 10 minutes) to attempt to have a daily bowel movement. It is also important to respond, without delay, to any urge to defecate.

The squatting position facilitates bowel function and can be emulated by using a footstool. The patient with weakened abdominal muscles can augment bowel function by leaning forward and applying firm pressure on the lower abdomen or by massaging the abdomen. Massage strokes should start from the proximal end of the large bowel and proceed up the ascending colon, across the transverse colon, and down the descending and sigmoid colon.

Pharmacological Interventions In general, laxatives and enemas should not be a part of routine bowel management. Those who have used laxatives for years require education about the harmful effects. Often a review of the bowel log demonstrates that laxatives are ineffective in relieving the symptoms of constipation over the long term. Patients who need to avoid straining or who have megacolon may need laxatives or enemas. In most patients, however, laxatives should be used only occasionally to prevent the complications associated with constipation.

The choice of laxative is determined by numerous factors: the cause of the problem, the specific symptoms, coexisting medical conditions, current medications, cost, and patient preference. For most elderly individuals who require long-term therapy, the best choices are bulk laxatives or hyperosmolar agents. Bulk laxatives can be effective in patients who cannot get enough fiber in their diet. They do not interfere with the absorption of calcium, iron, fat-soluble vitamins, or digoxin in elderly patients. Bulk agents with psyllium have the added benefit of lowering serum cholesterol. As with dietary fiber, these agents should be avoided in patients who are bed-bound, and in those with swallowing difficulties or who have intestinal stricture or megacolon.[33]

Hyperosmolar laxatives are good choices if bulk-forming agents are inappropriate, ineffective, or poorly tolerated, and if gastrointestinal motility is not significantly impaired. Lactulose and sorbitol are hyperosmolar agents that increase fluid in the colon and promote formation of a soft stool. The chief side effects are abdominal bloating and gas pains, but these can be minimized by gradually increasing the dose. These laxatives can be rather slow acting, but are often effective long-term agents for the frail elderly. Sorbitol is substantially less expensive and as effective as lactulose.[32] Compared to stimulant laxatives, hyperosmolar agents contribute to a more rapid return to normal bowel function. Polyethylene glycol (Golytely) is a hyperosmolar laxative that is often used to prepare the bowel prior to colonoscopy or barium enema.[33]

Most stimulant or irritant laxatives are not appropriate for long-term use because of the risk of damage to the colon and electrolyte imbalance. They are particularly effective for soft fecal masses in the rectum and for individuals with impaired GI motility secondary to narcotics or anticholinergics. Senna is safe for the elderly. Even individuals over age 80 do not have significant losses of intestinal protein after six months of daily use.[33]

Stimulants are popular, but they can have a more toxic long-term effect than other laxatives. Castor oil, aloe, and phenolphthalein (Ex-Lax, Feen-a-Mint) should be avoided entirely because safer choices are available. The elderly often used the latter despite its side effect profile (impaired vitamin D and calcium absorption, dermatitis, photosensitivity reactions, and Stevens-Johnson syndrome). The FDA has taken phenolphthalein off the market because of its link to cancer in laboratory mice.

Emollient laxatives include mineral oil and the docusate salts. Mineral oil, although effective, should be avoided in the elderly because of the risk of aspiration. Long-term use can cause interference with absorption of fat-soluble vitamins and risk of leakage through the anal sphincter. Stool softeners are popular, but unproven as laxatives. They are often recommended in bed-bound patients with hard, dry stool, in patients who must avoid straining, and as an adjunct to bulk agents. These agents should be avoided with large amounts of soft stool in the colon.

Saline laxatives work by osmotically drawing water into the small bowel and stimulating peristalsis. They are popular because the bowel is emptied within a few hours. Individuals with poor renal function should avoid magnesium, phosphate, or sulfate-based salts.

Bisacodyl and glycerin suppositories provide rapid effect. They work best when stool is present in the rectum. Suppositories are best used as an adjunct to a bowel program. Common side effects are cramping and local irritation.

Enemas are reserved for cases that do not respond to other approaches. Soapsuds and phosphate enemas are irritating to the rectal mucosa and should be avoided. Normal saline or tap water enemas (105 degrees F), no more than 500 ml, are probably the best choice. To avoid perforation, it is safest to have the enema administered by someone other than the patient.

The major complications of constipation are fecal impaction and increased risk of colorectal cancer.[36] Impaction can cause symptoms of malaise, fatigue, and cognitive problems, as well as urinary retention, bowel and bladder incontinence, anal fissures, hemorrhoids, stercoral ulcer, and intestinal obstruction. Watery leakage around impacted stool can lead to an incorrect diagnosis of diarrhea and treatment that exacerbates the problem. A mass of stool in the rectum can impair sensation and lead to the need for larger volumes of stool to stimulate the urge to defecate, thus contributing to megacolon. Valsalva maneuvers caused by straining during defecation can cause transient ischemic attacks and syncope, especially in the frail elderly.

◼ Cancer in the Gastrointestinal Tract

Cancer in the gastrointestinal tract is second to lung cancer as a cause of cancer-related mortality. GI cancers are responsible for more than 25% of all cancer deaths among the elderly.

Esophageal Cancer

Cancer of the esophagus is rather uncommon (about 4% of GI cancers), but quite lethal. In the approximately 12,300 Americans diagnosed in 1996, there were over 11,000 deaths. Esophageal cancer usually occurs after the age of 50 and it seems to be associated with lower socioeconomic status.[37]

Squamous cell carcinoma is the most common esophageal cancer. It is more common in males than females, and black males have four times the rate of white males. A long history of smoking and a history of heavy alcohol intake are the most significant environmental factors associated with squamous cell carcinoma. Adenocarcinoma of the esophagus is becoming increasingly common and now accounts for over 20% of esophageal cancers. It is more common in white males and usually arises from Barrett's epithelium.[6]

Clinical Presentation   Both squamous cell carcinoma and adenocarcinoma present with progressive dysphagia and weight loss. Occasionally, the patient may present with chest pain or aspiration pneumonia. Esophagoscopy is preferred to diagnose early, potentially treatable tumors. The larynx, trachea, and bronchi should also be checked because of the risk with smoking.[6]

Clinical Management   Less than 5% of those diagnosed with esophageal cancer survive five years. By the time diagnosis is made, the cancer involves more than half of the esophagus and has often spread outside the esophagus. Surgery is the treatment of choice if the cancer is localized. Squamous cell carcinoma is initially radiosensitive and is occasionally cured. The prognosis for adenocarcinoma is equally bleak. This cancer is not radiosensitive and early metastasis is common.[6]

Since the prognosis for patients with esophageal cancer is so poor, early detection is key. The APN must have a high index of suspicion for patients with risk factors. In addition to teaching patients about the risks associated with alcohol and smoking, the nurse should also emphasize the importance of reporting any problems with swallowing.

Stomach Cancer

Stomach cancer occurs twice as often in males and rarely occurs before the age of 60. The prevalence of gastric cancer has decreased markedly in the past 60 years, with about 22,000 new cases annually and 14,000 deaths. The decrease in the incidence of stomach cancer is associated with fewer mutagens (from dried, smoked, and salted foods) and more antioxidants (from fresh produce) in the diet. There is also a striking correlation with the decline in *H. pylori* infection that parallels the decline in gastric cancer.[15]

Pathophysiology   About 85% of gastric cancers are adenocarcinomas of two main types. Intestinal gastric cancer is usually seen in the antrum and is associated with type B antral gastritis. Diffuse gastric cancer causes a thickening of the stomach and is associated with type A gastritis and pernicious anemia.[15]

Clinical Presentation   Stomach cancer is asymptomatic when it is superficial and surgically curable. As the tumor progresses, patients may complain of epigastric pain, anorexia, early satiety, and occasional nausea. Dysphagia is often associated with tumors of the cardia, while nausea and vomiting are more pronounced in lesions of the pylorus.[37]

Diagnosis   Early diagnosis of gastric cancer is critical to successful management. About 80% of cancers that are detected before the lesion goes beyond the submucosa can be cured. The clinician needs to have a high index of suspicion for elderly individuals complaining of anorexia or presenting with significant weight loss or iron-deficient anemia. Double-contrast radiography is the simplest way to evaluate complaints of dyspepsia, but esophagoscopy is better for detecting early cancer. Esophagoscopy is the approach of choice in evaluating gastric ulcers and when only one procedure can be tolerated.[15,37]

Clinical Management   Surgery offers the one possibility for cure of gastric cancer, but only about 30% of adenocarcinomas are detected early enough to cure. These tumors are radioresistant and radiation is used for palliation only. Chemotherapy is helpful in fewer than 50% of cases. The five-year survival rate for adenocarcinoma is 20%.[37]

Although gastric lymphomas are the cause of less than 15% of stomach cancers, it is important to identify them since they are more responsive to treatment. MALT causes as many as half of all gastric lymphomas. These lymphomas are associated with *H. pylori* infection and eradication of the organism is the first step in successful treatment. In some cases, eradication of the organism has brought about cure of the cancer. Surgery and/or chemotherapy and radiation therapy achieve five-year survival rates of 40–60% with localized high-grade tumors.[15,37]

Colorectal Cancer

Colorectal cancer is the second leading cause of cancer death and the leading cause in women over the age of 75. In 1996, 133,500 new cases of colorectal cancer were diagnosed, with close to 55,000 deaths. The incidence rises throughout life, nearly doubling for each decade past the age of 50. The overall five-year survival rate is 57%, but is somewhat worse in the elderly.[37,38]

Pathogenesis   Adenocarcinomas cause 95% of colorectal cancers and virtually all of these malignancies arise from adenomatous polyps. On the other hand, probably less than 1% of all polyps ever become malignant. It takes approximately 5–10 years for early polyps to develop into invasive cancer and the risk increases with the size of the polyps. Polyps over 2.5 cm in size have about a 10% chance of containing invasive cancer.[27]

Etiology and Risk Factors   Although significant hereditary factors increase the risk of developing colorectal cancer, the great majority of such cancers are most likely related to environmental factors. Familial adenomatous polyposis causes less than 1% of all colorectal cancers and is rare in the elderly. This condition requires total colectomy since virtually all patients develop cancer before the age of 40.[39]

Hereditary nonpolyposis colon cancer causes no more than 6% of colorectal adenocarcinomas and usually appears before the age of 50. Heredity may also contribute to the sporadic form of colorectal cancer. Sporadic adenocarcinoma constitutes over 90% of colorectal cancers.[37,39]

Patients with inflammatory bowel disease have a higher risk of colorectal cancer and the risk increases with the duration of the disease. Radiation therapy for cervical cancer is associated with an increased risk for colorectal cancer 15 years after treatment. Cholecystectomy might lead to a slight increase in right-sided bowel cancer in women. Breast cancer is often identified as a risk factor for colorectal cancer, but the most rigorous studies suggest that this is not the case.[40]

Environmental factors are responsible for 85–90% of colorectal cancers in the United States and many of these could be prevented by diet and lifestyle changes. Upper socioeconomic groups, especially those in urban areas, have higher rates of colorectal cancer. There is a positive correlation between bowel cancer and high caloric intake and consumption of red meat and fat. Populations with high rates of elevated cholesterol and coronary artery disease also have higher rates of colorectal cancer. Consumption of alcohol may increase risk for adenomatous polyps, the precursors of cancer. Long-term cigarette smoking is also associated with increased risk of colorectal cancer.[39,40]

Lack of leisure-time exercise and sedentary occupations are both associated with increased risk for colorectal cancer. Workers who are exposed to solvents, abrasives, fuel oil, dyes, and grinding wheel dust are also at higher risk.[40]

Clinical Presentation   The presenting symptoms of colorectal cancer depend on the site of the lesions. Proximal (right-sided) tumors may not cause any early symptoms since the stool is liquid at that point and the colon is wider. Occult bleeding may occur, which can cause anemia and symptoms of fatigue. Iron-deficient anemia requires endoscopic or radiologic evaluation.[38]

Colorectal cancer in the transverse or descending colon often causes narrowing and the patient presents with symptoms of abdominal cramping or obstruction. Delay in diagnosis and treatment can lead to perforation. Diagnosis is made by abdominal radiography and the constricting lesion often has the appearance of an apple core.[37]

Patients with colorectal cancer in the rectosigmoid area may present with hematochezia, tenesmus, or narrow "pencil" stools. Patients with rectal bleeding or a change in bowel habits need a digital examination and sigmoidoscopy. The presence of obvious hemorrhoids should not deter further evaluation.[37]

Treatment   All polyps found during colonoscopy should be removed by electrocauterization. Malignant polyps and more invasive carcinomas need more extensive surgery. Surgery is the only curative treatment. Radiation and chemotherapy may offer a slight benefit as adjuvant therapy in advanced lesions.[38]

Recurrence is common but usually occurs in the first four years. Early detection of colorectal cancer is important because five-year survival rates for Dukes' stages A and B are over 80%.[37]

Screening   Despite improved outcomes with early detection, screening for colorectal cancer remains somewhat controversial.[41,42] This is, in part, because of the lack of sensitivity and specificity of the inexpensive Hemoccult test and the expense and discomfort of barium enema and endoscopic examination. Colorectal tumors tend to bleed intermittently, which can cause false negatives. Sensitivity is improved and specimens are usually collected on three different days. Certain foods, supplements, and medications can also cause false results.[37,38]

The American Cancer Society (ACS) recommends annual digital rectal examinations and testing for occult blood for older adults with average risk. In addition, the ACS recommends flexible sigmoidoscopy every three to five years. If a polyp is found on sigmoidoscopy, the entire colon should be examined.[38] Although some studies have shown significant reduction in mortality from colorectal cancer with large-scale screening, the overall survival rates were unchanged.[42]

Prevention   Since most colorectal cancer is associated with environmental factors, the APN has the opportunity to focus on prevention. Fortunately, the recommendations are consistent with those for overall good health. A diet high in red meat is a moderate risk factor, while vegetables, fruit, fiber, folate, and calcium all offer a degree of protection. A physically active lifestyle is moderately protective. A high-fat diet, alcohol, cigarette smoking, obesity, and high sucrose consumption are all associated with a modest risk for colorectal cancer. Aspirin and NSAIDs offer moderate protection that appears to be independent of more intense evaluation for bleeding caused by the drugs.[40] Of course, the risk for bleeding from the latter, especially in the elderly, might outweigh the benefit. At this point, NSAIDs (including aspirin) should not be used solely for prevention of colorectal cancer, but this information should be considered when making a clinical decision to use these medications for other purposes.

References

1. Triadafilopoulos G, Sharma R. Features of symptomatic gastroesophageal reflux disease in elderly patients. *Am J Gastroenterol.* 1997;92(11):2000–2011.
2. Middlemiss C. Gastroesophageal reflux disease: a common condition in the elderly. *Nurse Prac.* 1997;22(11):51–59.
3. Hall KE, Wiley JW. Age-associated changes in gastrointestinal function. In: Hazzard WR, Blass JP, Ettinger WH, et al., eds. *Principles of Geriatric Medicine and Gerontology.* 4th ed. New York: McGraw-Hill; 1999:835–842.
4. Goyal RK. Diseases of the esophagus. In: Fauci AS, Braunwald E, Isselbacher KJ, et al., eds. *Harrison's Principles of Internal Medicine.* 14th ed. New York: McGraw-Hill; 1998:1588–1596.
5. Castell DO, Richter JE, Spechler SJ. Achieving better outcomes for patients with GERD. *Patient Care.* 1996;30(8):21–42.

6. Pineau BC, Wu WC. Disorders of the esophagus. In: Hazzard WR, Blass JP, Ettinger WH, et al., eds. *Principles of Geriatric Medicine and Gerontology.* 4th ed. New York: McGraw-Hill; 1999:843–853.

7. Johnson DA. Medical therapy of GERD: current state of the art. *Hosp Pract.* 1996;31(10):135–148.

8. Robinson M. Gastroesophageal reflux disease. *Postgrad Med.* 1994;95(2):88–90, 93–94, 99–102.

9. Collen MJ, Abdulian JD, Chen YK. Gastroesophageal reflux disease in the elderly: more severe disease that requires aggressive therapy. *Am J Gastroenterol.* 1995;90(7):1053–1057.

10. Kahrilas PJ. Gastroesophageal reflux disease. *JAMA.* 1996;276(12):983–988.

11. Friedman LS, Peterson WL. Peptic ulcer and related disorders. In: Fauci AS, Braunwald E, Isselbacher KJ, et al., eds. *Harrison's Principles of Internal Medicine.* 14th ed. New York: McGraw-Hill; 1998:1596–1616.

12. Podolski JL. Recent advances in peptic ulcer disease: *Helicobacter pylori* infection and its treatment. *Gastroenterol Nurs.* 1996;19(4):128–136.

13. Raiha I, Kemppainen H, Kaprio J, et al. Lifestyle, stress, and genes in peptic ulcer disease: a nationwide twin cohort study. *Arch Intern Med.* 1998; 158(7):698–704.

14. Eastwood GL. Is smoking still important in the pathogenesis of peptic ulcer disease? *J Clin Gastroenterol.* 1997;25(Suppl 1):S1–S7.

15. Roufail WM. The stomach and duodenum. In: Hazzard WR, Blass JP, Ettinger WH, et al., eds. *Principles of Geriatric Medicine and Gerontology.* 4th ed. New York: McGraw-Hill; 1999:885–866.

16. Werdmuller BF, van der Putten AB, Loffeld RJ. The clinical presentation of ulcer disease. *Neth J Med.* 1997;50(3):115–119.

17. Laine L, Fendrick AM. *Helicobacter pylori* and peptic ulcer disease: bridging the gap between knowledge and treatment. *Postgrad Med.* 1998;103(3):231–238, 243.

18. Ofman JJ, Etchason J, Fullerton S, et al. Management strategies for *Helicobacter pylori*-seropositive patients with dyspepsia: clinical and economic consequences. *Ann Intern Med.* 1997;126(4):280–291.

19. Pound SE, Heading RC. Diagnosis and treatment of dyspepsia in the elderly. *Drugs Aging.* 1995;7(5):347–354.

20. NIH Consensus Development Panel on *Helicobacter pylori* in peptic ulcer disease. *JAMA.* 1994;272(1):65–69.

21. Cave DR, Hoffman JS. Management of *Helicobacter pylori* infection in ulcer disease. *Hosp Prac.* 1996; 31(1):63–75.

22. The European *Helicobacter pylori* Study Group: current European concepts in the management of *Helicobacter pylori* infection, the Maastricht consensus report. *Gut.* 1997;41(1):8–13.

23. Hawkey CJ, Tulassay Z, Szozepanski L, et al. Randomised controlled trial of *Helicobacter pylori* eradication in patients on non-steroidal anti-inflammatories: HELP NSAIDs. *Lancet.* 1998;352:1016–1021.

24. Fay M, Jaffe PE. Diagnostic and treatment guidelines for *Helicobacter pylori*. *Nurse Pract.* 1996;21(7):28–34.

25. Centers for Disease Control and Prevention. Knowledge about causes of peptic ulcer. *JAMA.* 1997;278(21):1731.

26. Malfertheiner P, Labenz J. Does *Helicobacter pylori* status affect nonsteroidal anti-inflammatory drug-associated gastroduodenal pathology? *Am J Med.* 1998;104(3A):35S–40S.

27. Zimmerman HM, Curfman K. Acute gastrointestinal bleeding. *AACN Clin Iss.* 1997;8(3):449–458.

28. Nankhonya JM, Datta-Chaudhuri ML, Bhan GL. Acute upper gastrointestinal hemorrhage in older people: a prospective study in two neighboring districts. *J Am Geriatr Soc.* 1997;45(6):752–754.

29. Segal WN, Cello JP. Hemorrhage in the upper gastrointestinal tract in the older patient. *Am J Gastroenterol.* 1997;92(1):42–46.

30. Griffin MR. Epidemiology of nonsteroidal anti-inflammatory drug-associated gastrointestinal injury. *Am J Med.* 1998;104(3A):23S–29S.

31. Kurata JH, Nogawa AN, Noritake D. NSAIDs increase risk of gastrointestinal bleeding in primary care patients with dyspepsia. *J Fam Prac.* 1997;45(3):227–235.

32. Romero Y, Evans JM, Fleming KC, et al. Constipation and fecal incontinence in the elderly population. *Mayo Clin Proc.* 1996;71(1):81–92.

33. Harari D. Constipation in the elderly. In: Hazzard WR, Blass JP, Ettinger WH, et al., eds. *Principles of Geriatric Medicine and Gerontology.* 4th ed. New York: McGraw-Hill; 1999:1491–1505.

34. Read NW, Celik AF, Katsinelos P. Constipation and incontinence in the elderly. *J Clin Gastroenterol.* 1995;20(1):61–70.

35. Friedman LS, Isselbacher KJ. Diarrhea and constipation. In: Fauci AS, Braunwald E, Isselbacher KJ, et al., eds. *Harrison's Principles of Internal Medicine.* 14th ed. New York: McGraw-Hill; 1998:236–244.

36. Jacobs ES, White E. Constipation, laxative use and colon cancer among middle-aged adults. *Epidemiology.* 1998;9(4):385–391.

37. Mayer RJ. Gastrointestinal tract cancer. In: Fauci AS, Braunwald E, Isselbacher KJ, et al., eds. *Harrison's Principles of Internal Medicine.* 14th ed. New York: McGraw-Hill; 1998:568–578.

38. Cheskin LJ, Schuster MM. Colonic disorders. In: Hazzard WR, Blass JP, Ettinger WH, et al., eds. *Principles of Geriatric Medicine and Gerontology.* 4th ed. New York: McGraw-Hill; 1999:881–888.

39. Kim EC, Lance P. Colorectal polyps and their relationship to cancer. *Gastroenterol Clin N Am.* 1997;26(1):1–17.

40. Sandler RS. Epidemiology and risk factors for colorectal cancer. *Gastroenterol Clin N Am.* 1996;25(4):717–735.

41. Early DS, Marshall JB. Is routine screening for colorectal cancer justifiable? These gastroenterologists say YES! *Postgrad Med.* 1997;102(1):48–52.

42. Koretz RL. Is routine screening for colorectal cancer justifiable? This gastroenterologist says NO! *Postgrad Med.* 1997;102(1):49–60.

CHAPTER **12**

Gynecological Problems of Postmenopausal Women

Valerie T. Cotter

Introduction

Life expectancy for women in the United States has risen dramatically over the past century. The average life expectancy for women is 79 years; women age 65 can expect to live to be 84 years old.[1] The three leading causes of death for women over age 65 are heart disease, cancer, and stroke.[1] Women today can expect to live one-third of their lives after menopause. Women in their postmenopausal years (aged 60 and beyond) look forward to this stage of life for personal growth and maturation, but also may confront significant disability from chronic conditions like osteoporosis, heart disease, and cancer.

Gynecological care should emphasize the range of options for older women including health promotion and preventive care that decrease morbidity. Women should be empowered to become partners in their own health care and health-care decision making. This chapter discusses age-related gynecological changes, current screening guidelines for breast and cervical cancer, available therapy, vaginitis, and sexually transmitted diseases.

Reproductive Age Changes

Physical changes with aging are the culmination of heredity, lifestyle, and hormonal alterations. The loss of estradiol, produced by the ovaries, results in a variety of changes in postmenopausal women. The number and severity of symptoms vary among women, but frequently involve vaginal and urinary tract changes, vasomotor instability, and insomnia.

With loss of estrogen, the mucosal lining of the vagina loses vascularity and rugae and the vaginal wall loses strength.[2] The resulting pelvic relaxation contributes to the development of cystocele or rectocele. Furthermore, loss of subcutaneous fat and elastic tissue leads to shrinkage in the labia majora and minora. The ovaries and fallopian tubes also atrophy and are usually not palpable on bimanual exam. Vaginal secretions decrease, often resulting in vaginal irritation, discomfort, and dyspareunia. Vaginal pH is more alkaline and infections are therefore more common. Hypoestrogenic changes in the urethra and bladder contribute to increased urinary frequency, urgency, and a greater susceptibility to urinary tract infection (UTI). Breast size diminishes as glandular tissue is replaced by fat.

Vasomotor instability, or hot flash, is a frequent symptom in menopause, but may persist for longer than five years. A rapid rise of luteinizing hormone causes a surge in body surface heat, followed by a fall in body temperature. This intense flushing of the chest, neck, and face can last for 5 to 12 minutes and concludes with perfuse perspiration. Vasomotor instability most frequently occurs at night and can lead to insomnia.

Normal physiologic changes increase susceptibility to vaginal discharge and infections, especially atrophic vaginitis in postmenopausal women. Symptoms of scant watery vaginal discharge, vulvar itching or irritation, and dyspareunia suggest atrophic vaginitis. The vaginal mucosa is thinned and erythematous on examination. Treatment with an estrogen cream applied vaginally for one to two weeks, followed by less frequent application, once or twice weekly thereafter, can be prescribed.

Sexuality

Despite limited study of sexuality in older adults, sexual interest and activity continue into the seventh, eighth, and ninth decade. Hormonal changes in menopause may contribute to sexual alterations and decreased libido, as shown in Figure 12–1.[2]

Although women may report increased time to achieve lubrication, pain during intercourse, and decreased genital sensitivity, women are nevertheless reluctant to discuss sexual concerns, fail to recognize the possible connection between sexual change and menopause, and simply cease sexual activity. A discussion about sexual habits, part-

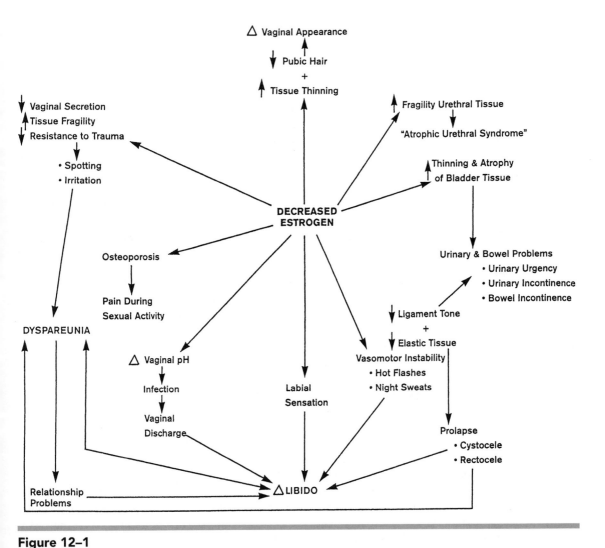

Figure 12–1

Hypoestrogenic effects that can cause sexual alterations.

Adapted from: Hefland SL, Powers J. Sexual dysfunction in the menopausal woman: hormonal causes and management issues. *Geriatr Nurs*. 1996;17:161–165.

ner(s) and relationship issues, physical signs or symptoms, and problems or satisfaction with sex life is an important part of any comprehensive history.[3] Determining the underlying reasons for change in sexual activity is an essential part of assessment, diagnosis, intervention, and teaching.

 ## Individualized Assessment

A complete history should be taken with special emphasis on the symptoms of hypoestrogenism; sexual function and relationship issues; and a history of osteoporosis; heart disease; thromboembolic disorders; hormone-related cancers of the breast, endometrium, or ovaries; liver or gallbladder disease; seizure disorders; or migraine headaches. Include a comprehensive reproductive history with data on menarche, obstetric history, age of menopause, sexually transmitted diseases (STDs), last pelvic exam, previous clinical breast examination (CBE) and breast self-examination (BSE), and results of previous Papanicolaou (Pap) smear and mammogram. Review current prescription and over-the-counter (OTC) medications, herbal therapies, dosages, reasons for use, and side effects; note drugs in the past that caused negative interactions or unpleasant effects.

Physical Examination

A gynecological examination begins with measurement of height, weight, and blood pressure. Perform the breast exam to identify masses, dimpling, nipple retractions, thickening, discharge, or abnormal lymph nodes. Examine the external genitalia, urethra, and Bartholin's glands, noting any lesions, discharge, or swelling. The vagina and cervix are examined noting signs of atrophic vaginitis, cystocele, prolapsed vagina, or rectocele. The Pap smear (using a wooden or plastic spatula) and an endocervical brush should be obtained. If the vagina is too small for a speculum, blind swabbing or vaginal aspiration is not recommended. During bimanual exam, assess the uterus and adnexa; any adnexal mass is highly suspicious of malignancy. Retrovaginally, the rectal exam is performed to detect adnexal or rectal masses. The left

lateral position may make the pelvic examination and Pap smear more comfortable for older women with musculoskeletal problems.

 ## Gynecological Screening in Older Women

Breast cancer screening guidelines include mammography, CBE, and SBE. The United States Preventive Services Task Force (USPSTF) currently recommends biennial mammography for women aged 50 to 70, but provides no guidelines beyond age 70.[4] The American Cancer Society and the National Cancer Institute advise annual mammography with no upper age limit. The American Geriatrics Society (AGS) recommends annual or at least biennial mammography until age 75, and biennially or at least every three years thereafter, with no upper age limit, as well as annual CBE and monthly SBE.[5] Mammography is unnecessary with progressive functional limitations from comorbid conditions negatively affecting life expectancy, such as advanced heart failure, steroid- or oxygen-dependent chronic obstructive pulmonary disease, or a known terminal diagnosis.[5]

Recommendations for periodic pelvic examination and Pap smear screening in older women are controversial. The AGS recommends regular Pap smear screening at one- to three-year intervals until age 70 and screening with at least two negative Pap smears one year apart for a woman of any age who has never had a Pap smear.[6] Support for or against screening women older than 70 years, who have been regularly screened in previous years is limited.[6] The USPSTF advises that regular Pap tests and pelvic examinations in women after age 65 who have had normal tests and regular screening is probably not indicated.[4]

Treatment Options for Postmenopausal Symptoms

Treatment of physiologic postmenopausal changes can be achieved through lifestyle modifications, complementary therapies, and prescription medications. Lifestyle modifications include exercise, healthy diet, weight management, stress reduction, and smoking cessation. Complementary products like foods and supplements containing soy, vitamins E and B complex, primrose oil, valerian root, and St. John's Wort are widely used by women. Though scientific data supporting the use of these complementary products are limited, they may provide an overall increase in quality of life.

Soy food products contain isoflavones, phytochemicals similar to estrogen that bind to estrogen receptors in the body and exert both estrogenic and antiestrogenic effects, as well as metabolic activities, such as antioxidant effects and protein synthesis. They are found in varying amounts in soy food products. The following isoflavone content is contained in a 100 g portion: 151.17 mg in green, raw soybeans; 148.61 mg in soy flour; 60.39 mg in miso soup (dry); 22.70 mg in extra-firm steamed tofu; and 16.30 mg in tofu yogurt.[7] A meta-analysis of 38 published controlled clinical trials of soy protein consumption suggested a 10% reduction in

cholesterol levels with 25 g per day (50 mg/day isoflavones).[8] In October 1999, the U.S. Food and Drug Administration (FDA) permitted the marketing claim that 25 g/day of soy protein, as part of a diet low in saturated fat and cholesterol, may reduce the risk of heart disease. There is, however, inadequate data to suggest the efficacy of isoflavones in reducing hot flashes and vaginal dryness, or the amount needed to prevent osteoporosis.[7]

Hormone therapies involve the administration of unopposed estrogen replacement therapy (ERT) or estrogen and progesterone hormone replacement therapy (HRT). They can be recommended for the treatment of specific menopausal symptoms on a short-term basis (less than five years), and long-term for the prevention and treatment of osteoporosis and for the possible reduction of the risk of coronary artery disease (CAD). Specific HRT treatment regimens are presented in Table 12–1.[9]

Table 12–1   HRT Regimens

Active Ingredient(s) Natural	Brand Name(s)	Form and Route of Administration	Strength
Estradiol (17-Beta estradiol)	Estrace	Oral tablet, vaginal cream	0.5 mg, 1 mg, 2 mg 0.01% (0.1 mg/g)
	Climara	Transdermal (applied once per week)	0.05 mg/day, 0.1 mg/day
	Estraderm	Transdermal (applied twice per week)	0.05 mg/day, 0.1 mg/day
	Vivelle	Transdermal (applied twice per week)	0.0375 mg/day, 0.05 mg/day, 0.075 mg/day, 0.1 mg/day
	Alora	Transdermal (applied twice per week)	0.0375 mg/day, 0.05 mg/day, 0.075 mg/day, 0.1 mg/day
	Fempatch	Transdermal (applied once per week)	0.025 mg
Estradiol valerate	Generic available	Intramuscular	10 mg/ml, 20 mg/ml, 40 mg/ml
Estradol cypionate	DepoEstradiol cypionate	Intramuscular	1.5 mg/ml
Estropipate	Ogen Ortho-est	Oral tablet Oral tablet	0.375 mg, 1.5 mg, 3 mg 0.375 mg, 1.5 mg
Estrone	Generic available	Intramuscular	2.5 mg/ml
Esterified estrogens	Estratab Menest	Oral tablet Oral tablet	0.3 mg, 0.625 mg, 1.25 mg, 2.5 mg 0.3 mg, 0.625 mg, 1.25 mg, 2.5 mg

Table 12–1 *(continued)*

Conjugated equine estrogen			
	Premarin	Oral tablet,	0.3 mg, 0.625 mg, 0.9 mg, 1.25 mg, 2.5 mg
		vaginal cream	0.625 mg/g
	Premarin intravenous	Intravenous, Intramuscular	25 mg/dose
Conjugated equine estrogen combination products			
	Prempro	Oral tablet	0.625 mg + 2.5 mg medroxyprogesterone acetate
	Premphase*	Oral tablet	0.625 mg + 5 mg medroxyprogesterone acetate
Synthetic			
Medroxyprogesterone acetate	Provera	Oral tablet	2.5 mg continuous dosage 5 mg, 10 mg for 12 to 14 days/month
Ethinyl estradiol	Estinyl	Oral tablet	0.02 mg, 0.05 mg, 0.5 mg
Quinestrol	Estrovis	Oral tablet	100 mg
Dienestrol	DV	Vaginal cream	0.01%
	Ortho-Dienestrol	Vaginal cream	0.01%
Chlorotrianisene	Tace	Liquid-filled capsule	12 mg, 25 mg
Natural progesterone			
(Micronized progesterone)	Prometrium	Oral tablet	100 mg continuous dosage
	Crinone	Vaginal insert	4%
	ProGest	Transdermal cream	

*Premphase is available in blister cards of 28 tablets; 0.625 mg conjugated equine estrogen and 5 mg medroxyprogesterone acetate is added to 14 of the 28 tablets.
Source: Witt DM, Lousberg TR. Controversies surrounding estrogen use in postmenopausal women. *Ann Pharmacotherapy.* 1997;31:745–745. Reprinted with permission.

Before recommending any form of HRT, an individualized assessment should cover menopause-related symptoms and the associated health benefits and potential risks (Figure 12–2).[10] A CBE, pelvic examination and Pap smear, and mammography should all be obtained prior to initiating HRT and yearly thereafter if continuing with HRT. Absolute contraindications for HRT include breast cancer (increased risk of breast cancer is not an absolute contraindication), endometrial cancer, unexplained vaginal bleeding, active liver disease or chronic severe liver disease, and recent vascular thrombosis. Potential contraindications include migraine headaches, seizure disorders, and history of gallbladder disease, thromboembolic events, thrombophlebitis, endometriosis, or familial hyperlipidemia.

Potential risks of HRT are well documented. The major risk associated with increased dosages and duration of estrogen therapy without progestins is endometrial cancer. Progestins prevent the development of endometrial hyperplasia and eliminate or decrease risk of endometrial cancer. Combined estrogen and progestin should be given

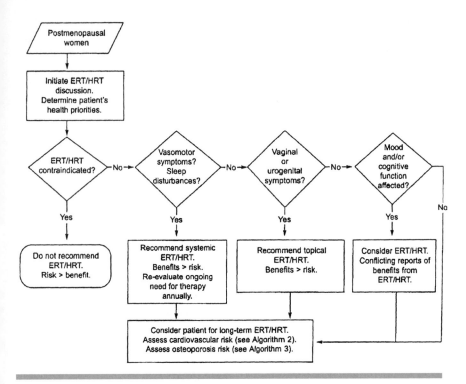

Figure 12–2
Assessment of menopause-related symptoms.
Source: North American Menopause Society. A decision tree for the use of estrogen replacement therapy or hormone replacement therapy in postmenopausal women: consensus opinion of the North American Menopause Society. *Menopause.* 2000;7(2):76–86.

to women taking estrogen for prolonged daily use. With cyclic progesterone and continuous estrogen, periodic uterine bleeding can complicate the recognition of endometrial cancer.

The connection between estrogen and breast cancer risk is still under investigation. Although HRT has not been directly linked to cancer, data are conflicting regarding these relationships. Prolonged use of estrogen and the combined estrogen-progesterone regimen increase risk.[11,12] In the Nurses' Health Study, a 43% increase in breast cancer deaths occurred in women who took HRT for more than 10 years.[13]

Raloxifene (Evista) is a selective estrogen receptor modulator with antiestrogenic effects on breast

and endometrial tissue and estrogenic effects on bone. It has been effective in preventing and treating postmenopausal osteoporosis; however, its effect on CAD is unknown. In a study of women taking raloxifene for osteoporosis, the risk of breast cancer was decreased 76% during three years of treatment.[14] The most common side effects are hot flashes and leg cramps. All HRT, including raloxifene, has other adverse effects including fluid retention, blood pressure elevation, breast tenderness, gallstones, glucose intolerance, and headaches.

Hormone replacement therapy is effective in women with vasomotor (hot flashes, night sweats), vaginal, or urogenital symptoms (vaginal dryness, dyspareunia, dysuria, urinary urgency and frequency, and recurrent UTIs; urinary incontinence has not been shown to be responsive to estrogen replacement). Oral, patch, or topical forms of estrogen provide symptomatic relief.

Determining whether a woman is a candidate for long-term use of HRT for osteoporosis or CAD is complex and requires patient participation in decision making. An algorithm for recommending HRT for the prevention of osteoporosis in postmenopausal women is presented in Figure 12–3.[10] Treatment of osteoporosis with HRT is recommended in:

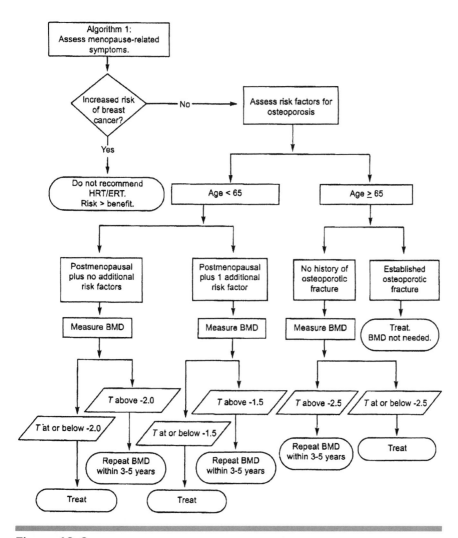

Figure 12–3
Assessment of osteoporosis risk.
Source: North American Menopause Society. A decision tree for the use of estrogen replacement therapy or hormone replacement therapy in postmenopausal women: consensus opinion of the North American Menopause Society. *Menopause.* 2000;7(2):76–86.

1. Postmenopausal women aged 65 years and older with no history of an osteoporotic fracture and a dual-energy x-ray absorptiometry (DXA) femur T score at or below –2.5 and

2. Postmenopausal women with an established osteoporotic fracture.[10]

See chapter 13 for additional management options for osteoporosis.

In postmenopausal women with CAD, findings from the Heart and Estrogen/progestin Replacement Study (HERS) suggest that HRT does not reduce risk of recurrent heart disease.[15] For women with CAD taking HRT for more than one year, it may be reasonable to continue treatment until trial data are available.[10] An algorithm for recommending HRT in women with cardiovascular risk is presented in Figure 12–4.[10]

 Vaginitis and Sexually Transmitted Diseases

The three most common diseases causing vaginitis and vaginal discharge are bacterial vaginosis (BV), trichomoniasis (caused by the protozoan *T. vaginalis*), and candidiasis (caused by yeast, such as *Candida albicans*). Causes of vaginitis are identified through pH and microscopic examination of vaginal secretions, in addition to the clinical exam-

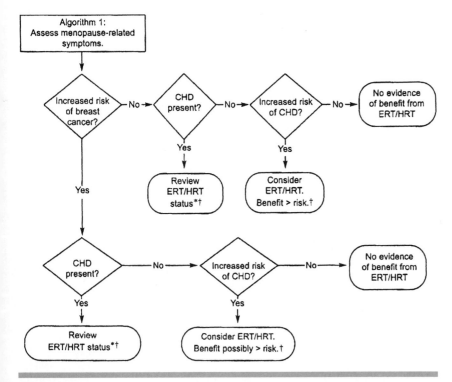

Figure 12–4
Assessment of cardiovascular risk.
Source: North American Menopause Society. A decision tree for the use of estrogen replacement therapy or hormone replacement therapy in postmenopausal women: consensus opinion of the North American Menopause Society. *Menopause.* 2000;7(2):76–86.

ination. Elevated pH over 4.5 is seen in BV or trichomoniasis. To prepare the sample for microscopic examination, dilute vaginal secretions in one to two drops of 0.9% normal saline solution on one slide and 10% potassium hydroxide (KOH) solution on another. If an amine (fishy) odor is detected immediately after applying KOH, BV is most likely. Under the microscope, the motile *T. vaginalis* or clue cells of BV are usually identified on the saline slide and the yeast or pseudohyphae of *Candida* identified on the KOH slide.

Bacterial vaginosis is caused by *Gardnerella vaginalis, Mycoplasma hominis,* and other anaerobic bacteria, which replace the normal lactobacilli in the vagina. Many women notice a thin, grayish discharge with a strong odor, especially after intercourse. It is not considered an STD, and treatment of the sex partner is not indicated. Recommended treatment is with metronidazole (Flagyl) 500 mg orally twice daily for seven days or clindamycin (Cleocin) cream 2%, 5 g intravaginally at bedtime for seven days or metronidazole gel 0.75%, 5 g intravaginally twice daily for five days.[16] Women should be advised to avoid alcohol during treatment with metronidazole and for 24 hours thereafter.

Vulvovaginal candidiasis (VVC) is diagnosed clinically by pruritus and erythema, and often a white discharge. Candidiasis can occur concomitantly with STDs or following antibacterial systemic or vaginal therapy. The Centers for Disease Control (CDC) recommendations for a variety of creams, suppositories, and oral regimens are presented in Table 12–2.[16] OTC preparations, including butaconazole (Femstat 3), clotrimazole (Gyne-Lotrimin), miconazole (Monistat), and tioconazole (Monistat) should be advised only for women previously diagnosed with VVC or who have a recurrence of symptoms. If symptoms persist after use of an OTC product, or with recurrence within two months, clinical evaluation is necessary. Routine treatment of sex partners is unnecessary, but may be considered for women who have recurrent infection and for men who have symptomatic balanitis or penile dermatitis.

Trichomoniasis is an STD, often symptomatic in women, but not in men. *T. vaginalis* characteristically causes a diffuse, malodorous, yellow-

Table 12–2   Recommended Regimens for Treatment of VVC[16]

Intravaginal agents:
Butoconazole 2% cream 5 g intravaginally for 3 days,
OR
Clotrimazole 1% cream 5 g intravaginally for 7–14 days,
OR
Clotrimazole 100 mg vaginal tablet for 7 days,
OR
Clotrimazole 100 mg vaginal tablet, two tablets for 3 days,
OR
Clotrimazole 500 mg vaginal tablet, one tablet in a single application,
OR
Miconazole 2% cream 5 g intravaginally for 7 days,
OR
Miconazole 200 mg vaginal suppository, one suppository for 3 days,
OR
Miconazole 100 mg vaginal suppository, one suppository for 7 days,
OR
Nystatin 100,000-unit vaginal tablet, one tablet for 14 days,
OR
Tioconazole 6.5% ointment 5 g intravaginally in a single application,
OR
Terconazole 0.4% cream 5 g intravaginally for 7 days,
OR
Terconazole 0.8% cream 5 g intravaginally for 3 days,
OR
Terconazole 80 mg vaginal suppository, one suppository for 3 days.

Oral agent:
Fluconazole 150 mg oral tablet, one tablet in single dose.

green discharge that causes vulvar irritation. Treatment of both the patient and sex partner(s) is recommended with metronidazole (Flagyl) 2 g orally in a single dose or metronidazole 500 mg twice daily for seven days.[16] Patients should avoid sex until the therapy is completed and patient and partner(s) are asymptomatic.

Chlamydia trachomatis infection is the most prevalent STD among sexually active adolescents and young adults. It may cause vaginal discharge or genitourinary tract infection; however, symptoms may be absent, mild, or nonspecific. While it is uncommon among older women, it should be considered in a sexually active woman. Annual screening is recommended in women older than 24 years with the following two risk factors: 1) lack of condom use, and 2) new or multiple partners in the preceding three months.[16] Urine and cervical sample tests using the DNA-based polymerase chain reaction method is the preferred diagnostic test. Treatment of the patient and sex partner(s) involves the following options: azithromycin (Zithromax) 1 g orally in a single dose, doxycycline (Doryx, Monodox, Vibramycin) 100 mg orally twice daily for seven days, erythromycin base 500 mg orally four times daily for seven days, erythromycin ethylsuccinate (EES) 800 mg orally four times daily for seven days, or ofloxacin (Floxin) 300 mg orally twice daily for seven days.[16]

Gonorrhea in women often does not produce recognizable symptoms, but may include cervical discharge, urethritis, infection of the Bartholin's glands, pelvic symptoms and signs, abnormal vaginal bleeding, acute exudative pharyngitis, or proctitis. In suspected cases, cultures from genital, anal, or pharyngeal sites are mandatory. Patients with gonorrhea often are coinfected with chlamydia and should be treated routinely with medication (doxycycline or azithromycin) effective against both STDs.[16] The following regimens are recommended for treatment of the patient and sex partner(s) with uncomplicated gonococcal infections of the cervix, urethra, and rectum:

1. Cefixime (Suprax) 400 mg orally in a single dose,

2. Ceftriaxone (Rocephin) 125 mg intramuscularly in a single dose,

3. Ciprofloxacin (Cipro) 400 mg orally in a single dose,

4. Azithromycin (Zithromax) 1 g in a single dose, or

5. Doxycycline (Doryx, Monodox, Vibramycin) 100 mg orally twice daily for seven days.[16]

Syphilis, an STD caused by the bacterium *Treponema pallidum*, can lead to serious systemic disease and death. Women who have syphilis may present with signs and symptoms of primary infection (ulcer or chancre at the infection site), secondary infection (rash, skin lesions, and adenopathy), or tertiary infection (e.g., neurosyphilis, cardiovascular syphilis, opthalmic disease).

For diagnosing early syphilis, Darkfield microscopic examination or direct fluorescent antibody tests of lesion exudate or tissue are definitive. Two serologic tests are diagnostic for latent syphilis. The nontreponemal antibody tests are the Venereal Disease Research Laboratory (VDRL) and Rapid Plasma Reagent (RPR). Reactive results are reported quantitatively in the form of a titer. The fluorescent treponemal antibody absorbed (FTA-ABS) and microhemagglutination assay for antibody to *T. pallidum* (MHA-TP) are two treponemal tests. The treponemal tests are designed to confirm the diagnosis of a reactive nontreponemal test and usually remain reactive regardless of treatment. Penicillin G (e.g., benzathine, aqueous procaine, or aqueous crystalline) is the preferred drug for treatment of all stages of syphilis; dosage and length of treatment depend on the stage and clinical manifestations of disease.[16] Patients who have primary or secondary syphilis and are penicillin allergic should be treated with either doxycycline 100 mg orally twice daily for two weeks or tetracycline 500 mg orally four times a day for two weeks.[16]

The most common sexually transmitted genital ulcer is caused by herpes simplex virus (HSV) infection, a recurrent, incurable viral disease. Serotypes HSV-1 and HSV-2 have been identified; genital HSV-1 causes most first episodes of genital herpes and HSV-2 infection is the most common in recurrences. Patients with mild or unrecognized infections that shed virus intermittently may be unaware that they have infection. Other patients with their first-episode genital herpes infection may suffer severe disease symptoms. Systemic antiviral drugs partially control symptoms; however, they do not cure the virus or affect the risk, frequency, or severity of symptoms of recurrences. Management includes antiviral therapy and counseling regarding genital herpes, sexual transmission, and methods to reduce transmission.

Treatment guidelines vary depending on whether the patient is having a first episode of genital herpes or a recurrence. For HSV-1 genital infection, the following medications are recommended:

1. Acyclovir (Zovirax) 400 mg orally three times daily for 7–10 days,
2. Acyclovir 200 mg orally five times daily for 7–10 days,
3. Famciclovir (Famvir) 250 mg orally three times daily for 7–10 days, or
4. Valacyclovir (Valtrex) 1 g orally twice daily for 7–10 days.[16]

Current CDC guidelines for episodic recurrent infection and daily suppressive therapy can be accessed at the website aepo-xdv-www.epo.cdc.gov/wonder/PrevGuid/p0000480/p0000480.htm.[16]

Education

Women with atrophic vaginitis and vaginal infection should receive educational counseling about preventive measures, such as avoiding douches, genital deodorants, nylon undergarments, and irritating soaps and bubble baths. Completing the entire treatment regimen and abstaining from intercourse during treatment should be advised.

All patients should be given information about prevention of STDs and safer sex practices. Safer sex practices include the use of a latex condom, limiting the number of sexual partners, and engaging in activities that do not involve the exchange of body fluids, such as cuddling, massage, and mutual masturbation.[3] The CDC recommendations for the use of male and female condoms are listed in Table 12–3.[16]

Table 12–3 CDC Guidelines for Proper Use of Condoms[16]

- Use a new condom with each act of sexual intercourse.
- Carefully handle the condom to avoid damaging it with fingernails, teeth, or other sharp objects.
- Put the condom on after the penis is erect and before any genital contact with the partner.
- Ensure that no air is trapped in the tip of the condom.
- Ensure adequate lubrication during intercourse, possibly requiring the use of exogenous lubricants.
- Use only water-based lubricants (e.g., K-Y Jelly, Astroglide, AquaLube, and glycerin) with latex condoms. Oil-based lubricants (e.g., pertroleum jelly, shortening, mineral oil, massage oils, body lotions, and cooking oil) can weaken latex.
- Hold the condom firmly against the base of the penis during withdrawal, and withdraw while the penis is still erect to prevent slippage.

Female Condoms

Laboratory studies indicate that the female condom (Reality)—a lubricated polyurethane sheath with a ring on each end that is inserted into the vagina—is an effective mechanical barrier to viruses, including HIV. Other than one investigation of recurrent trichomoniasis, no clinical studies have been completed to evaluate the efficacy of female condoms in protection from STDs, including HIV. If used consistently and correctly, the female condom should substantially reduce the risk for STDs. When a male condom cannot be used appropriately, sex partners should consider using a female condom.

Conclusion

Older women experience age-related gynecological changes that may have a negative impact on their sexual and genitourinary function. Treatment of physiologic postmenopausal symptoms can be achieved through lifestyle modifications, complementary therapies, and HRT. Long-term use of

HRT for osteoporosis or CAD is complex and requires active patient participation in the decision-making process. Primary care to postmenopausal women must include cancer screening, health education and counseling, and appropriate treatment.

References

1. US Bureau of the Census. *Statistical Abstract of the United States. Vital Statistics of the United States: 1999.* Washington DC: US Bureau of the Census; 1999.

2. Hofland SL, Powers J. Sexual dysfunction in the menopausal woman: hormonal causes and management issues. *Geriatr Nurs.* 1996;17:161–165.

3. Letvak S, Schoder D. Sexually transmitted diseases in the elderly: what you need to know. *Geriatr Nurs.* 1996;17:156–160.

4. US Preventive Services Task Force. *Guide to Clinical Preventive Services. Report of the U.S. Preventive Services Task Force.* Baltimore: Williams & Wilkins; 1996.

5. American Geriatrics Society Clinical Practice Committee. Breast cancer screening in older women. *J Am Geriatr Soc.* 2000;48:842–844.

6. American Geriatrics Society, Clinical Practice Committee. AGS position statement: screening for cervical carcinoma in older women. May 2000. Accessed February 14, 2001. Available at: http://www.americangeriatrics.org/products/positionpapers/cer_carc_2000.

7. The North American Menopause Society. The role of isoflavones in menopausal health: consensus opinion of the North American Menopause Society. *Menopause: J N Am Menopause Soc.* 2000:7(4):215–229.

8. Anderson JW, Johnstone BM, Cook-Newell ML. Meta-analysis of the effects of soy protein intake on serum lipids. *N Engl J Med.* 1995;333:276–282.

9. Witt DM, Lousberg TR. Controversies surrounding estrogen use in postmenopausal women. *Ann Pharmacother.* 1997;31:745–754.

10. The North American Menopause Society. A decision tree for the use of estrogen replacement therapy or hormone replacement therapy in postmenopausal women: consensus opinion of the North American Menopause Society. *Menopause: J N Am Menopause Soc.* 2000;7(2):76–86, 2000.

11. Collaborative Group on Hormonal Factors in Breast Cancer. Breast cancer and hormone replacement therapy. *Lancet.* 1997;350:1047–1059.

12. Schairer C, Lubin J, Troisi R, Sturgeon S, Brinton L, Hoover R. Menopausal estrogen and estrogen-progestin replacement therapy and breast cancer risk. *JAMA.* 2000;283(4):485–491.

13. Colditz GA, Hankinson SE, Hunter DJ, et al. The use of estrogen and progestins and the risk of breast cancer in postmenopausal women. *N Eng J Med.* 1995;332:1589–1593.

14. Cummings SR, Eckert S, Krueger KA, et al. The effect of raloxifene on risk of breast cancer in postmenopausal women: results from the MORE randomized trial. *JAMA.* 1999;281(23):2189–2197.

15. Hulley S, Grady D, Bush T, et al. for the Heart and Estrogen/progestin Replacement Study (HERS) Research Group. Randomized trial of estrogen plus progestin for secondary prevention of coronary heart disease in post-menopausal women. *JAMA.* 1998;280: 605–613.

16. Centers for Disease Control and Prevention. 1998 Guidelines for treatment of sexually transmitted diseases. *MMWR. Morb Mortal Wkly Rep.* 1998;47 (No. RR-1): 1–116. Available at: http://aepo-xdv-www.epo.cdc.gov/ wonder/PrevGuid/p0000480/p0000480.htm. Accessed February 14, 2001.

13

Musculoskeletal Problems

Johanna Yurkow
Jean Yudin

Introduction

Osteoporosis, rheumatoid arthritis, and osteoarthritis are disorders that are very common in the elderly population. Symptoms and clinical features of these disorders can often make diagnosis and management difficult. This chapter defines these disorders and outlines the clinical course to assist the practitioner in making an accurate diagnosis and an individualized plan of care.

Osteoporosis

Definition

Osteoporosis is a condition characterized by the loss of bone mass and density. In 1993, the Consensus Development Conference on Osteoporosis defined osteoporosis as "a systemic skeletal disease characterized by low bone mass and microarchitectural deterioration of bone tissue with a consequent increase in bone fragility and susceptibility to fracture."[1] The World Health Organization defines osteoporosis by bone mineral density (BMD) measurements, stipulating that osteoporosis occurs when bone mass is reduced greater than 2.5 standard deviations below peak adult mean.[2] Osteopenia, a precursor to osteoporosis, refers to a bone mass loss that is between 1 and 2.5 standard deviations below peak adult mean. Osteoporosis is classified as one of two types: postmenopausal osteoporosis (type I) and senile osteoporosis (type II).

Postmenopausal osteoporosis is related to accelerated bone loss in women, which occurs in the first two decades following menopause. Affecting mainly trabecular bone, the most common fracture sites for type I osteoporosis are crush fractures of the vertebrae (compression fractures) and fractures of the distal radius. Senile osteoporosis (type II) is related to impaired production of 1,25-dihydroxy vitamin D, and occurs primarily after the age of 75. It affects both trabecular and cortical bone with the most common fracture sites being multiple wedge fractures of the vertebrae and hip fractures.

Prevalence and Significance

Osteoporosis is typically a disease of aging with disability and mortality related to osteoporotic fractures primarily concentrated in the older population. Osteoporosis is a crippling and painful bone disease and the most common skeletal disorder affecting older adults. The direct health-care costs related to osteoporosis and resultant disorders are estimated to be $14 billion a year. Thus, identification, prevention, and treatment of osteoporosis are major health-care concerns. In women, the incidence of osteoporotic fractures, primarily hip and vertebral, increase near the time of menopause. Hip fracture incident rates accelerate approximately 10 years later as comorbidities and dysfunction related to other disease entities affect gait, cognition, and other conditions that affect the rate of falls and injuries.[3] In patients with hip fractures, about 12–20% die within one year after the fracture, and 20–50% of the survivors are unable to return to independent living.[4] Osteoporosis is typically seen as a disease of women; however, hip-fracture rates in men rise exponentially starting at age 75, with men suffering more than 75,000 hip fractures annually, one-third the rate of women.[3]

Pathophysiology

The two major causes of osteoporosis are calcium deficiency or lack of absorption caused by a diet low in calcium, and estrogen deficiency secondary to menopause. Secondary causes include cigarette smoking, prolonged steroid use, excessive caffeine, prolonged inactivity, endocrine disorders (primarily those affecting the parathyroid), liver disease, alcoholism, specific malignancies, and related bone disorders. Bone mass, 75–80% genetically predetermined, changes over the life span of an individual with peak bone mass occurring in the third decade. Shortly after peak bone mass is achieved, a slow rate of bone loss occurs beginning well before the onset of menopause. For about a decade following menopause, bone loss accelerates at a rate of approximately 3–7% a year due to the associated estrogen deficiency. Beginning in the seventh decade, bone loss continues at a rate of approximately 1–2% a year. Men also lose bone with age, most of it from the vertebral spine.

Mechanisms that contribute to bone loss in men (as well as women) are secondary hyperparathyroidism related to calcium deficiency. Parathyroid hormone, a strong stimulator of bone reabsorption when chronically elevated, increases in an attempt to maintain serum calcium levels. Furthermore, the decreased function of the skin and lessened exposure to sunlight leads to a reduced absorption of calcium and from vitamin D deficiency. Finally, increased reabsorption seen with aging (and menopause in women) is compounded by decreased osteoblast activity.

Clinical Presentation

The clinical presentation of osteoporosis includes loss of height (measuring against height at age 30), dorsal kyphosis or dowager's hunchback caused by vertebral collapse, back pain, and history of fractures.[5] Due to the porous and spongy nature of osteoporotic bone, vertebral fractures may be the result of normal activities such as bending and may affect primarily the twelfth thoracic and first lumbar vertebrae. Trauma may result in fractures of the distal radius when arms are extended to protect from a fall. Hip fractures occur primarily during falls, but may be incurred during normal walking or weight bearing. In some situations, the client may fall after the fracture has actually occurred. Spinal fractures are the most common osteoporosis-related fractures, with more than 700,000 occurring in the United States each year.[6]

History

Obtaining a history requires skilled investigation of family history, lifestyle patterns, and physical complaints. Family history is important because bone mass is 75–80% predetermined. Note the age and type of fractures that have occurred in family members, as well as outcomes and any resultant disability. Having a parent or sibling with osteoporosis is a definite risk factor, and may require stringent adherence to preventive measures. A review of general lifestyle habits is necessary and includes type and frequency of exercise, measures to increase safety and prevent falls, and dietary habits and vitamin supplementation. Comorbidities that contribute to falls need to be identified, as well as any specific indicators of osteoporosis. Note any history of fracture, the age at which it occurred, and the amount of trauma experienced. A loss of height, greater than two inches from age 30, associated with back pain may indicate vertebral compression. Note the severity and location of pain to determine the effects of previous fractures or areas of vertebral fracture that may require further assessment or treatment.

Physical Examination

A thorough physical examination will uncover comorbidities and their contribution to dysfunction. The primary focus in a physical examination for presence of osteoporosis is functional status and the presence of pain.

Diagnostic Tests

Diagnostic testing is essential to determine the presence and extent of osteoporosis and to identify the most appropriate treatment option. Unless certain treatment options are clearly known, diagnostic testing, which can be both costly and uncomfortable for certain patients, should not be performed.

Testing is not warranted with terminal, end-stage conditions, in situations where patients are likely to refuse treatment, or where the information obtained will not change the course of treatment.

Until recently, the simplest and least expensive diagnostic test has been x-ray visualization of porous bone. This method, however, is ineffective in identifying early osteoporotic changes, unless at least a 30% bone loss has already occurred. The best predictor of osteoporotic fracture and a more reliable method to determine the presence of osteoporosis, other than clinical observation or simple x-ray, is BMD measurement or bone mass measurement.

The National Osteoporosis Foundation recommends BMD measurements in the following situations: estrogen deficiency, osteopenia, long-term glucocorticoid therapy, and asymptomatic primary hyperparathyroidism. The most commonly used method of BMD measurement is the dual-energy x-ray absorptiometry (DXA). Measurements are typically taken of the hip, AP spine, lateral spine, and wrist. Fracture is thought to be 10 times greater in those whose measurements fall in the lowest quartile, as compared to those that fall in the highest quartile. Ultrasonography is sometimes considered as a simpler, portable method for residents of long-term care facilities.

A number of laboratory tests are available to determine the presence of secondary causes of osteoporosis. Ionized calcium, serum and urine protein electrophoresis, alkaline phosphatase, 25(OH)D, T4, TSH, bioavailable testosterone, and prolactin identify or rule out the presence of primary hyperparathyroidism, multiple myeloma, Paget's disease, osteomalacia, hyperthyroidism, and hypogonadism.

Interventions

Appropriate interventions and care plans depend on several factors including personal preferences, comorbidities, overall condition, prognosis, and contraindications to specific therapies. To be successful, these must be individualized and satisfactory to the client in order to promote adherence.

Lifestyle Modifications

General lifestyle modifications in cases of osteoporosis include smoking cessation, reducing or eliminating alcohol and caffeine intake, avoiding a sedentary lifestyle, increasing activity, and dietary modifications. Exercise is paramount to prevent further bone loss related to immobility and to reduce serious falls through general improvement in muscle and balance. Individualized exercise programs should focus on weight-bearing exercises, ambulation, and safety. Weight-bearing and muscle-toning exercises, such as walking and low-impact aerobics, should be done at least three times a week, starting slowly and gradually increasing, based on individual ability and tolerance. A structured program geared toward older adults, or consultation with a physical therapist for evaluation of rehabilitation potential and plan of care, may be helpful.

Based on an assessment, dietary recommendations should be aimed at prevention of further bone loss and increased well being. A normal weight is important; obesity strains muscles, bones, and joints. The diet should be high in natural sources of calcium from green leafy vegetables and dairy products. A nutritional consultation may be necessary for further evaluation and appropriate supplementation.

Pharmacological Interventions

Osteoporosis can be treated three ways pharmacologically, through calcium and vitamin D supplementation, hormone replacement therapy (HRT), or its alternatives. Calcium and vitamin D supplementation should be instituted following nutritional consultation and counseling, and only after natural sources of these nutrients have been optimized in the diet. Recommendations are 1200–1500 mg/day of calcium and 800–1200 IU/daily of vitamin D (to increase absorption) in divided doses, depending on customary intake of natural calcium (which should be promoted). This regimen requires education concerning regular bowel function since constipation is often associated with calcium supplementation.

HRT is indicated in estrogen-deficient women without contraindications and should be administered with progestin if the uterus is intact. The selective estrogen receptor modulator (SERM) raloxifene can be administered to those who cannot take HRT or when high risk of adverse effects is anticipated. Contraindications to HRTs include known or suspected breast cancer, known or suspected estrogen-sensitive neoplasm, undiagnosed abnormal genital bleeding, active thrombophlebitis or thromboembolic disorders, or significant history of thrombotic disease, hypersensitivity to the hormones, and untreated hypertension. For a comprehensive review of HRT, see Chapter 12.

Either alendronate or salmon calcitonin are most commonly used in situations when HRT is not indicated. The preferred administration route for salmon calcitonin is through nasal inhalation, alternating nostrils with each dose. Certain guidelines must be maintained when taking alendronate, including taking it 30–60 minutes before meals and other medications with 8 oz of water and then to stand or sit for 30 minutes following administration. Failure to follow these dosing instructions may cause such severe digestive reactions as irritation, inflammation, or ulceration of the esophagus. Alendronate is contraindicated in those with poor pill-swallowing ability, significant gastroesophageal reflux disease, large hiatal hernia, high gastric ulcer, frequent heartburn, hypocalcemia, and creatinine clearance < 35 cc/min.[6]

Management of Coexisting Morbidities

Paramount to the treatment of osteoporosis is the management of resultant and associated symptoms, which often lead to immobility. Three problems require maximum attention: impaired function, acute back pain, and prevention of falls and injury. Efforts to improve function should increase general well being, overall mobility, and independence. Patients with obvious deformities should be referred to physical and occupational therapy, especially for any assistive devices. These must be fitted appropriately to prevent further disability and to promote correct use. Assistive devices should not be purchased at a supply store without proper evaluation and recommendations. Deformities can lead to soft-tissue pain which is often treated successfully with rehabilitation modalities and nonpharmacological measures. Weight-bearing exercises may be prescribed, and education provided on posture, mobility, and safety issues.

With debilitating acute back pain, the patient should still remain mobile, but cautioned to take short rest periods periodically throughout the day. Nonsedating analgesics can be prescribed to relieve pain and promote activity. Rehabilitation services prove invaluable in prescribing a mobilization and exercise program tailored to current functional status and necessary for improved muscle strength. Any type of restrictive device, such as a corset or back brace, should be used only as long as necessary and removed once pain has subsided.

Of utmost importance in the management of osteoporosis are mechanisms that reduce the risk of falls. Falls are multifactorial and require an extensive and comprehensive evaluation to determine their cause. Decreased muscle strength, skeletal and muscle deformity which alter the center of gravity, and pain are often the precipitants of falls in persons with osteoporosis. Again, a structured program of rehabilitation provides muscle strengthening and improved balance, both of which contribute to a reduction in falls.

Education

For the patient with osteoporosis, education focuses on maintaining function, reducing pain, and preventing injury. Dietary recommendations need to be reviewed and a diet prescribed that is easy to follow and to maintain. The diet should be balanced, emphasize weight reduction if appropriate, and include as many natural sources of calcium and vitamin D as possible.

Nonpharmacological means of pain reduction should always be attempted, for example, topical agents and heat. If analgesics are prescribed, patients need to be well versed concerning efficacy and side effects. Assistive devices must be properly fitted and used. It is important to teach how to fall safely and to get up in a manner that minimizes further risk of injury.

Anticipated Outcomes

Expected outcomes center on arresting bone loss through exercise, diet, and medication. A treatment plan suitable to the patient's lifestyle provides the most optimal outcomes. Treatment measures should be selected on the basis of the lowest risk profile and the highest benefit. Prevention of injury is key in order to avoid a downhill spiral of dysfunction associated with fractures and other injuries during older adult years.

Referrals

Osteoporosis demands an interdisciplinary approach to comprehensive services aimed at optimal function. Key referrals are usually for rehabilitation and mental health, because of critical lifestyle changes and emotional issues concerning decreased function.

Rheumatoid Arthritis

Definition/Classification

Rheumatoid arthritis (RA) is a chronic, polyarticular, systemic disease of unknown etiology characterized by an inflammatory reaction in the synovial membrane that results in destruction of the joint cartilage and supporting structures. This chronic erosion and destruction accounts for the typical joint deformities that accompany the disease, including rheumatoid nodules and radiographic abnormalities. Rheumatoid arthritis is categorized as either standard or elderly onset rheumatoid arthritis (EORA).

Prevalence and Significance

Like osteoporosis, RA is a disease that primarily affects women. Of the 6 million Americans who are affected, 75% are women. Age of onset can be from infancy to the ninth decade, with the inci-

dence increasing with age. Peak onset usually occurs between the ages of 35 and 45. In addition to the physical and emotional prices it exacts, RA also presents a sizable financial hurdle: $8.7 billion, with an average annual direct cost of medical care for a single patient estimated at over $4,000.[7]

Pathophysiology

The etiology of rheumatoid arthritis is unknown, but is thought to be multifactorial. Infection, autoimmunity, and genetic factors are etiological possibilities. Diagnostically, the pathophysiological findings in rheumatoid arthritis consist of inflammatory synovitis with resultant erosion of the adjacent bone. The rheumatoid joint produces destructive enzymes that become active in the synovium.

Rheumatoid arthritis passes through four distinct phases. In stage I, synovitis, or joint inflammation, is initiated with resultant swelling of the synovial lining and production of excessive synovial fluid. In this stage, no destructive changes are noted on x-ray. In stage II, granulation inflammatory tissue is formed where the synovium meets the cartilage. This granulation inflammatory tissue, or pannus, eventually enters the joint capsule and subchondral bone. Some mild x-ray findings are evident at this stage, with slight subchondral bone and/or cartilage destruction. Generally some limitation of joint movement also occurs, but no obvious joint deformity. Fibrous connective tissue eventually replaces the pannus in stage III, occluding the joint space. Decreased joint motion, malalignment, and deformity result. X-ray evidence of cartilage and bone destruction is apparent. In the final phase, total joint immobilization results as the fibrous tissue calcifies with extensive muscle atrophy and soft-tissue lesions. Nodules may be present. X-ray examination reveals fibrous and bony alkylosis.

History

A comprehensive history is important to augment the physical findings so typical of rheumatoid arthritis. In the early stages of the disease, general symptoms of poor health may be noted. Questions should be related to general well being, as well as more specifically to joint function and overall activity, mobility, and independence. Any fatigue, malaise, pain, and fever should be noted. Joint stiffness, noting the time of day and duration of the stiffness, is helpful in differentiating rheumatoid arthritis from other musculoskeletal disorders, along with identification of symmetry or asymmetry of affected joints. Identify any functional problems associated with these functional changes, and question the patient about the presence of musculoskeletal deformities and nodules. With disease progression, a more in-depth history will be needed related to the extra-articular disorders typically found in later stages of the disease.

Clinical Presentation/Physical Examination

Clinically, patients present with an acute or gradual onset of pain, swelling, and stiffness of multiple joints. Related symptoms of fatigue, malaise, low-grade fever, anorexia, and weight loss may develop. Specific to the joint, pain, warmth, edema, and limitations of joint are likely; presentation is usually symmetrical, although asymmetry is possible. Prolonged morning joint stiffness is a positive indicator. Most patients suffer intermittent periods of active disease alternating with periods of complete remission. A few suffer with prolonged, unrelenting, and progressive symptoms. More common than the seropositive arthritis found in any age with rheumatoid arthritis are the seronegative findings in those that develop rheumatoid arthritis over the age of 60 (EORA). EORA is much milder than the RA that develops at a younger age. The synovitis manifested in EORA affects fewer joints, usually the moderate-sized joints such as the shoulders, knees, or wrists, rather than the smaller joints of the hands and feet as seen with standard rheumatoid arthritis. The onset of EORA may occur over a much shorter period of time, beginning in a few days to a week, with morning stiffness being severe.

The most common extra-articular finding with rheumatoid arthritis is the development of rheumatoid nodules, which occur in approximately 25% of cases. The nodules are thought to be the result of small-vessel vasculitis. They are firm and nontender, and present subcutaneously over the bony prominences during later stages of the disease. These deformities are characteristic of rheumatoid arthritis and are most common in the swan-neck deformities of the hand caused by hyperextension of the proximal interphalangeal joints, and boutonniere deformities caused by a flexion deformity of the interphalangeal joints. Ulnar drift, also a very common finding, occurs as the fingers drift toward the ulna. Other extra-articular findings are systemically produced and include synovial cysts, episcleritis (inflammation of the loose connective tissue between the sclera and the conjunctiva), pericarditis, and pulmonary fibrosis.

Diagnostic Tests

No single laboratory test is conclusive for rheumatoid arthritis; however, several studies are essential to an accurate diagnosis. A complete blood count (CBC) rules out anemia (normochromic, normocytic anemia or anemia of chronic disease with low serum iron or low serum iron-binding capacity), which is commonly seen in rheumatoid arthritis. In a patient with very active disease and on corticosteroid therapy, the leukocyte count may be elevated, although white blood cell counts (WBC) are usually normal. Thrombocytosis may be apparent in those with very active disease. The erythrocyte sedimentation rate (ESR) is usually elevated, but also typically increases with age. Serum rheumatoid factor assay, a circulating antibody, is positive in most cases of rheumatoid arthritis, although it is sometimes found in healthy individuals. An elevated rheumatoid factor may be present with connective tissue diseases, liver disease, sarcoidosis, syphilis, and tuberculosis. Most typically, however, it is seen in higher concentrations with rheumatoid arthritis.

In addition to laboratory tests, other diagnostic measures may be useful. X-ray findings are limited in the early stages of the disease because they reveal only bone demineralization and soft-tissue swelling. Later, x-rays show other structural changes, including narrowing of the joint space, destruction of articular cartilage, erosion, subluxation, malalignment, and ankylosis.

Synovial fluid analysis reveals several indices of RA: increased volume and turbidity, increased protein content, slightly reduced glucose content with decreased viscosity, and elevated WBC.

Interventions

Treatment goals are directed toward relief of the acute inflammatory manifestations of the disease, preventing musculoskeletal dysfunction, correcting deformities and extra-articular aspects of the disease, and education related to lifestyle changes. In developing an individualized plan of care, many factors need to be considered. It is important to know earlier levels of function and general lifestyle, psychosocial aspects related to age, occupation, home situation, current functional status, stage of the disease, and the results of treatments attempted in the past. In most cases, a team approach is needed to develop a plan that is individualized and successful. Team members may include rehabilitation specialists, orthopedic services, and mental health and social work professionals.

Lifestyle Changes

Initially, efforts related to lifestyle changes should be geared toward pain relief and optimization of functional status. Especially during the most active phases of the disease, a healthy balance between rest and therapeutic exercise is of utmost importance. Patients should be cautioned to rest periodically during the day and to participate in an activity program that is structured and therapeutic. They should be dissuaded from the mistaken belief that strenuous exercise delays or prevents deformity. Isotonic and isometric exercises are helpful in preventing deformities, improving range of motion, and promoting muscular strength. Nonpharmacological measures should be utilized to decrease pain and increase function, including superficial heat for subacute problems, deep heat (ultrasound), cold for inflamed joints and tendons, TENS units, and positioning techniques that allow maximum participation in the prescribed exercise program.

Splinting is useful in the prevention and correction of deformities caused by muscle spasms and contractures and to rest an inflamed joint. Splinting should be done by a professional, most often a physical therapist, and the splinting guidelines followed carefully by the patient. Splints must be removed periodically to provide skin care and range of motion, and need to be reapplied as prescribed.

In addition to rest and exercise, nonpharmacological pain relief measures, and splinting, the patient should adhere to a generally healthy lifestyle that encourages weight control, smoking cessation, and a diet low in caffeine and high in nutrients.

Pharmacological

Pharmacological management of rheumatoid arthritis consists of aspirin/nonsteroidal anti-inflammatory drugs (NSAIDs), corticosteroid therapy, and remission-inducing agents.

Aspirin/NSAIDs   Aspirin, used as an anti-inflammatory agent, forms the foundation for pharmacological treatment of rheumatoid arthritis. It should be given with meals in the enteric-coated form. High doses are needed for the desired effect; thus, it is poorly tolerated in many patients. Long-term, high dosages may result in elevated liver enzymes, gastrointestinal upset/bleeding, and tinnitus. Salicylate levels must be monitored on a regular basis with periodic evaluation of symptoms.

Currently, NSAIDs are a more desirable mainstay of therapy for rheumatoid arthritis. NSAIDs may be given alone or in combination with aspirin. Usually, NSAIDs control the most bothersome symptoms associated with RA including joint stiffness, swelling, and pain. Gastrointestinal complaints are the most common symptoms associated with NSAID use. If neither aspirin nor NSAIDs are tolerated, then a course of Tylenol (with great caution in older adults) may be attempted for pain relief.[8]

Corticosteroids   Corticosteroids are successful in decreasing joint erosion and suppressing inflammation, and are most appropriate for those with active disease, major functional deformities, and disabilities. Corticosteroids may be given orally or intra-articularly for long-term or immediate relief of pain. Adverse effects are well known and a thorough discussion of the risks and benefits of corticosteroid use should be discussed with the patient. Repeated injections are associated with the breakdown of bone and joint collapse. Other side effects include cataracts, glaucoma, gastrointestinal bleeding, osteoporosis, weight gain, glucose intolerance, risk for infection, and poor healing. Intra-articular injection may provide relief for pain and swelling for one to six weeks following a one- to two-day increase in pain. The identified joint should be infection free at the time of injection and no joint should be injected more than three times.

Remission-Inducing Agents   Antimalarials, penicillamine, and chrysotherapy (gold therapy) are considered remission-inducing agents, and are indicated when more conservative treatments have been unsuccessful. The exact mechanism of action is unknown. Cryotoxic drugs, primarily methotrexate, have been used successfully to control the inflammation and pain of rheumatoid arthritis. Side effects include cirrhosis, hepatitis, leukopenia, and thrombocytopenia. Remission-inducing agents carry a high side-effect risk, and follow-up and monitoring needs to comply with guidelines for the specific agent used. Again, the risks and benefits should be discussed with the patient and a commitment to long-term treatment with these agents should be elicited.

Surgical Management

Despite the array of drug therapies for rheumatoid arthritis, joint deformities and disabilities nevertheless occur due to the progressive and debilitating nature of the disease. These changes result in painful impairments to mobility and function. Regardless of treatment compliance, close monitoring, and follow-up, surgical intervention may still be warranted. Surgeries may include synovectomy (removal of the inflamed synovial lining), arthrodesis (fusion of the diseased joint), osteotomy (removal of a joint), and implant arthroplasty (joint replacement). Surgical intervention generally relieves pain and increases joint stability and mobility. Broad spectrum antibiotics, used sys-

temically and as irrigations, have made joint replacements common and relatively safe. Hip and knee replacements are performed most often, but elbow, wrist, and ankle joints may also be replaced. Prior to any joint replacement, the patient needs to understand the procedure and the importance of intensive follow-up rehabilitation. Complications include thrombophlebitis, shock, pain, and dislocation. Understanding and compliance with postoperative instructions minimize the chance of these occurrences. Postoperative rehabilitation is generally necessary for four to six months.

Management of Coexisting Morbidities

Rheumatoid arthritis is a complicated systemic disorder with numerous comorbidities requiring interdisciplinary management. Common extra-articular manifestations include vasculitis, lymphadenopathy, and ocular problems. Vasculitis is an early manifestation of rheumatoid arthritis and is thought to be responsible for myopathy, peripheral neuropathy, cardiopulmonary involvement, and ischemic ulceration of the skin. Vasculitic leg ulcers may be present in the 5% who develop Felty's syndrome (rheumatoid arthritis, splenomegaly, and neutropenia) with occasional massive splenic enlargement.

Lymphadenopathy is present in 25% of individuals suffering from rheumatoid arthritis, with signs and symptoms often suggestive of lymphoma. Splenomegaly is present to a much lesser extent. Recurrent infections and problems associated with healing present particularly difficult problems for patients with rheumatoid arthritis.

Ocular manifestations frequently occur when rheumatoid arthritis develops at an early age, but may also be present in those with later onset. Sjögren's syndrome involves destruction of the exocrine glands, including tear and salivary glands. Eye symptoms such as dryness, sensations of grittiness, and photophobia are likely. Sjögren's syndrome may also contribute to such oral problems as fissuring, dysphagia, gingivitis, and caries. Treatment focuses on the localized eye or oral problems and reevaluation of the regimen for rheumatoid arthritis.

Although rare, cardiac problems can occur. These usually result from rheumatoid granulomas that contribute to arrhythmias, aortitis, aortic regurgitation, and pericarditis. Pulmonary involvement is very rare.

Education

Community education should be directed toward early identification and timely evaluation for treatment. Patients need daily routines that decrease fatigue and provide for optimal functioning. Activities should be planned around morning joint stiffness, with certain activities delayed until later in the day when joint mobility is greater, and fatigue and pain lessened. To the extent possible, nonpharmacological measures to reduce pain should be encouraged, with emphasis on those measures best suited to individual routines and preferences. These measures include heat and cold modalities, transcutaneous electrical nerve stimulation (TENS) units, positioning, whirlpool baths, relaxation techniques, joint protection, biofeedback, meditation, and hypnosis.

Patients must be fully knowledgeable concerning the pharmacological treatments, expected outcomes, and anticipated side effects. It is essential to know when to notify a primary health-care provider concerning unanticipated side effects or other adverse outcomes. In general, medication schedules require strict adherence. For best results, regular reviews of medication regimens are warranted with follow-up visits.

Anticipated Outcomes

Ongoing evaluation of persons with rheumatoid arthritis should address the issues of pain management, joint mobility and deformity, generalized function, compliance with recommendations for independent activity, and progression of the disease. Patients should demonstrate basic understanding of the disease, treatments utilized, pharmacological measures and side effects, and any needs for adjustment and support through formal and informal means. Patients with rheumatoid arthritis are likely to utilize an array of care settings throughout their illness, including inpatient and outpatient rehabilitation, and home care. Appropriate assistive and splinting/support

devices should be familiar and available to the patient. Patients need support during periods of remission as well, although remissions are less likely with EORA. It is important for patients to understand that remissions do not represent cure and that reoccurrences are to be expected.

Referrals

Referrals depend on the stage, degree, and impact of the illness. In most cases, rehabilitation is warranted to develop an individualized plan of care, fitting for assistive devices and splinting, education, and continued follow-up to address resultant deformities and changes in functional status. Other referrals may include orthopedic surgeons, pharmacists, and professionals able to provide psychological support.

Table 13–1 Comparison of Osteoarthritis and Rheumatoid Arthritis

Osteoarthritis	Rheumatoid Arthritis
Considered a degenerative process, often begins after age 40	Considered an inflammatory process, often begins ages 25–50
Develops slowly	Develops suddenly, often over weeks to months
Cartilage is affected	Synovial membrane is affected
Affects some joints, rarely elbows and shoulders	Affects many joints, including elbows and shoulders
Stiffness decreases within half hour	Stiffness lasts for at least one hour
Often occurs asymmetrically	Often occurs symmetrically
Usually no joint inflammation	Joint inflammation is typical
Usually no feeling of illness associated with the disease	Patient often feels ill: fever, weight loss, fatigue, depression
No change in blood work associated with disease	Rheumatoid factor and elevated ESR can be present

Osteoarthritis

Definition

Arthritis is a general term referring to more than 100 different conditions affecting the joints. Generally, these conditions fall into two categories: osteoarthritis or degenerative arthritis, resulting when cartilage is damaged and bone undergoes abnormal changes; and inflammatory arthritis resulting from inflammation in the joints (see Table 13–1).

Prevalence and Significance

Osteoarthritis (OA) is the most common form and affects 12% of the general population. Among older adults 65 and above, well over half are affected. The leading cause of disability in the United States, OA has numerous economic implications, including cost-related needs for home care and physical therapy, and medications. The impact of OA on physical function is considerable, affecting ambulation, stair climbing, and basic activities of daily living. Osteoarthritis is seen worldwide, although risk and appearance vary among ethnic groups. OA of the hips is common in the United States but the risk is lower in Asia and some Middle Eastern countries. Asians appear to have a higher incidence of OA of the knee than Caucasians before age 45. OA occurs more frequently in males; after age 55, it develops more often in females. The hip is affected more often in men; hands, fingers, and knees more often in women. Osteoarthritis can be classified as primary or secondary: primary osteoarthritis has no known cause, whereas secondary OA occurs in response to other mechanisms including infection, injury, and metabolic disorders.[9]

Pathophysiology

Joints, comprised of bone, cartilage, synovial membranes, and synovial fluid, provide flexibility, support, and protection. Cartilage, a tough, slippery tissue covering the ends of bones at the joint, serves as a cushion allowing easy movement of bones. The entire joint is surrounded by the synovial membrane filled with synovial fluid, which acts as a lubricant. A capsule surrounds the entire synovial membrane and provides protection to the joint. Synovial fluid supplies nutrients and oxygen to cartilage, which is composed of proteoglycans and collagen. These proteins have waterbinding qualities; cartilage is, in fact, mostly water. Collagen forms a mesh and gives support and flexibility to the joint.

Osteoarthritis occurs as cartilage is destroyed. In early stages of the disease, cartilage surfaces swell and proteoglycans are lost. As the disease progresses, inflammation occurs around the synovium, tissue is lost, and cartilage loses its elasticity. Eventually, as much cartilage is lost, the bones within the joint are unprotected. Such deterioration of the cartilage leads to formation of bone spurs causing the joint to appear misshapen.

Osteoarthritis affects specific joints, especially in the fingers, feet, knees, hips, and spine. Wrists, elbows, or shoulders are rarely affected. Weight-bearing joints, such as the knees, hips, and spine are increasingly affected in both sexes with age. Joint effects differ depending on location.

Osteoarthritis of the fingers occurs most often in older women. Usually, the distal interphalangeal joints (Heberden's nodes) and the proximal interphalangeal joints (Bouchard's nodes) are involved. Considerable disability occurs as knees become enlarged and painful with advancing disease. Osteoarthritis of the hip may cause pain in the groin, buttocks, or hips with radiation to the knee (confusing during a workup). Typically, osteoarthritis causes a limp with walking, as the affected leg is rotated to decrease pain. Osteoarthritis of the spine affects disc cartilage. Pain, muscle spasms, or decreased mobility are frequent symptoms, along with numbness and muscle weakness as the disease progresses.

Clinical Presentation

The clinical presentation of osteoarthritis includes pain, morning stiffness, mild joint swelling, and increased temperature in the joint. Patients may present with symptoms including pain or stiffness, swelling, crepitus, or inflammation associated with one or more joints.

Pain associated with OA usually begins gradually and progresses over several years. The pain can be described as variable; it may increase or decrease in severity. It often worsens with activity or overactivity, or after periods of inactivity. Many experience the worst pain in the morning after resting joints for several hours. Patients may describe the need to "loosen up" joints before getting out of bed or moving about. Some report pain that worsens by the end of the day. Swelling occurs when synovial membranes become irritated. Bone spurs often add to the appearance of a swollen joint, and crepitus may occur as bones rub together. The most common findings in primary osteoarthritis are Heberden's nodes and Bouchard's nodes.

History

An accurate history is important in the diagnosis of osteoarthritis. Family history of OA is suggestive and all relevant risk factors should be identified. Age, female sex, ethnic/racial background, genetic predisposition, knee injury, and physical labor are positive for the development of OA.[10] Obesity, defined as 20% over ideal weight, places an increased stress on joints and exacerbates osteoarthritis once deterioration has begun.

Since osteoarthritis affects function, a thorough evaluation of ability to perform activities of daily living should be addressed. As many medical conditions have symptoms of joint pain, stiffness, and swelling, it is important to distinguish osteoarthritis by reviewing risk factors and carefully eliciting a description of symptoms. Multiple co-existing diseases or cognitive impairment may impede accurate diagnosis. Often pain and decreased function are regarded as age appropriate by the patient and family. Osteoarthritis may occur in conjunction with other arthritic conditions, especially rheumatoid arthritis. Chondrocalcinosis or pseudo-gout may exacerbate osteoarthritis as it often affects joints not damaged by osteoarthritis, including wrists, elbows, and shoulders. Finally, a thorough review of treatments is required, including prescribed and over-the-counter medications and physical therapy modalities.

Physical Examination

Physical examination should focus on both the general exam and musculoskeletal assessment. General examination includes vital signs, organ systems affected by rheumatic diseases, including integument (hair loss), respiratory (chest expansion may be affected by thoracic spine arthritis), and neurologic exam. The exam should not be limited to painful joints but also include all other joints. Note any tenderness and deformity.

Diagnostic Studies

Synovial fluid may be withdrawn from an affected joint; in OA the results indicate noninflammatory fluid. Radiographs (x-rays) show joint-space narrowing with subchondral sclerosis in the early phase of osteoarthritis. As the disease progresses, marginal osteophytes, subchondral bone cysts, and subluxation is seen on x-ray.[11] In the more advanced stages, loose bodies and subchondral bone collapse are evident. Laboratory findings are usually normal although researchers have begun to identify blood tests that may be a useful biomarker for osteoarthritis.

Intervention

Although cure is unrealistic, osteoarthritis can be treated in a variety of ways, including drugs, alternative therapies, and surgery. Treatment is based on minimizing the sequelae of the disease, alleviating pain, and retaining and maintaining function. Often, a combination of individualized treatments is most effective.

Lifestyle Modifications

Obviously, treatment begins with prevention. Risk factors such as obesity, joint injury, and repetitive or stressful movements to the joint should be identified and steps taken to alter these situations. Excess weight is the most common cause of pressure on joints. Thus, a weight loss plan, exercise program, and behavior modification aimed at weight loss decrease stress to joints, especially in knees and feet.

Regular exercise also relieves pain and stiffness associated with osteoarthritis, as well as increases muscle strength, flexibility, and general endurance. The types of exercise best suited for OA include range of motion or stretching, strengthening, and low-impact exercise. Daily stretching exercises reduce joint stiffness and improve flexibility. Strengthening exercises to maintain or build muscle around joints and enhance stability should be included. Weight lifting, especially one- to two-pound weights, two to three times per week, can be beneficial. Examples of endurance or low-impact exercises include walking, swimming, or bicycling. These allow for smooth, rather than jerky, movements to the joint. Swimming is excellent for individuals with osteoarthritis in the hips or knees.

The use of heat and cold for pain and stiffness is potentially beneficial. Heat usually relaxes and warms muscles before exercise; cold reduces pain by numbing the area. Heat may be provided with heating pads, hot tubs, warm pools, or just a hot shower. Patients must never apply heat or cold directly to the skin or use either treatment for more than 20 minutes. In general, acute pain or inflammation responds best to cold, while chronic pain improves with heat.

Canes, splints, or braces may offer joint protection. During any exercise, shoes that absorb shock should be worn. Acupuncture is increasingly popular for pain associated with OA; however, controlled studies have not shown clinically significant improvement.

Pharmacological Treatment

Drugs are often used in conjunction with non-pharmacologic therapies such as weight loss or exercise. Prior to prescribing any medication, comorbidities, age, and potential drug interactions must be considered.

Topical Pain Relievers   Topical agents temporarily relieve muscle or joint pain. Most such agents (usually in the form of ointments or creams) contain combinations of salicylates, skin irritants (which cause feelings of cold, warmth, or itching), or capsaicin, which blocks the release of substance P from nerve endings. Complaints of stinging or burning may occur with first use, but this usually subsides after several days. Mild to moderate arthritis pain is usually treated first with acetaminophen. It is most effective when used regularly, rather than occasionally. Studies have shown it to be as effective as naproxen or ibuprofen in treating knee OA, with fewer side effects when used in therapeutic doses of 4 g/day.[12] Acetaminophen does not reduce inflammation, but the source of pain in OA generally is not inflammation. Renal function must be monitored with any long-term use, especially in those individuals with liver disease or alcoholic cirrhosis.

NSAIDs   Nonsteroidal antiflammatory drugs are the most commonly prescribed drugs for treatment of osteoarthritis. When analgesics fail to relieve pain, NSAIDs in their lowest effective dose are initiated. Many NSAIDs are available and response varies among individuals. NSAIDs block prostaglandins, the substance that dilates blood vessels causing inflammation and pain. An initial trial of a nonacetylated salicylate (Trilisate) may be indicated; if that is ineffective for control of pain, then a more potent NSAID should be initiated. Other NSAIDs include aspirin, ibuprofen, and naproxen. Relief from pain may not be noticeable for one to two weeks after starting a NSAID. Side effects and duration of action must be carefully monitored, since all NSAIDs can damage mucosal lining of the stomach, causing ulceration and gastrointestinal (GI) bleeding. The elderly are more likely to experience these side effects,[13] along with perforation, nephrotoxicity, and hepatotoxicity.[14] Additionally, central nervous system effects include dizziness, confusion, cognitive impairment, and memory loss. Any patient for whom NSAIDs are being considered must have a thorough history for peptic ulcer disease, cigarette smoking, alcohol use, and other pain relievers, especially other NSAIDs.

Because of the risk of GI damage, misoprostol (Cytotec) or H_2 blockers are often prescribed with a NSAID. Misoprostol, however, may cause diarrhea and abdominal cramps. H_2 blockers reduce GI symptoms, but do not prevent the ulceration associated with NSAIDs. A new class of drugs, called COX-2 inhibitors, more specifically block cycloxygenase production in the joints, rather than in the gastric lining, thus greatly reducing the risk of gastric ulceration and hemorrhage. With use of any NSAIDs, renal and liver function and blood count must be established at baseline, one month after initiating therapy, and then on a routine basis.

Intra-articular Injections   Corticosteroid injections reduce pain and inflammation and are most beneficial during acute joint flares. Benefits usually last up to four weeks; however, because steroids may also cause adverse effects, long-term use is limited. Hyaluronic acid derivatives are also used as injectables to relieve symptoms of OA, but they do not alter disease progression. Hyaluronic derivatives produce an anti-inflammatory, analgesic, and lubricating effect. The mechanism of action is not completely understood. Injections may be given weekly for three weeks, and provide generally better pain relief than a corticosteroid injection.

Alternative Therapies   Two natural substances found in the synovial fluid of the knee, glucosamine and chondroitin sulfate, have been found useful in small studies of pain relief and improved function. No double-blind trials reporting long-term results are available. Other alternative therapies, such as antioxidants, may alter progression of OA, but need further investigation.

Invasive Therapies

Surgery may be the only route for pain relief, especially if other modalities have failed. Removal of bone and cartilage fragments from a joint by arthroscopy may relieve pain in shoulders and knees. Joint lavage may also be used for the removal of debris and inflammatory material.[15] Joint replacement surgery is most frequently performed to repair hips and knees, but may be appropriate for ankles, wrists, and toes as well. A successful joint replacement relieves pain and restores joint movement.

Osteotomy is frequently used, and mostly for younger people experiencing OA in hip or knee joints. Osteotomy realigns or reshapes joints by removing small pieces of offending bone. Debridement is also performed to remove loose or torn fragments. Pain is relieved by bringing healthy articular cartilage into position.

Education

For the patient with osteoarthritis, education focuses on reducing pain and maintaining function. A healthy diet should be maintained, emphasizing weight reduction if needed. The diet should include calcium and vitamin D, and vitamins C, E, and beta-carotenes have also been suggested.

Nonpharmacologic means of reducing pain have been reviewed and should be part of the regimen. These include topical agents, heat, and cold. Regular weight-bearing exercise helps protect joints and should be adjusted to the individual's abilities. Estrogen may promote healthy joints in women. Individuals with osteoarthritis should evaluate occupational stresses adjusting a work area or exchanging tasks may reduce repetitive shocks to affected joints. Assistive devices must be properly fitted.

Anticipated Outcomes

Outcomes center around managing pain, modifying risk factors including obesity, and incorporating exercise effectively into the patient's lifestyles.

Referrals

Although many people with osteoarthritis live full lives, others experience serious losses of mobility and function, making activities such as walking or dressing painful and difficult. Elderly persons are especially susceptible to the emotional ramifications of osteoarthritis. They may feel symptoms of pain are part of the natural process of aging or fail to discuss limitations in mobility for fear it will lead to institutionalization. Psychological variables play an important role in determining the extent of pain and incapacity in persons with arthritis. It is important to help any individual diagnosed with osteoarthritis to learn as much about their disease as possible. Arthritis education and support groups and the local chapter of the arthritis foundation can provide valuable information. The American Geriatrics Society has recently published guidelines for pain control. Modifying risk factors, engaging in a healthy exercise program, complying with physical therapy modalities, and following recommendations for drug use lead to better pain management, increased function, and a more optimistic outlook.

References

1. Scheiber LB, Torregrosa L. Postmenopausal osteoporosis: when—and how—to measure bone mineral density. *Consult Primary Care*. 2000;40(4):781–789.
2. *The WHO Study Group: assessment of fracture risk and its application to screening for postmenopausal osteoporosis*: Technical Report Series, No. 843. Switzerland: World Health Organization; 1994.
3. Edwards BJ, Perry HM. Age-related osteoporosis. In: Perry HM, ed. *Clinics in Geriatric Medicine: The Aging Skeleton*. Philadelphia: W.B. Saunders; 1994:575–588.
4. Staarts DO, Beier M, Cantrell L, et al. *Osteoporosis: Clinical Practice Guidelines*. Washington, DC: American Health Care Association; 1998.
5. Beck L. Nursing management of adults with degenerative, inflammatory, or autoimmune musculoskeletal disorders. In: Beare PG, Myers JL, eds. *Adult Health Nursing*. Philadelphia: Mosby; 1994:1583–1623.
6. Dowd R, Cavalieri RJ. Help your patient live with osteoporosis. *Am J Nurs*. 1999;99(4):55–60.
7. Ramsburg KL. Rheumatoid arthritis. *Am J Nurs*. 2000;100(11):40–43.
8. Sewell KL. Rheumatoid arthritis in older adults. In: Loeser RF, ed. *Clinics in Geriatric Medicine: Musculoskeletal and Connective Tissue Disorders*. Philadelphia: W.B. Saunders; 1998:475–494.
9. Ross C. A comparison of osteoarthritis and rheumatoid arthritis: diagnosis and treatment. *Nurse Pract*. 1997; 22(9):20–39.
10. Felson DT. Prevention of hip and knee osteoarthritis. *Bull Rheum Dis*. 1998;47(4):1–4.
11. Ling SM, Bathon JM. Osteoarthritis in older adults. *J Am Geriatr Soc*. 1998;46:216–225.
12. Towheed TE, Hochberg MC. A systematic review of randomized controlled trials of pharmacological therapy in osteoarthritis of the knee, with an emphasis on trial methodology. *Semin Arthritis Rheum*. 1997;26(5):755–770.
13. Davies NM, Jamali F, Skeith KJ. Nonsteroidal antiinflammatory drug-induced enteropathy and severe chronic anemia in a patient with rheumatoid arthritis. *Arthritis Rheum*. 1996;39(2):321–324.
14. Furst DE. Are there differences among nonsteroidal antiinflammatory drugs? *Arthritis Rheum*. 1994; 37(1):1–9.
15. Creamer P, Hochberg MC. Osteoarthritis. *Lancet*. 1997;350:503–508.

PART **3**

Functional and Clinical Problems Associated with Frailty

14

Falls

Tim Baum
Elizabeth Capezuti
Gerald Driscoll

◾ Overview

Problem

Falling is a normal part of life. During walking, playing games, or attempting new activities, falls occasionally occur without mishap. With aging, the consequences of falling become more severe. Muscles are less responsive, and the nervous system is slower to react; soft tissues bruise and bones can break. Recovery from injuries takes longer. Falls in older adults are not a brief interruption in activity as they are for younger persons, but potentially life-threatening events. Falls may be simply the first sign of a single problem or part of a more complex combination of multiple pathologies, treatments, and environmental factors. Falls can result in functional decline, hospitalization, or death. The cost to families and society is enormous. Risk reduction and appropriate intervention reduce the frequency and severity of falls, thereby decreasing mortality, morbidity, functional decline, and cost to society.

A fall is the process of descending "freely by the force of gravity."[1] Clinicians and researchers operationally define a fall as "inadvertently coming to rest on the ground or another lower level, with or without loss of consciousness or injury."[2] Falls occur each year in about 25% of older persons living in the community and as many as 50% of those in long-term care.[3,4]

Sequelae

Falls are the sixth leading cause of death in older adults.[4] In a 32-month retrospective analysis of admissions to a level 1 trauma center, only 14% of fall patients were over 65, but accounted for over 50% of the deaths.[5]

Several studies demonstrated that injury is a common result of falls, and contributes significantly to morbidity and mortality in the elderly. Among pedestrian falls, the average age was 65 with 55% requiring medical attention.[6] Over a one-year period, more than half of a group of 96 older adults living within the community who ambulated without aids fell. Five percent of these falls resulted in fractures and 9% in soft-tissue injuries.[7] Of 911 persons hospitalized for fractures of the proximal femur, 66% were greater than 80 years old and 96% were related to a fall.[8]

Studies also confirm the association between nonfatal falls and functional deterioration and institutionalization.[4] In a group of older, community-residing African Americans treated in an emergency department for fall-related injury, 43% continued to have pain or functional impairments eight weeks after the fall.[9] Among community-residing elders, a fall increases the risk of long-term admission to a nursing home.[10] Repeated falls further increase the incidence of hospital admissions and nursing home placements.[11,12] In one study, half of the fall injuries occurring in the home resulted in nursing home admissions.[13]

Falls also impose a high cost to society. The estimated total cost of fall injuries in the United States in the elderly was $20 billion in 1995 and is projected to rise to $32 billion for the year 2020, with the increase due in part to baby boomers reaching retirement age.[14]

Pathophysiology and Cause of Falls

Frequency of falling in older adults is sometimes attributed to "multisystem stability disorder" arising from the "accumulated effect of multiple disorders superimposed on age-related changes."[15] These multiple disorders, or risk factors, have been studied extensively in order to predict and reduce falls and their sequelae. Numerous retrospective and prospective studies have identified characteristics correlated with falls. Risk factors for falls are usually categorized as either intrinsic (those characteristics that are personal), or extrinsic (characteristics of context or environment).[16]

Intrinsic Risk Factors

Personal or intrinsic factors include presence of chronic disease, age-related physical and mental changes, acute health problems or acute exacerbation of chronic disease, and the concomitant effects of medications used in the course of treatment. These contribute to falls either by affecting gait and balance, or by inhibiting judgment of the individual.

Physical   Generally, falls are associated with poor gait or balance.[17–20] Gait and balance are the functional manifestations of three neural mechanisms: sensory (perception), motor (action), and central integration or coordination of the two.[21–23] These neural mechanisms are, in turn, affected by age: body sway increases with a loss of righting reflexes, feet are not lifted as high, and stride length decreases.[24] Neural mechanisms can also be affected by chronic diseases of the neurological or musculoskeletal systems,[19] for example, orthostatic hypotension, syncope, cardiac arrhythmias, peripheral neuropathies, visual disturbances, weakness, central nervous system (CNS) disorders, dementia, arthritis, ischemic brain events, parkinsonism, or seizure.[25]

Sensory impairments of vision and hearing, often related to common health problems or age-related changes, potentially impair gait and balance and are associated with increased likelihood of falling.[18,26–28] Age-related vision changes include decreased pupil size and ability to respond to darkness. With increased lens opacity there is a reduction in depth perception, color discrimination, and adjustment to glare. Age-related diseases such as macular degeneration, glaucoma, and cataracts diminish visual acuity.[24]

Loss of sensory function in the lower extremities, demonstrated by reduced vibratory, touch, discriminative, or position sense, is also implicated in fall risk.[18,29] With age, proprioceptive abilities decrease, leading to less postural stability.[29]

Instability also occurs with declining muscle strength.[29] Both upper and lower extremity impairment is correlated with increased falls.[28] Motor function is negatively affected by peripheral neuropathy,[30] and weakness of hips, knees, and ankles also increases fall risk.[18]

Surrounding soft tissues (skin, fat, and muscles) often lessen the impact of a fall and thereby reduce the likelihood of injury, especially in persons with greater skinfold thickness or body weight.[30–32] In a sample of community-residing older adults who fell, cognitive impairment, multiple chronic conditions, impairments in balance and gait, and low body mass index were associated with serious injury.[33]

Numerous studies indicate a direct relationship between fracture risk and osteoporosis.[34] Indirect indicators of osteoporosis, such as small frame, female gender, and European or Asian descent, are frequently cited.[13,35,36]

Psychological   Mental state and cognitive ability form the interface between the environment and mechanisms controlling gait and balance. When judgment about ability or the environment are impaired or ignored, the risk of falls increases. Illness, whether physical or psychological, and the associated medications, all can easily affect judgment. Falls are associated with anxiety, depression,[28] and dementia.[37] Mini-Mental State Examination scores less than 24 and Geriatric Depression Scales with 10 or more depressed responses more than double fall risk.[17] Inattentiveness or rushing to get things done is implicated in many falls among community-dwelling ambulatory older adults.[7,38]

Pharmacologic   To the above risk factors must be added the effects of drugs on a variety of systems, many affecting both integrative and cognitive functioning. In numerous studies concerning the effects of medication on falls, it is difficult to separate whether risk factors for falls are the medications or the problems for which the medications were prescribed. Nevertheless, a variety of drugs are associated with falls, including sedatives, antidepressants, vasodilators,[39] insulin and oral hypoglycemics, antihypertensives,[25,40] anticholinergics, psychotropics, opiates and their derivatives, and Tylenol PM.[41,42] Polypharmacy itself is often implicated in falls,[43] with incorrect administration of drugs found in as many as 50% of community-dwelling older adults who fall.[44] Alcohol consumption can impair protective responses and result in increased risk of hip fracture.[45,46]

Of all medications, psychotropics have the highest correlation with falls[47] and probably double the risk. Psychotropic drug use was the most significant risk factor for falls among ambulatory nursing home residents.[48]

Some estimate that 33% of falls in the nursing home and 13% of community falls are due to psychotropics. Of these, antidepressants seem to contribute most to increased fall risk.[49] Significantly increased risk of hip fracture is associated with long-acting hypnotics, anxiolytics,[47] tricyclic antidepressants (TCAs), and antipsychotics, as well as dose-related increases in fracture risk in these classes of medications.[42]

For many years selective seratonin reuptake inhibitors (SSRIs) were assumed to have less fall risk than TCAs; however, recent work suggests that all antidepressants are associated with increased fall risk[50] and injury.[51] It is possible that in both studies, older adults with the greatest fall risk were given SSRIs preferentially over TCAs, because of problems such as orthostatic hypotension or arrhythmias for which TCAs are less preferred.[52] By contrast, a large retrospective study found not only a dose relationship with SSRIs and falls, but also differences within this class of drugs. Fluoxetine showed no significant increase in the risk of fracture, paroxetine almost doubled

it, and sertraline was in the middle.[53] To further confound these findings, two recent meta-analyses assessing depression treatments found no difference in the efficacy of TCAs versus SSRIs.[54,55]

Other drugs are also associated with falls. The hypotensive effects of certain cardiovascular drugs would seem to implicate them as risk factors for falls, although no evidence is clearly supportive. In fact, thiazides may help prevent hip fractures by increasing bone density.[49] Similarly, debate continues concerning increased fall risk with hypoglycemic agents and analgesics.[47]

Many studies confirm a relationship between increased fall risk and a number of medications.[47,49] Explanations include drug interactions, greater error associated with more medications, more fall-related diagnosis, or the cumulative effect of each additional medication.[49]

Finally, it is the interplay between these various systems that puts older adults at greater risk for falls. Most falls are due to multiple factors, some chronic and others related to acute changes in health status. Table 14–1 summarizes the intrinsic risks factors that should be considered in any evaluation of fall risk.

Table 14–1   Intrinsic Risk Factors for Falls

Chronic Illnesses/Symptoms/Signs
Functional
Inability to move leg(s) or arm(s) independently
Unilateral weakness
Physical/cognitive inability or lack of knowledge to use assistive device correctly
Cardiovascular
Postural (orthostatic) hypotension
Aortic stenosis
Congestive heart failure
Arrhythmias
Anemia (e.g., iron deficiency usually secondary to GI blood loss, B_{12} deficiency, anemia of chronic disease)
Musculoskeletal
Arthritis (osteo, polymyalgia rheumatica)
Foot disorders   *(continues)*

Table 14–1   Intrinsic Risk Factors for Falls   (*continued*)

Osteoporosis
Disuse or deconditioning syndrome
Osteomalacia
History of fracture
Post-amputation
Proximal muscle weakness
Myopathy

Neuromuscular
Stroke
Parkinson's disease
Huntingdon's disease

Neurosensory
Impaired vision (cataracts, glaucoma, macular degeneration, and/or presbyopia)
Impaired hearing
Polyneuropathy secondary to diabetes, peripheral vascular disease, or alcoholism
Pain, especially of joints

Other neurological
Cerebellar disorders
Shy-Drager syndrome
Multiple sclerosis
Cervical spondylosis
8th cranial nerve tumor

Psychiatric
Dementia
Depression
Post-stroke

Acute Illnesses/Symptoms/Signs

Functional
New-onset of weakness or incapacity in movement of extremity(ies)
Recent, rapid decline in functional status (IADLs or ADLs)

Hypovolemia
Low plasma volume
Anemia
Venous stasis
Blood loss
Severe diarrhea

Cardiovascular
Postural (orthostatic) hypotension
Vasovagal response
Carotid sinus syncope
Vasodepressor syncope (fatigue, hunger, heat)
Acute heart failure

New-onset arrhythmias
Acute myocardial infarction
Aortic stenosis/hypertrophic cardiomyopathy
Carotid artery compression

Respiratory
Tussive syncope (syncope related to unrelenting cough)
Pneumonia
Massive pulmonary embolism
Pulmonary tamponade
Hypocapnia due to hyperventilation
Hypoxia

Neurological
Transient ischemic attacks/recent stroke
Seizures
Vestibular dysfunction
Glossopharyngeal neuralgia

Autonomic neuropathies
Diabetic
Uremic
Toxic
Amyloidosis

Musculoskeletal
Fracture (hip, vertebral compression)
Sprain

Gastrointestinal
Defecation syncope
Acute abdomen (cholecystitis, pancreatitis, appendicitis, diverticulitis)
Diarrhea
Vomiting
Blood loss

Genitourinary
Post-micturition syncope
Urinary tract infection
New-onset incontinence

Metabolic
Hypo/hyperthyroidism
Hypoglycemia
Anemia
Hypokalemia
Dehydration
Hyponatremia
Acidosis
Hypocapnia (hyperventilation)

Table 14–1 *(continued)*

Psychiatric
Delirium (often indicative of underlying acute physical illness)
Anxiety
Hysterical fainting (conversion reaction)
Recent, post-stroke personality change

Medications

Polypharmacy/drug–drug interactions

Vestibulotoxic drugs
Aminoglycoside antibiotics

Cancer chemotherapeutic drugs

Quinine drugs

Central nervous system drugs
Ototoxic drugs (aspirin)
Psychotropics
Hypnotics/sedatives
Antidepressants
Dopamine agonists

Circulatory drugs
Diuretics
Antihypertensives
Vasodilators (nitrates)
Alpha blockers
Beta blockers
Antiarrhythmics

Behavioral Symptoms

Poor judgment regarding personal safety
Cautiousness due to fear of falling
Risk-taking or impulsivity (may be secondary to stroke or impaired cognition)
Tendency to stand quickly, especially from bed or immediately after a meal
Effort to remove physical restraint
Propensity to climb over or around side rails
Disinterest or inability to use recommended assistive device

Sources: Bickley LS. *Bates' Guide to Physical Examination and History Taking.* 7th ed. Philadelphia: Lippincott; 1999.

Grisso JA, Capezuti E, Schwartz A. Falls as risk factors for fractures. In: Arcus R, Feldman D, Kelsey J, eds. *Osteoporosis.* San Diego: Academic Press; 1996.

Rubin RH, Voss C, Derksen DJ, Gateley A, Quenzer RW. *Medicine: A Primary Care Approach.* Philadelphia: W.B. Saunders; 1996.

Extrinsic Risk Factors

Extrinsic risk factors include environmental hazards and specific situations or activities. Activities most frequently associated with falling occur when older persons are performing "usual" activities, such as rising from a chair or ambulating.[20,56,57]

Environment   The literature on environmental hazards focuses mainly on community-residing older adults and matters related to inappropriately placed furniture or objects, scatter rugs, slippery surfaces,[20,58,59] unstable furniture, high beds, shiny floors, footwear, and dim lighting.[60] Studies of environment usually involve asking about the cause of falls, and are therefore subject to interviewer bias and recall of respondents.[13]

A recent study suggests that only the absence of bathroom grab bars increases the risk of injury-related falls for all groups over 65.[13] Risk increased in certain subgroups, for example, cognitive deficits more than doubled fall-injury risk in the absence of slip-resistant flooring. In those older than 85, poorly placed light switches increased risk ninefold; women's risk increased twofold with high cabinets; men's risk increased fivefold with cords or wires in the living room. Throw rugs, usually associated with increased fall risk, actually decrease the number of falls by covering other hazards like wires or slippery floors. The risk of fall-related serious injury is increased when falls occur on a hard surface.[35,61] A sevenfold increase for injury in those older than 85 may be the result of an unpadded (no carpet) fall.

Many falls are also attributed to collisions in the dark, temporary hazards, and inappropriate use of assistive devices.[62] Poor judgment or impulsive tendencies may contribute just as much to a fall as environmental hazards (see Table 14–1 for a summary of behavioral symptoms that increase fall/injurious fall risk). Outside the home, most extrinsic falls occur on uneven or slippery surfaces.[6] Fractures and other injuries from falls increased after an ice storm in one metropolitan area.[63] (See Table 14–2 for a list of extrinsic risk factors.)

Table 14–2   Extrinsic Risk Factors in the Home

In General
Poor lighting
Slippery floors
Low seating
Unstable furniture
Shiny floors
Thick pile carpeting
High shelving

Bathroom
No grab bars
Low toilet seats

Bedroom
High bed
No hand rail or other transfer enabler

Stairs
No hand rails
Worn treads
Stairs not visibly different than adjoining floor
Stair edge not clearly defined

Situations   Most injurious falls in young and middle-aged adults are associated with rapid movement and forward propulsion with major impact to the wrist and a resulting wrist fracture. In contrast, injurious falls in older persons generally occur while standing still, during transfer, or while walking slowly with little forward momentum.[64] Risk of hip fracture is significantly increased in women falling sideways, straight down, or on or near the hip, as opposed to backwards which decreases risk of hip fracture.[65,66] Fallers who grabbed or hit an object before landing, and those who landed on their hand, were less likely to sustain a hip fracture.[61]

Screening and Evaluation

The first two steps in fall reduction and prevention of serious sequelae are

1. Early detection through screening of those at risk

2. Implementation of an effective intervention

Despite much research, there is no agreed upon approach for either screening or intervention.

Subjective Information

The greatest predictor of the occurrence of a fall is history of a previous fall.[67] Patients should be asked about prior falls, near falls, and any associated circumstances. Fear of falling should also be explored because it is also an indication of fall risk.[68]

Falls are often symptoms of undetected or untreated illnesses.[5,69] Table 14–1 lists acute illnesses that may lead to a fall. It is critical to assess and to identify injuries related to a fall, as well as to identify any underlying illnesses, which may be the cause of the fall. This can be difficult when adults have more than one identifiable medical condition that could be a risk factor for falling.[70] Sudden onset of repeated falls is usually a sign of underlying acute pathology, such as infection, hypoglycemia, or dehydration.[69] Atypical presentations and nonspecific complaints further complicate assessment.

Evaluation begins with a detailed history of where, when, and how the fall occurred. Table 14–3 provides a list of possible "rule-outs" to consider based on specific circumstances of the fall. Further questioning should elicit clues as to which intrinsic and extrinsic factors may have precipitated the fall, or the interaction among these factors. A medication review should include not only prescribed medication, but also over-the-counter drugs, botanicals, supplements, illicit drugs, and alcohol use. A diet history and analysis of liquid intake also needs to be done. The physical exam should identify and rule out intrinsic causes.

Table 14–3 Causes of Falls

If This Event Was Associated With the Fall	Suspect This
Flexion of head backward	Basilar artery dysfunction
Excessive coughing	Tussive syncope (laryngeal vertigo)
Hunger prior to fall	Vasodepressor syncope Hypoglycemia
After a large meal	Post-prandial syncope
Urination	Slipped in urine
After urination (especially after getting out of bed to void)	Post-micturition syncope
After large bowel movement	Defecation syncope Vasovagal response
Nausea, vomiting	Vasodepressor syncope Benign positional vertigo Vestibular neuronitis (acute labyrinthitis) Meniere's disease Drug toxicity (aminoglycosides, ETOH intoxication)
Tinnitis, hearing loss	Benign positional vertigo Drugs (aspirin, streptomycin, gentamicin) Meniere's disease Acute labyrinthitis Acoustic neuroma 8th cranial nerve tumor (unilateral hearing loss)
Turning head suddenly	Carotid artery compression
Inability to turn head (limited neck mobility)	Herniated cervical disc Degenerative cervical intervertebral discs/bony spurring Cervical vertebrae arthritis

Dizziness with position change	Orthostatic hypotension
	    Inadequate vasoconstrictor reflexes (peripheral neuropathies, antihypertensive & vasodilator drugs, prolonged bed rest)
	    Hypovolemia (GI bleeding, trauma, vomiting, diarrhea, diuretics, polyuria)

Dizziness	Cardiovascular disorder
	    Arrhythmia
	    Hypotension
	    Autonomic insufficiency (drugs, diabetes)
	    Severe anemia
	    Volume depletion (dehydration)
	Neurosensory disorders
	    Diabetes
	    Cervical spondylosis
	    Cerebellar disease
	Metabolic disturbances
	    Hypoglycemia
	    Hypoxia
	    Hypercapnia

(*continues*)

Table 14–3   Causes of Falls   *(continued)*

Vertigo	Vestibular disease
	Peripheral lesions
	Benign positional vertigo
	Ototoxic drugs (aspirin, streptomycin, gentamicin)
	Acute labyrinthitis, vestibular neuronitis
	Meniere's disease
	Acoustic neuroma
	Central lesions
	Multiple sclerosis
	Vertebrobasilar insufficiency/ basilar artery disease
	Drugs (sedatives, anticonvulsants)
Syncope	Vasodepressor syncope
	Postural hypotension
	Cough, micturition, defecation syncope
	Cardiovascular
	Arrhythmia
	MI
	Massive pulmonary embolism
	Seizures
Hyperventilation	Anxiety
	Conversion reaction
	Hypocapnia/metabolic acidosis
Chest pain/palpitations	Arrhythmia
	MI
	Postural hypotension due to hypovolemia
Proximal muscle weakness	Myopathy
	Hypothyroidism
	Hypokalemia
	Polymyalgia rheumatica
	Osteomalacia
	Disuse/deconditioning syndrome
Delirium	Dementia
	Hypoglycemia
	Infection (respiratory, UTI), fever
	Hypoxia
	Drug reaction
	Sensory deficits
	Sleep deprivation
Vision related (e.g., unable to see obstacle)	Cataracts
	Glaucoma
	Macular degeneration
	Presbyopia
	Inappropriate glasses
While ambulating (gait problems)	Proximal muscle weakness
	Drugs
	Arthritis
	Parkinsonism

Table 14–3   *(continued)*

	Paraplegia
	Cerebellar dysfunction
	Peripheral neuropathy
	Foot disorders
	Footwear
	Slippers, uneven floor surfaces
	Assistive devices
Using stairs	Vision
	Foot disorders
	Footing (unable to lift foot adequately)
	Improper step spacing
	Step visually similar to adjoining floor
	Step edge poorly defined

Sources: Abrahms WB, Beers MH, Berkow R, eds. *Merck Manual of Geriatrics.* Rahway, NJ: Merck & Company; 1995.

Bickley LS. *Bates' Guide to Physical Examination and History Taking.* 7th ed. Philadelphia: Lippincott; 1999.

Grisso JA, Capezuti E, Schwartz A. Falls as risk factors for fractures. In: Arcus R, Feldman D, Kelsey J, eds. *Osteoporosis.* San Diego: Academic Press; 1996.

Rubin RH, Voss C, Derksen DJ, Gateley A, Quenzer RW. *Medicine: A Primary Care Approach.* Philadelphia: W.B. Saunders; 1996.

Objective Information

Physical Examination   The most important part of the physical exam is the assessment of gait and balance, but many of the tools have been developed as part of research protocols and are time consuming and require training. The Berg Balance Scale,[71] for example, requires 20 minutes to administer and requires performance of assorted movements. A shorter, simpler test with similar reliability is the Mathias "Get Up and Go."[72] The patient sits in a straight-backed, high-seat chair and is instructed to get up, stand still momentarily, walk 10 feet, return to the chair, and sit. The clinician notes abnormal gait, balance, coordination, and muscle strength. Although no norms have been established, timing the activity helps with successive comparisons.[73] Decreased stride length and increased time between strides may be a stabilizing adaptation to fear of falling.[74] In evaluating gait, note if the person becomes short of breath or complains of chest pain or palpitations. If so, perform a thorough cardiovascular and chest examination including changes in vital signs with position change and exercise.

A modified Romberg test can be used to assess balance. The patient is put through four maneuvers (feet comfortably apart, feet together, heel to instep, and heel to toe) with eyes open and then with eyes closed. The patient is asked at each point, "Are you steady?"[75]

A simpler tool is the Functional Reach Test which may be more useful than a complete neurological and musculoskeletal exam. The patient stands upright with one shoulder and arm against a wall. The same arm is extended straight out against the wall and parallel to the floor. Mark the position of his/her fist on the wall. Keeping the arm against the wall and parallel to the floor, have the patient reach as far forward as possible without moving his/her feet. Again, mark the position of his/her fist. Distances less than six inches between these two marks indicates an increased risk of falls.[76] Balancing on one leg for at least five seconds shows a correlation with low risk of injurious falls.[77]

In addition to gait and balance, a thorough head and neck, musculoskeletal, neurological, and foot examination helps reveal potentially treatable areas of dysfunction and weakness that can contribute to fall risk. The sensory exam should include evaluation of vibratory sense in upper and lower extremities (checking for peripheral neu-

Table 14–4   Physical Examination of an Older Person's Fall Risk

Functional Tests
    Berg Balance Test
    Get Up and Go Test
    Modified Romberg Test
    Functional Reach Test

VS: pulse, blood pressure, including orthostatics
Skin: ecchymosis
Head: evidence of trauma
Eyes: visual acuity and fields
Ears: hearing
Neck: thyroid
Lungs: absent or adventitious sounds
(refer to Table 14–9)
Cardiovascular: rhythm, murmurs, gallops
Musculoskeletal: range of motion of joints
(goniometer)
Neurologic:
    Cranial nerves
    Cerebellar function
    Motor system especially strength
        Hip abduction, adduction, extension
        Knee extension and flexion
        Ankle plantar and dorsiflexion
    Sensory systems
        Vibratory sense
Mental/affective function
    Mini-Mental State Examination
    Geriatric Depression Scale
    Alcoholism screening — CAGE questions:
      1. Have you ever felt you should Cut down on
         your drinking?
      2. Have people Annoyed you by criticizing
         your drinking?
      3. Have you ever felt Guilty about your
         drinking?
      4. Do you have a drink first thing in the morning
         to steady your nerves (an Eye opener)?

Laboratory/Diagnostic
    As indicated
    Consider bone mineral density

ropathy), vision (acuity and visual fields), and hearing. Testing of motor functioning should focus on assessment of joint range of motion (flexibility) and muscle strength. If range of motion is limited, document the angle of motion, preferably with a goniometer. To evaluate muscle strength, include hip abduction, adduction, and extension; knee extension (quadriceps) and flexion (hamstring); and ankle plantar and dorsiflexion. See Table 14–4 for a summary of all aspects of the physical examination.

Mental/Affective Function Testing   As indicated, formal cognitive and affective function should be evaluated. Indicators of increased fall risk include a Mini-Mental State Examination score less than 24, a Geriatric Depression Scale with 10 or more depressed responses,[17] or one positive CAGE question (the mnemonic for alcoholism screening):

1. Have you ever felt you should Cut down on your drinking?

2. Have people Annoyed you by criticizing your drinking?

3. Have you ever felt Guilty about your drinking?

4. Do you have a drink first thing in the morning to steady your nerves (an Eye opener)?[78]

Laboratory/Diagnostic Testing   Any laboratory or diagnostic tests should be tailored to the suspected underlying causes of the fall, for example, possible anemia, electrolyte imbalance, dehydration, or arrhythmia. Screening for osteoporosis using bone mineral density techniques is important. Clearly, accurate information is needed to evaluate the risks and benefits of any decision to employ hormonal replacement therapy.[79] Table 14–5 provides a method for assessing such hip fracture risk in postmenopausal women.[31]

Assessment   The "Get Up and Go" test, coupled with a history of falls, may be the only information needed for the primary-care provider to diagnose high risk for falls. Beyond test of balance and gait, assessment should focus on any specific pathologies associated with high risk for falls (see

Table 14–5 Weighing the Risk Factors for Hip Fracture

Risk Factor	Risk Weight
History of maternal hip fracture	1
Previous hyperthyroidism	1
Current use of long-acting benzodiazepines	1
On feet < 4 hours per day	1
Inability to rise from chair	1
Resting pulse rate > 80 beats/minute	1
Height > 165 cm at age 25	1/6 cm[a]
Self-rated health	
Fair	1
Poor	2
Decrease in weight since age 25	
20–40%	1
41–60%	2
Decreased calcaneal bone density[b]	1

[a] For every 6 cm beyond this height, risk weight increases by 1.

[b] For every 0.10 g/cm² (1 SD) below the mean of 0.41 g/cm² for calcaneal bone density measures, risk weight increases by 1. Bone density measures taken at other sites, such as the trochanter or femur, may be used as a proxy by applying 1 risk weight for each SD below the mean.

Adapted from: Col NF, Eckman MH, Karas RH, et al. Patient-specific decisions about hormone replacement therapy in postmenopausal women. *JAMA.* 1997;277:1140–1147.

Table 14–1: Intrinsic Factors). The next step is to implement individualized interventions for specific risk factors.

 Prevention

Based on the assessment, interventions should be tailored to the specific intrinsic and extrinsic risk factors. Much effort is directed toward reducing all falls, despite the fact that the majority of falls do not result in injury. It is suggested that fall-related serious injury, not falls per se, is the significant outcome measure and, thus, preventive actions should focus on risk factors for injurious falls only.[57,80,81,82] A prudent course, however,

would be to address risk factors for all falls. Risk for falls and injuries is often due to several factors and the best intervention strategy is usually multifactorial.[3,4]

Addressing Intrinsic Factors

The value of interventions aimed at intrinsic factors is not always immediately evident. A study of community-living adults over 70[4] showed only a modest reduction in falls when medication, behavioral instructions, and exercise were addressed. Although the one-year cost of intervention per participant was $925, total health-care cost per capita was $2,000 less than the controls.[83]

Physiologic

Underlying Medical Illness Specific medical conditions contributing to risk for falls/injury should be addressed or referred for further evaluation and treatment. For example, medications implicated in postural hypotension (drop in systolic blood pressure [SBP] greater than 20 mm Hg or a standing SBP less than 90 mm Hg) can be decreased or changed. Older adults can be taught to rise slowly, sitting on the edge of the bed before getting up. Hand clenching and ankle flexion can also improve blood return and reduce venous pooling. Recommendations for underlying medical illnesses are in Tables 14–1 and 14–3.

Pharmacologic Modifying drug use may decrease fall risk by over 40%;[2] in particular, reducing number of medications, assessing the risk and benefit of each medication, and using those medications with the shortest half life, least centrally acting or least associated with hypotension, and at the lowest effective dose.[84] Medication review includes a check for appropriateness, usage, and compliance. Those on sedatives and hypnotics should be provided information regarding the negative side effects associated with both long- and short-term usage. Sleep problems should be addressed with non-pharmacological interventions.[85]

Exercise   Any attempt to reduce falls must address gait and balance, the most important factors involved in fall risk. Repeatedly, exercise has been shown to reduce falls and the risk factors associated with falls. A meta-analysis of seven controlled clinical trials, the Frailty and Injuries: Cooperative Studies of Intervention Techniques (FICSIT), concluded that exercise reduced fall risk.[86]

Many studies confirm the value of exercise, including programs of moderate intensity that focus on the lower extremities;[87] strength and balance retraining exercises;[88] weight training;[89] and progressive resistive exercise led by a physical therapist using elastic bands.[90] These exercise programs target persons with specific problems (e.g., post hip fracture) and have demonstrated varying outcomes (e.g., reduced falls or improved gait, balance, and mobility). Any exercise program needs to be based on an appropriate assessment and exercise prescription.

Analysis of the FICSIT interventions suggest that balance training delays the onset of first falls.[86] Balance training, however, mostly conducted by physical therapists, is involved and time consuming. Alternatively, Tai Chi improves balance and delays onset of a first fall.[91]

Anything that keeps elders active may improve mobility and balance, thereby preventing immobility-induced fall risk. Examples include dancing, sports, low-impact aerobics, walking with modest uphill and downhill grades, stationary bike, treadmill, and water aerobics. For those with specific mobility deficits, interventions are focused on improving safe functioning. Attention is given to transfers, correct use of assistive devices, wheelchair safety, and mobility in bed.

Psychological   Similar to underlying medical illnesses, mental health problems such as depression and anxiety should be treated or referred to a specialist (geropsychiatric advanced practice nurse or geropsychiatrist). Poor judgment and/or unsafe behaviors associated with dementia or stroke are often amenable to environmental interventions described in the next section.[92]

Addressing Extrinsic Factors

Most falls are related to extrinsic factors.[8] Although environmental modifications aimed at safety are required by government mandate and other regulatory or accrediting bodies, increased fall risk among institutionalized and hospitalized older adults is often associated with high beds and inappropriate seating.[92,93] Since many intrinsic factors are not reversible, fall prevention efforts aimed at

Table 14–6   Home Safety Checklist

Eliminate Dangers in the Home
Clear walkways
Provide adequate lighting, easy to turn on or automatic
Light switches within reach and at both ends of hall or stair
Hand rails
Step contrast
Knobs on first and last steps
Outside stairs with nonslip surfaces (plastic treads or textured paint)
Cords stapled out of way
Eliminate throw rugs (or use rubber backing)
No high waxing
Nonskid appliques in tub or shower
Hand rails at tub and toilet securely fastened to studs, not drywall or plaster
Appropriate footwear

Avoid Unsafe Behavior
Climbing on stools or ladders
Walking on wet wooden decks and steps
Walking on snow or ice
Working overhead

Practice Safe Behaviors
Develop an alert plan should a fall occur
Learn how to fall
Rise slowly from lying and sitting positions
Sit correctly on toilet, i.e., lower oneself onto the toilet after legs are against the seat; place hands on rails and then sit down slowly
Avoid excessive straining when defecating or urinating
Do one thing at a time

environmental contributors among community-residing, institutionalized, and hospitalized older adults are critical.

At Home   For those living independently, a home safety checklist, described in Table 14–6, is helpful. Encourage the conduct of periodic self-assessments by patient or caregiver since behaviors and environment can change over time.[62]

Interventions aimed at extrinsic risk factors produce positive results. Following free home inspection and modification for 4,000 Australian elders, the total number of falls decreased by 63%. Trained inspectors offered free home safety audits, night lights, and information pamphlets. Modifications cost participants no more than $30 and included floor treatments and grab rails. Recruitment was done at gatherings frequently attended by older people.[94]

Environmental Interventions for Fall Prevention

Reducing extrinsic risk factors requires careful analysis of common aspects of the environment, such as chairs and beds. Many products promote safe transfer, comfortable seating, and prevent falls and fall-related injuries.[92,95,96] Table 14–7 provides a summary of environmental interventions.

Table 14–7   Environmental Interventions for Fall Prevention

Prevent Falls from Bed

A. Prevent "rolling-out"/discourage transferring without assistance
   1. Define bed perimeters
      a. Mattresses with "bumpers" (elevated edges)
      b. Rolled blankets under mattress edge
      c. "Swimming noodles" (hard, round, foam cylinder, 6' × 6") under fitted sheet at mattress edge
      d. Full-length "body" pillows, long immobilization bags, or other long cushions
      e. ½- or ¼-length padded siderail

2. Promote comfort
   a. Mattress firmness individualized according to needs (firm, pressure-relieving, etc.)
   b. Pillows/cushions and leg separator pads, and/or molded foam cushions to facilitate positioning
   c. Full-length "body" pillows, long immobilization bags, or other long cushions
   d. Periodic assistance with position changes
   e. Use of urinal/bedpan
   f. Easy to use, bulb call bell
   g. Individualized elimination rounds
   h. Appropriate, scheduled pain management
   i. Address sleep disorder, consider nonpharmacologic intervention

B. Encourage Safe Transfers
   1. Transfer enablers: trapeze, uni/bilateral bed handle, bed grab bar, transfer pole with handrail that rotates 360 degrees, quarter or half side rail (with narrow vertical bars to prevent head/limb entrapment)
   2. Bed height adjusted (manual, electric, hydraulic) to patient/resident's lower leg length
   3. Bedside commode (without wheels) placed on person's stronger side, and specific to height
   4. Use of assistive ambulatory devices, e.g., walker, cane
   5. Easily accessible call bell or bulb (pressure sensitive)
   6. Cordless press-on light at bedside, with pull cord for light within reach when in bed, or use motion sensor light
   7. Nonskid mat

C. Reduce injury risk
   1. Use very low platform or very low adjustable height bed (electric/hydraulic)
   2. Use mat (4' × 6–8') with nonslip surface, eggcrate mattress, nonskid, rubber-backed rugs at bedside
   3. Hip pads or padded pants
   4. Sheepskin siderail pad, bumper, bumper with see-through window, or bumper wedge on siderail
   5. Bed alarms

(continues)

Table 14–7   Environmental Interventions for Fall Prevention   *(continued)*

Prevent Falls from Chair

A. Provide individualized seating
1. Hemi-height wheelchair individually adjusted to leg length for wheelchair mobility
2. "Size" chair to individual, e.g., pediatric vs. extra large
3. Leg/foot pedal extensions and/or leg panels
4. Accommodate postural alignment needs: wedge cushion, lateral supports, arm trough, half tray, head extension

B. Promote comfort
1. Firm support cushion inserts for wheelchairs or other chairs without adequate support
2. Pressure-relieving seat cushions
3. Well-padded recliners, including cushions to fit chair to individual
4. Frequent change of position and accommodation of needs for elimination

C. Reduce injury risk
1. Wheelchair anti-tippers
2. Chair alarms

Prevent Falls While Walking

A. Encourage safe walking
1. Use night lights
2. Remove clutter from pathways
3. Provide adequate signage for toilets

B. Reduce risk of injury
1. Wear padded clothing/accessories, e.g., "bike" pants, hip pads, helmets
2. Padded/carpeted floor surfaces
3. Appropriate prescription and use of assistive devices in good working order
4. Use of hormonal replacement therapy, calcium/vitamin D supplementation, biphosphonates, or aminobiphosphonates plus calcium

Adapted from: Capezuti E, Talerico KA, Strumpf N, Evans L. Individualized assessment and intervention in bilateral siderail use. *Geriatr Nurs.* 1998;19(6):322–330.

Jones D, Rader J. *Individualized Wheelchair Seating for Older Adults: An Important Link to Restraint-Free Care.* Mt. Angel, Ore: Benedictine Institute for Long Term Care; 1998.

Strumpf NE, Robinson JP, Wagner JS, Evans LK. *Restraint-Free Care.* New York: Springer Publishing Company; 1998.

Preventing Falls From Bed   For the immobile, first address comfort needs with frequent changes in position (at least every two hours). Comfort needs include appropriate pain management, as well as individualized attention to elimination.[97,98] Bed bumpers on mattress edges, full-body pillows, or rolled blankets under mattress edges remind residents of the bed boundaries, and unlike metal side rails, such devices do not cause skin trauma.[99]

Many falls occur with attempts to transfer to and from bed, chair, or toilet. The height of the bed is crucial to safe standing. For shorter persons (less than five feet), the bed may be too high for safe transfer; thus, low beds that can be manually or electrically adjusted to promote transfer are recommended.[93,100] A nonskid mat placed at the side of the bed and toilet can reduce the likelihood of slipping on urine or water.[92] Reducing falls in the bathroom depends on securely fastened grab bars, as well as a toilet seat individually adjusted for height. Low-voltage "night" lights, lights that are easy to turn on, or lights that automatically illuminate with motion, can help prevent nighttime falls.

In addition to bed height, assistive devices (canes, walkers) should be placed within easy reach of the bed. A trapeze may be helpful to assist in transferring out of bed; however, a trapeze requires full shoulder mobility and adequate upper extremity strength. Transfer "enablers," including transfer poles, bars, or raised quarter or half-length side rails directly attached to or adjacent to the top of the bed, promote safe standing.[95,96] These may also serve as assistive bed-mobility devices. Reducing the distance to the bathroom (placement of a bedside commode) or reducing out-of-bed trips to the bathroom (urinal and bedpan use) are also helpful. Those with hand weakness who require human assistance to use a bedpan, commode, or bathroom may benefit from call bells sensitive to very light pressure or open monitors to the nursing station.

For persons with a history of climbing around or over side rails, especially those at high risk of injury (e.g., history of hip fracture or those with osteoporosis), reducing injury risk with a very low bed height is essential. Placing the mattress on the floor or use of low-height platform beds can be problematic since it may make it difficult for caregivers to provide assistance. Instead, beds that can be manually, electrically, or hydraulically adjusted down to a few inches off the floor and to 26 inches above the floor are recommended.[92]

Falling onto a hard surface increases the risk of serious injury;[61] thus, for those at high-risk for injury, a bedside cushion, such as an exercise mat or an "eggcrate" foam mattress, is useful. Padded pants or hip cushions may also reduce injury.[101-105]

Preventing Falls From Chairs   The primary goal of any chair is to provide comfortable, individualized seating. The most obvious way to decrease fall risk from a wheelchair is to spend as little time there as possible. Wheelchairs are designed for transport, not continuous seating; sling seats do not provide adequate support for long periods of sitting. Inserts are available to increase the support of the chair, and pressure-relieving seat cushions are often necessary if more than a couple of hours per day are spent in a chair. Many products are available to adapt the chair to individual seating needs.[95,96] For example, "pediatric" wheelchairs are available for very small people and extra-wide chairs for the obese. If weak upper extremities prevent wheelchair mobility, "walking" in the wheelchair can be facilitated with a "hemi-height" wheelchair adjusted to the lower leg length. Propelling the wheelchair forward with the legs is a safe alternative to walking for some people and promotes muscle strengthening of the lower extremities.[106] Leg and foot-pedal extensions as well as leg panels can be individually fitted on the wheelchair to promote leg comfort for those who cannot push the chair with their legs. Anti-tippers can prevent unwanted tipping of the chair forward or backward.

Other interventions to prevent falls from a chair or wheelchair include individualized seating to accommodate postural variation. For those unable to hold themselves upright, strategies involve propping the body in a variety of ways. A wedge can be inserted under the legs, tilting the person backward slightly and preventing forward leaning. A wedge seat may also prevent sliding from the chair. Similarly, leaning to the side is corrected with lateral supports or a solid seat. Stroke victims with hemiplegia with side arm weakness may develop shoulder subluxation when arms are allowed to dangle over the side of the chair. Such weakness may also contribute to poor balance when walking resumes. An arm trough or half tray prevents this problem. A head extension can be added or a reclining chair used for those unable to keep head erect. Rocking and glider chairs may be useful to dissipate the energy of pacers and those in constant motion as seen in those with dementia.

While alarms can help to monitor activities, caregivers must be close by and able to respond (often in less than 30 seconds) to prevent a fall. Chair alarms can be sensitive to changes in position or an alarm unit can be attached to the chair with a clip attached to personal clothing. Alarms in hospitals and nursing homes can decrease the incidence of falls.[24]

No matter how comfortable the chair, changing position, range of motion exercise, and, if possible, standing or walking at least twice a day are essential.

Fall Prevention Programs in Nursing Homes
Institutional fall prevention programs include nursing protocols and practitioner interventions. High-risk fallers are sometimes identified with flagged charts, markers on rooms or beds, or armbands. The aim is to make all staff aware of fall risk. Nursing protocols deal mostly with reducing extrinsic factors and interventions to help those with functional deficits. Standing orders or policies may address needs for use of the bathroom, commode, bedpan, or urinal, or other specific interventions must be based on individual needs.

Up until the late 1980s, physical restraints represented the "one-size-fits-all" approach to fall prevention in American nursing homes. The use of a restraint often replaced the assessment process of unraveling the complex multifactorial etiology of individual fall risk. Similarly, bilateral, full-length side rails were viewed as the simple solution to preventing falls from bed.[92,107] The Nursing Home Reform Act (Omnibus Budget Reconciliation Act [OBRA], 1987) was passed in 1987 as a mechanism to reduce, if not eliminate, the use of physical restraint in nursing homes. In

1997, the Health Care Financing Administration (HCFA) issued guidelines to nursing homes directing them that side rails were also restraints and care plans needed to address individual safety needs.[108] Nursing home staff can no longer rely on the traditional approach of "one intervention fits all fall prevention needs."

A major impetus for examining the effect of restraints/side rails is the growing number of associated injuries and deaths. Nursing home residents are not only subject to fall-related injuries, but also to injuries and fatalities that occur while attempting to remove restraints or to ambulate while restrained. The most common mechanism of restraint-related death is by asphyxiation, resulting from gravitational chest compression when suspended by a vest restraint from a bed or chair.[109,110,111] Similarly, incidents of head and body entrapment within side rails have resulted in serious injuries and death.[112,113]

Neither physical restraints nor side rails have ever been shown to decrease fall or injury risk. In one nursing home study, a significant association was demonstrated between restraint use and fall-related serious injury after controlling for other risk factors.[36] Another study examining restraint use in confused ambulatory nursing home residents found an increased risk of falling among restrained residents compared to nonrestrained residents.[107] Since implementation of the Nursing Home Reform Act, physical restraint use has been reduced from 41% in 1989 to 15.6% in January 1998.[114,115] Several studies examining the effect of restraint reduction have demonstrated no increase in falls, injurious falls, or both.[116–122] Moreover, there is ample evidence that fall and fall-related injury rates can be reduced without the use of restraints.[3]

One novel approach used in a dementia unit to reduce fall injury was insertion of plastic hip protectors inside pants resembling "bicycle shorts." These protectors significantly reduced hip fractures.[123] Other designs to diminish impact on the greater trochanter are under development.[124]

An elimination protocol for confused persons with mobility problems and risk of falling reduced falls during those shifts when there was compliance with the assessment and elimination protocol.[125] A randomized trial of a consultation service to reduce falls conducted in 14 Tennessee nursing homes[3] also demonstrated the effectiveness of individualized interventions to reduce fall risk.

Acute Management of Falls

Encountering the Person Who Has Fallen

When someone falls, the practitioner should be aware of the possible common injuries and immediately perform an assessment to rule out those injuries. Musculoskeletal injuries predominate in falls, with hip fractures being the most common.[126] Head and neck injuries are next with delayed subdural hematoma three times more likely to develop in the elderly.[127] Dislocation injuries to the cervical spine related to hyperflexion, as well as shoulder and hip dislocations, are also common following falls in the elderly.[128]

Initial Evaluation   Priorities are an initial assessment to determine any needs for basic life support for airway, breathing, and circulation, followed by an evaluation of disability and identification of injuries. Caution should be exercised in moving the elderly fall victim until a complete and thorough examination has been performed to rule out cervical or thoracic spine injury.

Once stability is established, a quick but thorough physical examination is performed, along with a past and present medical history, medication history, time of last meal, and presence of pain. Ask what happened. Was there a preceding event such as syncope, palpitations, or chest pain? Review the record or ask to determine a significant medical or psychiatric history or problem that could have caused the fall.

Physical Examination   The physical examination should be a concise head-to-toe examination. Begin by forming a first impression of what may have happened. This is an almost instant process that involves surveying the area of the fall and determining the presence of obstacles or hazards, possible mechanisms of injury, and whether additional help is necessary.[129]

Table 14–8   Presentation of Subdural Hematomas

Acute	Chronic
Signs/symptoms in first 24 hours	Signs/symptoms days to weeks later
Early loss of consciousness	Persistent or recurring headache
Changes in level of consciousness	Blurred vision, double vision
Localized motor/sensory deficits	Somnolence
Nausea/vomiting	Confusion or disorientation
Cushing's response:	Slurring or other speech impediment
Increased systolic blood pressure	Changes in personality
Increased respiratory rate	Hemiparesis or hemiparalysis
Decreased pulse rate	Hemianesthesia

Adapted from: Abrahms WB, Beers MH, Berkow R, eds. *Merck Manual of Geriatrics.* Rahway, NJ: Merck & Company; 1995.
McSwain NE, ed. *Pre-Hospital Trauma Life Support.* Akron, Oh: Emergency Training; 1990.

Assess level of consciousness and determine vital signs. Begin pulse oximetry (POX) monitoring if possible and appropriate. If there is history of diabetes or hypoglycemia, check blood glucose levels. Vital signs should be monitored on a continuous basis as the elderly often have small physical reserves and are less able to tolerate the effects of shock related to an injury sustained in a fall.[130] Initial blood pressure monitoring can be established by palpating the radial, femoral, or carotid arteries. A palpable radial pulse indicates an SBP of 80 mm Hg or greater; a palpable femoral pulse indicates an SBP of at least 70 mm Hg, and a palpable carotid pulse indicates an SBP of at least 60 mm Hg.[131] In the nursing home, begin monitoring vital signs at least every 15 minutes for the first hour, then every 30 minutes for the next hour, followed by every hour for the next two hours.

Perform a systematic musculoskeletal examination. The examiner should slide hands along the entire body with a firm but gentle pressure. Feel for deformities or bleeding, and watch the face for expressions of pain that may be elicited during the exam. Such deformities or grimaces aid in identifying any sites of injury and help focus the exam.

Inspect the head, ears, eyes, nose, and throat, looking for lacerations, bruising, bleeding, or discharge from the face, scalp, ears, nose, or mouth. Check for tracheal deviation, indicative of a pneumothorax, by pressing an index finger into the side of the sternal notch. A distinctive crackling sound of air in the soft tissues of the neck indicates subcutaneous emphysema, possibly from a ruptured larynx or trachea.

Point tenderness of the cervical/thoracic vertebrae, muscle spasm, and midline deformities suggest a spinal injury. The lack of point tenderness does not rule out the possibility of a spinal injury. Therefore, if there is any suspicion of spinal or related injuries, stabilize the head.

Because subdural hematomas are more likely to occur in the elderly, changes in neurological function may occur (Table 14–8). These changes may be abrupt or gradual over days to weeks. For this reason, any fall in which a head injury is suspected should also raise the suspicion for a possible closed head injury[132] or cervical spine injury.[133]

Continue by examining the chest and abdomen, assessing for symmetrical movement and point tenderness. Observe for rapid, shallow breaths and the use of accessory muscles indicative of a rib fracture or respiratory distress. Auscultate anteriorly and posteriorly to evaluate lung sounds (Table 14–9).

POX measurements of 93% or less may indicate the need for adjunctive oxygenation. Compression over the sternum may elicit pain over a possible fracture site, which may also be helpful in differentiating chest pain related to a rib fracture from other possible causes of chest pain as outlined in Table 14–10.

Table 14–9   Evaluation of Lung Sounds

Respirations	Breath Sounds	Adventitious Sounds	Possible Diagnosis
Gasping and labored	Loud, difficult to hear, or normal	Wheezes or crackles	Asthma, heart failure, airway obstruction
Rapid and shallow	High pitched and loud	Wheezes or absent	Shock, cardiac problems
Difficulty breathing when supine	Normal	Inspiratory crackles, wheezes	Heart failure, lung infection, asthma
Stertorous (snoring)	Harsh and loud	Absent	Stroke, skull fracture, drug or alcohol intoxication
Slowed breathing	Shallow, difficult to hear due to poor inspiratory effort	Absent	Stroke, head injury, chest injury
Shallow and painful	Decreased or absent	Possible pleural rub, gurgling	Pleural effusion, pulmonary edema

Adapted from: Abrahms WB, Beers MH, Berkow R, eds. *Merck Manual of Geriatrics*. Rahway, NJ: Merck & Company; 1995. Bickley LS. *Bates' Guide to Physical Examination and History Taking*. 7th ed. Philadelphia: Lippincott; 1999.

Palpate the abdomen. An abdomen that is firm, distended, or tender to palpation should alert the practitioner to possible internal bleeding, peritonitis, or bowel obstruction. Voluntary or involuntary guarding, rigidity, and rebound tenderness are a strong indicator of inflammation or hemorrhage; palpation should be avoided as it can aggravate hemorrhage or other injuries. Auscultation of the abdomen may reveal distant or absent bowel sounds, which may aid in the diagnosis of an abdominal injury, but is usually not helpful in determining injury alone.

Pelvis and proximal femur fractures are common injuries resulting from falls in the elderly. Palpate the pelvis by applying pressure to the iliac crests bilaterally and manipulating the hips with a gentle anterior/posterior motion. Those with pelvic injuries, especially to the ramus, often complain of an urgent need to urinate.[131] Note any pain or crepitus. Hip fractures involve the proximal head of the femur.

The involved extremity is almost always shorter than the uninvolved extremity and externally rotated. A dislocated hip is usually internally rotated and slightly flexed.[134]

Lower-extremity fractures include the distal tibia and proximal fibula. This injury is commonly the result of an eversion of the ankle and can also result in the classic Maisonneuve fracture where the tibial injury is usually an avulsion fracture of the medial malleolus.[135]

Fracture of the proximal humerus is often the result of a fall onto the acromioclavicular joint while an individual is carrying something. The fall is absorbed on the deltoid region of the humerus resulting in a fracture. A dislocation of the involved shoulder often accompanies this fracture with pain and tenderness as the presentation. A large bruise may be evident in the area of the fracture, even early in the injury, and may spread into the pectoral region.

Table 14–10   Evaluation of Chest Pain

Differential Diagnosis	Onset	Location	Signs and Symptoms	ECG Findings
Myocardial infarction Unstable angina	Minutes to hours	Substernal, may radiate to neck, jaw, and left arm	SOB, anxiety nausea/vomiting, dizziness, lightheadedness	ST elevations
Aortic dissection	Sudden	Anterior chest, may radiate to back	Decreased femoral pulses, pulsus para-doxus, decreased BP in arm	ST elevation ST depression Nonspecific
Pneumothorax	Sudden	Unilateral chest	Pleuritic pain, dyspnea, decreased breath sounds, tracheal deviation	R wave progressions in V1–V6 or QRS axis shift
Pulmonary embolism	Sudden	Substernal	Pleuritic pain that worsens with breathing, tachypnea, dyspnea, hemoptysis, rales	Inferior ST elevation or V1–V3 ST shifts
Pericarditis or pericardial tamponade	Hours to days	Retrosternal to left precordial	Friction rub, pulsus paradoxus with pericardial tamponade	ST elevation

Adapted from: Ewald GA, McKenzie CR, eds. *Manual of Medical Therapeutics*. Boston: Little, Brown; 1995.

The righting reflex is an attempt to break a fall by extending the arm and dorsiflexing the hand.[132] This may result in either a proximal humerus fracture, or a Colles' fracture, of the distal radius and ulna. The Colles' fracture often produces an obvious deformity called the dinner fork deformity, which presents with a dorsal depression and volar wrist fullness.

Treatment Interventions   Once the initial head-to-toe exam has been completed, treatment of injuries begins. Cervical stabilization is necessary for any suspected head injury as a result of a fall. Unresponsiveness almost always indicates cervical spine injury, requiring full immobilization with cervical spine stabilization. Other indications for cervical spine immobilization are listed in Table 14–11.

Alignment and immobilization of angulated limbs in a position of comfort is necessary to reduce pain and decrease the risk of additional damage to the injury site. Splint all fractures so that the joints above and below the injury site are immobilized. Upper-extremity fractures should be "sling and swathed" to provide support. Place the injured extremity in a sling and then secure the sling to the chest wall using a binder. Fractures of the hip and pelvis require long-board immobilization to provide complete stabilization. In the nursing home, it is best to allow injured residents to remain in a supine position on the floor until emergency care arrives. Lower-extremity fractures should be splinted so as to immobilize both the knee and ankle joints, as well as the fracture sight. Monitor the extremity distal to the fracture for motor and sensory function and for

Table 14–11   Certain Indications
for Cervical Spine Immobilization

Facial lacerations or deformities

Ecchymosis

Cervical/thoracic spine tenderness

Headache

Nausea/vomiting

Dizziness/lightheadedness

Changes in level of consciousness

Changes in motor or sensory function

Increases in systolic blood pressure with a concurrent
decrease in respiration

Changes in breathing patterns

Adapted from: Ewald G, McKenzie C, eds. *Manual of Medical
Therapeutics*. Boston: Little, Brown; 1995.

McSwain NE, ed. *Pre-Hospital Trauma Life Support*.
Akron, Oh: Emergency Training; 1990.

Bowman W. *Outdoor Emergency Care*. Lakewood, Co:
National Ski Patrol; 1993.

Singletary N. Keep ahead of head injuries. *Ski Patrol Mag*.
1998;14(4):2–4.

circulation. Decreased or absent neurologic function
or circulation indicates nerve or vessel involvement
and should be treated as a true emergency.

With head fractures or injuries, and difficulty
breathing or complaints of chest pain, provide oxygen with a non-rebreather mask at 15 liters of flow.
An electrocardiogram should be performed as soon
as possible to rule out acute cardiac changes. Vital
signs and POX monitoring should be ongoing.

Monitor the patient/resident carefully for signs
of shock. Hypovolemia, from bleeding into the
injury site, is a common occurrence with injury to
the abdomen, hip fractures, and injuries to the
aorta. Indications of shock are a decrease in blood
pressure and an increase in both heart rate and respiration. The priority is aggressive control of hemorrhage, followed by treatment for shock. In the
nursing home, this may be limited to elevating legs
and feet to improve circulation. Volume expanders
such as 0.9% sodium chloride or Ringer's lactate
may also be infused if protocols permit.

Extrication and Transport   Fall-related injuries
require timely and appropriate treatment. Whether
in the nursing home or elsewhere, decisions regarding preparation and transport are based on
information gathered during the assessment. Specialized diagnostics simply may not be available.
In a nonacute-care facility, the protocol for dealing with injury in most cases likely entails calling
911, fire/rescue, or a contracted ambulance company for transfer to the nearest emergency department (ED).

Prior to extrication following a serious fall-
related injury, immobilization devices such as cervical collars, backboards, and splints may be needed.
In the event of suspected cervical injury, do not
apply these devices unless specifically trained to do
so. Simply maintain head stabilization in an anatomically correct position by applying equal pressure
with both hands to the mandible bilaterally. Position
yourself above the patient/resident with both hands
in an inferior and dorsal position to the ears. Support the occipital region of the head with the
third and fourth fingers of each hand. Once this
stabilization is initiated, it should be maintained
until a cervical collar is in place and the head is
fully immobilized.

Once a decision for transport to the ED has
been made, provide complete documentation to
the transport team and telephone a report to the
triage nurse at the ED. Table 14–12 provides a list
of documentation that may be included. This provides invaluable baseline information for the ED
staff and aids in assessing not only the injury, but
also its underlying etiology.

Evaluation of the Fallen Elder in the ED   The role
of the nurse practitioner in the ED is twofold:

1. to identify and treat injuries related to a fall

2. to identify and treat the problems contributing
   to a fall[41,136]

Treatment of elderly patients who present in the ED,
with their multiple illnesses, atypical presentations,
nonspecific complaints, and varying pathologies is
often difficult and challenging. The patient needs to
be treated as an ill elderly patient who has fallen,
rather than as an elderly fall patient.

Table 14–12 Transport Documentation

Patient/resident's face sheet
Insurance information
Allergies
Chief complaint
Mechanism of injury
PMH/PSH
Medication sheets
Recent ECG
Recent physical exam
Ambulation history including assistive devices
Recent MMSE scores
Admitting diagnosis
Recent progress notes
Recent labs and diagnostics
Prosthetics, eyeglasses, hearing aids, and dentures

Conclusion

Falls are often dismissed as an inevitable result of aging. Continued education of the public and health-care personnel is needed about the cost of falls to individuals and society, the benefits of interventions to reduce the frequency and severity of falls, the unnecessary use of restraints and side rails for safety, the importance of exercise and physical activity, and proper evaluation, treatment, and follow-up after a fall injury.

References

1. Mish FC, ed.: *Webster's Ninth New Collegiate Dictionary*. Springfield, MA: Merriam-Webster; 1989.
2. Rubenstein LZ, Robbins AS, Josephson KR, Schulman BL, Osterweil D. The value of assessing falls in an elderly population: a randomized clinical trial. *Ann Intern Med*. 1990;113(4):308–316.
3. Ray WA, Taylor JA, Meador KG, et al. A randomized trial of a consultation service to reduce falls in nursing homes. *JAMA*. 1997;278(7):557–562.
4. Tinetti M, Baker D, McAvay G, et al. A multifactorial intervention to reduce the risk of falling among elderly people living in the community. *N Engl J Med*. 1994; 331:821–827.
5. Mosenthal AC, Livingston DH, Elcavage J, Merritt S, Stucker S. Falls: epidemiology and strategies for prevention. *J Trauma: Inj Infect Crit Care*. 1995; 38:753–756.
6. Gallagher E, Scott V. The STEPS project: participatory action research to reduce falls in public places among seniors and persons with disabilities. *Can J Public Health*. 1997;88(2):129–133.
7. Berg W, Alessio H, Mills E, Tong C. Circumstances and consequences of falls in independent community–dwelling older adults. *Age Ageing*. 1997;26(4):261–268.
8. Norton R, Campbell AJ, Lee-Joe T, Robinson E, Butler M. Circumstances of falls resulting in hip fractures among older people. *J Am Geriatr Soc*. 1997; 45:1108–1112.
9. Grisso JA, Schwarz DG, Wolfson V, Polansky M, LaPann K. The impact of falls on an inner city elderly African-American population. *J Am Geriatr Soc*. 1992;40:673–678.
10. Tinetti ME, Williams CS. Falls, injuries due to falls, and the risk of admission to a nursing home. *N Engl J Med*. 1997;337(18):1279–1284.
11. Kiel DP, O'Sullivan P, Teno JM, Mor V. Health care utilization and functional status in the aged following a fall. *Med Care*. 1991;29:221–228.
12. Wolinski DF, Johnson RJ, Fitzgerald JF. Falling, health status, and the use of health services by older adults: a prospective study. *Med Care*. 1992;30:587–597.
13. Sattin RW, Lambert-Huber DA, DeVito CA, et al. The incidence of fall injury events among the elderly in a defined population. *Am J Epidemiol*. 1990;131(6): 1028-1037.
14. Englander F, Hodson T, Terregrossa R. Economic dimensions of slip and fall injuries. *J Forensic Sci*. 1996;41(5):733–746.
15. Tinetti ME, Speechley M. Prevention of falls among the elderly. *N Engl J Med*. 1989;320(16):1055–1059.
16. Rawsky E. State of the science: review of the literature on falls among the elderly. *Image J Nurs Scholar*. 1998;30(1):47–52.
17. Graafmans W, Ooms M, Hofstee H, et al. Falls in the elderly: a prospective study of risk factors and risk profiles. *Am J Epidemiol*. 1996;143(11):1129–1136.
18. Lord SR, Ward JA, Williams P, Ansrey KJ. Physiological factors associated with falls in older community dwelling women. *J Am Geriatr Soc*. 1994;42:1110–1117.
19. Studenski S, Duncan PW, Chandler J, et al. Predicting falls: the role of mobility and nonphysical factors. *J Am Geriatr Soc*. 1994;42(3):297–302.
20. Topper AK, Maki BE, Holliday PJ. Are activity-based assessments of balance and gait in the elderly predictive of risk of fallings and/or type of fall? *J Am Geriatr Soc*. 1993;41(5):479–487.
21. Owen DH. Maintaining posture and avoiding tripping: optical information for detecting and controlling orientation and locomotion. *Clin Geriatr Med*. 1985; 1(3):581–599.

22. Sabin TD. Biologic aspects of falls and mobility limitations in the elderly. *J Am Geriatr Soc*. 1982; 30(1):51–58.

23. Wolfson LI, Whipple R, Amerman P, Kaplan J, Kleinberg A. Gait and balance in the elderly: two functional capacities that link sensory and motor ability to falls. *Clin Geriatr Med*. 1985;1(3):649–660.

24. Tideiksaar R. *Falling in Old Age: Prevention and Management*. 2nd ed. New York: Springer; 1996.

25. Demerest G, Osler T, Clevenger F. Injuries in the elderly: evaluation and initial response. *Geriatrics*. 1992;45:36–42.

26. Oliver D, Britton M, Seed P, Martin FC, Hopper AH. Development and evaluation of evidence based risk assessment tool (STRATIFY) to predict which elderly inpatients will fall: case-control and cohort studies. *BMJ*. 1997;315(7115):1049–1053.

27. Rudberg MA, Furner SE, Dunn JE, Cassel CK. The relationship of visual and hearing impairments to disability: an analysis using the Longitudinal Study of Aging. *J Gerontol Med Sci*. 1993;48(6):M261–M265.

28. Tinetti ME, Inouye SK, Gill TM, Doucette JT. Shared risk factors for falls, incontinence, and functional dependence: unifying the approach to geriatric syndromes. *JAMA*. 1995;273(17):1348–1353.

29. Hurley M, Rees J, Newham D. Quadriceps function, proprioceptive acuity and functional performance in healthy young, middle-aged and elderly subjects. *Age Ageing*. 1998;27(1):55–62.

30. Buchner DM, Larson EB. Falls and fractures in patients with Alzheimer-type dementia. *JAMA*. 1987;257:14.

31. Col NF, Eckman MH, Karas RH, et al. Patient-specific decisions about hormone replacement therapy in postmenopausal women. *JAMA*. 1997;277:1140–1147.

32. Grisso JA, Kelsey JL, Strom BL, et al. Risk factors for falls as a cause of hip fracture in women. *N Engl J Med*. 1991;324:1326–1331.

33. Tinetti ME, Doucette J, Claus E, Marottoli R. Risk factors for serious injury during falls by older persons in the community. *J Am Geriatr Soc*. 1995;43(11):1214–1221.

34. Grisso JA, Capezuti E, Schwartz A. Falls as risk factors for fractures. In: Arcus R, Feldman D, Kelsey J, eds. *Osteoporosis*. San Diego: Academic Press; 1996:599–611.

35. Nevitt MC, Cummings SR, Hudes ES. Risk factors for injurious falls: a prospective study. *J Gerontol*. 1991;46(5):M164–M170.

36. Tinetti ME, Liu WL, Ginter SF. Mechanical restraint use and fall-related injuries among residents of skilled nursing facilities. *Ann Intern Med*. 1992;116(5):369–374.

37. Capezuti E, Talerico KA. Review article: physical restraint removal and falls and injuries. *Res Pract Alzheimer's Dis*. 1999;2:338–355.

38. Lundin-Olsson L, Nyberg L, Gustafson Y. Attention, frailty and falls: the effect of a manual task on basic mobility. *J Am Geriatr Soc*. 1998;46:758–761.

39. Jech A. Preventing falls in the elderly. *Geriatr Nurs*. 1992; Jan:43–44.

40. Leipzig RM, Cumming RG, Tinetti ME. Drugs and falls in older people: a systematic review and meta-analysis: II. cardiac and analgesic drugs. *J Amer Geriat Soc*. 1999;47:40–50.

41. Baraff LJ, Della Penna R, Williams N, Sanders A. Practice guideline for the ED management of falls in community-dwelling elderly persons. *Ann Emerg Med*. 1997;30(4):480–492.

42. Leipzig RM, Cumming RG, Tinetti ME. Drugs and falls in older people: a systematic review and meta-analysis: I. psychotropic drugs. *J Am Geriatr Soc*. 1999;47:30–39.

43. Ross J. Iatrogenesis in the elderly: contributors to falls. *J Gerontol Nurs*. 1991;17:19–23.

44. Vernon G. Medication iatrogenesis in the elderly: common yet preventable. *Nurse Pract*. 1994;19:27–28.

45. Grisso JA, Kelsey JL, Strom BL, et al. Risk factors for hip fracture in black women. *N Engl J Med*. 1994; 330(22):1555–1559.

46. Grisso JA, Chiu GY, Maislin G, Steinmann WC, Portale J. Risk factors for hip fractures in men: a preliminary study. *J Bone Mineral Res*. 1991;6(8):865–868.

47. Hanlon J, Cutson T, Ruby C. Drug-related falls in the older adult. *Top Geriatr Rehabil*. 1996;11(3):38–54.

48. Thapa PB, Brockman KG, Gideon P, Fought RL, Ray WA. Injurious falls in nonambulatory nursing home residents: a comparative study of circumstances, incidence, and risk factors. *J Am Geriatr Soc*. 1996;44(3):273–278.

49. Cumming R. Epidemiology of medication-related falls and fractures in the elderly. *Drugs Aging*. 1998; 12(1):43–53.

50. Thapa PB, Gideon P, Cost TW, Milam AB, Ray WA. Antidepressants and the risk of falls among nursing home residents. *N Engl J Med*. 1998;339:875–882.

51. Liu B, Anderson G, Mittmann N, et al. Use of selective serotonin-reuptake inhibitors of tricyclic antidepressants and risk of hip fractures in elderly people. *Lancet*. 1998;351:1303–1307.

52. Verlhac B, Wolmark Y, Forette B. Elderly patients, use of antidepressants, and hip fractures [letter]. *Lancet*. 1998;352:401.

53. Lapane KL, Gambassi G, Hume A, Sgadari A, Mor V. Which antidepressants increase the risk of femur fracture in long term care? Paper presented at: Annual Meeting of the American Geriatric Society and American Federation of Aging Research; May 9, 1998.

54. McCuster J, Cole M, Keller E, Ballavance F, Berard A. Effectiveness of treatments of depression in older ambulatory patients. *Arch Intern Med*. 1998; 158:705–712.

55. Mittmann N, Herrmann N, Einarsonn T, et al. The efficacy, safety, and tolerability of antidepressants in late life depression: a meta-analysis. *J Affective Disord*. 1997;46:191–217.

56. Van Dijk PT, Meulenberg OG, Van de Sande HJ, Habbema JD. Falls in dementia patients. *Gerontol.* 1993;33(2):200–204.

57. Gurwitz JH, Sanchez-Cross MT, Eckler MA, Matulis J. The epidemiology of adverse and unexpected events in the long-term care setting. *J Am Geriatr Soc.* 1994; 42(1):33–38.

58. Hornbrook MC, Stevens VJ, Wingfield DJ, et al. Preventing falls among community-dwelling older persons: results from a randomized trial. *Gerontol.* 1994;34(1):16–23.

59. Northridge ME, Nevitt MC, Kelsey JL, et al. Home hazards and falls in the elderly: the role of health and functional status. *Am J Public Health.* 1995;85: 509–515.

60. Brady R, Chester F, Pierce L, Salater S, Radziewicz R. Geriatric falls: prevention strategies for the staff. *J Gerontol Nurs.* 1993;19(9):26–32.

61. Nevitt MC, Cummings SR, Hudes ES. Type of fall and risk of hip and wrist fractures: the study of osteoporotic fractures. *J Am Geriatr Soc.* 1993;41(11):1226–1234.

62. Connell B, Wolf S. Environmental and behavioral circumstances associated with falls at home among healthy elderly individuals. *Arch Phys Med Rehabil.* 1997;78(2):179–186.

63. Smith RW, Nelson DR. Fractures and other injuries from falls after an ice storm. *Am J Emerg Med.* 1998; 16(1):52–55.

64. Cummings SR, Nevitt MC. A hypothesis: the causes of hip fractures. *J Gerontol.* 1989;44:M107–111.

65. Hayes WC, Myers ER, Morris JN, et al. Impact near the hip dominates fracture risk in elderly nursing home residents who fall. *Calcified Tissue Int.* 1993;52(3): 192–198.

66. Nevitt MC, Cummings SR. Type of fall and risk of hip and wrist fractures: the study of osteoporotic fractures. *J Am Geriatr Soc.* 1993;41(11):1226–1234.

67. Fleming B, Pendergast D. Physical condition, activity pattern, and environmental factors in falls in adult day care facility residents. *Arch Phys Med Rehabil.* 1993; 74:627–630.

68. Howland J, Lachman ME, Peterson EW, et al. Covariates of fear of falling and associated activity curtailment. *Gerontol.* 1998;38:549–555.

69. Miceli DLG, Waxman H, Cavalieri T, Lage S. Prodromal falls among older nursing home residents. *Appl Nurs Res.* 1994;7(1):18–26.

70. Rubenstein L, Josephson K, Robbins A. Falls in the nursing home. *Ann Intern Med.* 1994;121(6):442–451.

71. Shumway-Cook A, Gruber W, Baldwin M, Liao S. The effect of multidimensional exercises on balance, mobility, and fall risk in community-dwelling older adults. *Phys Ther.* 1997;77(1):46–57.

72. Mathias S, Nayak U, Isaacs B. Balance in elderly patients: the "Get Up and Go" Test. *Arch Phys Med Rehabil.* 1986;67:387–389.

73. Fleming K, Evans J, Weber D, Chutka D. Practical functional assessment of elderly persons: a primary-care approach. *Mayo Clin Proc.* 1995;70(9):890–910.

74. Maki BE. Gait changes in older adults: predictors of falls or indicators of fear? *J Am Geriatr Soc.* 1997; 45(3):313–320.

75. O'Brien K. Getting around: a simple office workup to assess patient function. *Geriatrics.* 1994;49:38–42.

76. Duncan P, Weiner D, Chandler J, Studenski S. Functional reach: a new clinical measure of balance. *J Gerontol.* 1990;45:M192–M197.

77. Vellas BJ, Wayne SJ, Romero L, et al. One-leg balance is an important predictor of injurious falls in older persons. *J Am Geriatr Soc.* 1997;45(6):735–738.

78. Ewing JA. Detecting alcoholism, the CAGE questionaire. *JAMA.* 1984;252:1905.

79. D'Epiro NW. HRT: new data, continuing controversies. *Patient Care Nurse Pract.* 1998;1:18–20, 25–28, 31–34.

80. Ginter SG, Mion LC. Falls in the nursing home: preventable or inevitable? *J Gerontol Nurs.* 1992; 18(11):43–48.

81. Evans LK. Research on falls: implications for practice. In: Funk P, Tornquist E, Champagne M, Wiese, R, eds. *Key Aspects of Elder Care Managing Falls, Incontinence, and Cognitive Impairment.* New York: Springer Publishing; 1992:129–131.

82. Misener M, Matteson MA. Fall-related injury in nursing home residents [Abstract]. *Gerontol.* 1993;33 (special issue 1):276.

83. Rizzo JA, Baker DI, McAvay G, Tinetti ME. The cost-effectiveness of a multifactorial targeted prevention program for falls among community elderly persons. *Med Care.* 1996;34(9):954–969.

84. Tinetti ME, Speechley M, Ginter SF. Risk factors for falls among elderly persons living in the community. *N Engl J Med.* 1988;319(26):1701–1707.

85. McDowell JA, Mion LC, Lydon TJ, Inouye SK. A nonpharmacologic sleep protocol for hospitalized older patients. *J Am Geriatr Soc.* 1998;46:700–705.

86. Province M, Hadley E, Hornbrook M, et al. The effects of exercise on falls in elderly patients: a preplanned meta-analysis of the FICSIT trials. *JAMA.* 1995;273:1341–1347.

87. Connelly D, Vandervoort A. Improving muscle strength in the frail elderly. *Can Nurs Home.* 1996;7(4):24, 26–30.

88. Campbell A, Robertson MC, Gardner MM, et al. Randomized controlled trial of a general practice program of home based exercise to prevent falls in elderly women. *BMJ.* 1997;315(7115):1065–1068.

89. Sherrington C, Lord S. Home exercise to improve strength and walking velocity after hip fracture: a randomized controlled trial. *Arch Phys Med Rehabil.* 1997;78(2):208–212.

90. Chandler J, Duncan P, Kochersberger G, Studenski S. Is lower extremity strength gain associated with improvement in physical performance and disability in frail, community-dwelling elders? *Arch Phys Med Rehabil*. 1998;79(1):24–30.

91. Wolf SL, Barnhart HX, Ellison GL, Coogler CE, Horak FB. The effect of Tai Chi Quan and computerized balance training on postural stability in older subjects. *Phys Ther*. 1997;77(4):371–384.

92. Capezuti E, Talerico KA, Strumpf N, Evans LK. Individualized assessment and intervention in bilateral siderail use. *Geriatr Nurs*. 1998;19(6):322–330.

93. Capezuti E, Lawson WT. Falls, physical restraints and liability issues. In: Iyer P, ed. *Nursing Home Malpractice*. Phoenix, Az: Lawyers and Judges Publishing; 1999:205–249.

94. Thompson PG. Preventing falls in the elderly at home: a community-based program. *Med J Aust*. 1996; 164(9):530–532.

95. Rader J, Jones D, Miller LL. Individualized wheelchair seating: reducing restraints and improving comfort and function. *Top Geriatr Rehabil*. 1999;15:34–47.

96. Strumpf NE, Robinson JP, Wagner JS, Evans LK. *Restraint-Free Care*. New York: Springer Publishing; 1998.

97. Cruise PA, Schnelle JF, Alessi CA, Simmons SF, Ouslander JG. The nighttime environment and incontinence care practices in nursing homes. *J Am Geriatr Soc*. 1998;46:181–186.

98. Schnelle JF, Cruise PA, Alessi CA, Al-Samarrai N, Ouslander JG. Individualizing nighttime incontinence care in nursing home residents. *Nurs Res*. 1998;47: 197–204.

99. Donius M, Rader J. Siderails: rethinking a standard practice. In: Burggraf V, Barry R, eds. *Gerontological Nursing Current Practice and Research*. Thorofare, NJ: Slack; 1996:225–232.

100. Capezuti L. Legal liability issues and physical restraints. *HCFA's Nat Restraint Reduction Newsl*. 1997;5(3):1–2, 9.

101. Lauritzen JB, Askeguard V. Protection against hip fracture by energy absorption. *Danish Med Bull*. 1992;39(1):91–93.

102. Lauritzen JB, Petersen MM, Lund B. Effect of external hip protectors on hip fracture. *Lancet*. 1993;341:11–13.

103. Ross JE, Wallace RB, Woodworth G, et al. The acceptance of elderly of a hip joint protective garment to prevent hip fractures: Iowa FICSIT Trial. Paper presented at: Second World Conference on Injury Control; May 20, 1993; Atlanta, Ga.

104. Ross JE, Huston J. The development of a hip joint protective garment [Abstract]. *Gerontol*. 1993;33 (special issue 1): 239.

105. Wallace RB, Ross JE, Huston JC, Kundel C, Woodworth G. Iowa FICSIT Trial: the feasibility of elderly wearing a hip joint protective garment to reduce hip fractures. *J Am Geriatr Soc*. 1993;41(3):338–340.

106. Simmons SF, Schnelle JF, MacRae PG, Ouslander JG. Wheelchairs as mobility restraints: predictors of wheelchair activity in nonambulatory nursing home residents. *J Am Geriatr Soc*. 1995;43:384–388.

107. Capezuti E, Strumpf N, Evans LK, Maislin G. Outcomes of nighttime physical restraint removal for severely impaired nursing home residents. *Am J Alzheimer's Dis*. 1999;14:157–164.

108. *Side Rails Guidance*. Department of Health and Human Services, Health Care Financing Administration; February 4, 1997.

109. Miles SH, Irvine PI. Common features of deaths caused by physical restraints. *Gerontol*. 1991; 31(11):42.

110. Miles SH, Irvine PI. Deaths caused by physical restraints. *Gerontol*. 1992;32(6):762–766.

111. Weakley-Jones B, Wernert J. Accidental deaths in the aged by protective devices. *J Kentucky Med Assoc*. 1986;84:397–398.

112. Burlington DB. Entrapment hazards with hospital bed side rails. FDA Safety Alert. Rockville, Md: Food and Drug Administration, Public Health Service, Department of Health and Human Services; August 23, 1995.

113. Parker K, Miles SH. Deaths caused by bedrails. *J Am Geriatr Soc*. 1997;45:797–802.

114. Castle NG, Mor V. Physical restraints in nursing homes: a review of the literature since the Nursing Home Reform Act of 1987. *Med Care Res Rev*. 1998;55:139–170.

115. Health Care Financing Administration. *HCFA's Restraint Reduction Newsletter*. 1998;6:(Fall).

116. Cali CM, Kiel DP. An epidemiologic study of fall-related fractures among institutionalized older people. *J Am Geriatr Soc*. 1995;43:1336–1340.

117. Capezuti E, Strumpf N, Evans L, Grisso JA, Maislin G. The relationship between physical restraint removal and falls and injuries among nursing home residents. *J Gerontol Med Sci*. 1998;53A:M47–M53.

118. Ejaz FK, Jones JA, Rose MS. Falls among nursing home residents: an examination of incident reports before and after restraint reduction programs. *J Am Geriatr Soc*. 1994;42(9):960–964.

119. Evans LK, Strumpf NE, Allen-Taylor SL, et al. A clinical trial to reduce restraints in nursing homes. *J Am Geriatr Soc*. 1997;45:675–681.

120. Kramer JD. Reducing restraint use in a nursing home. *Clin Nurse Spec*. 1994;8:158–162.

121. Stratmann D, Vinson MH, Hardin SB. The effects of research on clinical practice: the use of restraints. *Appl Nurs Res*. 1997;10:39–43.

122. Werner P, Cohen-Mansfield J, Koroknay V, Braun J. The impact of a restraint-reduction program on nursing home residents. *Geriatr Nurs.* 1994;15(3): 142–146.

123. Buckler J, Dutton T, MacLeod H, Manuge M, Nixon M. Use of hip protectors on a dementia unit. *Physiother Can.* 1997;49(4):297–299, 310.

124. Robinovitch SN, Hayes WC, McMahon TA. Energy-shunting hip padding system attenuates femoral impact force in a simulated fall. *J Biomech Eng.* 1995;117(4):409–413.

125. Bakarich A, McMillan V, Prosser R. The effect of a nursing intervention on the incidence of older patient falls. *Aust J Adv Nurs.* 1997;15(1):26–31.

126. Sartoretti C, Sartoretti-Schefer S, Ruckert R, et al. Comorbid conditions in old patients with femur fractures. *J Trauma: Inj Infect Crit Care.* 1997;43(4):570–577.

127. Dandan I. Trauma in the elderly patient. *Top Emerg Med.* 1992;14(3):39–46.

128. Rozycki GS, Maull KI. Injuries sustained by falls. *Arch Emerg Med.* 1991;8:254–252.

129. Dobson J. New patient assessment expedites proper care. *Ski Patrol Mag.* 1998;14(4):2–4.

130. Abrahms WB, Beers MH, Berkow R, eds. *Merck Manual of Geriatrics.* Rahway, NJ: Merck & Company; 1995.

131. Auerbach P, ed. *Wilderness Medicine: Management of Wilderness and Environmental Emergencies.* St. Louis, Mo: Mosby; 1995.

132. Blake A. Falls in the elderly. *Br J Hosp Med.* 1992; 47(4):268–272.

133. Singletary N. Keep ahead of head injuries. *Ski Patrol Mag.* 1998;14(4):8–10.

134. Bowman W. *Outdoor Emergency Care.* Lakewood, Co: National Ski Patrol; 1993.

135. Jones T. Distal tibia and proximal fibula fracture in an elderly woman. *J Emerg Med.* 1996;14(4):497.

136. Keil DP. The evaluation of falls in the emergency department. *Clin Geriatr Med.* 1993;9(3):591–595.

CHAPTER

15

Sensory Impairment

Marie Boltz

Definition and Scope of Concern

The sensory organs are a primary interface with the environment. Thus, sensory changes in the older adult can have a profound impact on independence, social interaction, and lifestyle. Vision, hearing, taste, smell, and touch all may be affected by the aging process, but vision and hearing are the most dramatic and have the greatest effect on health and function. In addition, as many as 75% of the elderly have significant visual and hearing losses not reported to their practitioner.[1] Diligent screening for these problems is essential.

The practitioner must assess each sensory organ systematically and carefully consider other age-related changes producing less specific alterations in the senses. Assessment of the sense organs is often complicated by the presence of coexisting disease processes such as Parkinson's disease, stroke, dementing illness, and diabetes mellitus. Medications used by older people may also cause iatrogenic sensory problems. Sensory decrement varies among and within individuals, requiring an individualized assessment and plan.

The goal of care is to prevent and correct pathology as well as to identify mechanisms for maximal function and quality of life. To that end, this chapter presents the age-related changes in vision, hearing, smell, taste, and touch and pertinent contributing factors to sensory alterations. Assessment and interventions for common problems are also described.

Age-Related Changes and Pathophysiology

Vision

Structural Changes in the Eye Among the more obvious changes are graying of the eyebrows and eyelashes, and wrinkling and loosening of the skin around the eyelids. The eyes sink deeper with

limited upward gaze due to loss of orbital fat. Reduced tear secretion may cause discomfort and irritation, often relieved by "artificial tears."

The number of endothelial cells in the cornea is decreased, resulting in diminished and limited awareness of injury or infection. A grayish-yellow ring surrounding the iris, that is caused by an accumulation of lipids, also commonly surrounds the cornea.

The lens becomes less transparent, hydrated, and elastic. As a result, accommodation, the process of focusing an image in the retina, is more difficult and presbyopia, or farsightedness, results. Increased density of the lens causes increased scattering of light and sensitivity to glare. The lens also becomes progressively yellowed and opaque, with reduced discrimination for blue–green colors.

The iris loses its pigment with age, and eyes appear gray or light blue in many older persons. The pupil becomes smaller and constricts more slowly.

In the posterior cavity, the vitreous gel liquefies and collapses, leading to condensation and debris known as floaters. Although clinically insignificant, they can be annoying.[2]

Functional Changes in the Eye Changes in eye structure decrease the amount of light reaching the retina and cause decreases in visual acuity, tolerance to glare, and peripheral vision. Glare is common in the elderly, along with poor adjustment to darkness. Many older adults frequently give up night driving because adaptation to light and darkness decreases. These changes may also contribute to a greater risk for falls. Loss of peripheral vision may limit social interaction, as well as cause hazardous driving.[3]

Visual Impairment—Classification Most older adults encountered in clinical practice display varying degrees of vision loss. Impairment can vary from day to day, depending on environmental conditions.

The following range of terms are used to describe alterations in normal vision:[4]

- Blindness
- Legally blind
- Severely visually impaired
- Low vision
- Visually impaired
- Partially sighted

While the terms *blind* and *blindness* suggest no ability to see, more precisely a person is *legally blind* if, with best correction, vision does not exceed 20/200 or the visual field is no greater than 20 degrees in the better eye (a full visual field is 180 degrees).

Severe visual impairment is usually defined as the inability, with best correction, to read newspaper print. Visual impairment is also such that it interferes with the independent performance of activities of daily living (ADLs).

Partially sighted, low vision, and *visually sighted* indicate some degree of functional vision. These visual disorders, however, cannot be corrected with eyeglasses or contact lenses. Low-vision specialists can maximize remaining vision through visual aids and environmental modification.

Visual Impairment—Incidence

The prevalence of visual disability increases with age, with almost 95% of the over-75 population requiring correction to maintain visual function. Approximately one in five Americans age 85 and older, and 12% of persons age 75–85, have severe visual impairments.[5]

Although it affects many older adults, visual impairment is often unrecognized and misunderstood. Failure to assess vision, especially in persons with cognitive changes, and to correlate loss of vision with functional impairment, contributes to poor detection and treatment. The effects of untreated visual impairment and blindness include stress, lower life satisfaction, predisposition to falls/injuries, and depression.[6,7] The advanced practice nurse (APN) should provide assessment, counseling, intervention, and referral aimed to enhance visual function in the older adult. A list of resources for the blind and visually impaired can be found in Table 15–1.

Table 15–1   Resources for the Blind and Visually Impaired

Governmental and private agencies provide low-vision services including special devices, independent home-living instruction, and orientation and mobility training.

Selected resources:

- American Foundation for the Blind, 11 Penn Plaza, Suite 300, New York, NY 10001. (1-800-232-5463)
- National Association for Visually Handicapped, 22 West 21st Street, New York, NY 10010 (212-889-3141)
- National Library Service for the Blind and Physically Handicapped, Library of Congress, Washington, DC 20542 (1-800-424-8567)
- National Center for Vision and Aging, The Lighthouse, 111 East 59th Street, New York, NY 10022 (1-800-334-5497)

Among the visual disorders associated with aging, cataract has the greatest incidence in persons over age 65, followed by senile macular degeneration, diabetic retinopathy, and glaucoma.

Problems of Vision

Cataract   A cataract is an opacity of the crystalline lens. In the early stages, improvements in near vision may occur because increased lens density temporarily improves refraction. The most common subjective finding, however, is progressive, unilateral, or bilateral painless loss of vision. Examination reveals haziness of the lens, inability to see the fundus in detail, and a reduced red reflex.

Referral for surgical removal of the cataract is the treatment of choice, depending on individual need. Surgery is influenced by functional level, the location of the cataract, and degree of visual impairment. When the cataract is extracted, improvement in visual acuity is dramatic unless coexisting retinal disease negatively affects the prognosis.

Follow-up is required to monitor the surgically implanted lens or use of contact lenses or eyeglasses. Functional status should also be closely observed and independent activity supported.

Glaucoma Glaucoma refers to an increase in intraocular pressure. Primary open-angle glaucoma, also known as simple, ordinary, or chronic glaucoma, is caused by obstruction in the aqueous outflow system, causing an increase in intraocular pressure and destruction of nerve fibers. Subjective findings are not reported until late in the disease and include loss of peripheral vision, or "tunnel vision," pain in and around the eye, cloudy vision, and halos around lights. Objective findings include high intraocular pressure, degeneration and cupping of the optic disc, atrophy of the optic nerve head, and loss of visual field.

Referral to an ophthalmologist, with ongoing annual evaluation, is required. Medications decrease the secretion of aqueous fluid and enhance aqueous outflow. Noncardioselective beta blockers, alpha agonists, miotics, carbonic anhydrase inhibitors, sympathomimetics, and cholinesterase inhibitors are commonly used antiglaucoma agents (Table 15–2).[8]

Closed-angle glaucoma is a sudden increase in intraocular pressure due to mechanical obstruction of the outflow channels. Although a relatively uncommon disease (less than 5% of all cases of primary glaucoma), it is important to recognize and treat early. Symptoms include severe pain (in or around the eye or over the fifth cranial nerve area) with nausea, vomiting, and prostration. Vision becomes blurred or foggy and colored halos appear around lights as the cornea assumes a "steamy" appearance. The pupil is fixed and large. Ciliary injection is apparent with conjunctival venous engorgement. The optic disc can swell within 24 hours and complete visual loss can occur in just a few days. This ophthalmologic emergency requires immediate referral to lower intraocular pressure with topical medications and intravenous or oral hyperosmotic agents. A peripheral iridectomy may be necessary.

Age-Related Macular Degeneration (AMD) AMD is the second leading cause of blindness. "Wet" (or exudative) AMD occurs when tiny blood vessels grow rapidly beneath the retina, leaking blood and causing scar tissue to form. Wet AMD is responsible for severe visual loss. The "dry" form, which accounts for 70–80% of AMD, is caused by a breakdown or thinning of tissues in the macula. Visual loss in dry AMD is moderate.[9]

Subjective findings of AMD include loss of central vision (scotoma), impairing reading, and impaired object recognition. Side vision and mobility remain intact. Affected persons may find it very difficult to perform simple activities demanding sharp vision, such as reading, sewing, or drawing. Objective findings include an abnormal response on the Amsler grid and the appearance of dreusen upon fundoscopic exam. Early referral to an ophthalmologist is for possible photocoagulation treatment, which may be very effective. Unfortunately, most cases are discovered late in the disease and are therefore untreatable. Follow-up and referral to low-vision therapies nevertheless assist in maintaining or restoring function and independence. Low-vision devices are described in Table 15–3.

The APN must teach older adults ways to slow the progression of AMD, such as increasing the consumption of carotenoids, wearing ultraviolet lenses, and not smoking or drinking alcohol to excess.[9]

Diabetic Retinopathy Diabetic retinopathy brings early damage to the retinal capillaries, progressive growth of abnormal cell vessels, and leaking and hemorrhage of the retinal vasculature into the vitreous body. The subjective finding is central vision impairment. Fundoscopic exam reveals white exudates, microaneurysms, and possible retinal detachment. Primary treatment is aimed at controlling blood glucose levels.

Sjögren's Syndrome Sjögren's is described as a combination of any two of the following entities: keratoconjunctivitis sicca (KCS), xerostomia, and rheumatoid arthritis or other connective tissue disease.

KCS is a nonspecific condition due to deficient production of tears. In addition to Sjögren's syndrome, KCS can be caused by hyperplasia of the lacrimal glands or congenital absence. Other sys-

Table 15–2   Commonly Prescribed Anti-Glaucoma Agents

Generic Name	Trade Name	Category	Indication
Brimondine Tartate	Alphagan	Alpha agonist	Open-angle glaucoma/ocular hypertension
Brinzolamide 1%	Azopt	Carbonic anhydrase inhibitor (sulfonamide)	Open-angle glaucoma and ocular hypertension
Levobunolol Hel .25%	Betagan	Noncardioselective beta-blocker	Open-angle glaucoma
Timolol .25%	Betimol	Noncardioselective beta-blocker	Open-angle glaucoma
Betaxolol .5%	Betoptic	Cardioselective beta-blocker	Open-angle glaucoma where beta blockers alone are inadequate
Dorzolamide HCI 2%/ Timolol maleate .5%	Cosopt	Alpha agonist/ carbonic anhydrase inhibitor	Adjunct in open-angle glaucoma
Acetazolamide	Diamox	Carbonic anhydrase inhibitor	Refractory open-angle glaucoma
Decumcarium bromide	Humorsol	Cholinesterase inhibitor	Refractory open-angle glaucoma
Apraclonidine .5%	Iopidine	Alpha agonist	Adjunct in open-angle glaucoma
Carbachol hydroxprophy Methylcellulose	Isopto carbachel	Carbonic anhydrase inhibitor	Open-angle glaucoma unresponsive to pilocarpine
Methazolamide	Neptazane	Carbonic anhydrase inhibitor	Adjunct in open-angle glaucoma
Carteolol	Ocupress	Carbonic anhydrase inhibitor	Adjunct in open-angle glaucoma
Pilocarpine sustained release	Ocusert Pilo	Miotic	Adjunct in open-angle glaucoma
Pilo carpine	Pilocar	Miotic	Chronic open-angle glaucoma
Dipivefrin HCI	Propine	Sympathomimetic	Open-angle glaucoma
Timolol	Timoptic	Noncardioselective beta blocker	Open-angle glaucoma
Latanoprost	Xalaton	Prostaglandin agonist	Open-angle glaucoma in patients who have failed to respond to other treatment

temic diseases such as sarcoidosis, leukemia, or lymphoma also cause KCS.

Sjögren's is almost always a bilateral disease. Symptoms evolve insidiously and include redness, dryness, itching, burning, photophobia, and a foreign-body sensation. Symptoms often appear only in times of increased tear demand such as crying or environmental irritation. Conjunctivae usually appear normal, but may be gray and lusterless. Symptomatic treatment of KCS associated with Sjögren's syndrome requires instillation of artificial tears and lubricants as often as necessary.

Conjunctivitis   Conjunctivitis is the most common cause of acute red eye. Etiology can be bacterial, viral, chlamydial, rickettsial, fungal, allergic,

Table 15–3 Low-Vision Devices

Optical Low-Vision Devices

Magnifying spectacles: designed for close vision. The person needs to hold the reading material very close.

Hand magnifiers: can be bought in a drug store. The person can hold reading material at a normal distance.

Stand magnifiers: rest on the reading material.

Telescopes: are used for distance magnification. They may be hand held or mounted on spectacles.

Closed-circuit television: uses adjustable magnification and contrast, produces an enlarged image in a television screen.

Non-Optical Low-Vision Devices

- Enlarged telephone dials
- Voice-recognition telephone service
- Check-writing guide
- Machines that scan print and read aloud
- Talking books
- Large-print books, newspapers, and magazines
- High-contrast watch faces
- Large playing cards
- Computers that talk and use voice-recognition software

traumatic, parasitic, or of unknown origin. Although the conjunctiva is rich in blood vessels and lymphoid tissue, pain fibers are few. Therefore, symptoms include vague discomfort, scratchiness, or burning. In contrast, corneal inflammation is characterized by severe pain. Exudate is typically present and may be thin and watery (viral disease), purulent (bacterial disease), or white and stringy (allergic disease). Vision may be blurred from secretions floating over the cornea, but testing generally demonstrates that visual acuity is unaffected. Conjunctival injection is present in varying degrees. Pupillary size and corneal reflex are normal. Palpable preauricular nodes may be present, especially in viral infections. Visual and bacterial conjunctivitis may be associated with a coexisting upper respiratory infection.

Diagnosis is made by history, exam, and conjunctival culture. Treatment is aimed at the cause, usually with antibiotic ophthalmics for bacterial conjunctivitis, the most common cause of acute red eye in the older adult.

Corneal Trauma and Infection   Symptoms include eye pain, reflex blepharospasm, and photophobia. Ciliary injection (fixed dull red or violet vessels on the conjunctiva) is present and vision is often blurred. Discharge is rare, except with a purulent bacterial ulceration, which requires prompt referral and treatment to prevent scarring.

Giant Cell Arteritis   Giant cell arteritis is also known as temporal arteritis, cranial arteritis, and Horton's arteritis. Symptoms may include unilateral or bilateral temporal, occipital, or fronto-occipital head pain and tenderness. Visual changes range from no loss to sudden loss of vision. Diplopia and ptosis may also be present in jaw muscles, making chewing uncomfortable. Nodules are occasionally palpable on affected vessels.

An elevated erythrocyte sedimentation rate (usually greater than 80 mm per hour) is a characteristic feature of the disease. Further consultation is generally needed. Temporal artery biopsy is the most reliable diagnostic test. Ongoing evaluation is needed to assess response to the usual treatment of long-term steroids.[1]

Retinal Detachment   Retinal detachment presents with a sudden appearance of many floaters, a blind spot, blurred vision, or shadowy lines. Patients often describe the sensation of a curtain closing over the eye. Prompt referral is required to prevent macular involvement and complete loss of vision. Laser photocoagulation, performed on an outpatient basis, may repair small retinal tears. Other treatments include cryoprexy, the use of extreme cold, to cause scar formation and seal the edge of a retinal tear, or vitrectomy performed under general anesthesia. Most detached retinas can be repaired, with half of these repairs resulting in the full return of vision.

Senile Entropion and Ectropion   These two disorders are not usually threatening but cause discomfort and changes in body image. Entropion is a complete inversion of the lower lid due to weakening and wasting of the muscle fat and skin around the orbit. Complaints are of irritated, watery eyes. Generally, referral is indicated to assess for surgery or cautery to prevent keratitis and corneal ulceration. Temporary relief can be obtained by extending the lid outward with a short strip of adhesive tape.

Senile ectropion is outward turning of the eyelid margin, resulting from facial paralysis or atrophy of eyelid tissues. Surgical treatment is performed to shorten the lid and improve muscle tone.

Field Disturbance Associated with Stroke   Hemianopsia, or visual loss in half of the visual field, is readily evident with confrontation. Field cuts are caused by vascular accidents or pressure in the optic nerve and may occur in both right halves or in either the lower or upper fields. Changes in ADL function and negotiation of the environment suggest a field cut; for example, ignoring items placed either to the right or left side. Activities such as traveling and reading, especially if there is an inferior hemianopsia defect in the lower half of the visual field, are often limited. Low-vision therapists can recommend environmental modification, special glasses, adaptive equipment, and safety education.[10]

Hearing

Structural Changes in the Ear   Age changes of the external ear include drying and sagging of the auricle with increased wrinkling. Continued deposition of cartilage causes the earlobe to elongate and alters the shape of the auditory canal. The tragus of adult males becomes longer and coarser and tends to be embedded with dry cerumen. Some degeneration occurs in the bony joints of the middle ear, but does not affect sound transmission. Thickening of the tympanic membrane and a slight decrease in the intensity of the light reflex are normal age-related changes.

The most significant age-related changes occur in the inner ear, where degeneration of the vestibular structure occurs, affecting speech, equilibrium, and sensitivity to sound. Loss of hair cells and

myelinated nerve fibers, and atrophy of the cochlea, the organ of corti, and the stria vascularis cause decreased hearing and equilibrium.

Functional Changes   Some hearing loss is inevitable with advancing age. In the United States, it is estimated that 13 to 14 million people have hearing loss affecting daily function. Institutionalized older adults have greater impairments than those living in the community. Approximately 30% of community-residing older adults above age 65 have hearing impairments as compared to 90% in institutions.[10]

Presbycusis   Adults with normal hearing perceive sound at a frequency of 300–3500 Hz. With aging, hearing for higher frequency sounds (1500–4000 Hz) is lost. Long-term exposure to noise affects hearing for low-frequency sounds.

Presbycusis is a common, slowly progressive, symmetrical sensorineural hearing loss. Word discrimination and comprehension are affected by reduced speech perception and high-tone hearing loss. Older adults take longer to process information in the higher auditing centers and have more difficulty understanding accelerated speech. In addition, consonants such as "t," "f," and "g," which have high frequencies, are difficult to hear.

Conductive Hearing Loss   Conductive hearing loss results from any interference in vibration through the external and middle ears. Such hearing loss can be caused by accumulated cerumen, otitis media, otosclerosis, eardrum perforation, or radiation. Subjective findings include intact speech discrimination and enhanced hearing in the presence of extraneous noise. Complaints of low-pitched tinnitus are also reported.

Persons with conductive hearing losses usually speak softly and have occlusions of cerumen. Accumulated wax can be removed with over-the-counter eardrop preparations such as Debrox. The drops soften wax, which is then followed by lavage. Instillation of mineral oil into the ear canal for 24 hours, followed by a gentle lavage of hydrogen peroxide and water, also is effective.

Sensorineural Hearing Loss   Sensorineural hearing loss can be caused by noise damage, heredity, tumors around the acoustic nerve, Meniere's disease, complications of arteriosclerosis, and Paget's disease. Presbycusis, an age-related cause of sensorineural hearing loss, was discussed previously.

Subjective findings, in addition to decreased hearing acuity, may include high-pitched tinnitus, anxiety, depression, social isolation, and mental status changes. Affected persons may be observed lip-reading, unable to communicate unless with face-to-face contact.

Otosclerosis, which causes a conductive hearing loss when the ossicular chain is fixated, also causes sensorineural loss with bony capsule fixation.

Numerous medication toxicities lead to hearing loss, including aminoglycosides, antibiotics, ethacrynic acid, furosemide, and aspirin. Except for aspirin, removal of the offending agent does not reverse the sensorineural loss.

Paget's disease may contribute to conductive and sensorineural hearing losses. Referral to an Ear, Nose, and Throat (ENT) specialist and radiological studies are warranted. Hearing loss may also be associated with hypothyroidism.

Communication difficulties caused by permanent hearing loss should be carefully evaluated to determine any reversible causes. Audiologic evaluation is essential with chronic hearing loss to identify needs for amplification and aural rehabilitation. Types of hearing aids include postauricular (behind the ear), eyeglass, body (amplifier is carried by the individual), and all-in-the-ear (tympanette inserts in the ear canal). Depending on the level of impairment, hearing aids may be placed in one or both ears (binaural). Binaural aids localize sound and improve speech reception threshold and discrimination. A trained audiologist provides the necessary expertise to conduct testing and fitting of hearing aids.[11,12]

Tinnitus   Although it may be present without hearing loss, tinnitus is an annoying symptom that is also associated with both conductive and sensorineural hearing deficits. A sensation of hissing and buzzing or ringing, high pitched with sensorineural loss and low pitched with conductive loss, are common. Tinnitus is associated with otosclerosis, trauma, tumors, ototoxic drugs, diabetes mellitus, Meniere's disease, and labyrinthitis. Symptoms may be alleviated through biofeedback, competing noise, or masking device producing a narrow band of sound at a frequency similar to tinnitus.

Taste and Smell

Atrophic changes in the tongue with associated diminishment of taste occur naturally with aging. Salivary secretion decreases, thus decreasing the solubilization of flavoring agents. Taste acuity may be diminished as upper dentures cover secondary taste sites.[13] In addition, olfactory loss is thought to affect the sense of taste. More research is needed to determine how taste changes with age.[14]

Rhinorrhea and stomatitis can adversely affect taste due to interference with taste receptors on the tongue. Rhinorrhea also affects olfaction, which influences taste. When these conditions are treated, problems with taste also correct. Damage to the hypoglossal nerve may alter taste as well. Experimentation with seasonings and spices may make food more palatable.

Touch and Vibration

Knowledge of age-related changes to the tactile senses is scarce. Studies suggest a loss of vibratory sense at the ankle. Peripheral neuropathy secondary to diabetes mellitus results in inability to sense light touch in distal portions of the extremities. Paresthesias and decreased sense of hot and cold are often noted. Gabapentin (Neurontin) or carbamazepine (Tegretol) may alleviate the discomforts of paresthesias. Education is required regarding prevention of injury and infection.

Toxin-induced peripheral neuropathy also impairs tactile sensation. Antineoplastic agents or other toxins resulting in limited sensation to touch may destroy peripheral nerve endings. Peripheral nerve damage occurs as well with arterial insufficiency, usually evidenced by diminished or absent pulses; cool, thin, shiny, and taut skin; decreased hair distribution; nail changes; and gray pallor. Referral to a vascular surgeon and prevention of stasis ulcer are standard approaches for the APN. In all of these conditions, extreme safety precautions and safety counseling are required to prevent injury.

Kinesthesia

Aging does not generally affect the kinesthetic sense, that is, where the body is in space. Some older people experience an absence or decrease in position sense of the large toe. Meniere's disease, dementia, and stroke, all of which interfere with a sense of balance, righting reflex, and proprioception, affect kinesthesia. Immobilized patients are most at risk for kinesthesic distortion. Regular exercise with full range of motion promotes proprioceptive and vestibular function. Natural mobility, such as frequent transfers from chair to chair and a consistent, customized walking program, are also beneficial.

Sensory/Perceptual Overload Pain

Sensory-perceptual overload is defined as an increase in sensory stimulation, which results in a loss of the normal ability to discriminate patterns. Feeling out of control may be expressed, along with evidence of sudden mental status changes, restlessness, irritability, anxiety, postural changes, muscular tension, hallucinations, and withdrawal.[10] Potential sources of overload include incessant use of the intercom and noise from staff and equipment.

Alleviation of symptoms requires identifying environmental factors that are most disturbing and modifying the environment accordingly. Input from patients, family members, and simple trial and error should be utilized.

Sensory/Perceptual Deprivation

Sensory/perceptual deprivation signifies an absence or lessening of meaningful patterning. Immobility, lack of meaningful activity, and diminished social contact are all associated with sensory deprivation. Clinical presentation can be the same as sensory perceptual overload. Approaches, aimed at promoting mobility, function, and control over the

environment, are also applicable. Prescribed adaptive equipment should be used consistently as prescribed (including aural and visual devices). Social interactions and activity programs need to be sensory rich; for example, opportunities for preferred and varied tastes, horticultural experiences, or pet therapy. Structured exercise also promotes mental agility, proprioception, and vestibular function. Following the person's preferred routine and promoting menu selection, choice of clothes, and activities will help the patient organize and control the stimuli and thereby increase its relevance.

Assessment of the Senses

History

Even minor changes in the sensory modalities of vision, hearing, smell, taste, and touch can represent a primary problem in the sense organs or systemic pathology. In addition to diagnostic significance, there is considerable prognostic value in determining sensory impairments and any functional losses.[15]

Patients do not always report sensory changes; thus, the clinician must be an adept interviewer, listener, and detective. Any reported changes in ADLs deserve particular attention, as well as changes in patterns of social interaction.[16] These can then be linked to a systematic review of systems and analysis of sensory alterations.

Patient Profile   Data on the living environment, routine/activity, social interaction, and nutrition provide rich information that may indicate change in the sensory organs.[17] Occupation, past or present, may suggest contact with environmental factors (e.g., sustained exposure to noise pollution) affecting sensory function.

Activity pattern should be scrutinized for social contacts and time spent out of the home/room. Failure to engage in activities may be the result of a hearing deficit. A decision to no longer drive at night may be due to waning visual acuity and intolerance of glare.

Questions such as "Would you describe your health as excellent, good, fair, or poor?" and "Do you feel young, middle-aged, or old?" often disclose a diminished life satisfaction, which may relate to sensory losses. Older people with sensory impairments are more likely to feel older and in poorer health.[18]

Any description of a sensory problem should be accompanied by further questions about coping patterns, both internal (spirituality, sense of humor, positive attitude) and external (family and professional support). Internal and external coping resources appear to support a positive outlook on life, despite certain losses.[19]

Obtain a 24-hour nutritional intake to determine any changes in appetite and food preferences. Deficits in taste and smell, poor dentition, problems swallowing and chewing, or ill-fitting dentures may be disclosed. Analysis of the nutritional content of the diet needs to be assessed; especially for any vitamin and mineral deficits. A limited intake of protein can result in vitamin A deficiency, leading to visual disturbances.

Past Health History/Family History   The frequency, results, and last date of vision and hearing testing and dental care should be noted. Describe any related illness, treatment, and residual effects. Diabetes, hypertension, cerebral vascular accident, arteriosclerosis, and arthritis suggest the possibility of visual or auditory problems. Chemotherapy for cancer may have caused a permanent peripheral neuropathy. Familial tendencies exist for glaucoma, senile macular degeneration, and cataracts.

A thorough history of past and current medications is essential, as many drugs cause sensory problems. Table 15–4 lists medications that are commonly prescribed for older adults with potential adverse effects to the eyes, ears, nose, and mouth.

Review of Systems   In conducting a review of systems, any of the following are potentially indicative of sensory pathology:

- increased tearing: may be due to impaired drainage of the ductal system
- pain in and around the eye, cloudy vision, "halos" around lights: symptoms of late, chronic glaucoma or acute glaucoma

- loss of visual acuity
- diplopia, inflammation, pain, and photophobia

The following symptoms of potential visual loss should be explored:

- change in performing any ADLs
- difficulty recognizing faces
- difficulty managing utensils and spills
- impaired mobility: bumping into objects, difficulty walking, falls
- squinting or tilting head to the side
- difficulty reading, writing, or driving
- difficulty identifying colors
- tinnitus, vertigo, or ear pain

Determine the onset of hearing loss, if possible. Presbycusis tends to be chronic and progressive. Obtain a description of the hearing loss; for example, ability to hear conversation, difficulty with background noise, and so on. Environmental factors (such as ability to cope with background noise) needs to be discussed. Determine any adaptations to hearing changes (e.g., lip reading or environmental modifications) and their effectiveness. Explore the presence of mental status changes (depression), other physical complaints, and social isolation. The Hearing Handicap Inventory for the Elderly Screening (HHIES) questionnaire is a useful screening tool for use in cognitively intact older adults.[20] Changes in taste and smell and altered appetite should be included in the history.

Ascertain the presence of pins-and-needles sensations or difficulty differentiating hot and cold. The presence of pain should be further explored by evaluating the onset, location, duration, relieving factors, associated symptoms, and intensity.

Physical Exam

The Eye   Examination of the eye begins with a determination of visual acuity. For an accurate evaluation, the light source should originate behind the person. The Snellen chart tests visual accuracy at 20 feet. Newspaper or other reading material should be used to determine near vision. Visual acuity is an indicator of second cranial nerve function (barring

Table 15–4 Iatrogenic Problems of the Eyes, Ears, Nose, and Mouth Caused by Medications Commonly Taken by Older People

Health Problem	Medication		Side Effects			
	Generic Name	Trade Name	Eye	Ear	Nose	Mouth
Arthritis	Choline magnesium Trisalicylate	Trilisate		Tinnitus, decreased hearing		
	Ketoprofen	Orudis	Blurred vision	Tinnitus		
	Naproxen	Naprosyn		Tinnitus		
	Oxaprozin	Daypro	Blurred vision, photosensitivity	Tinnitus		
Heart disease	Digoxin	Lanoxin	Blurred or yellow vision	Tinnitus		Anorexia
	Pentoxifylline	Trental	Blurred vision			
Glaucoma	Cholinergics		Miosis, diminished light adaptation		Rhinorrhea	Increased salivation
Hyperlipidemia	Gemfibrozil	Lopid	Blurred vision			
	Lovastatin	Mevacor	Blurred vision			Altered taste
Hypertension	Furosemide	Lasix		Tinnitus, decreased hearing		Dry mouth
	Hydrochlorothiazide	Hydrodiuril	Photosensitivity	Tinnitus, decreased hearing		Dry mouth
	Indapamide	Lozol	Blurred vision			
	Metoprolol	Lopressor	Blurred vision	Earache, tinnitus		
Infection	Ciprofloxacin	Cipro	Photosensitivity			
	Gentamycin	Garamycin	Blurred vision			
	Levofloxacin	Levaquin	Photosensitivity			
	Sparfluxacin	Zagam	Photosensitivity			
Mood disorder	Fluvoxamine	Luvox				Taste perversion
	Mirtazapine	Remeron			Rhinitis	Taste perversion
	Paroxetine	Paxil				Dry mouth
	Venlafaxine	Effexor	Blurred vision			Dry mouth
Seizures	Carbamazepine	Tegretol	Lens opacity			Dry mouth
	Gabapentin	Neurontin	Visual disturbance, nystagmus			

an opacity of the lens which negatively affects acuity). A confrontation test is then used to provide a gross estimate of the visual field. Teller acuity cards, which were developed to test visual acuity in children aged 1–12 months, can be useful with cognitive impairment.[20]

The Amsler grid is utilized to assess for age-related macular degeneration (AMD). Place the grid on the wall at eye level, 12 inches from the examinee, and instruct the patient to look at the center dot, one eye at a time. If lines are missing, or appear distorted or wavy, AMD should be considered.

Assess the external eye for excess tearing, discharge, swelling, entropion, and ectropion. Note drainage and injection of the sclerae and conjunctivae. Pupils may appear smaller in size, unequal, and irregular in shape in older adults. Reaction to light, reflecting third cranial nerve function, should be symmetrical and equal, but may not be brisk.

The shape and clarity of the cornea remain unchanged with age and abnormalities require ophthalmologic evaluation. When testing the corneal reflex (fifth cranial nerve function), prolonged stimulation may be necessary to achieve a response. Once elicited, however, the response should be brisk and consensual.

Inspect for cataracts prior to fundoscopic examination. Some cataract development is expected in most persons over 70 years of age. A cataract may partially or totally block the red reflex and visualization of the fundus. A centrally placed cataract may appear as a milky white opacity when viewed through the pupil. Some cataracts present as areas of diffuse dark pigmentation or as spider webs.

The retina and optic disc appear paler than in younger adults and arteries and veins are in the typical ratio of 2 to 3.[2] Tortuosity and silver wire appearance are indicative of an atherosclerotic process. Signs of macular degeneration include altered pigmentation and configuration in and near the macula.

Fundoscopic recognition of hypertension, arteriosclerosis, and diabetes are critical for early recognition, referral, and treatment. Narrowing and constricting of the vessels with hemorrhages and exudates present characterize retinal hypertension and arteriosclerosis. Diabetic retinopathy presents with white or waxy exudates and microa-

neurysms around the macula. Presence of cataracts or glaucoma is suggestive of diabetes mellitus, which needs further screening.

The eye examination should also include tenometry, a measure of intraocular pressure, in glaucoma. Normal intraocular pressure is 10–21 mm Hg, with any reading over 21 mm Hg viewed suspiciously.

Behavioral and functional changes indicative of visual problems may be observed, especially in the long-term care setting. These include bumping into objects, straining to watch television, changes in ADL/IADL activity, and social withdrawal.

The Ear   Inspect the external ear for lesions, dryness, or exudates and the canal for cerumen, scarring, and infections. During otoscopic examination, visualize the tympanic membrane, ossicles, and light reflex. The presence of a bulging tympanic membrane, injection, and a very diminished or absent light reflex is not normal for the aging process.

Hearing loss can be assessed with questions asked out of the range of vision that require more than a "yes" or "no" answer. To determine functional hearing, observe the patient with others, watching television, or using the telephone. Hearing reflects eighth cranial nerve function. The Weber and Rinne tests provide a gross assessment of hearing, as well as the finger rub and finger snap tests. If presbycusis is present unilaterally, the Weber lateralizes to the unaffected ear and Rinne demonstrates a normal ratio of air to bone conduction with a generalized decrease in total hearing. Gross hearing can also be evaluated using a Welch-Allyn audioscope. Referral for an audiological evaluation should be the standard approach for all patients demonstrating hearing deficits.

Smell and Taste   To assess smell and taste, ask the older adult to identify odors and tastes with eyes closed. Cloves, cinnamon, oranges, ammonia, and coffee are useful olfactory stimuli. Mint, oil, sugar, water, salt water, and lemon juice are useful taste tests. The palate needs to be cleansed between tastes.

Data from a baseline assessment of smell and taste may indicate a need for further patient education. For example, with altered taste perception, dietary counseling may be required to ensure intake that is palatable and nutritionally sound.

Touch and Vibration   Small objects, sampled from a closed paper bag, can be used to assess touch. Light pinpricks or a brush with cotton on the skin are a measure of somatic sensation. Vibratory sense should be tested in the upper and lower extremities. Hands and feet should be warm when testing for vibration. Testing on the malleoli is more reliable than testing on the toes.

Kinesthesia   To evaluate kinesthesia, observe sitting and standing balance and recovery from a disequiliberating force, such as a gentle shove on the shoulder. Note any nystagmus. During testing, reassure the patient and provide safety precautions.

Unilateral Neglect   Unilateral neglect is defined as lack of awareness or inattentiveness to one side of the body, usually resulting from a problem with the processing of sensory information. Prognostically, it is a predictor of poorer outcomes following stroke. Assess the patient in real-life situations in order to evaluate impact on function, safety, and body image:

- bumping or injuring affected side
- allowing affected limb to remain poorly positioned or misaligned
- pocketing of food in affected side of the mouth
- ignoring food on one side of the plate
- bathing, dressing, and grooming only the unaffected side

Integrated Functioning   Assessment of sensory changes also includes evaluation of function. Customary routine, lifestyle, and level of activity suggest whether any sensory alterations are adversely affecting general health and functioning. Answers to questions such as "How has your life changed?" "How would you like it to change?" and "What is the potential for increased function?" can be revealing. Responses can be especially valuable in developing an individualized plan and evaluating its effectiveness.

 ## The Senses: Implications for the Practitioner

Appreciation for the impact of sensory alterations on function and quality of life is essential. The APN provides prompt evaluation and treatment for common, uncomplicated problems, and referral of complex clinical presentations to the relevant physician or other health-care providers, while simultaneously providing support and counsel to the patient. The APN frequently functions as a consultant to long-term care and other facilities striving to provide a culture of autonomy, independence, and dignity.

Special attention to sensory/perceptual alteration can mean greater attention by long-term care and other facilities to programs and environments that are enabling. Living situations dedicated to continued growth and involvement in life are achievable goals.

 ## References

1. Kane R, Ouslander J, Abrass I. *Essentials of Clinical Geriatrics*. New York: McGraw-Hill; 1997.
2. Smith SC. Aging, physiology and vision. *Nurse Pract For*. 1998;9(1):19–22.
3. Wood JM, Troutbeck R. Elderly drivers and simulated visual impairment. *Optom Visual Sci*. 1995;72(2):115–124.
4. Lawrence K, ed. *Geriatric Patient Education Resource Manual*. Gaithersburg, Md: Aspen; 1996.
5. Braus P. Vision in an aging America. *Am Demographics*. 1995;17(6):34–38.
6. Rovner BW, Zisselman PM, Shmvely-Dulitzki Y. Depression and disability in older people with impaired vision: a follow-up study. *J Am Geriatr Soc*. 1996;44:181–184.
7. Ivers R, Cumming R, Mitchell P, et al. Visual impairment and falls in older adults: the Blue Mountains Eye Study. *J Am Geriatr Soc*. 1998;46(1):58–64.
8. Butler RN, Faye EE, Guazzo E, et al. Keeping an eye on vision: primary care of age-related ocular disease. *Geriatrics*. 1997;52(8):30–41.
9. Elfervig LS. Age-related macular degeneration. *Nurse Pract For*. 1998;9(1):4–6.
10. Matteson MA, McConnell ES, Linton AD. *Gerontological Nursing*. Philadelphia, W.B. Saunders; 1997.
11. Humes LE, Halling D, Caughlin M. Reliability and stability of various hearing-aid outcome measures in a group of elderly hearing-aid wearers. *J Speech Hearing Res*. 1996;39(5):923–935.

12. Tolson D. Age-related hearing loss: a case for nursing intervention. *J Adv Nurs.* 1997;26:1150–1157.

13. Schiffman SS. Taste and smell losses in normal aging and disease. *JAMA.* 1997;278(16):1357–1362.

14. Nordan S, Monsch AV, Murphy C. Unawareness of smell and loss in normal aging and Alzheimer's disease: discrepancy between self-reported and diagnosed smell sensitivity. *J Gerontol.* 1995;50(4):187–192.

15. Reuben DB, Mui S, Damesyn M, et al. The prognostic value of sensory impairment in older persons. *J Am Geriatr Soc.* 1999;47(8):930–935.

16. Resnick H, Fries B, Verbrugge L. Windows to their world: the effect of sensory impairments on social engagement and activity time in nursing home residents. *J Gerontol.* 1997;52(3):S135–S144.

17. Stevens JC, Cruz LA, Marks LE, et al. A multimodal assessment of sensory thresholds in aging. *J Gerontol.* 1998;53(4):262–272.

18. Klempen G, Verbrugge LM, Merrill SS, et al. Impact of multiple impairments on disability in community-dwelling older people. *Age Aging.* 1998;27(5):595–604.

19. Kleinschmidt J. Older adults' perspectives on their successful adjustment to vision loss. *J Visual Impairment Blindness.* 1999;Feb:69–81.

20. Abyad A. In-office screening for age-related hearing and vision loss. *Geriatrics.* 1997;52(6):45–46.

16

Nutritional Problems

Sara Lisa Sheiman

Introduction

The prevailing goal of gerontology is maturity with enjoyment, gratification, comfort, and optimal health. Good nutrition is an essential component of health care, and should be the target of primary, secondary, and tertiary intervention. Unfortunately, geriatric nutrition is not widely understood or recognized by the health-care system or the public as differing from nutrition for the general population.

Both obesity and weight loss in the older person are associated with poor health outcomes. Poor diet and malnutrition are linked to chronic disease, decreased functional status, increased length of hospitalization, and increased mortality.[1] Decreased albumin and cholesterol are associated with malnutrition and increased mortality in older adults.[2]

The prevalence of nutritional deficiencies in the older population is not completely known. This is related to diversity of the population, lack of information regarding nutritional requirements beyond age 51, and need for better assessment tools to screen and diagnose nutritional deficiencies. One source suggests that up to 65% of older patients are protein-energy undernourished at admission or acquire nutritional deficits while hospitalized.[3] Nutritional data for the outpatient older population is limited, but nutritional deficiencies occur more frequently in frail and functionally dependent older adults than in those who are independent in the community. A metaanalysis of malnutrition in different elderly groups in the United Kingdom found community prevalence to be 5–10%, with an increase of 30–60% for homebound and hospitalized older patients.[4] In a cross-sectional study of 202 nursing homes on the east coast of the United States, 9.9% of the residents sampled had weight loss.[5]

For most people, eating is a pleasurable experience and a time to socialize. With aging, diet restrictions associated with chronic disease may limit food choices. In addition, certain physiologic age changes may bring bloating, gas, heartburn, reflux, and other discomforts. As taste, smell, and dentition are diminished, food textures and sensations may not be appreciated. Fine and gross motor incoordination and difficulty with chewing and swallowing may interfere with the social pleasure of eating food and even lead to fatigue and isolation.

Much nutritional information comes from nonprofessional sources, especially the media. Older adults often erroneously extrapolate such information. Many widely cited reports are based on studies of younger, healthier age groups, or represent a single dietary problem or disease, as with cholesterol and heart disease. Some information can actually be harmful to the frail older adult. To make matters worse, nutritional recommendations explicit to an older population are not included in most nursing and medical school curricula. Thus, diets for independent community-dwelling older persons with diabetes or coronary heart disease are also prescribed for frail, thin, nursing-home residents.

Greater awareness of geriatric nutrition is crucial with increasing life expectancy and desire for optimal levels of health. Population-appropriate recommendations, nutrition screening, and individualized nutrition prescriptions are essential. Gerontological advanced practice nurses (APNs) have a key role in educating the community, both professional and nonprofessional.

Risk Factors Associated with Poor Nutrition

Similar to many geriatric syndromes, the etiology of nutritional deficiencies is multifactorial. Aging itself may be a risk factor for nutritional problems. Three major classifications of risk factors exist:

Table 16–1   Risk Factors Associated with Nutritional Deficiencies

Physiological	Psychological	Social
COPD	Depression	Poverty
CHF, ASCVD	Despair	Isolation
DM	Delusion	Mobility
Hypo/hyperthyroid	Delirium	Abuse
Osteoporosis	Psychosis	Neglect
Hypercalcemia	Paranoia	Expensive drugs
CVA (stroke)	ETOH abuse	
Parkinson's disease	Drug abuse	Bereavement
Motor disorders	Excessive pacing	
Cancer	Excessive wandering	
Dementia	Fixation on diet prescriptions	
Collagen vascular disorders	Psychiatric medication	
HIV		
TB		
Nausea/vomiting		
Malabsorption		
Dysphagia		
Reflux		
Intestinal ischemia		
Constipation/ diarrhea		
Obesity		
Poor dentition		
Periodontal disease		
Xerostomia		
Sensory deficits: taste/smell sight/hearing		
Medications		
Increased metabolic rate: tremor		

Sources: Egbert AE. The dwindles: failure to thrive in older patients. *Nutr Rev.* 1996;54(1):S25–S30.

Lipschitz DA. Approaches to the nutritional support of the older patient. *Clin Geriatr Med.* 1995;11(4):715–725.

Wallace JI, Schwartz RS. Involuntary weight loss in elderly outpatients: recognition, etiologies and treatment. *Clin Geriatr Med.* 1997;13(4):717–735.

1. Physiological
2. Psychological
3. Social (Table 16–1)

Physiological factors include acute and chronic diseases and age-related phenomena resulting in increased caloric utilization or decreased caloric intake. Caloric losses occur with limited ability to eat, chew, or swallow, sensations of satiety, or diminished cues to eat. Obesity also suggests nutritional deficiency with a diet high in sugar and fat and low in nutrients. Identifying psychological and social risk factors is important. These may be the direct cause of nutritional problems exacerbating disease or worsening morbidity.

Very restrictive diet prescriptions may be an iatrogenic source of weight loss and anorexia. Any recommendation to limit calories, cholesterol, fat, and sugar in an individual over 70 years must be carefully made. This is particularly important when body weight is below normal.

Medications, both prescription and over the counter, can interfere with nutrition. Drugs may impair taste, cause anorexia, and produce gastrointestinal upset, malabsorption, or drug-related nutritional deficiencies secondary to binding nutrients and vitamins. Table 16–2 lists medications often associated with weight loss, anorexia, and nutritional deficiencies. Finally, a risk factor assessment is incomplete without an examination of living arrangement and the economic situations of the older person.

Physiologic Age-Related Body Changes

Physiologic changes associated with aging contribute to the older person's risk for nutritional problems. Almost every system must be considered (Table 16–3) when evaluating weight loss, anorexia, and nutrition. Taste and smell decline with age. Saliva flow decreases, producing xerostomia. Gustatory papillae atrophy, resulting in diminished taste for sweet and salty foods and an increased preference for tartness. Nerve damage, polyps, chronic allergies, colds, and smoking are suspected reasons for alter-

Table 16–2 Drugs Associated with Nutritional Problems and Anorexia

Cardiac:	Angiotensin II receptor blockers/angiotensin converting enzyme inhibitors
	Calcium channel blockers
	Beta blockers
	Hydralazine
	Reserpine
	Antiarrhythmics
	Furosemide
	Spironolactone
	Lanoxin
	Cholestyramine
Antidepressants:	Selective serotonin reuptake inhibitors (some may stimulate appetite)
Antipsychotics:	Lithium
	Phenothiazines
Antiparkinsons	
Anticonvulsants	
Antihistamines	
Antibiotics/anti-infectives	
Narcotics	
Theophylline	
Antineoplastics	
Baclofen	
Laxatives	
Antirheumatics	
Nonsteroidal anti-inflammatories	
Allopurinol	
Colchicine	
Nutritional supplements:	Ascorbic acid
	Zinc
	Tocopherol
	Ferrous sulfate

Sources: Egbert AE. The dwindles: failure to thrive in older patients. *Nutr Rev.* 1996;54(1):S25–S30.

Morley JE. Anorexia in older persons: epidemiology and optimal treatment. *Drugs Aging.* 1996;2:135–155.

Table 16–3 Age Changes Associated with Nutrition and Anorexia

I. **Body composition**
- increased fat mass
- decreased muscle mass (sarcopenia)
- decreased bone mass (osteopenia)

II. **Skin**
- decreased capacity for cholecalciferol synthesis

III. **Gastrointestinal system**
- decreased gastric motility
- increased gastric emptying time
- increased gastric pH
- decreased portal circulation
- decreased number of hepatocytes
- decreased absorptive surface area of small intestine

IV. **Taste**
- decreased production and flow of saliva
- decreased and atrophy of gustatory papillae
- decreased ability to taste sweets and salt

V. **Smell (anosmia)**
- possible nerve damage
- mucosal changes

VI. **Endocrine/hormone and immune milieu**
- increased CKK
- increased homocysteine
- decreased calcium
- change in hormonal environment, i.e., insulin, glucagon, lipids, amino acids

VII. **Central nervous system/brain**
- change in neurotransmitters, i.e., opioid, serotonin, oxytonin, ACTH
- atrophy in CNS: hypothalamus, amygdala, prefrontal cortex, brainstem

VIII. **Cardiac/renal/pulmonary changes associated with age and disease**

ations in olfaction, which declines markedly with Alzheimer's dementia and Parkinson's disease.[6]

Changes in body composition include a decrease in muscle mass and increase in fat, along with alterations in bone density. These changes appear responsible for a reduction in the basal metabolic rate (BMR).

Hormones and neurotransmitters concerned with appetite and satiation are altered with aging, including cholecystokinin, homocysteine, gastrin, glucagon, somatostatin, opioid, and serotonin neurotransmitters, adrenal corticotropin releasing hormone, oxytocin, estrogen, testosterone, progesterone, insulin, and thyroid hormones.[6,7] However, the role and action that these hormones and neurotransmitters exert on appetite and weight are unknown.

A combination of changes in the gastrointestinal system result in reflux, heartburn, constipation, bloating, and cramping. Gastric motility slows and emptying time increases. The pH in the stomach increases and the absorptive surface area of the small intestine decreases. Liver size decreases, the number of hepatocytes decline, and after age 20, portal blood flow decreases by 0.3–1.5% per year.[8]

 ## Nutritional Requirements for Older Adults

Recommended daily allowances (RDA) for persons above 51 years of age do not exist. In the absence of data, the nutritional requirements for those 51 years and above are used for all older adults. Table 16–4 provides these RDAs; however, the provider must be cautious in extrapolation to older adults. Careful evaluation of risk factors, age-related body changes, and health and disease profiles must precede any dietary prescription.

A modest research base suggests that specific micro- and macro-nutrient supplementation is needed by older adults to compensate for age-related losses, insufficient production of nutrients, and increased requirements associated with disease.

Debate exists regarding protein requirements. Currently, the RDA are 0.8 g/kg/day. It is also suggested, however, that the requirement should be increased to 1.5 g/kg/day because of greater risks for malnutrition during illness and hospitalization.[3] Decreased albumin is associated with pressure ulcer development; in the absence of protein, healing can be delayed. Although exact protein needs for older adults are now known, an albumin level consistently

Table 16–4 Recommended Daily Allowances (RDAs) for Persons 51 Years and Older

Nutrient	Men	Women
Protein (g)	60	46
Vitamin A (mcg RE)*	1000	800
Vitamin D (mcg)	400	400
Vitamin E (mcg)	10	8
Vitamin K (mcg)	80	65
Vitamin C (mg)	60	60
Thiamin (mg)	1.2	1.0
Riboflavin (mg)	1.4	1.2
Niacin (mg NE)†	15	13
Vitamin B_6 (mg)	2.0	1.6
Folate (mg)	0.2	0.18
Vitamin B_{12} (mcg)	2.0	2.0
Calcium (mg)	1000	1500 §
Phosphorus (mg)	800	800
Magnesium (mg)	350	280
Iron (elemental) (mg)	10	10
Zinc (mg)	15	12
Iodine (mcg)	150	150
Selenium (mcg)	70	55

*Retinol equivalents.
†IU
§ Postmenopausal, not receiving estrogen.
NE = Niacin equivalents
Source: Food and Nutrition Board. *Recommended Dietary Allowances.* 10th ed. National Academy of Sciences: Washington DC; 1989.

below 3.5% g/dl indicates protein malnutrition. Monitoring of protein, albumin, and prealbumin levels are useful guides, remembering that indices change with acute and chronic disease and hydration status.[9]

Calcium intake in older adults needs to be individualized. Lactose intolerance may be a barrier to adequate intake; furthermore, calcium absorption may be decreased with aging. Decreased absorption may be due to gastrointestinal resistance to the action of 1,25 dihydroxyvitamin D_3, related to decreased vitamin D receptors and atrophic gastritis impairing calcium bioavailability.[7] The recommendation for calcium supplementation in postmenopausal women is 1,000–1,500 mg/day.[10] Dosages need to consider coexisting diseases, for example, history of kidney stones, hyperparathyroidism, or certain cancers.

Vitamin B_{12} (cobalamine) malabsorption is increased secondary to atrophic gastritis, diet, and pernicious anemia. B_{12} deficiency can cause anemia and exacerbate dementia, depression, fatigue, and anorexia. In older adults, B_{12} supplementation is instituted when serum levels fall to 150–250 pmol/L.[11] Oral, parenteral, or intranasal administration is individualized. With serum levels above 300 pmol/L, supplementation can be oral. Intranasal administration is more costly and useful only after serum B_{12} has been repleted parenterally.

Vitamins B_6 and folate supplementation is often suggested for older adults, because of their association with cardiovascular benefits, immunity, and antibody response. Hyperhomocysteinemia, a risk factor for cardiovascular disease, can be modified with folate and B complex vitamins.[7,12] Folic acid dosage is typically 400 µg/day to 1000 µg/day. The RDA for B_6 is 2.0 mg/day to 25 mg/day; however, repletion secondary to deficiencies from nutrient–drug interactions is typically 50 mg/day.

Requirements for vitamin C, E, copper, and zinc are controversial. The RDA for vitamin C is 60 mg/day. Vitamin C (ascorbic acid) is required for optimal phagocytic function. Severe deficiency, such as in scurvy, is associated with poor wound healing and skin conditions in all age groups. The current practice of mega dosing with vitamin C to hasten wound healing is not empirically supported.[13] Vitamin C has been implicated in anorexia and gastric irritation.[6] Therefore, risk/benefit ratios need to be evaluated prior to prescribing high doses of vitamin C.

Zinc supplementation is also controversial. Zinc deficiency is also linked to poor wound healing; however, zinc excess is associated with depressed neutrophil function and lymphocytic response, as well as copper deficiency. Decreased copper results in impairment of peritoneal macrophages.[13,14] Although mega doses of zinc are often used with pressure ulcers, no studies demonstrate effectiveness of the treatment.

Vitamin E is associated with antioxidant action, improved immunity, memory preservation, and cardiovascular benefits. Supplementation of 400–1200 mg/day appears harmless. Vitamin E may act as a blood thinner, warranting careful monitoring with any anticoagulation or antiplatelet therapy.

Supplementation with iron may cause the gastrointestinal side effects of anorexia, constipation, and diarrhea. Unless a documented iron-deficiency anemia is present, iron should not be prescribed without an adequate workup. Determining the underlying cause of iron deficiency is important; typically, iron does not improve deficiency from chronic diseases. Iron may be effective in conjunction with epoetin in anemia from renal disease and certain anemias secondary to chronic disease. Such uses, however, remain very limited at this time.

In conclusion, vitamin supplementation in older adults is controversial due to limited evidence of effectiveness. Some supplementation may be beneficial, but mega doses may well have adverse effects.

Obesity

Obesity occurs when energy intake exceeds energy expenditure. Obesity is defined by body mass index (BMI) exceeding 30%. BMI is calculated by dividing weight in kilograms by height in meters squared. Obesity in older adults differs from younger adults who have an increase in both fat mass and fat-free mass. Older adults have increased fat mass, but low fat-free mass. Since BMI classifications are based on younger adults, indices must be carefully interpreted in older adults who have changes in bone and muscle mass. Virtually no studies of obesity in older adults exist; therefore, we know little about weight gain or loss, caloric restriction, morbidity, and mortality related to excessive weight.

The pathogenesis of obesity in the general population is multifactorial. Genetic, neurologic, psychologic, endocrine, and environmental factors all have varying roles. Medications, including antidepressants, tranquilizers, narcoleptics, beta-adrenergic agents, steroids, and hormones, have been associated with appetite stimulation. Lifestyle and eating habits clearly influence energy consumption and expenditure, and it is assumed that changes in activity and mobility with age influence development of obesity. Obesity is linked to increased morbidity and is also associated with diabetes, coronary heart disease, cancer, hypertension, hyperlipidemia, arthritis, and gallstones. When addressing obesity in older adults, one must consider age, comorbidity, lifestyle, and risks and benefits to caloric restrictions.

Drugs that suppress appetite in younger populations can be divided into several categories:

1. Those affecting the catecholinergic system (amphetamines, phenteramine, and phenylpropanolamine)
2. Those affecting the serotonergic system (fenfluramine and dexfenfluramine)
3. Those affecting the GABA receptors (biculine)
4. Those affecting peptinergic receptors (naloxone)
5. Those with serotonergic and catecholinergic effects (sibutramine)
6. Those affecting fat metabolism (orlistat).

Since catecholamines and GABA agents have central nervous system, cardiovascular, and peripheral vascular effects, they are not recommended for use in older adults. Chromium, ephedrine, anabolic steroids, and orlistat are also not recommended; ephedrine is associated with stroke, arrhythmia, and cardiac arrest. No carefully controlled studies of appetite suppressants have been conducted with older adults.

Any dietary restrictions or appetite suppressant requires careful assessment and clinical judgment. Lifestyle strategies aimed at increasing energy expenditure, decreasing fat mass, and increasing fat-free mass (bone and muscle density) are strongly encouraged. Exercise—aerobic and anaerobic, active and passive—and sensible eating with attention to basic food groups appears the safest method of treating obesity in older adults.

■ Dysphagia

Dysphagia causes weight loss and also contributes to morbidity and mortality in older adults. Two types of dysphagia, oropharyngeal and esophageal, are based on location of the abnormality. Odyno-phagia refers to painful swallowing. Dysphagia and Odynophagia can occur together or separately.[15]

Oropharyngeal dysphagia is a problem of transfer, occurring when a bolus of food does not move easily from the mouth into the esophagus. The pathology is above or proximal to the esophagus, usually secondary to a structural defect or neuromuscular problem linked to the brainstem. About 80% of patients with oropharyngeal dysphagia have a neuromuscular disorder.[16]

With oropharyngeal dysphagia, difficulty occurs in initiating a swallow and symptoms may be localized to the oropharynx. Liquids are implicated more frequently with oropharyngeal than esophageal dysphagia. Symptoms may include nasal regurgitation, cough during swallowing, dysarthria, or a wet hoarse voice.

Esophageal dysphagia usually affects the swallowing of solids and is a problem of transport. Normally, it takes 2–3 seconds for liquids and 8–10 seconds for solids to be transported through the esophagus. With esophageal dysphagia, transport time is lengthened as a result of mechanical obstruction (structural defect) or peristaltic contraction (neuromuscular effect).

Esophageal dysphagia causes a sensation of food sticking retrosternally or in the epigastric area. For diagnostic purposes, it is helpful to determine whether the problem is intermittent or progressive, the type of foods or liquids that cause difficulty, and any association with heartburn. Table 16–5 lists the causes of dysphagia in older adults.

Evaluation and Management of Dysphagia

Dysphagia increases with age. It is a symptom with multiple pathologies and requires thorough investigation. The history is an essential and crucial tool in the correct evaluation of dysphagia. Figure 16–1 provides an algorithm for determining the cause of dysphagia. Management depends on the etiology.

History

- ■ Medical, dental, and surgical (head, neck, throat, oral lung, esophagus)
- ■ Family history

Table 16-5 Common Causes of Dysphagia in Older Adults

Oropharyngeal

I. Central & Peripheral Nervous System Lesions and Muscular Diseases

Cerebrovascular accidents
Parkinson's disease
Amyotrophic lateral sclerosis
Multiple sclerosis
Bulbar poliomyelitis
(Poly)neuropathies
Myasthenia gravis
Muscular dystrophies
Endocrine myopathy

II. Structural Lesions

Carcinoma
Cricoid webs
Postsurgical scarring
Inflammatory lesions
Anterior cervical osteophytes

III. Upper Esophageal Sphincter (UES) Disorders

Hypertensive UES
Abnormal relaxation of the UES
Abnormal opening of the UES

Esophageal

I. Motility Disorders

Achalasia
Ineffective esophageal motility
Scleroderma
Esophageal spasm
Nutcracker esophagus
Hypertensive lower esophageal sphincter (LES)

II. Mechanical Lesions

Carcinoma
Stricture (peptic or medication induced)
Lower esophageal ring (Schatzi's) or webs
Esophagitis
Diverticula
Vascular compression

- Medication review
- Attempt to classify as oropharyngeal or esophageal: other neurologic symptoms, weakness, paresis, speech problems, hoarseness, does the food stick in the pharynx or esophagus?
- Is the dysphagia with solids or liquids or both?
- Is the dysphagia acute (over one month) or progressive?
- Is the dysphagia intermittent or continuous?
- Nutritional history
- Diet history

Review of Systems

- Weight loss, weakness, fatigue, appetite
- Mental status: dementia, psychiatric, depression, psychosis
- HEENT (head, eyes, ears, nose, throat): oral problems, oral sores, dentures, drooling, pain
- Endocrine: diabetes, thyroid
- Gastrointestinal: reflux, nausea, vomiting, heartburn, burping
- Cardiovascular: hypertension, chest pain during meals, dyspnea
- Pulmonary: tobacco, cough
- Neurologic: weakness; paresis; numbness of lips, tongue, or jaw; CVA

Physical Examination

- Complete physical examination with attention to head, oropharynx, neck, and neurologic system
- Perform a mental status exam with attention to motor activity, cognitive function, thought processes, and content and mood

Laboratory and Diagnostic Evaluation

- Blood work to rule out metabolic, endocrine pathology
- Barium swallow to assess swallow function and identify stricture, tumors, diverticula, webs

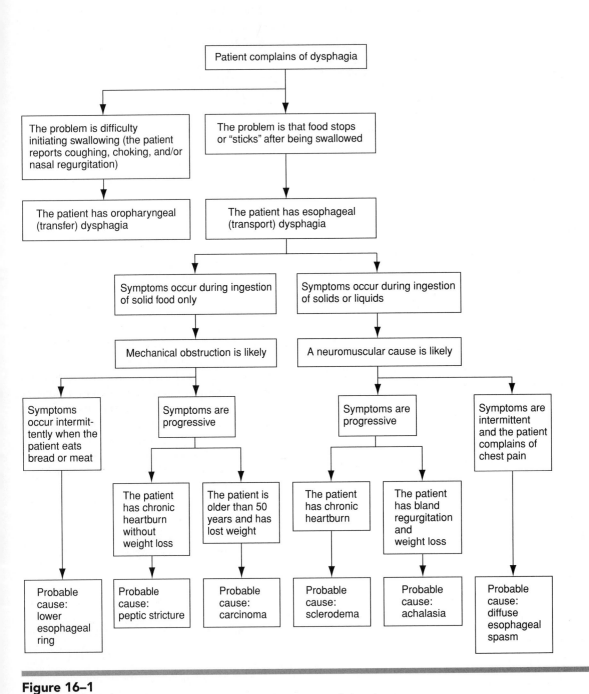

Figure 16–1

Using the clues in the history to determine the cause of dysphagia.

Source: Champion G, Richter JE. Esophageal dysphagia: Is the cause benign or potentially deadly? *J Crit Illness.* 1998;13:21.

- Endoscopy to visualize reflux esophagitis, Barrett's esophagus
- Barium swallow and endoscopy for visualization and biopsy, and assessment of motor function
- Esophageal manometry to diagnose esophageal motility disorders
- Chest x-ray for suspected aspiration
- Referral to speech therapist
- Referral to gastroenterologist, dentist, neurologist

Management of Dysphagia

Individualized management of dysphagia depends on clinical presentation, patient circumstances, and practitioner judgment. All treatable causes need to be addressed. Malignancy must be ruled out. A speech therapy evaluation with swallow therapy may be helpful to manage symptoms caused by neuromuscular problems. Postural maneuvers, muscle strengthening, and changing food consistency are techniques that can assure nutrition and minimal complication. If adequate nutrition cannot be met orally, enteral routes may be considered.

The following medications can cause esophageal injury; consider empirically stopping or substituting and treating for esophageal injury:

- Tetracycline
- Doxycycline
- Potassium
- Ascorbic acid
- Ferrous sulfate
- Nonsteroidal anti-inflammatory
- Corticosteroids
- Acetylsalicylic acid
- Quinidine
- Alendronate
- Theophylline

Gastroesophageal reflux disease (GERD) with peptic stricture or dysmotility is the most common reason for esophageal dysphagia.[15] Treatment of GERD includes lifestyle modification, medication, and esophageal dilatation.

Lifestyle changes include:

1. Proper chewing of food
2. Adequate dentition
3. Avoidance of foods that decrease lower esophageal sphincter (fatty foods, chocolate, peppermint, alcohol, some fruit juices)
4. Eliminating caffeinated foods (coffee, cola, tea) that increase acid secretion
5. Avoiding large meals that slow gastric emptying and switching to smaller, more frequent meals.

Administration of histamine 2 receptor antagonists and proton pump inhibitors can decrease acid secretion.

Dysmotility problems are also common. Achalasia is an idiopathic disorder with neurologic origins leading to decreased peristalsis and failure of the lower esophageal sphincter to relax. Reflux of solids and/or liquids occurs, bringing symptoms of chest pain and weight loss. Malignancy must be ruled out when these symptoms appear. Treatment of achalasia includes pneumatic dilatation, injection of botulism toxin, esophagotomy, and medication. Pneumatic dilatation is less expensive and requires a shorter hospital stay than esophagotomy; however, risk of perforation is about 5%. Injection with botulism toxin relieves symptoms for about 6–12 months, is less invasive than pneumatic dilatation and esophagotomy, and is becoming the treatment of choice in older adults.[17] Medication therapy includes smooth muscle relaxants and anticholinergics.

Esophageal cancer should be suspected when the dysphagia is acute, of short duration (less than 6 months), occurs with solids, and is accompanied by rapid weight loss. A history of smoking or heavy alcohol use may be other clues in making a differential diagnosis. Surgical resection may be possible; however, by the time symptoms develop, the cancer is typically incurable. Therefore, management is largely palliative, including radiation, chemotherapy, and stent placement.[17]

Cachexia

Cachexia is a syndrome manifested by anorexia, weight loss, metabolic alterations, and weakness. These occur secondary to increased metabolic demands, increased protein breakdown, altered protein synthesis, and increased cytokinin production. Cancer is the typical underlying cause; however, cachexia also occurs in end-stage cardiac and pulmonary disease, and rheumatoid arthritis. End-stage dementia is also associated with anorexia and cachexia. Cachexia differs from starvation, which is characterized by decreased metabolic rate, little alteration in protein breakdown, and initially, preservation of skeletal muscle.[6] With starvation or anorexia, a complicating end-stage disease is not usually present.

Cachexia associated with cardiac disease is related to an increased BMR, increased protein breakdown, altered hepatic protein synthesis, protein losses from enteropathy and early satiety, and nausea secondary to gastroparesis, autonomic neuropathy, and edema of the small bowel. Iatrogenic causes of anorexia also complicate this syndrome. Many cardiac medications have gastrointestinal side effects or cause dry mouth and altered taste.

Rheumatoid arthritis-associated cachexia is probably caused by increased tumor necrosis factor and interleuken, both of which are cytokinins implicated in anorexia. Increased BMR and decreased intake of protein, along with pain, fatigue, depression, and medication side effects add to the problem.

Normally, breathing expends about 36–72 calories per day. In chronic obstructive pulmonary disease (COPD), caloric expenditure increases 10 times this amount due to increased respiratory muscle effort and increased pulmonary resistance. Poor oral intake is also related to taste, fatigue, dyspnea, depression, early satiety, and medication side effects.

Cachexia occurs in older adults without identifiable cause, known as Idiopathic Senile Anorexia[18] or failure to thrive. Little is known about the risk factors, development, diagnosis, or treatment of this phenomenon. Potentially treatable causes of anorexia need to be evaluated, and failure to thrive should be a diagnosis of exclusion.[19]

Cancer is the most common condition associated with cachexia. Severity and progression varies with the cancer. Cachexia appears to be a paraneoplastic condition maintained by tumor necrosis factor. Altered glucose and lipid metabolism, and decreased gluconeogenesis, are also associated with cancer-related cachexia. A tumor enlarging in the gastrointestinal tract exacerbates pain, early satiety, nausea, and vomiting. Again, increased BMR, stomatitis, and medications greatly contribute to the problem.

Management of Cachexia

Management needs to be tailored to specific patient needs, as outlined below:

1. Treat underlying pathology if appropriate
2. Control pain
3. Manage depression
4. Early satiety: small frequent meals, limit foods that delay gastric emptying (highly fatty foods), consider drugs that increase gastric emptying (metoclopramide)
5. Consider fatigue: frequent rest periods, avoid awakening for treatments and medication if possible
6. Control nausea, vomiting, GI upset: acknowledge food and odor aversions, recognize medication side effects, consider reducing or eliminating anorexant medications, monitor for drug toxicity (lanoxin, theophylline, phenytoin, phenobarbital, valproic acid, mysoline, lithium), consider medication to reduce symptoms (compazine, tigan, metoclopramide)
7. Treat stomatitis and mucositis: viscous lidocaine
8. Control xerostomia: oral hygiene, sour candy and lemon drops, spray bottle with lemon water to increase salivation, artificial saliva preparations
9. Encourage nutrient-dense foods high in calories and proteins: supplement with commercially prepared puddings and milkshakes

10. Address psychosocial issues: social inter-action, meal availability and preparation

11. Consider medications that stimulate appetite (note that research has failed to demonstrate benefits)

Carefully consider enteral nutrition for noncur-able cancers and end-stage cardiac, pulmonary, and rheumatological disease. Tube feeding is associated with side effects, including aspiration, nausea, vomiting, diarrhea, constipation, and abdominal distention and cramping. Consider the risks and benefits; forcing nutrition in end-stage disease may only prolong a life of limited quality. In some cases, it may even hasten mortality secondary to complication.[20,21]

Nutritional Risk Assessment

Identifying risks for nutritional problems is an inte-gral part of the health evaluation. Signs and symp-toms are subtle and often attributed to age. Many tools exist for screening risk or identifying disease. Questionnaires, laboratory indices, and anthropo-metric measurements vary in cost, sensitivity, time to administer, and reliability. Nutritional assess-ment needs to be simple, easy to administer, cost effective, reproducible, and reliable. A stepwise approach should be incorporated into the initial visit of any older adult. The appropriate portions of an initial comprehensive history and physical examination for an older adult follows.

History

Inquire about involuntary weight loss, fit of cloth-ing, and change in appetite. If the patient is thin, is this usual? Are there illnesses that may lead to nutritional deficiencies, such as malabsorption syndromes, chronic diarrhea, wounds, fistulas, or abscesses? Is there an illness that limits the person from eating? Inquire about living and social ac-commodations, recent deaths of significant others, and financial status as clues to depression, social isolation, or inability to afford nutritional foods. Is the patient independent or dependent on others to shop or prepare meals? Ask about meals and snacks for a typical day. Ask the patient or care-giver whether nutritional problems exist.

Activities of Daily Living (ADLs) and Exercise History   Inquire about daily activities and mobil-ity, and any recent changes. Inquire about type, amount, and duration of exercise and any change in tolerance.

Review of Systems

- General: weakness, fatigue, alcohol and drug problems, pain
- Psychiatric: depression, sleep pattern, coor-dination, memory
- Hair: changes
- Eyes: vision changes
- Oropharynx: dentition, oral discomfort, dry mouth
- Cardiac: cardiac problems, chest pain, con-gestive heart failure, hypertension
- Pulmonary: COPD, oxygen therapy, tobacco, cough
- Gastrointestinal: nausea, vomiting, diarrhea, constipation, chewing or swallowing prob-lems, heartburn, reflux
- Hematological and endocrine: diabetes, thy-roid, anemia
- Genitourinary: fluid intake, renal problems, dialysis
- Musculoskeletal: range of motion, deformi-ties, atrophy, gout, arthritis, fractures
- Peripheral vascular: swelling, pain
- Skin: nail changes, rashes, pruritis, sores, lesions, bruises
- Neurologic: paresis, paresthesia, numbness, cerebrovascular accident (CVA)
- Medications: prescription, over the counter, herbal remedies, and vitamins

Physical Examination

- Anthropometric measures: height and weight
- Mental Status: consider Mini-Mental State Exam,[22] Geriatric Depression Scale[23]

Mini Nutritional Assessment
MNA®

Last name:	First name:	Sex:	Date:
Age:	Weight, kg:	Height, cm:	I.D. Number:

Complete the screen by filling in the boxes with the appropriate numbers.
Add the numbers for the screen. If score is 11 or less, continue with the assessment to gain a Malnutrition Indicator Score.

Screening

A Has food intake declined over the past 3 months due to loss of appetite, digestive problems, chewing or swallowing difficulties?
0 = severe loss of appetite
1 = moderate loss of appetite
2 = no loss of appetite ☐

B Weight loss during last months
0 = weight loss greater than 3 kg (6.6 lbs)
1 = does not know
2 = weight loss between 1 and 3 kg (2.2 and 6.6 lbs)
3 = no weight loss ☐

C Mobility
0 = bed or chair bound
1 = able to get out of bed/chair but does not go out
2 = goes out ☐

D Has suffered psychological stress or acute disease in the past 3 months
0 = yes   2 = no ☐

E Neuropsychological problems
0 = severe dementia or depression
1 = mild dementia
2 = no psychological problems ☐

F Body Mass Index (BMI) (weight in kg) / (height in m)²
0 = BMI less than 19
1 = BMI 19 to less than 21
2 = BMI 21 to less than 23
3 = BMI 23 or greater ☐

Screening score subtotal max. 14 points) ☐ ☐

12 points or greater — Normal – not at risk – no need to complete assessment

11 points or below — Possible malnutrition – continue assessment

Assessment

G Lives independently (not in a nursing home or hospital)
0 = no   1 = yes ☐

H Takes more than 3 prescription drugs per day
0 = yes   1 = no ☐

I Pressure sores or skin ulcers
0 = yes   1 = no ☐

J How many full meals does the patient eat daily?
0 = 1 meal
1 = 2 meals
2 = 3 meals ☐

K Selected consumption markers for protein intake
• At least one serving of dairy products (milk, cheese, yogurt) per day?   yes ☐ no ☐
• Two or more serving of legumes or eggs per week?   yes ☐ no ☐
• Meat, fish or poultry every day   yes ☐ no ☐
0.0 = if 0 or 1 yes
0.5 = if 2 yes
1.0 = if 3 yes ☐ ☐

L Consumes two or more servings of fruits or vegetables per day?
0 = no   1 = yes ☐

M How much fluid (water, juice, coffee, tea, milk...) is consumed per day?
0.0 = less than 3 cups
0.5 = 3 to 5 cups
1.0 = more than 5 cups ☐ ☐

N Mode of feeding
0 = unable to eat without assistance
1 = self-fed with some difficulty
2 = self-fed without any problem ☐

O Self view of nutritional status
0 = view self as being malnourished
1 = is uncertain of nutritional state
2 = views self as having no nutritional problem ☐

P In comparison with other people of the same age, how do they consider their health status?
0.0 = not as good
0.5 = does not know
1.0 = as good
2.0 = better ☐ ☐

Q Mid-arm circumference (MAC) in cm
0.0 = MAC less than 21
0.5 = MAC 21 to 22
1.0 = MAC 22 or greater ☐ ☐

R Calf circumference (CC) in cm
0 = CC less than 31   1 = CC 31 or greater ☐

Assessment (max. 16 points) ☐ ☐ ☐

Screening score ☐ ☐

Total Assessment (max. 30 points) ☐ ☐

Malnutrition Indicator Score

17 to 23.5 points ☐

Less than 17 points ☐

08.98 USA

Ref.: Guigoz Y, Vellas B and Garry PJ. 1994. Mini Nutritional Assessment: A practical assessment tool for grading the nutritional state of elderly patients. *Facts and Research in Gerontology.* Supplement #2:15-59.
Rubenstein LZ, Harker J, Guigoz Y and Vellas B. Comprehensive Geriatric Assessment (CGA) and the MNA: An Overview of CGA, Nutritional Assessment, and Development of a Shortened Version of the MNA. In: "Mini Nutritional Assessment (MNA): Research and Practice in the Elderly". Vellas B, Garry PJ and Guigoz Y, editors. Nestlé Nutrition Workshop Series. Clinical & Performance Programme, vol. 1. Karger, Bâle, in press.

® Société des Produits Nestlé S.A., Vevey, Switzerland, Trademark Owners

Figure 16–2

The Mini Nutritional Assessment (MNA) form is useful for initial screening.

- Function: ADLs[24] and Independent Activities of Daily Living (IADLs)[25]

- HEENT: alopecia, pale conjunctiva, nasolabial seborrhea, stomatitis, glossitis, swollen bleeding gums, fissured tongue, cheilosis, xerosis, teeth, denture fit, sores, pain, lesions

- Cardiac, pulmonary, GI: cachexia, increased use of accessory muscles, hepatomegaly, ascites, edema

- Musculoskeletal: deformities, atrophy, arthralgia, kyphosis, degenerative joints, muscular wasting, Tinetti Gait, and Balance Scale[26]

- Skin: dermatitis, xerosis, petechiae, ecchymosis, pressure ulcers

Laboratory and Diagnostic Evaluation

- Complete blood count (CBC) with platelets and differential, iron, mean corpuscular volume (MCV)

- B_{12}, folate

- Lipid profile

- Hepatic profile

- Electrolytes, calcium, phosphorous

- Blood urea nitrogen (BUN), creatinine

- Thyroid profile

- Protein, albumin

- Glucose

Among existing nutritional assessment tools, none have been extensively validated for older adults. For initial screening purposes the Mini Nutritional Assessment (MNA)[4] is easily included in a health visit. It incorporates the clinical, dietary, biochemical, anthropometric, and functional evaluations routinely obtained in an older person (Figure 16–2).

The Determine Your Nutritional Health Checklist, developed by Nutrition Screening Initiative (NSI), can be self-administered (Figure 16–3). Ten questions pertain to meals, foods and liquids, finances, health, and function. It serves as a useful alert to the patient, caregiver, and primary-care provider and can be used as an educational tool.

Indicators of Nutritional Risk

1. Weight loss: > 5 pounds in 1 month
   > 5% weight loss in 1 month
   > 7.5% in 3 months
   > 10% in 6 months

2. Change in function, health, or mental status

3. Score < 23.5 on MNA

4. Score < 2 on the Determine Your Nutritional Health Checklist

5. Laboratory indices: Degree of Malnutrition

Albumin	< 3.5 g/dL
Cholesterol	< 160 mg/dL
Transferrin	> 200 mg/dL: normal
	151–200 mg/dL: mild
	100–150 mg/dL: moderate
	< 100 mg/dL: severe
Prealbumin (transhytrin)	10–15 mg/dL: mild
	5–10 mg/dL: moderate
	< 5 mg/dL: severe
Total lymphocyte count	> 2,000 cell/mm: normal
	1,200–2,000 cell/mm: mild
	800–1,200 cell/mm: moderate
	< 800 cell/mm: severe

With the above information, determine whether a condition might exist that would explain the deficiency or weight loss. Determine if intake is adequate, food utilization is poor, or increased nutrient requirements exist. Laboratory indices that are sometimes used as nutritional indicators lack specificity with regard to malnutrition and may also reflect acute or chronic illness.

Hypoalbuminemia also occurs with acute and chronic disease, and possibly normal aging. It is not sensitive to early nutritional change, secondary to the prolonged half-life, approximately 20 days. Transferrin has a shorter half-life than albumin (days). It is an acute phase reactant to inflammation, infection, and iron transport. In the presence of iron deficiency and inflammation, it is elevated and therefore is not a sensitive indicator of malnutrition.[9] Prealbumin is also used as a marker of nutritional status. The half-life is 2–3 days and responds to nutrient imbalance within

The warning signs of poor nutritional health are often overlooked. Use this checklist to find out if you or someone you know is at nutritional risk.

DETERMINE YOUR NUTRITIONAL HEALTH

Read the statements below. Circle the number in the **yes** column for those that apply to you or someone you know. For each yes answer, score the number in the box. Total your nutritional score.

	YES
I have an illness or condition that made me change the kind and/or amount of food I eat.	2
I eat fewer than 2 meals per day	3
I eat few fruits, vegetables, or milk products.	2
I have 3 or more drinks of beer, liquor, or wine almost every day.	2
I have tooth or mouth problems that make it hard for me to eat.	2
I don't always have enough money to buy the food I need.	4
I eat alone most of the time.	1
I take 3 or more different prescribed or over-the-counter drugs a day.	1
Without wanting to, I have lost or gained 10 pounds in the last 6 months.	2
I am not always physically able to shop for, cook for, and/or feed myself.	2
TOTAL	

Total Your Nutritional Score. If it's—

0–2   Good! Recheck your nutritional score in 6 months.

3–5   You are at moderate nutritional risk. See what can be done to improve your eating habits and lifestyle. Your office of aging, senior nutrition program, senior citizens center, or health department can help. Recheck your nutritional score in 3 months.

6 or more   You are at high nutritional risk. Bring this checklist the next time you see your doctor, dietitian, or other qualified health or social service professional. Talk with them about any problems you may have. Ask for help to improve your nutritional health.

Adapted from: *Nutritional Screening Initiative: Incorporating Nutrition Screening and Intervention into Medical Practice: A Monograph for Physicians.* The American Academy of Family Physicians, the American Dietetic Association, and the National Council on the Aging.

Figure 16–3
The Determine Your Nutritional Health Checklist can be self-administered.

seven days. Like transferrin, prealbumin responds to inflammation, infection, and stress, but it is not sensitive to malnutrition.[9,27] Total lymphocyte count (TLC) is decreased in malnutrition. Again, this is a poor indicator of nutritional status since it can be increased or decreased in many pathologic processes.

Management

Addressing malnutrition and weight loss encompasses:

1. Understanding and treating underlying causes of malnutrition or weight loss
2. Dietary modification
3. Social and environmental modification
4. Pharmacological intervention

Treat Underlying Cause Determine first if malnutrition or weight loss is due to a pathologic process and if caloric intake is adequate. If possible, alteration in the medication regime can be attempted.

Dietary Modification

- Individualized diet/meal plans
- Alternate liquids and solids and hot and cold foods
- Provide soft-textured and finger foods
- Consider speech therapy evaluation
- A variety of nutritional supplements are on the market; cost and taste vary (Table 16–6)

Social and Environmental Modification

- Meals on Wheels: program available through Area Agency on Aging
- Geriatric day program with meals
- Assisted living facility with dining program
- Home health referral for meal preparation assistance
- Caregiver education/awareness:
  - attention to posture and positioning during meals
  - good lighting
  - attention to unappetizing odors and sights, especially in long-term care facilities where other residents have catheters, odors, tubes, incontinence, or unpleasant eating styles
  - attention to the dining environment: Is it too stimulating? unpleasant? noisy?

Pharmacological Intervention

Megestrol Acetate This is a synthetic derivative of a progestational agent that has been approved for appetite stimulation and weight gain in AIDS and cancer patients. One study demonstrated improved appetite and well being after 12 weeks of treatment.[28] A 12-week trial can be considered; side effects include fluid retention and thromboembolism. It is contraindicated in patients with history of heart failure, pulmonary embolism, and deep vein thrombosis. The recommended dose for cancer is 400–800 mg/day. No data is available about older adults; trial start at 40 mg twice daily, titrating up to 800 mg/day.

Cyproheptadine This is a serotonin agent with anecdotal evidence for increasing appetite, despite absence of support from the literature. Because of anticholinergic and antihistaminic actions, this drug is *not* recommended for older adults.[29]

Pentoxifylline Used for peripheral arterial disease, this drug decreases tumor necrosis factor and therefore was thought that it may improve appetite. No empiric support exists for improved appetite or weight gain in cancer.[29]

Melatonin This is a pineal hormone found to decrease tumor necrosis factor in advanced cancer patients with dosages of 20 mg/day.[30] Since harm to older adults is not documented, a trial can be considered.

Methylphenidate Hydrochloride This drug paradoxically acts as a CNS stimulant in older adults, thus increasing food intake. No careful studies have been performed; however, anecdotal success is cited. A trial can be considered. Starting

Table 16-6   Nutritional Supplementation

Oral Nutritional Supplements			
Product	Calories	Protein	
Carnation Breakfast	250/9 oz		Milk based
Great Shake	250/9 oz		Milk based
Shake Ups	250/9 oz		Milk based
Resource Shake	200/4 oz	6 g/4 oz	
Resource Pudding	250/4 oz	9 g/4 oz	
Sustacal Pudding	240/5 oz	6.8 g/5 oz	
Ensure Pudding	240/5 oz	6.8 g/5 oz	
Resource Plus Ice Cream	290/4.5 oz	9 g/4.5 oz	High caloric
Boost	250/8 oz		
Nu Basics	250/8 oz		
Ensure	250/8 oz		
Boost Plus	375/8 oz		High caloric
Nu Basics Plus	375/8 oz		High caloric
Ensure Plus	375/8 oz		High caloric
Resource Plus	375/8 oz		High caloric
Deliver 2.0	500/8 oz		Calorically dense
Novosource 2.0	500/8 oz		Calorically dense
Two Cal HN	500/8 oz		Calorically dense
Nu Basics 2.0	500/8 oz		Calorically dense
Boost HP	250/8 oz		High protein
Ensure HP	250/8 oz		High protein
Promote	250/8 oz		High protein
Sustacal	250/8 oz	8.8 g/8 oz	High protein
Resource Diet Shake	200/8 oz	8 g/8 oz	For diabetics
Glucerna	240/8 oz		For diabetics
Boost Bar	125/bar		Soft chewable
Resource Bar	125/bar		Soft chewable
Ensure Bar	125/bar		Soft chewable
Protein Powders: Can Be Added to Shakes, Soups, or Foods			
Promod		7.5/10 g powder	
Casec		8.8/10 g powder	
Prosource		7.5/10 g powder	

dose is 2.5 mg two to three times daily, 30 minutes prior to meals.

Corticosteroids   Glucocorticoids affect appetite and mood and may cause weight gain on a short-term basis. No studies demonstrate long-term weight gain and improved quality of life in older adults. Given the serious side effects, use for weight gain is controversial.

Oxandrolone   This is a testosterone analogue with anabolic activity that improves lean mass and possibly weight gain following extensive surgery, severe infection, trauma, AIDS, and severe burns.

It is FDA approved for the above indications. Side effects include liver abnormalities, CNS changes, and edema. Contraindications are prostate cancer, male breast cancer, hypercalcemia, and nephrosis. Adult dosage is 2.5 mg two to four times/day, up to 20 mg/day. A course of therapy is two to four weeks, repeated intermittently.[31]

Antidepressant Therapy Treatment of depression often improves appetite, mentation, and cognition with weight gain as an outcome. The newer selective serotonin reuptake inhibitors (mirtazapine, venlafaxine) have less gastrointestinal and anorexant side effects. Mirtazapine lists appetite stimulation as a side effect.

Enteral Nutrition

Enteral nutrition for anorexia of aging syndromes is a controversial medical practice "with recognized, although generally unacknowledged, iatrogenic effects."[20] Little data supports use in older adults. Furthermore, no data exists demonstrating long-term benefit in advanced or end-stage disease; for example, advanced dementia, end-stage COPD, severe congestive heart failure, other advanced cardiac diseases, and incurable cancers. The literature describes the risks and complications of enteral nutrition, the poor prognosis, and high morbidity and mortality.[21]

Many misconceptions exist regarding the effectiveness of enteral nutrition in geriatrics. Prevention of aspiration, healing of pressure ulcers and wounds, and treatment of infection and sepsis are often reasons for initiating enteral feeding. Nevertheless, enteral nutrition does not prevent aspiration; rather it increases it, especially in persons with advanced dementia, COPD, and cardiac disease.[21,32]

Although poor nutrition impedes wound healing, no data exists to demonstrate the benefit of enteral nutrition in healing pressure ulcers.[32–34] It is thought that the combination of poor health, concurrent illness, and chronicity cannot be overcome by enteral nutrition. In addition, the complications of aspiration pneumonia, infection, immobility, and incontinence create greater risks for pressure ulcer sepsis.

No support exists for the use of long-term enteral nutrition as a comfort measure in end-stage disease. More likely, the complications cause hardship and pain. If the maintenance of enteral lines result in physical restraints, discomfort is only worsened, and dignity and autonomy are seriously jeopardized. Comfort measures in end-stage disease and anorexia of aging, such as accepted and tolerated food and fluids, ice chips, glycerin swabs, positioning, and companionship are far more beneficial in their contribution to a peaceful and painless end.[35–38]

A few conditions may benefit from enteral nutrition, including CVA with dysphagia or other neurologic conditions with clear and intact mental status, malabsorption syndromes, mild to moderate dementia, and curable cancers or obstructions. Withdrawal of tube feeding needs to be an option when functional and mental status worsen, or the disease advances to the point where benefit is unlikely and quality of life is absent.

Enteral nutrition cannot be undertaken lightly. Comprehensive family and caregiver education and guidance regarding the risks, complications, long-term consequences, high morbidity and mortality, and limited benefits need to be explored. Misconceptions must be addressed, if possible by a team of informed and involved health-care providers. The APN must be aware of the risks and burdens of enteral nutrition, employ evidence-based practice, and act as resource person, mediator, and educator regarding the appropriate use of enteral feeding.

Routes for Enteral Nutrition

When appropriately prescribed, three routes exist for enteral nutrition:

1. nasogastric (NG)
2. jejunostomy (JT)
3. gastrostomy (GT).

The NG route is seldom used in older adults and never used on a long-term basis. Risk of aspiration is high. If implemented short term, placement should be verified prior to feeding, preferably radiographically, with strict aspiration precautions in place.

1. Prior to implementing enteral nutrition, determine that artificial feeding is indicated, will improve quality of life, and will not cause morbidity or mortality.

2. Initiating tube feeding:

   ■ Start "low and slow": good start rate is 30 cc/hr, or 120 cc q 4 hr bolus

   ■ Gradually increase rate via pump 10 to 15 cc/hr every 24–36 hours. May need to be slower

   ■ Increase via bolus 60 cc every 24–36 hours

   ■ Monitor for intolerance to feeding: vomiting, diarrhea, abdominal distention and bloating, coughing, choking, change in mental status, cramping

   ■ Monitor vital signs: blood pressure, heart rate, respirations, temperature

   ■ Check lungs for signs of aspiration

3. Check for Dobhoff tube placement prior to initiating feeding

4. Monitor feeding tube insertion site (nares, stoma) for signs of breakdown or infection

5. Check residual prior to start of feeding (difficult with JT site); do not supplement if residual is greater that 50–100 cc. Wait 1–2 hours and check residual again

6. Assess for abdominal distention, bowel sounds, pain prior to giving feedings

7. Observe aspiration precautions:

   ■ Elevate head of bed at 35–45-degree angle during and 1 hr post feeding

   ■ Turn tube feeding off prior to turning and positioning

8. Know nutrient drug interactions and contraindications

9. Monitor hydration and electrolytes weekly for the first month, then every 3–6 months

10. Water flushes 150–200 cc 3–6 times daily; individualize according to age, weight, clinical hydration status, and coexistent disease, especially CHF, SIADH, fever, sepsis, dehydration

11. Oral hygiene 3 times/day, more as necessary to prevent xerostomia and periodontal disease

12. Continue to offer foods orally if dysphagia is not a concern. This aids in normal lifestyle, oral hygiene, digestion, and elimination

13. Monitor for enteral nutrition complications (Table 16–7)

Figure 16–4
Protocols for enteral nutrition in older adults.

The JT route is also seldom used. It requires a catheter with a very narrow lumen, which easily obstructs and requires numerous replacements. Because of the narrowness and pliability of the catheter, it is impossible to check for retention by syringe aspiration. Although it is thought that aspiration occurs less frequently with the JT route, research does not support this idea. JT insertion is not indicated or practical in older adults with the exception of total gastrectomy.

GT is the most practical site for older adults. The procedure can be done percutaneously in the hospital or as an outpatient procedure. When enteral feeding is indicated, care must be taken to reduce complications. A protocol for implementing enteral nutrition is presented in Figure 16–4. Enteral feeding complications, their causes, and management are outlined in Table 16–7. Table 16–8 lists types of enteral nutrition supplements.

■ Nutrition in Long-Term Care

Nursing Facilities

Prompted by the history of abuse and neglect of nursing home residents, federal regulations were adopted by the Omnibus Budget Reconciliation Act, 1987 (OBRA) to ensure standards of nursing home care. These standards include:

1. Assessment of nutritional status and requirements in the comprehensive resident assessment

2. Assurance that the resident maintains acceptable parameters of nutritional status, such as body weight and protein levels, unless the clinical condition demonstrates that this is impossible

3. A therapeutic diet for any nutritional problem.

Additional standards must be met for long-term care facility accreditation by the Joint Commission on Accreditation of Healthcare Organizations (JCAHO). JCAHO standards for nutrition include:

1. Screening for nutritional risk

2. Assessing for nutritional intervention and counseling

3. Developing a plan of nutritional care

4. Prescribing nutrition products

5. Preparing, distributing, and administering food and nutrition products

6. Monitoring response to the nutritional care plan.

Separate standards exist for dementia special care units and subacute programs, related to the specific nutritional risk factors, assessments, and needs of these residents.

Table 16-7   Causes and Management of Enteral Nutrition (EN) Complications

Complication	Causes	Management
Aspiration	• Reflux/vomiting • Poor cough reflex • Unable to handle saliva • Too rapid infusion rate • Concurrent respiratory problems (COPD, CHF) • Improper NG placement • Body alignment: contractures kyphoscoliosis • Position during infusion head down, turning	• Aspiration alone is not an indication to recommend EN • Begin EN "low & slow" • Elevate head of bed • Change to pump feeding • Change to higher cal/cc formula and use lower infusion rate • Temporarily stop infusion • Monitor for residuals • Dry oral secretions (sal-tropine hycosamine) • Dry respiratory secretions (Albuterol nebs, guaifenesin) • Trial metclopramide to decrease reflux
Blockage	• Formula retained in tubes • Small lumen • Pill fragments • Improper placement of balloon	• Use infusion pump • Use elixers • Avoid giving medications together • Flush tube well
Leakage at stoma, skin irritation	• Internal tube migration causing obstruction • Gastrocutaneous fistula	• Use bumper to prevent retraction into stoma (internal migration occurs more commonly with Foley catheters) • Use of a clamping device • Consider radiographic study to evaluate for abscess/fistula • Avoid use of occlusive dressings

(continues)

Table 16-7   Causes and Management of Enteral Nutrition (EN) Complications   *(continued)*

Complication	Causes	Management
Diarrhea	• Infectious etiology • Malabsorption: high osmolarity • Low serum albumin • Lactose intolerance • Formula intolerance: rapid infusion • Obstruction: fecal, volvulus, pseudo-obstruction • Medication • More common with JT	• Rule out (R/O) infections • Lower rate of infusion (increase over 4–6 days as tolerated) • Change to lower osmolarity formula • Use ½-strength formula, gradually increase to full strength • Change to lactose-free formula • Raise albumin with protein supplement or higher protein formula • R/O fecal impaction/obstruction • Stop laxatives, elixirs made with sorbital • R/O drug toxicity • Banana flakes, kaoline pectate cholestramine (may cause tube blockage) • Bismuth subsalicylate, loperamide diphenoxylate hydrochloride
Dehydration, electrolyte imbalance	• Diarrhea/malabsorption • Vomiting • High osmolarity/HHNK (impaired glucose tolerance) • Concurrent illness/medications	• Treat diarrhea/vomiting • Change to isotonic formula • Increase free water • R/O concurrent illness, other metabolic processes
Vomiting	• Sepsis, metabolic shifts, pancreatitis • Obstruction/residual/volvulus • Delayed gastric emptying • Intolerance • Fecal impaction	• R/O sepsis/metabolic process • R/O retention/obstruction • R/O fecal impaction • Change formula (more isotonic) • Trial metclopromide, H_2 blocker, proton pump inhibitor
Restraints (physical/chemical)	• Incorrectly used by some to prevent self extubation • Dementia/delirium/agitation	• Should never be used to prevent self extubation • Need to evaluate benefit vs. burden of EN
Pressure ulcers	• Immobility • Diarrhea/incontinence • Use of restraints • Concurrent chronic disease • Low albumin	• Healing of pressure ulcers is not an indication for EN • No use of restraint • Attention to immobility • Address incontinence: good skin care and hygiene • Treat low albumin levels

Table 16-8 Enteral Nutrition Supplements

Intact Protein Diets			
Supplement	Calorie	Protein	
Isocal Osmolite Isosource Ensure Nutren 1.0	1 cal/cc	40 g/1000 cc	
Nutren 1.0 with Fiber Fiber Source Jevity Ultracal	1.0-1.06 cal/cc	40 g/1000 cc	Higher fiber
Isocal HN Isosource HN Osmolite HN Fiber Source HN	1.0 cal/cc	54 g/1000 cc	Higher protein
Comply Nutren 1.5 Ensure Plus Ensure Plus HN Isosource 1.5 Resource Plus	1.5 cal/cc		Increased caloric density
Nutren 2.0 Deliver 2.0 Novo Source 2.0 Two Cal HN	2.0 cal/cc	80 g/1000 cc	Calorically dense for fluid restriction
Glucerna Glytrol Diet Choice DM Diabetic Source Resource Diabetic	1.0 cal/cc	45 g/1000 cc	Lower carbohydrate for diabetics
Pulmocare Respalor Nutrivent Diet Nova Source Pulmonary	1.5 cal/cc	67.5 g/1000 cc	Lower carbohydrate high caloric/high protein for pulmonary management
Replete Promote Perative Trauma Cal	1.0–1.3 cal/cc	62.5 g/1000 cc	Higher protein/vitamins A, C, and zinc added
Renal Cal Nepro Amin-Aid	2.0 cal/cc	34.4 g/1000 cc	High caloric/low electrolyte, low fluid/ moderate protein
Suplena	2.0 cal/cc	30 g/1000 cc	High cal/low protein

(continues)

Table 16-8   Enteral Nutrition Supplements   *(continued)*

Elemental Diets			
Supplement	Calorie	Protein	
Crucial Diet Impact Perative Immu-Aid	1.5 cal/cc	94 g/1000 cc	High protein/high caloric/hypermetabolic states, diarrhea, burns, surger
Peptide Based Elemental Diets			
Criticare HN Peptamen Vivonex TEN Vital HN	1.0 cal/cc	40 g/1000 cc	Malabsorption, chronic pancreatitis, Crohns, hypoalbuminemia, chronic diarrhea, short bowel syndrome
Peptide Based High Protein			
Peptamen VHP Vivonex Plus Alitraa	1.0 cal/cc	40 g/1000 cc	Colitis/pressure sores
Peptide Based High Caloric			
Peptamen 1.5	1.5 cal/cc	60 g/1000 cc	Higher density/fluid restriction

Personal Care Homes (PCH)

Unlike nursing facilities, federal regulations do not govern PCHs. Each state institutes standards and policies for licensure of PCHs. In the state of Pennsylvania, for example, PCHs are required to comply with Personal Care Home Licensing Regulation (Title 55, PA CODE Chapter 2620), the Department of Public Welfare, and the Office of Social Programs. Offering three nutritionally well-balanced meals a day is the only standard regulation in Pennsylvania. No regulations exist addressing geriatric nutritional needs, screens, or assessments. Older adults in PCHs generally are at high risk for nutritional problems. Although not mandated at this time, nutritional screens and nutritional risk protocols should be standard in all PCHs.

 ## Conclusion

Screening for nutritional deficiencies are justified for many reasons.[39]

- Methods of improving nutrition are available

- Asymptomatic periods often exist during which detection and treatment of the nutritional deficiency reduces morbidity and mortality

- Treatment in the asymptomatic period usually produces results greater than delaying treatment until symptomatic

- Screening tests are available at reasonable costs

■ The incidence of nutritional deficiencies (e.g., weight loss, vitamin deficiency, obesity, anorexia) is sufficient to justify some screening costs.

The advanced practice nurse needs to be an advocate regarding screening for poor nutrition, reducing nutritional misconceptions, promoting nutritional risk programs in the community and assisted living settings, and educating all about the hazards of tube feeding.

References

1. Fabiny AR, Douglas DP. Assessing and treating weight loss in nursing home residents. *Clin Geriatr Med.* 1997;13(4):737–749.
2. Council for Nutritional Clinical Strategies in Long Term Care. *Anorexia in the elderly* [pamphlet]. 1999.
3. Sullivan D, Lipschitz D. Evaluating and treating nutritional problems in older patients. *Clin Geriatr Med.* 1997;13(4):753–767.
4. Guigoz Y, Vellas B, Garry PJ. Assessing the nutritional status of the elderly: the Mini Nutritional Assessment as part of the geriatric assessment evaluation. *Nutr Rev.* 1996;54:S59–S60.
5. Blaum CS, Fries BE, Fiatarone MA. Factors associated with low body mass index and weight loss in nursing home residents. *J Am Geriatr Soc.* 1995;50A:M162.
6. Morley JE. Anorexia in older persons. *Drug Aging.* 1996;2:134–155.
7. Blumberg J. Nutritional needs of seniors. *J Am Coll Nutr.* 1997;16:517–523.
8. Dvorak R, Starling RD, Calles-Escandon J, et al. Drug therapy for obesity in the elderly. *Drug Aging.* 1997; 11:338–351.
9. Lipkin EW, Bell S. Assessment of nutritional status: the clinician's perspective. In: Labbe F, ed. *Clinics in Laboratory Medicine.* 1993;13:329–350.
10. Celotti F, Bignamini A. Dietary calcium and mineral/vitamin supplementation: a controversial problem. *J Ind Med Res.* 1999;27:1–14.
11. Metz J, Bell AH, Flicker L, et al. The significance of subnormal serum vitamin B_{12} concentration in older people: a case control study. *J Am Coll Nutr.* 1997; 16:517–523.
12. Fallest-Stobl P, Kock D, Stein J. Homocysteine: a new risk factor for atherosclerosis. *Am Fam Phys.* 1997;56: 1607–1612.
13. Thomas DR. The role of nutrition in prevention and healing of pressure ulcers. *Clin Geriatr Med.* 1997;13: 497–511.
14. Fosmire GJ. Zinc toxicity. *Am J Nutr.* 1990;51: 508–512.
15. Castell DO. Eating and swallowing disorders. In: Hazzard WR, Bierman EL, Blass JP, et al., eds: *Principles of Geriatric Medicine and Gerontology.* New York: McGraw-Hill; 1994.
16. Champion G, Richter JE. Esophageal dysphagia: is the cause benign or potentially deadly? *J Crit Illness.* 1998;13:236–246.
17. Paterson WG. Dysphagia in the elderly. *Can Fam Phys.* 1996;42:925–932.
18. Fox KM, Hawkes WG, et al. Markers of failure to thrive among older hip fracture patients. *J Am Geriatr Soc.* 1996;44:371–376.
19. Verdery RB. Failure to thrive in older people. *J Am Geriatr Soc.* 1996;44:465–466.
20. Sheiman SL. Tube feeding in the demented nursing home resident. *J Am Geriatr Soc.* 1996;44:1268–1270.
21. Finucane TE, Christmas C, Travis K. Tube feeding in patients with advanced dementia: a review of the evidence. *J Am Med Soc.* 1999;282:1365–1369.
22. Folstein MF, Folstein SE, McHugh PR. Mini-mental state: a practical approach for grading the cognitive state of patients for the clinician. *Psychiatry Res.* 1975:12:189–198.
23. Yesavage JA, Brink TL, Rose TL, et al. Development and validation of a geriatric depression screening scale: a preliminary report. *Psychiatry Res.* 1983;17:37–49.
24. Katz S, Ford AB, Moskowitz RW, et al. Studies of illness in the aged. The index of ADL a standardized measure of biological and psychological function. *JAMA.* 1963;185:914–919.
25. Lawton MP, Brody EM. Assessment of older people: self-maintaining and instrumental activities of daily living measure. *Gerontologist.* 1996;9:179–186.
26. Tinetti IM, Williams WF, Mayeweski R. Fall risk index for elderly patients based on number of chronic disabilities. *Am J Med.* 1986;80:429–443.
27. Agarwahl N, Acevedo F, Leighton LS. Predictive ability of various nutritional variables effect mortality in elderly people. *Am J Clin Nutr.* 1998;48: 1173–1178.
28. Wallace JI, Schwartz RS. Involuntary weight loss in elderly outpatients: recognition, etiologies and treatment. *Clin Geriatr Med.* 1997;13:717–735.
29. Puccio M, Nathanson L. The cancer cachexia syndrome. *Sem Oncol.* 1997;24:277–287.
30. Lissoni P, Paolorossi F, Tancini G, et al. Is there a role for melatonin in the treatment of neoplastic cachexia? *Eur J Cancer.* 1996;32A:1340–1343.
31. Demling RH, DeSanti L. Oxandrolone, an anabolic steroid, significantly increases the rate of weight gain in the recovery phase after major burns. *J Trauma: Inj Crit Care.* 1997;43:47–51.

32. Peck A, Cohen CE, Mulville MN. Long term enteral feeding of aged demented nursing home patients. *J Am Geriatr Soc.* 1990;38:1195–1198.

33. Sheiman SL, Pomerantz JD. Tube feeding in dementia: a controversial practice. *J Nutr Health Aging.* 1998;2: 184–188.

34. Henderson CT, Trumbore LS, Mobarban S, et al. Prolonged tube feeding in long term care: nutritional status and clinical outcomes. *J Am Coll Nutr.* 1991; 11:309–325.

35. Billings JA. Comfort measures for the terminally ill: is dehydration painful? *J Am Geriatr Soc.* 1984;32: 563–564.

36. Fisher R, Nadon G, Shedletsky R. Management of the dying elderly patient. *J Am Geriatr Soc.* 1984; 32:563–564.

37. Sullivan R. Accepting death without artificial nutrition or hydration. *Gen Intern Med.* 1993;8: 220–223.

38. Volicer L, Rheaume Y, Brown J, et al. Hospice approach to the treatment of patients with advanced dementia of the Alzheimer type. *JAMA.* 1986;256: 2210–2213.

39. Frame PS, Carlson SL. A critical review of periodic health screening using specific screening criteria. *J Fam Pract.* 1975;2:29–35.

CHAPTER 17

Pressure Injury and Ulceration: A Holistic Context for Advanced Practice Nurses

Sarah H. Kagan

Alicia A. Puppione

Anna S. Beeber

Mechele Fillman

Joseph Adler

Ara A. Chalian

■ Pressure Ulcers in Older Adults

Pressure ulcers are often viewed as a complication of acute or chronic illness. The presence of pressure ulcers may also be seen as evidence of poor nursing care, although this viewpoint is not supported by research. The advanced practice nurse (APN) regards pressure ulcers as a clinical indicator of overall health. Hence, one must ask what else occurs in a particular patient's situation that contributes to the development of persistent pressure injury. Although pressure ulceration is theoretically preventable, it may still occur despite optimal nursing care and advanced technologies.[1]

The APN is often called on to assess and treat pressure ulcers, including acute and chronic wounds. In order to provide effective nursing care of the older adult with pressure ulcers, the APN must approach patient care within a holistic framework. This framework should include an integration of astute assessment, use of research-based interventions, and methodical evaluation of patient outcomes. This chapter examines specific issues of prevention, assessment, and treatment of the older adult with pressure ulcers.

■ Aging Skin

With age, the effects of time and exposure are visible on the skin and other soft tissue. The skin wrinkles, epidermis thins, dermal blood vessels recede, dermal-epidermal ridges flatten, and the skin appears thin and fragile.[2,3,4] The skin loses sensation and immune response, thus diluting the ability to feel the warning signs of pressure, as well as tissue resistance to pressure-related injury.[5] These age-related changes may increase the risk of ulceration due to pressure, shearing, drying, increased moisture, and friction.[2,3] Discussion begins by thinking of the skin as a "window" into a patient's physiologic condition and the epidemiological and economic impact of pressure ulcers.

■ Skin as a "Window" on the Person

The skin is the largest organ of the human body and serves as its first line of defense against disease. The integumentary system is often ignored as a diagnostic tool. The skin, as our largest organ, is a window for viewing the overall functioning of the entire body. It often heralds grave situations: impending shock is evident with pallor; liver disease appears as jaundice; adverse drug reactions surface as a rash; hypoperfusion is signaled by cyanosis; and advanced diabetes may be evident as a nonhealing ulcer. Individuals with pressure ulcers are often chronically ill and among the sickest patients.[6] New pressure ulcers may indicate comorbidity, malnutrition, and impaired function.[7] All clinicians working with older adults at risk for, or suffering from, pressure ulcers must be mindful of these varying relationships in using the cutaneous "window" of the person to plan and implement individualized, comprehensive care.[8]

Epidemiology

Pressure ulcers are a significant source of morbidity and mortality for older adults.[9] Tissue ulceration is a portal into the body's primary defense mechanisms, allowing microbes to gain access and affecting the compromised host at higher risk for a pressure ulcer.[5,10] Pressure ulcer development is associated with increased mortality.[11] Mortality increases fourfold when an older adult develops a pressure ulcer and sixfold when an ulcer is nonhealing.[2,12] The patient that develops a pressure ulcer during a hospital stay is at higher risk of death within a year.[7] Increased morbidity and mortality may be from the pressure ulcers, but more likely result from comorbid fragility.[5,7] Pressure ulcers prolong medical acuity and promote chronic illness in older adults.

In the United States, approximately 1 million people in hospitals and nursing homes have pressure ulcers,[9] and 70% of these patients are 65 years and over.[10,11,13] The financial implications and resource utilization for patients with pressure ulcers are substantial. Pressure ulcers increase the length of a hospital stay[2] and significantly increase Medicare costs postdischarge.[13] The care of patients with pressure ulcers costs $1.3 billion per year,[14] and the expense of one surgically treated pressure ulcer is estimated at over $60,000.[11]

Incidence and Prevalence

The Agency for Health Care Policy and Research (AHCPR) estimates that the incidence of pressure ulcers in acute-care facilities ranges from 2.7–29.5%.[14] Seven to eight percent of the international general population has a pressure ulcer.[9,14] Twelve percent of immobile older patients develop a pressure ulcer of stage two or greater within 10 days of hospital admission.[3] Elsewhere, it was found that 30% of subjects developed pressure ulcers during a two-week stay in a surgical intensive care unit.[11]

Pathophysiology

A pressure ulcer is any lesion caused by unrelieved external pressure resulting in the occlusion of blood flow, tissue ischemia, and cell death.[14,15] When this external pressure exceeds capillary refill pressure, the result is damage to skin, muscle, and underlying tissue, usually over a bony prominence.[14] This process results in tissue ischemia and eventual necroses, should external pressure remain above physiologic threshold.

Impaired mobility is the greatest risk factor and is a necessary condition for pressure ulcer development.[3] The bedridden individual with mobility impairment is at high risk for ulcerated tissue over the coccyx and sacrum.[3,11] Other sites of pressure ulcer development are the calcaneus, trochanter, scapulae, olecranon processes, malleoli, and occiput.[11] The chair-ridden individual often forms pressure ulcers over ischial tuberosities.

Staging Pressure Ulcers

The AHCPR and the National Pressure Ulcer Advisory Panel (NPUAP) encourage the use of a staging system to classify degree of tissue damage based on extent and depth of tissue injury.[14] Stage 1 ulcers are characterized by nonblanchable erythema of intact skin. It is important to note that stage 1 pressure ulcers are difficult to identify in darkly pigmented individuals and are usually indicated by discoloration, warmth, edema, induration, and hardness.[2,16] Stage 2 ulcers are partial-thickness lesions extending into the epidermis and dermis. Stage 3 pressure ulcers are defined as full-thickness skin loss involving the subcutaneous tissue. Stage 4 is characterized by extensive tissue damage, which extends to muscle, bone, or underlying structures. When eschar is present, staging is not possible until the devitalized tissue is removed and the base of the wound can be visualized. The staging system is useful in research and initial assessment, but is not useful to describe ulcer progression or healing.[2] Ulcers are not restaged during the healing process; rather they should be described anatomically and physiologically (i.e., a healing stage 3 sacral pressure ulcer with evidence of granulation tissue).

Unrelieved pressure above the physiologic threshold causes ischemia and eventual ulceration.[1] The amount of pressure is directly related to the time needed for ulceration to occur. The greater the pressure, the less time for ulceration to occur. Over the past decade, researchers have questioned this causal relationship as it relates to pressure ulcer prevention and treatment.[14,15,17] It may be too narrow and fail to account for host factors.[2] To evaluate the risk for, or the existence of, a pressure ulcer, individual physiologic and functional status must be assessed. Clinical evaluation of comorbid conditions is essential to understanding why one patient ulcerates and others do not, given similar primary risk factors. Impaired nutritional status, mobility, and vascular disease appear to increase risk for the development of pressure ulcers.

Through a holistic assessment and evaluation, the APN can build a plan of care for those patients who suffer from, or are at high risk for, pressure injury. The comprehensive assessment of the older adult should include an evaluation of both extrinsic and host factors. A systematic assessment of skin integrity should include an inspection of the skin and the underlying structures and careful palpation. Observation alone often does not yield enough information about the skin. Anatomic location, distribution, size, shape, type, and color of any lesions need to be included in a description of pressure ulcers.[4,15] For example, a pressure ulcer is usually over a bony prominence; an ulcer located elsewhere on the body indicates an alternative etiology, such as a fungal or viral infection.

Clinical Presentation

Clinical research supports the cost-effectiveness of intensive pressure ulcer prevention to reduce financial, social, and personal costs.[15,18] Clearly, the goal of pressure ulcer treatment is prevention. Through identification of at-risk individuals, APNs can initiate aggressive prevention strategies. Many risk-assessment tools have been developed to aid providers, but it is unclear how the use of these tools prevents pressure ulcers. The tools vary widely in sensitivity and specificity[15] and have varied results with regard to identification and effectiveness.

The Norton Scale[19] provides a mechanism for clinicians to evaluate overall physical condition, mental state, activity, mobility, and incontinence (many of the risk factors associated with pressure ulcers), but it fails to provide a physiological evaluation.[15] The Braden Scale[20] is more detailed than the Norton, but it, too, does not replace a complete assessment. Both scales use mobility, incontinence, mental status, and nutrition as predictors of pressure ulcers. The Braden Scale is used across settings, while both scales are used in long-term care. Assessing other risk factors that correlate with illness severity, like interaortic balloon pumps, are necessary, to evaluate pressure ulcer risk in acutely ill patients.[14] Both of the scales use the indicators of mobility, incontinence, mental status, and nutrition to identify those at-risk individuals. The Braden scale is more commonly used across settings, while both are used in long-term care settings.

In addition to the Braden and Norton scales, global measures of medical acuity, like the acute physiology score of the APACHE II, can be used to identify persons at risk for pressure ulcers.[2] These scales often evaluate independent risk factors for mortality, as well as overall medical acuity or risk for pressure ulcers.[7] Despite limitations, standard risk-assessment tools are a first step in routine and standardized evaluation.

Risk factors for pressure ulcers are often nonspecific and generally predict overall fragility.[7] Immobility is the greatest risk factor for pressure ulcer development, and limited activity level is another primary risk factor.[15] Lymphopenia, xerosis, and decreased body weight are independent risk factors for ulceration in hospitalized older adults with impaired mobility.[3] Pressure ulcers, malnutrition, immobility, and functional dependence are interrelated and associated with increased medical complications and death.[6] Severity of ulceration correlates with degree of malnutrition as measured by hypoalbuminemia.[21] Similarly, higher transferrin levels correlate with wound healing. In surgical patients, lower hemoglobin, hematocrit, and serum albumin levels, and the presence of diabetes mellitus perioperatively, is significant for future pressure ulcer development.[22]

The two critical determinants of ulceration are tissue tolerance for pressure and intensity and duration of pressure.[22] Certain person-specific characteristics are independent predictors for pressure ulcer development, such as incontinence, diabetes, stroke, increased age, and hypotension.[2] A combination of both intrinsic and extrinsic factors influence tissue response and tolerance to pressure.[17] The most common intrinsic factors placing individuals at higher risk are incontinence, malnutrition, and altered level of consciousness.[15] Other commonly cited intrinsic risk factors include increased age, decreased oxygen transportation/decreased arteriolar pressure, comorbidities, decreased mobility, and malnutrition.[3,14] The extrinsic factors most commonly associated with ulcer development include pressure, shear, friction, and moisture.[17] When intrinsic and extrinsic risk factors act in concert, critically, acutely, and chronically ill older adults are placed at extreme risk for pressure injury.[23]

Illness is an independent risk factor for ulceration in older adults. Older adults are at highest risk for developing pressure ulcers during acute illness and hospitalization.[2] Hospitalization has many negative sequela for older adults, including debilitation.[24] When older adults are debilitated, ability to resist injury and infection is severely compromised. Impaired resistance may account for the relationship between length of hospitalization and pressure ulcer incidence.[3,25] Certain concomitant diagnoses, such as hip fractures and cardiac surgery, place older adults at increased risk for pressure ulcer development because of the immobility and fragility associated with these conditions.[2,23,26] Chronic clinical illnesses, such as acute renal failure, are associated with poor wound healing and mortality.[27]

Malnutrition is independently associated with pressure ulcers and increased mortality.[27] The severely malnourished patient is at a higher risk for death, sepsis, infections, and increased length of hospital stay.[28] Hypoalbuminemia is a reliable prognostic indicator associated with pressure ulcer development and increased morbidity and mortality.[3,28,29] Lymphopenia and decreased body weight, as indicators of poor nutritional status, are independent risk factors for ulceration.[3] If increased nutrition is not supplied to the patient under severe physiologic stress, then an even higher risk for development of pressure ulcers results.[23,27]

 Goals of Treatment

Overarching goals of pressure ulcer treatment are predicated on prognosis and the individual's physiological capabilities. The principle maxim for local care is the maintenance of a clean, moist wound. When cure is the treatment goal, local care should focus on wound healing. For a chronic, nonhealing ulcer, comfort should be a top priority. Treatments should correlate with the goal and the individualized needs of the patient and family members, particularly so if family members are direct caregivers, as well as professional and nonprofessional caregivers and the institutional resources available.

Functional, Biological, and Chronological Age

Over a lifetime, environmental exposure, activity level, nutrition, and past or present illness can influence individual ability to respond to stress. Exercise, nutritional supplementation, and other health-promoting activities are linked with disease prevention and symptom reduction.[30,31] The long-term effects of health-promoting or health-detracting activities render chronological age a poor indicator of health or function. For example, a person may be 80 years old chronologically, but function as if 20 years younger. Similarly, the cumulative effects of chronic illness and environmental exposure may negatively affect persons in their 50s, giving them the appearance and physiological and functional capacity of persons who are much older. In any assessment, consider biological and functional ages in addition to chronological age.

Clinical Application of Theory and Research

Pressure Injury

Early identification of vulnerable individuals through standardized (albeit limited) tools and clinical judgment is paramount to effective pressure ulcer treatment. In situations where acute debilitation occurs, pressure ulcer reduction should be a primary treatment goal. Careful positioning and proper padding, to reduce the risk of pressure ulceration, is critical. More advanced technologies, such as a pressure reducing mattress, may be needed to care for the vulnerable patient, especially those unable to recover function and mobility quickly. Treatment goals should always be aimed at limitation of injury.

To achieve successful rehabilitation, local and systemic efforts must be employed in the treatment of pressure ulcers. The combined expertise of nursing, medicine, and physical and occupational therapists help to optimize patient positioning and mobility. Individuals with chronic mobility dysfunction require constant care to achieve effective pressure relief. Physical therapists determine if the individual patient has the strength, range of motion, and cognitive ability to shift his/her weight independently. If patients are unable to reposition themselves, the plan of care becomes more complex, requiring technological intervention to reduce pressure injury risk.

Local Care

Decisions related to the prevention and treatment of pressure ulcers should be consistent with the overall goals for individualized care. Based on specific patient needs, appropriate dressings are those that keep the ulcer base moist while allowing the surrounding tissue to remain dry. A dressing should protect the wound from exogenous sources of infection and further injury. Many options for wound-dependent dressings are available. In choosing the dressing, it must meet needs for cleansing, maintenance of moisture, and protection within the particular phase of wound healing. Selection also depends on the abilities of the caregiver and patient. Dressing

choice should be reevaluated frequently for wound condition and patient comfort in order for optimal patient outcomes. The AHCPR recommends topical antibiotics for ulcers that fail to heal after two weeks of optimal care.[14]

Support Surfaces

Pressure-reducing devices and an increasing array of sophisticated technologies minimize the effects of decreased mobility. Their effectiveness, however, has not been conclusively reported in the research literature.[3,32,33] The decision for use of pressure-reducing technologies must be guided by a careful cost–benefit analysis. Selection of a support surface should be guided by a holistic approach, including physiological, psychological, and economical needs of patients and treatment goals. A single technology will not heal a wound and can often be expensive and limit bed mobility.

Wound Healing

Wound healing occurs only if the patient is physiologically able to provide needed substrates; the wound is clean, moist, and infection free; and the source of ischemic injury is removed. In general, older adults have slow wound healing and are at higher risk for complications. Critical illness is widely associated with catabolism, muscle wasting, and nonhealing wounds.[5] Critical illness presents significant challenges to wound healing, as it increases nutritional needs, lowers the immune response, and stresses all body systems.[5,27,34] Severe stress results in metabolic changes and, without intervention, metabolic failure.[34] These stress-related metabolic changes further deplete the patient and impede wound healing. Age-related regression of blood vessels impedes wound healing and increases risks of hypoperfusion and hypoxia.[5]

Colonization

All stage 2 and greater pressure ulcers are colonized with bacteria.[14] Colonization refers to organism attachment to devitalized tissue, without invasion to viable tissue.[5] Healing occurs when the colonies are prevented from infecting the wound. Routine local care, dressing changes, and irrigation with a physiologic solution, like normal saline, helps reduce the risk of bacterial invasion. Studies have indicated pressure ulcers cannot heal with a bacterial load exceeding 100,000 organisms per gram of tissue.[14]

Infection

Wound infection occurs when organisms invade viable tissue and elicit an ineffective immune response.[5,14] Pressure ulcers must be free from infection in order for wound healing to occur.[5] Local wound care (i.e., wound cleansing and debridement) minimizes pressure ulcer colonization and promotes wound healing.[14] The presence of purulent drainage and foul odor (wound infection) indicate that more aggressive local care is necessary.[5,14] Clinically infected wounds require both topical and systemic antibiotics to reduce bacterial counts to a level that promotes healing.[5] Patients with progressive cellulitis, bacteremia, osteomyelitis, or other complications of wound infections should be treated with systemic antibiotic therapy.[14]

Nutritional Interventions

Optimal nutritional status is integral to wound prevention and healing. A nutritional assessment is essential to achieve ideal wound healing and clinical outcomes.[34] The patient with poor nutritional status has delayed or impaired wound healing.[6,28,35] Protein-calorie malnutrition alters tissue regeneration, inflammatory reaction and immune function.[28] Additionally, significant protein loss occurs with large or deep ulcers.[10] Adjunctive nutritional support is essential to ulcer prevention and wound healing in critically ill patients.[27]

In the chronically ill older adult, the relationship between nutritional intervention and wound healing is not as clear.[35] Chronically ill patients can have an increase in metabolic demands due to the inflammatory response noted in many disease states; thus, determination of basal metabolic rate can be especially useful. The increased production and release of cytokines accelerate muscle catabo-

lism resulting in weight loss and negative nitrogen balance.[27,36] In addition to increased caloric and fluid demands, a 13% increase in oxygen consumption occurs for each increase in degree (centigrade) in body temperature.[36] The association between malnutrition and poor wound healing is constant, but in chronic illness, decreased functional reserve further complicates the relationship.

Oxygen and nutrients are necessary for the body to produce and support fibroblasts during the proliferative phase of wound healing.[5,37] Vitamin C, vitamin A, riboflavin, iron, zinc, oxygen, and growth factors are necessary to produce the collagen required to fill wound cavities.[5,34] Collagen formation at ulcer edges increases markedly following vitamin C saturation at a dose of 1 g daily.[38] The stabilization of collagen cannot occur without ascorbic acid, which is necessary for the hydroxylation of proline to hydroxyproline.[28,34]

Laboratory Assessment

Obtain blood urea nitrogen and creatinine ratio to evaluate renal clearance, and serum electrolyte panel to determine hydration and electrolyte status. Hydration status is important because under- or overhydration affect visceral protein levels, as well as electrolytes, complete blood count, and weight. A complete blood count is useful to determine the presence of infection or anemia; lymphocyte counts are useful with regard to an immune response. A serum albumin level is indicative of visceral protein status for up to three weeks prior to pressure injury. Transferrin and prealbumin levels indicate the patient's nutritional status in the last 3 to 10 days. Serum transferrin, however, is sensitive to the increase in iron stores with aging, so a drop in transferrin level may be misleading. A common anemia in older adults is iron deficiency, which elevates transferrin levels. Prealbumin is not sensitive to iron stores.

General Medical Intervention

Both acute and chronic disease adversely affect the wound healing process.[5] Hence, to optimize ulcer treatment, clinicians should strive for systemic health. Promoting systemic health includes encouraging physical activity, ensuring systemic and local oxygenation, and providing supportive nutrition. Maintenance of adequate blood pressure is paramount for adequate local perfusion. In addition, control of comorbid diseases, especially those like diabetes that have microvascular implications, is necessary to encourage wound healing. Ensuring that the necessary substrates are available for wound healing often means providing vitamin supplementation.

Surgical Intervention

When customary interventions fail to heal a pressure ulcer, or the ulcer is of significant size, surgical intervention may be the best option. Generally only stage 3 and 4 ulcers require surgical intervention.[9] First-line surgical treatment is debridement of any grossly devitalized tissue.[9,14] Following debridement, usual clinical management includes dampening gauze dressings with normal saline to promote granulation at the wound base. The most common surgical procedures used on chronic pressure ulcers are skin grafts and tissue flaps.[9] Skin grafts, either split or full thickness, involve transfer of epidermis and dermis to provide superficial coverage.[9] Free tissue flaps, involving the transfer of skin and the underlying structures to fill the deficit left by ulceration, are the most common surgical procedures used to manage pressure ulcers.[9]

Resources and Collaboration

Guidelines

The AHCPR has two clinical practice guidelines dedicated to pressure ulcers. The first guides clinicians with the prediction and prevention of pressure ulcers.[15] The AHCPR issued a follow-up guideline dedicated to treatment of pressure ulcers.[14] Given an aging population and limited health-care resources, the NPUAP was formed in 1987 as an independent, nonprofit health-care organization.[17] The NPUAP is dedicated to the research, prevention, and management of pressure ulcers.[17] These two national resources should be

among the first to which any clinician turns for guidance in evidence-based care of patients at risk for, or suffering from, pressure ulcers.

Interdisciplinary Care

Patients with pressure ulcers often have very complex needs, usually requiring the collaborative expertise of many disciplines. Extensive tissue injury requires a long, multifaceted rehabilitation for complete healing. As part of an interdisciplinary team, nurses are often responsible for the diagnosis and treatment of most pressure ulcers. Dedication and accountability to preventive measures is key to reducing their number and severity. Education of all nurses, as well as nonprofessional staff and family caregivers, in pressure ulcer prevention and treatment, is essential to successful programs of prevention and treatment for older adults and vulnerable patients in any settings.

Comprehensive prevention and treatment of pressure ulcers often requires the expertise of multiple disciplines to reduce the occurrence of these painful and costly chronic wounds. Along with nursing, physical and occupational therapists work with patients to reduce the effects of shear and pressure. Assisting patients with rehabilitation, occupational and physical therapists increase mobility and decrease risk of ulceration. Registered dietitians assist to maximize nutritional status. To ensure successful restoration of health, the primary team must continue the dialog with physical and occupational therapy and nutrition support.

The complex needs of patients with pressure ulcers demand a coordinated, interdisciplinary approach for effective care. Nursing and internal or geriatric medicine outline and implement individualized first-line interventions and treatment plans. If first-line treatments fail, or if care needs are complicated by other dermatological disorders, then the expertise of dermatology may be beneficial. Infectious-disease physicians are occasionally needed to identify and treat superinfections that impair wound healing. Large, deep, or necrotic pressure ulcers usually require surgical intervention. Surgeons, particularly those trained in plastic and reconstructive techniques, and other surgical subspecialists must be included in teams dealing with complex or longstanding pressure ulcers. If cure is a treatment goal, the surgical team can assist the primary team and patient in choosing among surgical options including intra-operative sharp debridement and healing by secondary intent, primary closure, and local or free flap closure. General surgeons may also be helpful in determining the value of diverting colostomy to avoid fecal soiling, which clearly interferes with healing of pressure ulcers.

Conclusion

Prevention and treatment of pressure ulcers is best understood within the context of holistic, individualized nursing care. APNs, in collaboration with other health-care providers, can transition the focus of wound care from a rote, quantitative approach to one that is more naturalized and tailored to individual patient needs. The goals of pressure ulcer management should be prevention or minimization of tissue injury, provision of intrinsic and extrinsic factors needed for wound healing, rehabilitation, and patient comfort and education. APNs and colleagues in related specialty areas possess the skills and resources to lead changes in pressure ulcer prevention and management. Relying on evidence-based practice, aided by the practice guidelines outlined by the AHCPR and NPUAP, APNs can lead an interdisciplinary team approach to pressure ulcer treatment from a systematic, yet individualized, approach.

References

1. Kosiak M. Etiology and pathology of ischemic ulcers. *Arch Phys Med Rehabil*. 1959;40:62–69.
2. Allman RM. Pressure ulcer prevalence, incidence, risk factors, and impact. *Clin Geriatr Med*. 1997;13: 421–436.
3. Allman RM, Goode PS, Patrick MM, Burst N, Bartolucci AA. Pressure ulcer risk factors among hospitalized patients with activity limitation. *JAMA*. 1995;273:865–870.
4. Bickley L. *Bates' Guide to Physical Examination and History Taking*. Philadelphia: Lippincott; 1999: 145–161.
5. Flynn MB. Wound healing and critical illness. *Crit Care Nurs Clin N Am*. 1996;8:115–123.
6. Breslow RA, Hallfrisch J, Guy DG, Crawley B, Goldberg AP. The importance of dietary protein in healing pressure ulcers. *J Am Geriatr Soc*. 1993;41: 357–362.
7. Thomas DR, Goode PS, Tarquine PH, Allman RM. Hospital-acquired pressure ulcers and risk of death. *J Am Geriatr Soc*. 1996;44:1435–1440.
8. Happ MB, Williams CC, Strumpf NE, Burger SG. Individualized care for frail elders: theory and practice. *J Gerontol Nurs*. 1996;22:3:6–14.
9. Bryant RA, Shannon ML, Peiper B, Braden BJ, Morris D. Pressure ulcers. In: Bryant RA, ed. *Acute and Chronic Wounds: Nursing Management*. St. Louis, Mo: Mosby-Year Book; 1992.
10. Kaplan LJ, Pameijer C, Blank-Reid C, Granick MS. Necrotizing fasciitis: An uncommon consequence of pressure ulceration. *Adv Wound Care*. 1998;11: 185–189.
11. Baldwin KM, Ziegler SM. Pressure ulcer risk following critical traumatic injury. *Adv Wound Care*. 1998;11: 173–186.
12. Pase MN. Pressure relief devices, risk factors, and development of pressure ulcers in elderly patients with limited mobility. *Adv Wound Care*. 1994;7(2): 38–42.
13. Allman RM, Damiano AM, Strauss MJ. Pressure ulcer status and post-discharge health care resource utilization among older adults with activity limitations. *Adv Wound Care*. 1996;9:38–44.
14. Agency for Health Care Policy and Research, Public Health Service, U.S. Department of Health and Human Services. Treatment of Pressure Ulcers. *Clinical Practice Guideline Number 15*. 1994.
15. *Clinical Practice Guideline, Number 3: Pressure Ulcers in Adults: Prediction and Prevention*. Rockville, Md: Agency for Health Care Policy and Research, U.S. Department of Health and Human Services; 1992.
16. Lyder CH, Yu C, Emerling J, et al. The Braden scale for pressure ulcer risk: evaluating the predictive validity in black and Latino/Hispanic elders. *App Nurs Res*. 1999;12(2):60–68.
17. National Pressure Ulcer Advisory Panel. An introduction to the NPUAP. 2000. Available online: http://www.npuap.org.
18. Xakellis GC, Frantz RA, Lewis A, Harvey P. Cost-effectiveness of an intensive pressure ulcer prevention protocol in long-term care. *Adv Wound Care*. 1998;11:22–29.
19. Norton D. Calculating the risk: reflections on the Norton Scale. *Decubitus*. 1989;2(3):24–31.
20. Braden BJ, Bergstrom N. Predictive validity of the Braden Scale for pressure sore risk in a nursing home population. *Res Nurs Health*. 1994;17(6): 459–470.

21. Kaminski MV, Williams SD. Review of the rapid normalization of serum albumin with modified total parenteral nutrition solutions. *Crit Care Med.* 1990;18:327–335.

22. Lewicki LJ, Mion L, Splane KG, Samstag D, Secic M. Patient risk factors for pressure ulcers during cardiac surgery. *AORN J.* 1990;65:933–942.

23. Mainous MR, Block EFJ, Deitch EA. Nutritional support of the gut: how and why. *N Horizons.* 1994;2:193–201.

24. Creditor MC. Hazards of hospitalization of the elderly. *Ann Intern Med.* 1993;118(3):219–223.

25. Stotts NA, Deosaransingh K, Roll FJ, Newman J. Under utilization of pressure ulcer risk assessment in hip fracture patients. *Adv Wound Care.* 1998;11:32–38.

26. Garrett BM. The nutritional management of acute renal failure. *J Clin Nurs.* 1995;4(6):377–382.

27. Barton RG. Nutrition support in critical illness. *Nutr Clin Pract.* 1994;9(4):127–139.

28. Thomas DR. The role of nutrition in prevention and healing of pressure ulcers. *Clin Geriatr Med.* 1997;13: 497–511.

29. McCluskey A, Thomas AN, Bowles BJ, Kishen R. The prognostic value of serial measurements of serum albumin concentration in patients admitted to an intensive care unit. *Anesthesia.* 1996;51(8):724–727.

30. Maugh TH. Capsules. *Los Angeles Times.* May 24, 1999; Home Edition, Health Section: 3.

31. Mestel R.Vitals. *Los Angeles Times.* May 24, 1999; Home Edition, Health Section: 1–2.

32. Chalian AA, Kagan SH. Backside first in head and neck surgery? Preventing pressure ulcers in extended length surgeries. *Head Neck.* In press.

33. Ferrell BA. Pressure ulcer products and devices: are they safe, much less effective? *J Am Geriatr Soc.* 1998;46:654–655.

34. Bagley SM. Nutritional needs of the acutely ill with acute wounds. *Crit Care Nurs Clin N Am.* 1996;8:159–167.

35. Finucane TE. Malnutrition, tube feeding and pressure sores: data are incomplete. *J Am Geriatr Soc.* 1995; 43:447–451.

36. Sullivan D, Lipschitx D. Evaluating and treating nutritional problems in older patients. *Clin Geriatr Med.* 1997;13:753–768.

37. Adzick NS. Wound healing: biological and clinical features. In: Sabiston DC, Lyerly HK, eds. *Textbook of Surgery: The Biological Basis of Modern Surgical Practice.* 15th ed. Philadelphia: W. B. Saunders; 1997: 207–220.

38. Hunter T, Rajan KT. The role of ascorbic acid in the pathogenesis and treatment of pressure sores. *Paraplegia.* 1971;8:211-215.

18

Elder Abuse and Neglect

Laura Wagner
Sherry Greenberg
Elizabeth Capezuti

Introduction

Elder mistreatment is the last form of family violence to be acknowledged by society, having gained national attention at a congressional hearing in 1978. Spearheaded by public recognition of the problem, legislators enacted Adult Protective Service (APS) laws providing authority to social service agencies to investigate suspected cases of mistreatment, as well as funding for services to help elderly victims. All 50 states and the District of Columbia have APS statutes for identification, investigation, and in some states, services to alleviate abusive situations.[1]

Due to the high incidence of health problems associated with both age and mistreatment, elder mistreatment must be recognized as more than a social or law enforcement problem. It is also a health-care problem, one often with devastating and long-term ramifications, including death.[2] As a nexus of social, legal, and health concerns, elder mistreatment victims are best served by a network of services that encompass a variety of disciplines.

This chapter focuses on elder abuse and neglect and the implications for the gerontological advanced practice nurse (APN). Identification of those at risk, early detection of victims, and subsequent referral for assistance and/or ongoing surveillance are the key roles of APNs.

Prevalence

A survey of 2,020 randomly selected older persons residing in the Boston metropolitan area found that 3.2% reported being abused.[3] The National Elder Abuse Incidence Study (NEAIS) estimated in 1996 more than half a million new cases of elder mistreatment among community-dwelling older Americans.[4] Of this estimate, over five times as many incidents of mistreatment went unreported to local APS agencies. These numbers are lower than previous estimates because prior studies reported the total number of cases (versus total number of new cases). Nevertheless, a greater number of elder mistreatment cases are being reported to the APS agencies compared to previous years.[4] The NEAIS also found that female elders are abused at higher rates than male elders and that those over 80 years of age are mistreated two to three times their proportional numbers in the elderly population. About 90% of the incidents of mistreatment had a perpetrator known to the victim.

According to the American Medical Association, it is difficult to collect accurate data on the extent of elder mistreatment.[5] Elderly victims may feel embarrassed, intimidated, or overwhelmed. The victim or person reporting the abuse might also be fearful of the outcomes of such reporting. Unfortunately, individuals often do not recognize abuse or know to whom or how to report it.[5] The social isolation of some frail elders increases the risk and difficulty in identifying mistreatment, making it more difficult to uncover than child abuse. In contrast to children, many elders live alone and may interact only with other family members.

Relevant Pathophysiology

Definition and Types of Mistreatment

Elder mistreatment is defined as the abuse and neglect of older adults. It includes physical, psychological, and sexual abuse, caregiver neglect and self-neglect, and financial exploitation.[6] See

Table 18–1 for a list of the types of abuse, definitions, and prevalence. It is not uncommon for older adults to experience more than one of type of abuse simultaneously.[7] Physical abuse is the infliction of bodily injury to the older adult. It includes hitting, grabbing, pushing, slapping, improper use of physical restraints, or force feeding.[5,8] Any unexplained injury may indicate the possibility of physical abuse. Moreover, the identification of physical abuse is complicated by normal age changes, such as the bruising seen in the senile purpura associated with capillary fragility.[6]

Physical abuse is often accompanied by psychological abuse.[7] Psychological neglect includes verbal harassment and intimidation.[9] Emotional abuse may result in isolation of the elder from other persons, leading to feelings of depression, hopelessness, and helplessness. Complaints of psychological abuse may be vague and easily misinterpreted by health-care providers as the symptoms of other physical or emotional illnesses.[6]

Sexual abuse is identified less often than other forms of elder mistreatment.[10] Sexually abusive behavior is perpetrated by family members and caregivers, both in the home and institution. Sexual abuse encompasses numerous acts ranging from forced penetration to offensive sexual behavior. Rape, or sexual assault, has been defined in one state as sexual intercourse or unnatural sexual intercourse with a person during which one is compelled to submit by force and against his or her will, or compelled to submit by threat of bodily injury.[11] Legal definitions vary from state to state. Elder abuse victims generally do not report incidents of sexual assault, either because of a mental illness that prevents them from doing so or strong feelings of shame and humiliation.[11]

Caregiver neglect may be passive or active. Passive neglect is defined as neglect resulting in the lack of

Table 18–1   Types of Elder Mistreatment

Type	Definition	Examples
Physical abuse	Acts of violence resulting in pain or injury	Pushing, slapping, hitting, improper use of physical restraints
Emotional or psychological abuse	Infliction of mental anguish	Intimidation, yelling, insulting, threatening, silence, treating like an infant, isolation from others
Sexual abuse	Any form of intimate sexual activity without consent, including those who are unable to provide consent (dementia and mental retardation)	Rape, molestation, sexual harassment, forcing viewing of pornographic material
Financial exploitation	Misuse of elder's funds without his/her knowledge or consent	Withdrawal of money from bank accounts
Caregiver neglect	Malicious neglect by a caregiver of an older person's needs; failure to provide the elder with social stimulation	Leaving elder alone for long periods of time, inadequate provision of nutrition, misusing medications (e.g., oversedation)
Self-neglect	Disregard of one's personal well-being and home environment, possibly due to a mental health problem	Poor hygiene, manifestations of inadequately treated medical problems, poorly kept surroundings

information or resources needed to care for an older adult. This can occur when caregivers also have physical or psychological impairments. Active neglect is the malicious neglect of an older adult's needs. Such neglect usually results from disinterest, retaliation, or a desire to gain financially. In these situations, it is often difficult to obtain an accurate history of the injuries or even to gain entry into the home.

Self-neglect is defined as "an adult's inability, due to physical and/or mental impairments or diminished capacity, to perform self care tasks . . . to maintain physical health . . . general safety and/or manage financial affairs."[12,13] The causes include longstanding mental health problems, dementia, or fear of "outsiders."[6] In states where the APS statute includes self-neglect, it is the most frequently reported type of mistreatment.[14] It can be difficult to identify victims because often they are reclusive, suspicious, or territorial.[6] The self-neglector may not gain attention until a neighbor notices a problem such as a large accumulation of garbage around the house or garbage that has not been removed for months.

Financial exploitation involves misuse of an older adult's finances. It includes stealing money or possessions, and coercing the older person to sign contracts, change a will, or purchase items. Financial neglect is the failure to use the available funds necessary to meet an older adult's health needs and well-being.[5] In many cases, the victim lacks decisional capacity and competence to manage his or her financial affairs. Elders who are female, over 75, frail, and dependent on a caregiver are at high risk for financial abuse.[14] Signs of financial abuse may include sudden or unexplained withdrawal of money from accounts, or an extraordinary interest by family members in the victims' assets.

Theories of Elder Abuse

Theories regarding causality have emerged based on profiles of victims and perpetrators identified by APS agencies, researchers, and clinicians. For example, the "caregiver stress" or dependency theory of elder mistreatment is based on findings that the "average" victim is an older (> 80 years of age), physically and cognitively frail woman. The "average" perpetrator

is a middle-aged adult child providing some assistance to the victim.[4] According to the theory, the level of dependency by the victim on the caregiver is directly related to the risk of mistreatment. Case control studies, however, do not demonstrate that the victim's level of dependency increases the risk of elder mistreatment.[3,15] Rather, caregiver stress is a possible triggering event for mistreatment within a dysfunctional caregiving context.[16]

Several studies provide empirical support for the psychopathology of the abuser, manifested as a history of substance/alcohol addiction, untreated psychiatric illness, or criminal acts as the most likely contributors to physical or financial abuse.[15,17-20] In addition to the characteristics of the perpetrator, the relationship between victim and perpetrator are strongly correlated with elder abuse, especially those in codependency relationships.

Risk factors for self-neglecting elders include untreated mental illness, dementia, suspicious personality, and a poor social network.[6,13,21,22] The severing of relationships with family and friends can also be viewed as self-neglecting behavior.

Risk Factors

Most studies concerning risk factors for elder abuse are retrospective analyses and only a few identify causative risk factors associated with specific types of mistreatment. Furthermore, findings are inconsistent in the elder mistreatment literature.[18] The chief problem with many studies is that most factors are too vague to be clinically meaningful.

Several characteristics of the frail elder and the perpetrator may increase the risk of mistreatment. See Table 18–2 for a list of risk factors for elder mistreatment. In both national surveys and research studies, most perpetrators of abuse/exploitation tend to be the "problem relative or friend" and are more likely to be men.[4] In contrast to abuse, most perpetrators of neglect are women.[4]

Consequences

Adverse outcomes of elder mistreatment range from physical conditions such as pressure ulcers to

Table 18–2   Risk Factors for Elder Abuse

New, worsening, or prolonged cognitive or physical impairment

Increased age

Poverty

Psychopathology in family members/caretaker

   Substance abuse

   Mental illness

Shared living arrangement

Dependency

   Abuser dependent on victim for housing and finances

   Elder dependent on caretaker for assistance with activities

Lack of close family ties

Unsafe housing conditions

Cultural sanctions against seeking help to care for elder

Family history of violence

Isolation of the caregiver or victim

Caregiver stress

Financial strain or other stressful life events

mental problems like depression. Elder mistreatment affects both morbidity and mortality of the victim. Lachs and colleagues analyzed a cohort of community-dwelling older adults in New Haven to estimate the long-term survival of abused individuals.[2] The results of the New Haven Established Population for Epidemiologic Studies in the Elderly (EPESE) were completed after a 13-year follow-up period. Subjects seen for elder mistreatment at any time during the follow-up period had poorer survival scores than those subjects seen for self-neglect. The risk of death in those experiencing elder mistreatment and neglect was also elevated compared to others in the cohort.[2] This study clearly supports the need for long-term interdisciplinary intervention of elder mistreatment cases.

Implications for APN Practice

APN as Critical Gatekeeper

The chronic illnesses common to older persons bring them into frequent contact with primary-health-care providers, whether in provider's offices, clinics, emergency departments (EDs), inpatient hospital units, or the home. Older adults visit primary-care provider's offices more frequently than younger persons. Continued contacts with the older person over time place the APN in an ideal position to detect signs of mistreatment, as well as to identify potential victims. Although emergency room staff may witness the more obvious signs of abuse, the long-term APN–patient relationship affords greater opportunity to observe subtle changes in health status and thereby play a significant role in case detection.

For the last 20 years, many researchers and clinicians have accepted the "iceberg theory" of reporting mistreatment: only the most visible incidents of mistreatment are detected while most cases are neither identified nor reported. The NEAIS in 1998 validate this observation in its finding that 79% of elder mistreatment cases in 1996 were unreported to APS agencies.[4] Lack of reporting and identification challenges clinicians to increase awareness of elder mistreatment and improve detection of potential cases.

Unfortunately, few practicing health-care professionals have received training in elder mistreatment during their basic professional education. Thus, they may be unaware of obvious mistreatment, or may even be unconscious to the possibility of abuse. Any fracture or wound needs to be evaluated for cause. An evaluation of any child presenting to an ED with fractures, bruises, dehydration, or malnutrition, would have "mistreatment" included as part of the workup. On the other hand, similar injuries or conditions in an older adult may be attributed to "normal aging," despite evidence to the contrary.

Such disparities in treatment prompted the Joint Commission on the Accreditation of Healthcare Organizations (JCAHO) to approve the adoption of new standards. Hospital EDs are required to develop protocols and to provide annual training of personnel in the detection and treatment of elder mistreatment. Refer to Table 18–3 for an abbreviated version of the JCAHO standards.

Institutional Mistreatment

Information on elder abuse in long-term care is lacking because available data is often incomplete or aggregated. Many abusive acts are never even labeled as mistreatment.[23] Moreover, many residents and families fail to report abuse or mistreatment out of fear of reprisal or discharge. Data collection of elder mistreatment in nursing homes is particularly difficult because multiple agencies

Table 18–3 JCAHO Standards Addressing Victims of Possible Abuse or Neglect

1. Emergency departments/services have written policies and procedures relating to the handling of adult and child victims of alleged or suspected abuse or neglect.

2. There is a plan for education of appropriate staff about the criteria for identifying and handling possible victims of abuse.

3. The hospital has a role in the collection, retention, and safeguarding of specimens, photographs, and other evidentiary material released by the patient, and as legally required, notification of and release of information to the proper authorities.

4. The medical record includes documentation of examination, treatment given, any referrals made to other care providers and to community agencies, and any required reporting to the proper authorities.

5. A list is maintained in the emergency department/ service of private and public community agencies that provide or arrange for evaluation and care for victims of abuse and referrals are made as appropriate.

Source: Joint Commisssion on Accreditation of Healthcare Organizations. *Accreditation Manual for Hospitals, Vol I (Standards). Standards PE1.9 and PE6.2* Chicago, Il: Joint Commission on Accreditation of Healthcare Organizations; 1995.

are responsible for investigation, including APS, the ombudsman, state/local health departments, law enforcement agencies, and Medicaid fraud control units.

Older adults can be mistreated by professional and paraprofessional staff of hospitals, nursing homes, or congregate living facilities. Residents of the latter may be at particular risk, because boarding homes and assisted-living or personal care facilities are not well supervised by government or accreditation agencies.[24] Nursing home residents are also at special risk, as many do not have regular visitors who monitor their day-to-day care. In addition, nursing homes with system problems such as short staffing, limited resources, and inadequate supervision leave residents at greater risk for mistreatment.

Mistreatment in the long-term care setting also includes failure to follow a care plan, isolation of the resident from others, or abuse of property. The most common complaints of mistreatment in long-term care are neglect (pressure ulcers, malnutrition, nosocomial infection), theft, sexual assault and failure to honor resident rights.[8,10,25]

The perpetrator in nursing homes may be an individual staff member who physically or sexually abuses a patient, or may be more broadly defined as an institutional milieu that discourages the appropriate provision of care. For example, inadequate staffing levels may contribute to the use of physical restraints and limited ambulation, thus leading to serious problems such as contractures and pressure ulcers.

Reports of suspicious acts indicating institutional mistreatment should be made to the state's Long Term Care Ombudsman Program. The Federal Older Americans Act of 1976 mandated that each state establish ombudsman programs to investigate allegations of mistreatment in nursing homes.[8] Long-term-care ombudsmen investigate allegations of abuse in institutionalized settings such as nursing homes, adult daycare centers, and residential care facilities. Reports to other agencies (Department of Health, APS) may also be mandated by state laws and regulations. Law enforcement must be notified in alleged criminal acts such as sexual assault.[10] It is imperative that the

APNs in long-term-care settings work with the relevant agencies in any case of alleged mistreatment. Nursing home administrators should not delay in reporting the case while performing an internal review. The APN should play an instrumental role in orienting and training staff about detection and reporting of elder mistreatment.

Clinical Presentation

Relevant History

Identification of elder mistreatment begins with a comprehensive history. Any questioning must be sensitive to the varying types of elder mistreatment, including physical, psychological, and financial abuse, as well as neglect, both past and present. Caution is warranted, however, not to assume that mistreatment is actually occurring. Questions should be framed in a nonjudgmental and nonthreatening manner. General questions in the history may include:

- Are you afraid of anyone?
- Has anyone ever taken anything that was yours without asking?
- Have you ever talked about this with anyone before?

Table 18–4 provides specific questions for suspected types of mistreatment.

Other important areas for inquiry are more specific health-related questions, for example, complaints; past medical, surgical, and psychiatric histories; frequent visits to the ED; over-the-counter and prescription medications; habits such as smoking, alcohol, and illicit drug use; diet, including food, fluids, and any dietary restrictions; sleep pattern; environmental history; psychosocial history, including the home and safety environments; significant others; daily routine and activities; important experiences; religious beliefs; and outlook on life. The history should also include a thorough functional history and review of head-to-toe systems. Alterations in any of these may trigger signs of elder mistreatment. A thorough functional history includes asking if the patient is independent, dependent, or in need of assistance with any of the activities of daily living (ADLs) such as bathing,

Table 18–4 Questions for Suspected Types of Elder Mistreatment

Has anyone ever tried to hurt you in any way?

Have you had any recent injuries?

Has anyone ever touched you or tried to touch you without permission?

Suspected evidence of physical abuse (i.e., black eye) ask:

    How did that get there?

    When did it occur?

    Did someone do this to you?

    Are there other areas on your body like this?

    Has this ever occurred before?

Has anyone ever yelled at you or threatened you?

Has anyone been insulting you and using degrading language?

Has anyone ever made you do things you didn't want to do?

Do you live in a household where frustration or stress is exhibited?

Are you cared for by anyone who abuses drugs or alcohol?

Are you cared for by anyone who was abused as a child?

Who pays your bills? Do you ever go to the bank with him/her? Does this person have power of attorney?

Have you ever signed documents you didn't understand?

Are any of your family members exhibiting a great interest in your assets?

Are you alone a lot?

Has anyone ever failed you when you needed help?

Have you ever been tied down?

Are you afraid of anyone?

Has anyone ever taken anything that was yours without asking?

Has anyone ever talked with you before about this?

dressing, toileting, continence, transferring, and feeding, or with any instrumental activities of daily living (IADLs), such as grooming, taking medications, doing laundry, cleaning, traveling outside of walking distance, and managing finances. Changes, especially sudden changes in a person's ability to carry out any of these functions, may be the first indication of elder mistreatment. For example, a sudden inability or decreased ability to carry out ADLs or IADLs may be due to deterioration in health status, decrease in physical ability, or decreased cognition caused by possible elder abuse and/or neglect. Note any vague or implausible answers or explanations to questions.[26]

Once the potential victim has been assessed, the suspected abuser also must be questioned. During the interview, note inconsistencies in the histories. Questions should focus on a general description of what he/she knows about the client, the client's medical condition, the care required, what he/she expects of the client and what the client expects of him/her, exactly what he/she does for the client in terms of ADLs and IADLs, how a typical day is spent, if there are any difficulties, how he/she copes with caring for the client, and whether support system(s) or respite services are available. If financial abuse is suspected, additional questions should focus on whether the client's social security checks and other income are directly deposited in the bank, who owns the client's home or pays the rent, whose name is on the bank account(s), and if there is a power of attorney.[27] Questions should remain client-focused and asked as nonjudgmentally as possible so that the suspected abuser remains engaged in the conversation. Otherwise, the suspected abuser may feel threatened or become defensive. Note any signs of defensiveness. Keep in mind that a suspected abuser may be suffering from caregiver stress and in need of his/her own support systems and assistance, as opposed to having an actual intent to abuse the client. Note any vague or implausible answers or explanations to questions.[26]

Physical Examination

APNs should conduct a complete physical exam to assess for signs of possible mistreatment (Table 18–5). Clinical indicators of neglect include malnutrition, dehydration, pressure ulcers, contractures, and oversedation.[28] The APN should assess for bruises that appear new or at any stage of heal-

Table 18–5   Physical Exam Findings

General appearance
    Hygiene, cleanliness, and appropriateness of dress
Vital signs
    Orthostatic blood pressure
    Height and weight
Skin
    Facial injuries
    Bite marks
    Pressure ulcers
    Dehydration: dry and poor turgor
    Wrist or ankle lesions from inappropriate use of restraints
Head
    Injuries, hematomas, lacerations, and abrasions
Eyes
    Papilledema that may be related to a head injury sustained from a fall during an abusive episode
Breasts
    Excoriation and fungal infections
Musculoskeletal
    Pain, gait, fractures,
Neurological
    Impairments in strength, balance, gait, sensory perception
Genital/rectal
    Vaginal or rectal bleeding
    Vaginal or rectal discharge
    Genital, rectal, or urinary irritation, injury, infection, or scarring
    Presence of sexually transmitted disease

ing; burns, especially those that appear as an imprint of an object such as an iron, cigarette, or rope; or pressure areas that may suggest grabbing, pulling, or hitting. These should be described in terms of location, size, shape, length, width, depth, color, odor, evidence of infection, and approximate duration. One can approximate the original date of a bruise by its color: 0–2 days, swollen and tender; 0–5 days, red-blue; 5–7 days, green; 7–10 days, yellow; 10–14 days, brown; and 2–4 weeks, clear.[27] A description of the surrounding area(s) should be included as well. Bilateral bruises of the upper arms may result from forcibly holding, grabbing, or shaking a person. Bilateral bruises of the inner thighs suggest sexual assault. Whenever possible, photographs should be taken.

Fractures, dislocations, and sprains need to be explored within the context of other suspicious signs and symptoms of abuse. Imprint injuries (bruises that retain the shape of the object, such as a belt buckle, hand, or iron) are strong physical indicators of abuse. A physical restraint may be indicated by rope burns or marks on the ankles or wrists. Burns in an unusual location, such as the back, are highly significant.

Several studies demonstrate that older women are more likely, when compared to younger victims, to have injuries of the genitalia and increased frequency of vaginal lacerations or tears; one-quarter of such injuries require surgical repair. Decreased strength of the vaginal tissue, due to reduced estrogen in postmenopausal women, is the major contributor to genital tract trauma. Genital trauma may result in vaginal bleeding, as well as swelling, bruising, abrasions, and lacerations of the genital area.[29,30,31]

Psychological Assessment

Impairments of psychological/emotional status may be a precipitant or consequence of mistreatment. Specifically, the APN needs to screen for chronic mental disorders, dementia, depression, and delirium. APNs must evaluate potential victims for cognition, mood, affect, and behavior. Psychological abuse may lead to a wide range of mental/emotional behaviors, such as withdrawal, anger, aggressiveness, mood swings, anxiety, defen-

Table 18–6   Laboratory and Diagnostic Workup

Test	Indication
Complete blood count	Rule out anemia and infection
Chemistry profile, including albumin and protein levels	Rule out electrolyte imbalances, dehydration, malnutrition, and alterations in kidney and liver function
Vitamin B_{12} and folate levels	Rule out deficiencies
Thyroid function tests	Assess for hypothyroidism or hyperthyroidism
Serum levels of medications	Assess for medication overdose or subtherapeutic levels of drugs
Toxicologic screening	Assess for evidence of psychotropic agents and illicit drugs that were not prescribed
Cultures/swabs	Assess for unexplained venereal disease or genital infections
PAP smear	If needed during internal examination
Bone x-rays	Rule out fractures; look for potential misaligned fractures that may be healing or healed
Chest x-ray	Assess for worsening of chronic illness, such as congestive heart failure and chronic obstructive pulmonary disease

siveness, isolation, depression, demoralization, or fear.[7] In addition, it is important to assess for any evidence of the dynamics between victim and alleged perpetrator.

Changes in mental status may be due to physical causes related to neglect, such as malnutrition, misuse of medications, or dehydration. To assess for delirium, the APN must note new onset or fluctuating mental status and inattention, as well as disorganized thinking or altered level of consciousness.[32,33] A new onset of disorientation, confusion, or extreme lethargy may be the result of oversedation. It is very important to determine decisional capacity to remain in an abusive relationship with a perpetrator or to remain in a self-neglecting situation. Often it is necessary to collaborate with a psychiatric/mental health APN, psychiatrist, or psychologist for complex mental health evaluation or for assistance in evaluating competency or decisional capacity.

Laboratory and Diagnostic Testing

Diagnostic tests may be needed to evaluate pertinent findings and causes of delirium or apparent dementia. See Table 18–6 for tests and indications. Abnormal results may reveal causes for altered behavior or risk factors for mistreatment.[26]

Treatment of specific problems may result in more appropriate behavior and improved function, thereby lessening the burdens of care and the risk of mistreatment. Alternatively, the results of laboratory and diagnostic testing may indicate dehydration, malnourishment, over- or undermedication or other signs of mistreatment requiring immediate intervention.

◼ Evaluation and Referral

The diagnosis, management, and prevention of elder mistreatment should never occur in isolation, but rather involve interdisciplinary collaboration, including Adult Protective Services, nursing, medicine, social services, law enforcement, and case management. Across the country, a variety of service models have been developed to assess, evaluate, and prevent elder mistreatment.[34]

Hospital-Based Consultation

The ED may be the first place an abused elder encounters a health-care professional for treatment of an injury. A longitudinal study by Lachs and colleagues concluded that elderly victims of abuse have high rates of ED visits that frequently result in hospitalization. The implications of this study support the need for rigorous training for the detection and screening of elder mistreatment in EDs.[18]

The APN needs to determine emergency situations requiring immediate attention. More than 10% of 300 elder mistreatment victims seen in a community-based program required acute-care hospitalization.[6] When the mistreatment results in illness or injury requiring hospitalization, medical intervention is a priority. As the danger of recurrence of mistreatment upon return to the home is high, individuals representing resources within the hospital need to be contacted immediately. Early contact promotes a successful plan upon discharge. The hospital should not discharge a mistreated elder unless a safe place with sufficient supports has been secured.[35,36]

Some acute-care settings have elder abuse assessment teams providing both evaluation and discharge planning services.[37,38] Geriatric APNs and multidisciplinary inpatient geriatric consultation teams are also important resources. APNs should be familiar with state and county resources for elder mistreatment. In the absence of such resources, hospital social workers and discharge planners are usually available for patient follow-up.

Adult Protective Services

The primary agency responsible for investigation and case management of mistreatment is the county-based APS agency. APS has the legal responsibility and authority to investigate reports of abuse and neglect in the home, community, and institutions. In addition, APS provides services to its victims and works closely with medical professionals such as visiting nurse services (VNS) in order to enhance the victim's well-being and security.[5]

Table 18-7 Elder Mistreatment Statutes

State	APS Law	Minimum Year of Age	Reporting Requirement[1]	Penalty[2]	Reporter Protection[3]	Self-Neglect[4]	Services[5]
Alabama	1977	18	M-O	$500/6 months	L,C		E,T,H
Alaska	1988	18	M-O	M-PNS	L,C,E		T,CM
Arkansas	1977	18	M-N	M-PNS	L,C		E,T,CR,M,L
Arizona	1980	18	M	M-PNS	L,C	No	
California	1986	18	M-N	$1,000/6 months	L,C,E	No	CM,S,P,B,M
Colorado	1991	18	V	NA	L,C,E		CM
Connecticut	1977	60	M-N	$500	L,C		T,CM,CR,S,H,P,B,M
Delaware	1982	18	M-O	None	L,C		E,T,CM,S,H,B,M,L
District of Columbia	1985	18	M-O	$300	L,C,E	No	E,T,CM,S,P,B,M,L
Florida	1974	18	M-N	FNS/2 months	L,C,E		E,T,CR,CM,S,H,M,L
Georgia	1981	18	M-N	$1,000/1 year	L,C	No	P,B,M,L
Hawaii	1989	Adult	M-N	M-PNS	L,C		E,CR,CM,M
Idaho	1991	18	M-N	$300/6 months	L,C		CM,M
Illinois	1988	60	V	NA	L,C	No	T,CM
Indiana	1985	18	M-O	None	L,C,E		E,T,M
Iowa	1983	18	M-O	Civil damages	L,E		T,CM,CR,P
Kansas	1985	18	M-N	$1,000/6 months	L,C,E		T,CM,CR,H,B,M,L
Kentucky	1976	18	M-N	$250/1 year	L,C		E,T,M
Louisiana	1982	18	M-O	$500/6 months	L,C		T,CM
Maine	1981	18	M-N	$500*	L,C		E,T,CM,H,M
Maryland	1977	65	M-O	None	L,C		E,T,CM,P,L
Massachusetts	1983	60	M-N	$1,000	L,C,E	No	E,T,CM,S,P,M,L
Michigan	1982	18	M-O	$500 plus damages	L,C		CM,M,L
Minnesota	1980	18	M-O	Civil damages	L,C		E,T,CR,S,P,B,M,L
Mississippi	1986	18	M-O	$1,000/1 year	L,C,E		T,CM,CR,H,M
Missouri	1980	18	M-N	M-PNS	L,C		E,T,H
Montana	1975, 1983	60, 18	M-N	FNS	L,C,E		T,CM,CR,S,H,P,B,M,L
Nebraska	1988	18	M-N	M-PNS	L,C		

State	Year	Age	Reporting[1]	[3]	Penalty[2]	Protection[3]	Services[5]
Nevada	1981	60	M-N		1-6 years	L,C	CM,CR
New Hampshire	1978	18	M-O		M-PNS	L,C	T,CM,CR,M
New Jersey	1993	18	V		NA	L,C,E	CR,M,L
New Mexico	1989	18	M		None	L,C	E,CM,H,P,M,L
New York	1975	18	V		NA	L,C,	E,CM,H,M
North Carolina	1973	18	M-O		None	L	E,CM,S,P,B,M,L
North Dakota	1989	18	V		NA	L,C,E	CM,S,B,M,L
Ohio	1981	60	M-N		None	L,E	E,CM,S,H,P,B,M,L
Oklahoma	1977	18	M-O		M-PNS	L,C	E,T,CM,S,P,B,M
Oregon	1975, 1981	18, 65	M-N	No	None	L,C	T,CR
Pennsylvania	1987	60	V		NA	L,C,E	E,S,P,B,L
Rhode Island	1981	60	M-O	No	$1,000/1 year	L,C	T,CM,M,L
South Carolina	1974	18	M-N		$2,500/1 year	L,C,E	E,M,L
South Dakota	1976	18	V	No	NA	L	
Tennessee	1978	18	M-N		$500/3 months	L,C,E	E,CM,S,H,P,B,M,L
Texas	1981	18	M-O		M-PNS	L,C	E,T,CM,H,P,M,L
Utah	1985	18	M-N		M-PNS	L,C	E,CR
Vermont	1985	18	M-N		$500	L,C,E	T,CM,CR
Virginia	1974	18	M-N		$1,000	L,C	E
Washington	1984	60	M-N	No	None	L,C	CM
West Virginia	1981	18	M-O		$100/10 days	L,C	T,CM,P,M
Wisconsin	1983	60	V		NA	L,C,E	
Wyoming	1981	18	M-O		None	L,C	E,T,CM,P,M

The information in this table is based on a study conducted in 1993 and a review of each state's statute and amendments as of 1/1/96 (Westlaw computer-assisted legal research service).

[1]M = mandatory reporting; V = voluntary reporting; N = law specifically names nurses as mandated reporters; O = law does not name nurses specifically but names health-care professionals or anyone with the knowledge or cause to believe.

[2]Penalty = fine and/or jail term; M-PNS = misdemeanor, penalty not specified; FNS = fine not specified; * = report to professional licensing board; NA = not applicable for states with voluntary reporting laws.

[3]L = law guarantees protection from civil and criminal liability; C = law stipulates that reporting records, including the reporter's name, are confidential; E = law specifically prohibits retaliation by an employer against any employee who reports mistreatment.

[4]Each APS law includes self-neglect as a category with the exception of those listed as "no."

[5]Key to services: E = emergency intervention; T = 24 hour, statewide and/or toll-free telephone service; CR = central registry; CM = case management, including counseling and information and referral services; S = shelter; H = housing, relocation service, or respite; P = personal care, homemaker, and/or chore services; B = basics such as food, clothing, home energy assistance; M = medical and mental health services; L = legal services.

329

Community-Based Services

If assessment is inconclusive, other community agencies can give assistance with detection. For example, a home visit from a VNS can uncover the extent of a poor living situation suspected by the physician or nurse practitioner, and assist in the evaluation by APS. Additionally, each county is served by a local Area Agency on Aging providing a wide range of services to prevent or alleviate abusive or neglectful situations.

Legal Considerations

Laws/Protective Services

All states have statutes or APS laws addressing elder mistreatment.[39] Three types of state legislation address elder mistreatment: APS, elder abuse-specific statutes, and institutional elder abuse laws. State APS statutes provide APS agencies with the authority to investigate cases of mistreatment and, in some states, fund services to alleviate the abusive or neglectful situation.[40] Forty-two states require mandatory reporting of suspected mistreatment, with nurses specified as mandatory reporters in 23 states and "health care professionals, or anyone with the knowledge or cause to believe" in 16 others with mandatory reporting requirements.[1,40] Most mandatory reporting laws include civil and criminal penalties for failure to report, including fines of $100 to $1,000 and/or three months to six years imprisonment.[1,40,41] In some states, nurses cooperating with an investigation are protected from retaliation, discrimination, or disciplinary action by their employers.[1]

Table 18–7 contains a summary of the essential aspects of APS laws in each of the 50 states and the District of Columbia. Besides differences in reporting requirements, the statutes vary widely in purpose, definition, immunity, and confidentiality provisions; implementation agency; investigation procedures; and service components. It is imperative for APNs to know the laws specific to their state.

Despite adult protection laws, numerous controversies remain concerning mandatory reporting. Mandatory reporting requires the disclosure of suspected elder mistreatment regardless of victim wishes.[1] An elderly victim's refusal to accept services is also a barrier to intervention. Most frustrating are provider–patient relationships in which victims in an abusive environment insist on provider confidentiality. Failure to report the abuse and lack of consent are in direct opposition to the ethical principles of beneficence and autonomy.[8,39,42]

Documentation

Detailed, well-organized documentation is crucial when investigating any case of elder mistreatment. Although documentation may be a time-consuming process, it often proves crucial to the outcome of an elder mistreatment case. Because the written record serves both as a legal document and a care plan, records must be clear, comprehensive, and systematic. Records should include an objective description of the facts, rather than interpretation of behaviors or emotions. To the extent possible, document the client's own words and their interpretation of feelings.[5,43]

For the written record to withstand legal scrutiny, it must be legible without changes or omissions. Include all sources of information in the record, and provide the following data:

- Description of the abusive situation
- Complete medical and social history
- Physical examination detailing injuries, bruises, color, location, and measurements of the suspected injury
- Color photographs if necessary.

Any telephone or face-to-face conversations with professionals or family members need to be accurately and completely described, including where and what time the conversation occurred, and the full name, title, and relation to the victim.[5]

Prevention

APNs play an important role in the prevention of elder mistreatment, including identification of risk factors or employment of general preventive methods. These include taking steps to encourage the maintenance of friendship and support systems, community activity to the extent possible, care with regard to valuables, direct deposits of checks, and avoidance of living with those with known histories of violent behavior, alcohol abuse, or drug abuse.[44]

Prevention should also focus on caregiver stress, especially when the patient has cognitive impairment. A caregiver with untreated mental health problems, responsible for the daily care of a parent with moderate dementia, is at considerable risk for caregiver stress and potential abuse. Prevention includes arranging for respite, counseling, and treatment for the caregiver, and instruction regarding assistance as caregiving becomes too burdensome. In an acute-care setting, discharge planning should include a thorough evaluation of the caregiving situation, with attention to a respite plan or an alternative living arrangement. Prevention of elder mistreatment may also include provision to caregivers of information and assistance with alcohol or drug addictions.

In long-term-care settings, prevention should be directed toward staff members, especially those providing direct care to residents. Programs aimed at preventing staff burden include coping strategies with challenging residents and establishing support and stress management groups.[45] To promote better care, exemplary care needs to be rewarded at all levels. Interdisciplinary rounds and team meetings regarding care planning and consulting should include all levels of staff, especially when problems arise.[7] As staff members participate actively in the interdisciplinary team, they feel the value of their assessments, as well as their contribution to comprehensive care of the residents. This philosophy alone may help prevent abuse and neglect, especially inappropriate use of physical restraints and psychoactive drugs.

Conclusion

APNs play a critical role in the reduction or elimination of elder mistreatment through recognition and referral. No single provider is entirely responsible for assessment and intervention. A multidisciplinary approach, coordinated by APS and utilizing social workers, health-care providers, lawyers, and police officers can offer the most effective solutions to such devastating problems. Working cooperatively, we have a better chance to alleviate the suffering of mistreated elders.

References

1. Capezuti E, Brush B, Lawson WT. Reporting elder mistreatment. *J Gerontol Nurs.* 1997;23:24–32.
2. Lachs MS, Williams C, O'Brien S, et al. The mortality of elder mistreatment. *JAMA.* 1998;280:5, 428–432.
3. Pillemer K, Finkelhor D. The prevalence of elder abuse: a random sample survey. *Gerontologist.* 1998;28:51–57.
4. Administration for Children and Families, Administration on Aging. *The National Elder Abuse Incidence Study.* Rockville, Md: US Dept of Health and Human Services; September 1998.
5. American Medical Association. *Diagnostic and Treatment Guidelines on Elder Abuse and Neglect.* Chicago: American Medical Association; 1992.
6. Capezuti E, Yurkow J, Goldberg E. Meeting the challenge of elder mistreatment. *Nurs Dynamics.* 1995;4:1, 5–9.
7. Humphries-Lynch S. Elder abuse: what to look for, how to intervene. *Am J Nurs.* 1997;97:26.
8. Kleinschmidt KC. Elder abuse: a review. *Ann Emerg Med.* 1997;30:463.
9. Rosenblatt DE. Elder mistreatment. *Crit Care Nurs Clin N Am.* 1997;9:183.
10. Capezuti EA, Swedlow DJ. Sexual abuse in nursing homes. *Elder's Advisor: J Elder Law Post-Retirement Planning.* 2000;2:51–61.
11. Ramsey-Klawsnik H. Assessing physical and sexual abuse in health care settings. In: Baumhover LA, Beall SC, eds. *Abuse, Neglect, and Exploitation of Older Persons: Strategies for Assessment and Intervention.* Baltimore, Md: Health Professions Press; 1996:145–160.
12. Duke J. A national study of self-neglecting adult protective services clients. In: Tatara T, Rittman MM, eds. *Findings of Five Elder Abuse Studies.* Washington, DC: National Aging Resource Center on Elder Abuse; 1991:27–53.
13. Dyer CB, Pavlik VN, Murphy KP, et al. The high prevalence of depression and dementia in elder abuse and neglect. *J Am Geriat Soc.* 2000;48:205–208.
14. Salend E, Kane RA, Satz M, et al. Elder abuse reporting: limitations of statutes. *Gerontologist.* 1984;24:61–69.
15. Pillemer K, Suitor JJ. Violence and violent feelings: what causes them among family caregivers? *J Gerontol.* 1992;47:S165–S172.
16. Jones JS, Holstege C, Holstege H. Elder abuse and neglect: understanding the causes and potential risk factors. *Am J Emerg Med.* 1997;15:579–583.

17. Lavrisha M. What can nurses do about financial exploitation of elders? *J Gerontol Nurs.* 1997;23:49–50.

18. Lachs MS, Williams C, O'Brien S, et al. Risk factors for reported elder abuse and neglect: a nine-year observational cohort study. *Gerontologist.* 1997; 37:469–474.

19. Godkin MA, Wolf RS, Pillemer KA. A case-comparison analysis of elder abuse and neglect. *Int J Aging Hum Dev.* 1989;28:207–225.

20. Pillemer K, Finkelhor D. Causes of elder abuse: caregiver stress versus problem relatives. *Am J Orthopsych.* 1989;59:179–187.

21. Lachs MS, Berkman L, Fulmer T, et al. A prospective community-based pilot study of risk factors for the investigation of elder mistreatment. *J Am Geriatr Soc.* 1994;42:169–173.

22. Longres JF. Self-neglect among the elderly. *J Elder Abuse Neglect.* 1995;7:69–86.

23. Nieves-Khouw FC. Recognizing victims of physical and sexual abuse. *Crit Care Nurs Clin N Am.* 1997; 9:141–148.

24. Conlin MM. Silent suffering: a case study of elder abuse and neglect. *J Am Geriatr Soc.* 1995;43: 1303–1308.

25. Capezuti E, Siegler EL. The role of the academic nurse and physician in the criminal prosecution of nursing home mistreatment. *J Elder Abuse Neglect.* 1996; 8:47–58.

26. Lachs MS, Pillemer K. Abuse and neglect of elderly persons. *N Engl J Med.* 1995;332:437–443.

27. Quinn MJ, Tomita SK. *Elder Abuse and Neglect: Causes, Diagnosis, and Intervention Strategies.* 2nd ed. New York: Springer; 1997.

28. Fulmer T, Ashley J. Clinical indicators of elder neglect. *Appl Nurs Res.* 1989;2:161–167.

29. Ramin SM, Satin AJ, Stone IC, et al. Sexual assault in postmenopausal women. *Obstet Gynecol.* 1992;80:860–864.

30. Cartright PS, Moore RA. The elderly victim of rape. *South Med J.* 1989;82:988–989.

31. Muram D, Miller K, Cutler A. Sexual assault of the elderly victim. *J Interpersonal Violence.* 1992;7:70–76.

32. Inouye S, vanDyck C, Alessi C, et al. Clarifying confusion: the confusion assessment method. *Ann Int Med.* 1990;119:474–481.

33. Inouye S, Charpentier P. Precipitating factors for delirium in hospitalized elderly persons. *JAMA.* 1996;275:852–857.

34. Baron S, Welty A. Elder abuse. *J Gerontol Social Work.* 1996;25:33.

35. Chiplin AJ. Medicare discharge-planning regulations: an advocacy tool for beneficiaries. *Clearinghouse Rev.* 1995;29:152–156.

36. Conrad JR. Granny dumping: the hospital's duty of care to patients who have nowhere to go. *Yale Law Policy Rev.* 1992;10:463–487.

37. Beth Israel Hospital Elder Assessment Team. An elder abuse assessment team in an acute hospital setting. *Gerontologist.* 1986;26:115–118.

38. Matlaw JR, Spence DM. The hospital elder assessment team: a protocol for suspected cases of elder abuse and neglect. *J Elder Abuse Neglect.* 1994;6:23–34.

39. Greenberg SA, Ramsey GC, Mitty EL. Elder mistreatment. Case law and ethical issues in assessment, reporting, and management. *J Nurs Law.* 1999;6:76–84.

40. Tatara T. *An Analysis of State Laws Addressing Elder Abuse, Neglect, and Exploitation.* Washington, DC: National Center on Elder Abuse; 1995.

41. Formby WA. Should elder abuse be decriminalized? A justice system perspective. *J Elder Abuse Neglect.* 1992;4:121–130.

42. Lachs MS, Fulmer T. Recognizing elder abuse and neglect. *Clin Geriatr Med.* 1993;9:665–681.

43. Rosenblatt DE. Documentation. In: Baumhover LA, Beall SC, eds. *Abuse, Neglect, and Exploitation of Older Persons: Strategies for Assessment and Intervention.* Baltimore, Md: Health Professions Press; 1996:67–81.

44. Greenberg EM. Violence and the older adult: the role of the acute care nurse practitioner. *Crit Care Nurs Quart.* 1996;19:76–84.

45. Hudson B. Ensuring an abuse-free environment: A learning program for nursing home staff. *J Elder Abuse Neglect.* 1992;4:25–36.

CHAPTER **19**

Pain

Rosemary C. Polomano

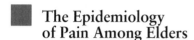

The Epidemiology of Pain Among Elders

Pain among elders is not a normal part of aging. In most cases, chronic pain in the elderly is a symptom of pathological processes caused by disease or other condition. Whatever the cause, pain experienced by elders is generally poorly controlled. Liebeskind and Melzack contend that, "pain is most poorly managed in those most defenseless against it — the young and the old."[1] Failure to appreciate the alarming number of elders who suffer from pain is a major factor contributing to ineffective pain management.

Until recently, knowledge about pain in elders was limited, but research now documents variations in estimates of pain among elders according to age groups, health status, level of independence, and living situations. Although differences in reports of pain may be affected by definitions of pain and willingness of subjects to report pain,[2] some 70–80% of elders experience pain at one time or another.[3] The incidence of pain in community-dwelling elders is about 25–50% with higher estimates, 45–80%, reported for long-term-care residents.[4,5,6] Approximately 78% of the young-old (60–69 years) have current complaints of pain, and about 64% of the healthy oldest-old (80–89 years and living independently) report some pain.[7] Elsewhere, 45% of hospitalized elders (80 years and older) complained of pain, with 19% experiencing moderate to severe pain.[8] Those most at risk are older adults with orthopedic problems (hip and other fractures). Pain present during hospitalization is likely to persist after discharge, which is significant for clinicians treating pain in home health- and long-term-care settings.

Persistent pain is often attributed to chronic musculoskeletal conditions, such as low-back pain, rheumatoid and osteoarthritis, neurologic prob-lems, and progressive cancer.[9,10] Each of these painful conditions is associated with specific mechanisms for tissue injury. Thus, an understanding of the pathophysiological processes of diseases and conditions causing pain, and the effects on psychosocial outcomes, are important for clinicians.

Physiology of Pain

The anatomical and physiological origins of pain provide the framework for assessing and treating pain. Pain may result from thermal, mechanical, and chemical activation of nociceptors, free nerve endings located in various body tissues and structures. Pain stimuli originating in the peripheral nerves are transmitted through specific fibers to pathways in the spinal cord and terminate in the thalamus. Sensory input from the thalamus is conveyed, in turn, to central areas of the brain where these painful stimuli are processed and perceived. Somatic pain arising from subcutaneous tissues of the skin, muscles, bones, and other support structures, and visceral pain from linings of body cavities and organs, result from activation of nociceptors. Characteristics of these types of pain, underlying pathophysiological mechanisms, and examples of acute and chronic pain syndromes experienced by elders are outlined in Table 19–1.

The most disturbing and complex pain, caused by damage to nerve fibers in the periphery or spinal cord and brain, is nerve injury or neuropathic pain. Distinctions between neuropathic versus somatic or visceral pain lie not only in mechanisms for the pain, but also in the responses to treatment. Neuropathic pain is believed to occur from direct damage to nerves, rather than from activation of nociceptors. It is a complex pain syndrome arising from nerve injury anywhere in the nervous system. Direct insults to nerves lead to very puzzling manifestations, such as persistent

Table 19–1   Pathophysiological Mechanisms and Examples of Acute and Chronic Pain Syndromes Experienced by Elders

Type of Pain	Physiologic Structures	Mechanism of Pain	Characteristics of Pain	Examples of Acute Pain	Sources of Chronic Pain
Somatic pain	Cutaneous: skin and subcutaneous tissues Deep somatic: bone, muscle, blood vessels, connective tissues	Activation of nociceptors	Localization of cutaneous pain: well localized Localization of deep somatic pain: less well defined Common descriptions: constant, achy	Postoperative incisional pain Pain at the insertion sites of tubes and drains Bone or hip fractures Skeletal muscle	Bony metastases Degenerative or osteoarthritis Rheumatoid arthritis Compression fractures from osteoporosis Back pain Peripheral vascular disease Chronic stasis ulcers
Visceral pain	Organs and the linings of body cavities	Activation of nociceptors	Localization: poorly localized, diffuse, deep Common descriptions: cramping, splitting	Chest and abdominal tubes and drains Bladder distention or spasms Intestinal distention Pericarditis Constipation	Organ metastases Spastic bowel Inflammatory bowel disease Hiatal hernia Chronic hepatitis
Neuropathic pain	Nerve fibers Spinal cord Central nervous system	Non-nociceptive Injury to the nervous system structures	Localization: poorly localized Common descriptions: shooting, hot-burning, fire-like, electric shock-like, sharp, painfully numb	Phantom limb pain Post-mastectomy pain Nerve compression	Diabetic neuropathy Herpes zoster-related pain Cancer-related nerve injury Chronic phantom limb pain Trigeminal neuralgia Central post-stroke pain Post-mastectomy syndrome

pain, even after an injury resolves, or pain disproportionate to the damage.[11,12] Central neuropathic pain can be due to a lesion or dysfunction in the central nervous system or thalamic pain from extrathalamic lesions. A classic example of central pain is post-stroke pain syndrome accompanying a cerebrovascular accident (CVA). Patients often report, or indicate through behavior, pain on the affected side of the body, although peripheral injury is not evident. Phantom limb is another example of central pain.

Typically, neuropathic pain is described as a very distressing sensation, such as hot or burning, fire-like, and constrictive. Paroxysmal firing, or ectopic discharge of damaged neurons, produces pain characteristically described as shooting or electric shock-like. Neuropathic pain is difficult to diagnose; however, sensory and sometimes motor deficits can be detected in the area of nerve damage. An understanding of the pathological process, along with a pain history and clinical exam, are essential for the diagnosis of neuropathic pain syndromes. Radiological evaluations with x-rays, computed tomography (CT) scans, and magnetic resonance imaging (MRI), while not conclusive for neuropathic pain, may demonstrate abnormal findings in areas of major nerves and nerve plexuses. Clinically, neuropathic pain is associated with the following abnormalities:[12]

- Alterations in sensory modalities such as touch, pressure, and thermal sensations
- Allodynia (pain evoked from stimuli that are generally not painful, such as touch)
- Dysesthesia (an unpleasant abnormal sensation, whether spontaneous or evoked)
- Hyperalgesia (exaggerated pain to stimuli that are normally painful)
- Hyperpathia (a painful syndrome characterized by increased reaction to a stimulus, especially a repetitive stimulus, as well as an increased threshold)
- Descriptions of the pain as lancinating, shooting, burning, fire-like, or painfully numb
- Motor weakness in the affected area

Barriers to Assessment and Control of Pain in the Elderly

Several barriers are responsible for inadequate assessment and undertreatment of pain among elders. Fortunately, many of these barriers have been identified, and advance practice nurses (APNs) are in a key position to work collaboratively with patients and professionals to clarify misconceptions about pain and its management.

Patient-Specific Barriers

First and foremost, clinicians must provide a climate in which patients can report pain and obtain relief. Elders have numerous misconceptions with regard to pain and pain therapies, particularly those with cancer-related pain. Misinformation held by family members must also be addressed, as family members often influence a patient's reports of pain and compliance with treatment.

Patient-related barriers are identified in the literature.[13–16] Therapeutic interventions, from pain assessment practices to education and counseling, must be directed toward these barriers:

- Inability to express pain due to altered cognitive function and mental status (e.g., dementia, delirium)
- Decreased perceptual acuity
- Fear of side effects from opioid analgesics or other analgesic medication (e.g., sedation, constipation, cognitive disturbance)
- Concerns about addiction
- Reluctance to report pain for fear that complaints will not be taken seriously
- Fear that worsened pain means worsening of disease
- Desire to be a "good patient" and not complain
- Lack of understanding about the impact of uncontrolled pain
- Persuasion by family members to avoid taking medication for pain

Health Professional Barriers

Health professionals caring for the elderly practice with numerous myths and misconceptions. Unfortunately, attitudes and beliefs about pain and analgesic therapies play a major role in limiting the use of effective pain medications. Nursing home residents, who experience the most pain, are often deprived of analgesic medications, often because they are unable to communicate pain, appear withdrawn, or the magnitude of pain is underestimated by care providers. This happens especially for the cognitively impaired, despite evidence that patients with altered cognitive states can accurately communicate their pain.[15,17] Self-reports of pain from the cognitively impaired may be just as valid as reports from those who are cognitively intact.[18] This problem is not limited just to cognitively impaired elders or those in long-term care facilities, but even in oncology outpatient settings as well, where older persons with cancer receive significantly less analgesic medications compared to younger adults.[19]

Among nurses (and others), lack of knowledge is a major challenge in the diagnosis and treatment of pain.[19,20,21] Unfounded concerns over tolerance, physical dependence, and addiction stem from confusion regarding the definitions of these terms. Tolerance is defined as resistance to the effects of a drug, whereby increased doses are needed over time to sustain the same effect. More often than not, an increased need for opioid analgesics is usually explained by worsening pain and variability in response to opioid analgesics. Although some tolerance to opioid analgesics occurs over time, this is not generally a clinical problem.

Physical dependence occurs with continued use of opioid analgesics, as opioid-agonists (morphine-like opioids) bind to the μ receptor. Over time, μ receptors become accustomed to opioids and when the opioid is abruptly withdrawn, activation of the autonomic nervous system brings about physical withdrawal. Patients with physical dependence can be safely weaned from opioid therapy, should their pain resolve or diminish. To prevent acute physiological withdrawal, opioid doses can be reduced no more than 10% each day. Tapering schedules should be individualized, however, as some patients require slower reductions in daily dosages.

Addiction is neither tolerance nor physical dependence; rather, it is a behavioral and social phenomenon rooted in drug abuse and craving. No published data support the likelihood of addiction among elders treated for pain. Occasionally, behaviors thought to be signs of addiction occur. These may include frequent requests or watching the clock for medication, preoccupation with pain, and emotional outbursts. Such behaviors most likely stem from opioids with insufficient analgesic efficacy or ineffective doses of short-acting opioids that are improperly administered.

Other barriers that contribute to the inadequate treatment of pain by health professionals include:

- Lack of appreciation for the magnitude of pain
- Inability to appreciate individualized responses to pain
- Lack of knowledge about the physiology of pain

- Belief that pain is a normal part of aging
- Belief that long-term pain is more tolerable over time
- Misconception that older people experience less pain than younger people
- Misinformation regarding the efficacy of less-potent analgesics
- Traditional and standardized approaches to pain
- Concerns over potential adverse effects from opioid and other analgesics (e.g., sedation, increased risk for self-injury such as falls)
- Fear of investigations or repercussions from drug enforcement agencies for prescribing opioids

Systems-Related Barriers

Health systems-related barriers impose significant limitations on clinicians' abilities to treat pain in elders effectively, especially in long-term-care facilities. Not only is pain poorly managed in long-term-care residents; interventions to enhance comfort care are hindered further by institutional factors.[5] Despite the selected, but growing and effective, use of nurse and pharmacist consultants from provider pharmacies, along with palliative care and hospice services, residents in long-term-care facilities still suffer from unrelenting pain. Stein and Ferrell provide a comprehensive review of factors that influence pain practices in long-term care.[5]

Barriers Encountered in Long-Term-Care Facilities

- Limited education of professional and non-professional staff
- Reluctance to refer patients to outside pain clinics or centers
- Limited drug formulary options for pharmacotherapy, especially for opioids
- Standardized protocols for analgesic therapy that encourage fixed doses and dosing intervals of analgesics without individualizing medication regimens

- Outdated policies and procedures for medication administration
- Limited staffing resources to assess pain and implement flexible analgesic therapy schedules
- Misinterpretation of restrictions imposed on practice by state regulations (e.g., the use of psychoactive drugs)

Overcoming these barriers to pain control require familiarity with evidence-based literature, ongoing education, and resocialization of clinicians concerning practices for pain management. The latter is best accomplished through collaboration among physicians, nurses, pharmacists, and other professionals, along with the nonprofessional staff and facility administrators. Evidence- and consensus-based guidelines published by authoritative agencies and organizations such as the American Geriatrics Society, Agency for Healthcare Research and Quality (AHRQ), and the American Pain Society can be powerful sources for changing practice.[6,22–24]

Pain Assessment and Evaluation

Numerous factors complicate the pain assessment process in the elderly. Validated age-specific pain assessment criteria and measurements exist and can be implemented in clinical practice; however, reluctance to appreciate the incidence and magnitude of pain hampers consistent use.

Acute Versus Chronic Pain

Distinctions between acute and chronic pain follow.

Acute Pain

- Always serves a biologic purpose
- Associated with physiological and autonomic responses

   ($\uparrow$ BP, $\uparrow$ HR, $\uparrow$ RR)
   Dilated pupils
   Perspiration
- Typically well described and localized

- Often presents with restlessness, apprehension, anxiety, or inability to concentrate
- Generally subsides with or without treatment

Chronic Pain

- Never serves a biological purpose
- Rarely associated with physiological and autonomic responses
- Poorly localized and described
- Rarely resolves on its own
- Can be progressive and debilitating
- Often associated with depression and altered mood states

Pain History

The American Geriatrics Society recommends use of a comprehensive pain assessment form when taking a pain history.[6] Figure 19–1 represents the dimensions of pain that should be evaluated as recommended by the American Geriatrics Society.[6] A pain history not only is important to understanding the pain experience, but also provides the necessary data for designing analgesic regimens and guiding psychosocial interventions. A comprehensive pain assessment and evaluation includes the following.

Pain Pattern   Assess whether pain is constant, intermittent, or both. Is pain associated with certain activities, ingestion of food, a particular time of day, or other factors? Is the pattern of pain predictable? Answers to these questions are especially useful for designing analgesic regimens. For example, pain that is moderate to severe, and both constant and intermittent, may require a regularly scheduled opioid analgesic and a short-acting supplemental or "rescue" analgesic available on a prn basis. Intermittent pain may be predictable, occurring at certain times of the day or in response to specific circumstances (e.g., getting out of bed in the morning), and treated accordingly.

GERIATRIC PAIN ASSESSMENT

Date: _____   Medical Record Number   _____

Patient's Name   _____

Problem List: Medications:

_____   _____

_____   _____

_____   _____

_____   _____

Pain Description:

Pattern: Constant   Intermittent   Pain Intensity:

Duration: _____   0   1   2   3   4   5   6   7   8   9   10

Location: _____   None   Moderate   Severe

Character:

Lancinating   Burning   Stinging   Worst Pain in Last 24 hours:

Radiating   Shooting   Tingling   0   1   2   3   4   5   6   7   8   9   10

Other Descriptors: None   Moderate   Severe

_____   Mood: _____

_____   Depression Screening Score: _____

_____   Gait and Balance Score: _____

_____   Impaired Activities:

Exacerbating Factors: _____

_____   _____

_____   _____

Relieving Factors: Sleep Quality: _____

_____   Bowel Habits: _____

_____

Other Assessments or Comments: _____

_____

Most Likely Cause of Pain: _____

Plans: _____

_____

_____

Figure 19–1

Example of a medical record form that can be used to summarize pain assessment in older persons.[5]

Breakthrough pain occurs at particular times, despite use of regularly scheduled or around-the-clock opioid analgesia. When breakthrough pain occurs at the duration end-point for long-acting analgesics, the dose can be increased (e.g., con-trolled-released morphine [MS Contin], oxycodone [OxyContin], and hydromorphone [Pallidone] or transdermal fentanyl system [Duragesic]). With short-acting opioids, consider increasing the dose, decreasing the dosing interval, or switching to a long-acting opioid. Unpredictable breakthrough pain can be managed with prompt administration of short-acting analgesics.

Aggravating or Precipitating Factors   Ask what makes the pain worse. What changes in lifestyle are affected by the pain (e.g., diet, sleep, getting out of bed, walking, and other activities of daily living [ADLs])?

Duration of Pain   How long has pain persisted?

Pain Relieving Factors   What relieves the pain?

Location of Pain   Pain can either be deep, superficial, or both. Position or location can be identified through the use of pictorial aids, where the patient shades areas of pain or points to painful areas showing extent of the pain. Pain can be:

1. Localized: confined to a specific area
2. Projected: pain along a specific nerve distribution
3. Radiating: diffuse pain in a particular location without clear delineation
4. Referred: pain that is perceived distant from the site of origin

Pain Intensity   Several pain rating scales are validated for older adults (Figure 19–2). [6, 25, 26] A numeric rating scale (NRS) from 0 to 10, with 0 representing no pain and 10 the worst pain, is the most popular measure. Those suffering from intense, unrelenting pain, or who are cognitively impaired, may have difficulty with a numeric scale. A categorical scale with limited word choices matched to a numeric rating is preferred by many elders. Choose the one that works for a particular patient and use it consistently.

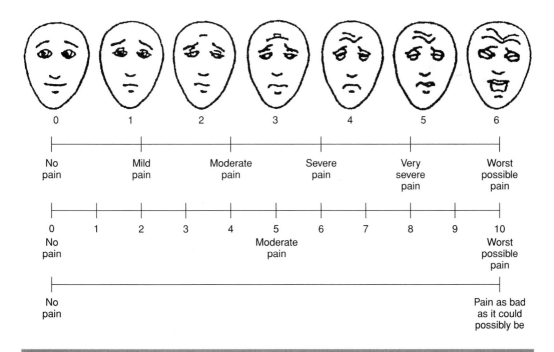

Figure 19–2
Examples of pain intensity scales for use with older patients. The Faces Rating Scale is shown at top.[27]

The Faces Rating Scale is useful with cognitive dysfunction. Representations of adult faces may be more acceptable for use in elders.[27]

Because intensity of pain varies, it may be helpful to quantify pain as average, present, worst, and least pain as outlined in a well-accepted pain measure, the Brief Pain Inventory (Figure 19-3).[28]

- Average pain intensity (API): A rating of the pain on the average or most of the time. The

API is useful to determine whether a regularly scheduled analgesic is needed to keep the pain under control, and to gauge the overall effectiveness of continuous or regularly scheduled analgesic therapy.

- Present pain intensity (PPI): A rating of the level of pain at the time the patient is asked. PPI levels can be obtained at various time points coinciding with an increase or

---

Brief Pain Inventory (Short Form)

Study ID # _____   Hospital # _____

Do not write above this line

Date: _____/_____/_____
Time: _____
Name:_____ _____ _____
            Last   First   Middle initial

1) Throughout our lives, most of us have had pain from time to time (such as minor headaches, sprains, and toothaches). Have you had pain other than these everyday kinds of pain today?   1. Yes   2. No

2) On the diagram, shade in the areas where you feel pain. Put an X on the area that hurts the most.

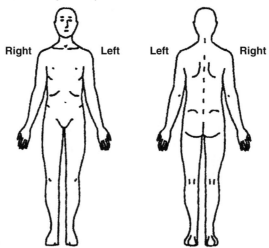

     Right   **Left**   **Left**   **Right**

3) Please rate your pain by circling the one number that best describes your pain at its **worst** in the past 24 hours.

   0   1   2   3   4   5   6   7   8   9   10
   No   Pain as bad as
   pain   you can imagine

Figure 19–3
The Brief Pain Inventory (short form) is a well-accepted measure.[28]

4) Please rate your pain by circling the one number that best describes your pain at its **least** in the past 24 hours.

| 0 | 1 | 2 | 3 | 4 | 5 | 6 | 7 | 8 | 9 | 10 |

No
pain

Pain as bad as
you can imagine

5) Please rate your pain by circling the one number that best describes your pain on the **average.**

| 0 | 1 | 2 | 3 | 4 | 5 | 6 | 7 | 8 | 9 | 10 |

No
pain

Pain as bad as
you can imagine

6) Please rate your pain by circling the one number that tells how much pain you have **right now.**

| 0 | 1 | 2 | 3 | 4 | 5 | 6 | 7 | 8 | 9 | 10 |

No
pain

Pain as bad as
you can imagine

7) What treatments or medications are you receiving for your pain?

_____

8) In the past 24 hours, how much **relief** have pain treatments or medications provided? Please circle the one percentage that most shows how much relief you have received.

| 0% | 10% | 20% | 30% | 40% | 50% | 60% | 70% | 80% | 90% | 100% |

No
relief

Complete
relief

9) Circle the one number that describes how, during the past 24 hours, **pain has interfered** with your:

A. General activity

| 0 | 1 | 2 | 3 | 4 | 5 | 6 | 7 | 8 | 9 | 10 |

Does not
interfere

Completely
interferes

B. Mood

| 0 | 1 | 2 | 3 | 4 | 5 | 6 | 7 | 8 | 9 | 10 |

Does not
interfere

Completely
interferes

C. Walking ability

| 0 | 1 | 2 | 3 | 4 | 5 | 6 | 7 | 8 | 9 | 10 |

Does not
interfere

Completely
interferes

D. Normal work (includes both work outside the home and housework)

| 0 | 1 | 2 | 3 | 4 | 5 | 6 | 7 | 8 | 9 | 10 |

Does not
interfere

Completely
interferes

E. Relations with other people

| 0 | 1 | 2 | 3 | 4 | 5 | 6 | 7 | 8 | 9 | 10 |

Does not
interfere

Completely
interferes

F. Sleep

| 0 | 1 | 2 | 3 | 4 | 5 | 6 | 7 | 8 | 9 | 10 |

Does not
interfere

Completely
interferes

G. Enjoyment of life

| 0 | 1 | 2 | 3 | 4 | 5 | 6 | 7 | 8 | 9 | 10 |

Does not
interfere

Completely
interferes

Figure 19–3 (continued)

decrease in the pain, or the peak action or duration of an analgesic in order to determine effectiveness.

■ Worst pain intensity (WPI): Indicates the highest level of pain when it is most severe. Ask patients to identify factors associated with increased levels of pain such as getting out of bed, ambulating, or with activities at different times of the day. WPI levels indicate the usefulness or effectiveness of "rescue" or supplemental analgesia.

■ Least pain intensity (LPI): It is helpful to know at what times or under what circumstances pain levels are at their lowest.

Character and Quality of the Pain   Several instruments using descriptive words have been validated with older adults. The Short-Form McGill Questionnaire (Figure 19–4) allows patients to report sensations and feelings and to rate pain intensity.[29] The first 11 words define the sensory component of pain and the last 4 capture its affective components. Aggressive attempts to manage the pain and evaluate the presence of psychological distress are critical for those patients who choose words indicative of moderate to severe pain. In these cases, ongoing efforts to manage both the pain and the psychological distress are warranted.

Those with neuropathic pain tend to select words like shooting, hot-burning, and stabbing. Word choices can be monitored with the initiation of adjuvant drug therapy, along with associated features of neuropathic pain such as painful numbness, vasomotor responses, and motor weakness.

Perception of Pain Relief   A pain relief scale is useful to determine perceptions of effectiveness of the analgesic medication(s), especially with analgesics having no or limited documented use for moderate to severe chronic pain (acetaminophen, propoxyphene, and codeine). Various scales for measuring pain relief are outlined in the AHRQ clinical practice guidelines for cancer pain.[23] Percentage rating scales, as in the Brief Pain Inventory,[28] might be confusing to elders because the numeric ratings are the opposite of those for pain intensity. Higher values on pain relief indicate a more favorable response, whereas higher values for pain intensity indicate greater pain. It is very easy and practical to simply ask patients if their pain relief is acceptable.

Pain Expressions and Behaviors   Behavioral cues may be a significant indicator of pain, especially among elders with dementia or delirium. Observe for grunting, groaning, facial grimacing, wrinkled forehead, body positioning and movements (fetal position, guarding or holding a part of the body, rubbing or massaging parts of the body, etc.), reluctance to move or change position, and ritualistic behaviors (rocking or pacing). Patients with neuropathic pain may experience cutaneous hypersensitivity to touch, pressure, heat, and cold. Some simply experience pain from the contact of clothing on sensitive areas of the body.

Pain Diaries or Pain Flow Sheets   Pain inventories or pain diaries enable clinicians to track patterns of the pain, as well as allow patients an avenue for self-expression concerning pain. A diary (depending on whether maintained by the patient or for more specific clinical purposes) should include date/time, pain intensity (if possible), vital signs (if acute pain), time-dependent analgesic administration, observations during ADLs, behaviors, general description, pertinent assessment data, and any other relevant information about the pain experience.

Pain in the Cognitively Impaired Elder

Assessing pain in cognitively impaired persons is clinically challenging. Does pain or its treatment exacerbate cognitive impairment? The coexistence of pain with depression and dementia makes assessment particularly difficult. Nevertheless, almost all elders with degrees of cognitive impairment or even dementia have some capacity for communicating pain, be it through facial expressions, unwillingness to move about, or other behaviors. In a random sample of 217 elderly subjects (average age 85 years) in 10 nursing home facilities, with varying degrees of cognitive impairment (Folstein Mini-Mental State Exam mean score of 12.1 ± 7.9), Ferrell and colleagues found

	NONE	MILD	MODERATE	SEVERE
THROBBING	0)	1)	2)	3)
SHOOTING	0)	1)	2)	3)
STABBING	0)	1)	2)	3)
SHARP	0)	1)	2)	3)
CRAMPING	0)	1)	2)	3)
GNAWING	0)	1)	2)	3)
HOT-BURNING	0)	1)	2)	3)
ACHING	0)	1)	2)	3)
HEAVY	0)	1)	2)	3)
TENDER	0)	1)	2)	3)
SPLITTING	0)	1)	2)	3)
TIRING/EXHAUSTING	0)	1)	2)	3)
SICKENING	0)	1)	2)	3)
FEARFUL	0)	1)	2)	3)
PUNISHING/CRUEL	0)	1)	2)	3)

Figure 19–4
The Short-Form McGill Pain Questionnaire allows patients to rate pain
intensity.[29]

that most (83%) were able to use at least one of
five pain intensity scales, while 32% rated pain on
all five.[15] The McGill Present Pain Intensity
Questionnaire had the highest completion rate.

When it is not possible to elicit subjective measurements of pain, ADLs, behaviors, and other

nonverbal cues should be observed. Data suggest
that independent activity or "elective" activities
such as ambulating, walking to the bathroom, rising from a sitting to standing position, and putting
on clothes may be more valid predictors of pain
than other self-report measures.[15,30]

Useful Strategies to Assess Pain in the Cognitively Impaired Elder

- Evaluate all possible physiological sources for pain associated with diseases and painful conditions.
- Determine the presence of pain prior to cognitive dysfunction.
- Obtain histories from family members, if possible.
- Observe the patient during ADLs.
- Observe nonverbal cues and behaviors.
- Assess pain with aids that are designed for the cognitively impaired (e.g., Faces Rating Scale).
- Consistently use the same pain scale, by the same health-care provider, where possible.
- Assess responses to a trial of analgesic medication.

Pain Management Therapies

Analgesic Therapy

When designing analgesic regimens for the treatment of either acute or chronic pain, it is important to consider the following factors:

1. Etiology (disease-related, condition-related, unclear, or unknown)
2. Physiological sources (somatic, visceral, neuropathic, or any combination)
3. Mechanism (e.g., inflammation, muscle spasm, visceral distention, nerve compression, or infiltration)
4. Trajectory (progressive or nonprogressive)
5. Severity (mild, moderate, or severe)
6. Degree of physical debilitation
7. Duration
8. Confounding psychological variables (depression and anxiety)
9. Cognitive or mental status
10. Physiological changes from aging

Table 19–2 highlights those physiological changes that occur with aging that are most likely to influence the pharmacodynamics of analgesic therapy.[31–37]

Management of Acute Pain

Postoperative Pain　　Inadequate relief of postsurgical pain is linked to negative postoperative outcomes.[22] Misconceptions about the use of conventional methods for pain control are responsible for their limited use for older persons. In general, the same modalities used for adults are also effective with elders. Numerous studies have shown that patient-controlled epidural analgesia and systemic patient-controlled analgesia offer the best outcomes for pain and recovery compared to more traditional prn nurse-administered analgesia.[22] Unfortunately, technology-supported pain care is underutilized for pain control in the elderly.

Severe postoperative pain has been associated with altered mental status. There appears to be a strong relationship between higher levels of pain at rest and delirium in the first three days following noncardiac surgery.[38] Consistent pain relief is critically important following surgery. Adequate management of postsurgical pain in the elderly leads to improvements in physiological variables such as neuroendocrine stress responses and pulmonary function.[39] Combinations of aggressive pain techniques that include regional analgesia tend to be most effective.

Patient-Controlled Analgesia　　Although patient-controlled analgesia (PCA) is an effective and safe method for pain control in the elderly,[40] the design of PCA regimens are debated. Because elders are more likely to experience a higher analgesic peak and a longer duration from opioid analgesics, careful attention to PCA self-administered demand doses and continuous or basal rate background infusions are critical.

Morphine remains the opioid of choice for PCA in both young and old. Compared to meperidine (Demerol), morphine is superior in relieving pain, despite potential side effects of nausea, mood disturbances, and unusual dreams.[41] Meperidine should be avoided in the elderly as it has an active metabolite, normeperidine, that accumulates with repeated doses. Toxic metabolites can also accumulate with morphine. Starting doses of morphine sulfate should be 0.5 to 1 mg per hour, with a demand or self-administered dose of 1 mg at an interval of

Table 19–2 Age and Its Effects on Managing Pain[6,31–37]

	Physiological Age-Related Changes	Preexisting Diseases and Conditions	Considerations with Pharmacotherapy	Assessment and Interventions
Mental Status	Normal changes • Decreased mental acuity • Increased response to sedating agents Abnormal changes • Short-term memory deficits • Slower processing of information and response	Dementia Alzheimer's disease Delirium Depression	Use caution with psychoactive agents. Select opioid agents with low side-effect profile for sedation (e.g., hydrocodone, oxycodone, and hydromorphone), as well as adjuvant agents (e.g., gabapentin and desipramine). Initiate therapy with one-half the usual starting doses for adults. Therapy with an SRI may be indicated if depression persists following adequate control of pain.	Perform baseline cognitive assessments and monitor for changes in mental status. Institute safety precautions. Use appropriate age-specific pain measures for the elderly and cognitively impaired. Use aids to facilitate memory deficits. Allow ample response times for patients who are slow to process information.
Hearing and Visual Acuity	Decreased visual acuity Increased drying of the eyes Hearing impairment	Glaucoma Cataracts	Avoid drugs that are contraindicated with glaucoma (e.g., agents with anticholinergic effects)	Instruct patients to report changes in vision. Use pain assessment measures and teaching materials that are easy to read. Modify the environment (e.g., proper lighting, reduce noise and external stimuli). Speak clearly and maintain eye contact. Use medication labels that can be read easily. Ensure proper functioning of hearing aids. Assess adherence to medication schedules. Request feedback to ensure patients understand medication schedules.
Musculo-skeletal	Degenerative joint disease Joint stiffness Decreased mobility	Osteoarthritis Rheumatoid arthritis Back pain Osteoporosis with or without compression fractures Bony metastases	Begin with nonopioid agents. Do not exceed daily recommended doses of > than 4,000 mg. Use NSAIDs appropriately for inflammatory pain. Discontinue therapy if analgesia is not effective. Consider opioids for moderate to severe pain from long-term effects of rheumatoid and osteoarthritis. Prescribe and administer effective supplemental analgesia for provoked pain associated with activity.	Routinely evaluate liver and renal function studies with long-term use of acetaminophen and NSAIDs. Assess radiological evaluations of skeletal structure (skeletal films, bone density studies). Promote independence with ADLs. Encourage exercise and physical therapy programs. Institute treatment with methods of cutaneous stimulation.

(continues)

Table 19–2 Age and Its Effects on Managing Pain[6,31–37] (continued)

	Physiological Age-Related Changes	Preexisting Diseases and Conditions	Considerations with Pharmacotherapy	Assessment and Intervention
Pulmonary	Decreased pulmonary reserves	COPD Emphysema	Use caution with opioid and other analgesic agents that cause sedation. For patients who are opioid-naive, initiate opioid therapy using one-half the usual starting dose for adults. Remember that the risk of respiratory depression from opioids is minimized if doses are escalated safely. Respiratory depression from opioids is rarely a problem for patients who are opioid-dependent and tolerant to their effects.	Obtain baseline assessments of respiratory status, especially for patients who are opioid-naive or debilitated, and closely monitor respiratory rates. Observe for early signs of respiratory insufficiency such as confusion or changes in breathing patterns. Encourage activity, and for patients who are bedridden, cough, turn, and deep breathing exercises.
Cardio-vascular	Reduced blood volume Decreased cardiac output and reserve Decreased circulation Conduction abnormalities	Congestive heart failure Hypertension Cardiac arrhythmias	Drug absorption, distribution, and excretion may be altered by cardiovascular changes associated with aging. Administer NSAIDs cautiously to patients with congestive heart failure due to a reduction in prostaglandins that are necessary to maintain renal perfusion. This increases the risk for fluid retention and peripheral edema. Reduction in renal function from NSAIDs may interfere with elimination of digoxin, increasing the risk for digitoxicity. Avoid tricyclic antidepressants if patients have cardiac conduction defects.	Observe for increased signs and symptoms of adverse effects from analgesics. Assess for peripheral edema and signs of worsening congestive heart failure. Be aware of drug interactions (e.g., quinidine and tricyclic antidepressants). Monitor digoxin levels and watch for signs of digitoxicity for patients taking NSAIDs. ECG should be done before initiating therapy with tricyclic antidepressants. Assess patients for dizziness or syncope.
Gastro-intestinal	Changes in salivary flow and dentition Decreased fluid intake Dehydration Decreased gastric emptying	Gastropathy or gastroparesis Constipation	Avoid NSAIDs in patients with a history of peptic ulcer disease. Avoid NSAIDs in patients concurrently taking anticoagulants (e.g., warfarin). Use opioids cautiously in patients who are dehydrated, as they may be more susceptible to opioid-related side effects.	For opioid and adjuvant therapy with tricyclic antidepressants: • Maintain adequate fluid intake • Encourage good oral hygiene practices • Institute aggressive bowel regimens

System	Physiologic Change	Condition		
Hepatic	Delayed hepatic metabolism of drugs		Avoid long-acting agents in patients with hepatic dysfunction. Use caution with opioids and adjuvant agents with long T½.	Administer lower doses of opioid analgesics with longer intervals between dosing. Monitor liver function tests.
Renal	Decrease renal filtration and renal clearance	Renal insufficiency	Consider doses of 400 mg of ibuprofen tid to reduce the risk of renal toxicity with long-term use. Avoid agents with toxic active metabolites that are excreted by the kidney (meperidine, proproxyphene).	Obtain baseline BUN, creatinine, and creatinine clearance prior to initiating therapy with NSAIDs, and monitor renal function closely for long-term NSAID use. Monitor digoxin levels and watch for signs of digitoxicity if patients are taking NSAIDs.
Urinary		Benign prostatic hypertrophy in men Urinary incontinence, stress incontinence in women	Patients who are opioid-naïve are most at risk for urinary retention. Use caution with anticholinergic agents (e.g., amitriptyline) that may cause urinary retention.	Monitor for adverse effects as a result of prolonged drug clearance. Monitor urinary output if patients are receiving postoperative systemic opioids or epidural analgesia. Instruct patients taking opioids or tricyclic antidepressants to report changes in urination, and be aware of signs of urinary tract infections.

10–15 minutes. For the oldest-old, 80 years or older, intermittent demand dosing alone is recommended until response to therapy can be evaluated.

Elders require intensive teaching on the use of PCA, preferably prior to surgery. In general, elders are reluctant to access demand doses because of fearfulness about medication effects or addiction. Concerns about opioid analgesics should be addressed both pre- and postoperatively.

Regional Analgesia   Epidural analgesia with either opioid or local anesthetics, or a combination of both, should be considered whenever possible. Epidural analgesia is associated with improved perfusion and pulmonary function, early mobilization, faster recovery of gastrointestinal function, reduced risk of thromboemboli, and lower incidence of chronic pain following surgery (e.g., postamputation phantom limb pain).[42] Elders may be at risk for respiratory depression, especially with epidural morphine. Fentanyl (Sublimaze) may be a better choice for the elderly as it is less likely to reach the central nervous system by rostral (vertical) spread. Local anesthetics, such as bupivacaine (Marcaine), have an effect on sensory and motor neurons and may cause orthostatic hypotension and lower motor weakness. Ropivacaine, selective for sensory nerves, may avoid motor effects.[43] Epidural local anesthetics can decrease the sensation of pressure, especially in the skin. Long-acting local anesthetics, for example, lidocaine, often given as a bolus epidural injection, can produce cognitive impairment if serum levels become toxic. Use of epidural analgesia with elders requires attention to the following points:

- Use with caution for men with preexisting bladder problems and benign prostatic hypertrophy because of greater risk for urinary retention.

- Administer lower concentrations of bupivacaine (Marcaine) (e.g., 0.05–0.0625% solutions) to minimize orthostatic hypotension and lower motor weakness.

- Note that elders who suffer from respiratory disorders may be at increased risk for respiratory depression.

- Assess cognitive status, which may be further compromised.

- Monitor respiratory rates for the first 24 hours of therapy.

- Assist patients while getting out of bed and ambulating.

- Reposition patients frequently while in bed.

- Assess urinary function.

Management of Chronic Pain

Despite the high prevalence of pain among elders, studies continue to document that older people receive fewer analgesics.[9,15,17] Guidelines on the management of pain in older persons from the American Geriatrics Society reflect the existing research on pain and present evidence- and consensus-based recommendations on effective pharmacological and nonpharmacological interventions.[6] There is no doubt that the management of cancer pain in elders is fraught with fear of overmedicating patients and lack of knowledge as to the appropriate use of analgesics. Specialized palliative care for elders has become a growing area of specialization. Abrahm examines the components of an effective pain program that includes decision-making criteria and strategies to reduce pain and manage adverse effects from analgesics at the end of life.[44] While concerns remain about analgesic use, especially opioids in the elderly, problems can be avoided with careful attention to initial dosing, timing of doses, side effect profiles, age-specific changes in hepatic and renal function, and environmental safety. Problems with opioid analgesics are most often caused by improper prescribing practices and inappropriate administration. Above all, the goal for analgesic therapy should be acceptable pain relief, not minimal drug doses.[24]

Cancer Pain   Despite the high incidence of pain, elders with cancer are less likely to receive aggressive pharmacotherapy, interventional techniques for pain control, and palliative care services.[45] In a multi-statewide effort to determine the prevalence of cancer pain and predictors of poor outcomes, 13,625 elders with cancer were evaluated from hospitalization to long-term care facilities using the Systematic Assessment of Geriatric Drug Use via Epidemiology (SAGE) database.[46] An alarming 25–40% of patients with cancer experienced daily pain. Lack of adequate analgesia and decreased use of adjuvant agents for cancer pain were associated with increased age. Patients of ethnic minorities were also more likely to be undermedicated. Additionally, as medication regimens for other health problems became more complex, the use of analgesic therapies was reduced. Preexisting nonmalignant pain problems, cognitive impairment, and depression were linked to poorer outcomes. A thorough examination of health-care practices in long-term care facilities for recognizing pain, eliciting self-report outcomes, and prescribing effective analgesic therapy showed an increased need for education and change in attitudes and opportunities for maximizing pharmacotherapy in the treatment of cancer pain.[46]

Patients with cancer not only experience pain from their disease, but must also contend with pain from preexisting conditions and cancer therapies. The complex nature of pain associated with cancer and other factors requires a thorough evaluation of all possible sources of pain. Figure 19–5 provides an algorithm for specific pain management practices. The World Health Organization has established a three-step analgesic ladder intended to guide the selection of pharmacological therapy based on varying levels of pain (Figure 19–6). The Management of Cancer Pain Guideline Panel outlines the advantages and disadvantages of specific pain therapies.[23]

Opioid Analgesics Opioid analgesics are indicated when chronic moderate to severe pain has not responded to nonopioid preparations. Elders with longstanding chronic pain usually require opioid therapy. Centrally acting opioid-agonists (e.g., codeine, hydrocodone, oxycodone, morphine, hydromorphone) have an affinity for μ receptors and are preferred over other opioid preparations. Opioids, such as mepridine (Demerol) and propoxyphene (active agent in Darvocet), are weak, and toxic metabolites from these drugs accumulate with repeated dosing. The toxic metabolite of

meperidine, normeperidine, can lead to seizures; cardiac toxicity may occur from the metabolite of propoxyphene.[37,41] Even with its serious limitations, propoxyphene is still overprescribed and it is no better in its analgesic efficacy than acetaminophen or aspirin.[37]

Guidelines for Opioid Therapy

- "Start low and go slow":[6] begin with lower doses of less-potent, short-acting opioids such as codeine, hydrocodone (Vicodin, Lotabs), oxycodone alone, or oxycodone + acetaminophen (Percocet, Roxicet, Endocet).

- Be aware of analgesic peak effects from opioids and duration: a trial of short-acting opioids at half the usual starting dose for adults should be initiated. Peak effects from the opioid may be heightened in elders and duration extended. Initial prescribing should allow for longer dosing intervals until response to the opioid has been evaluated.

- Avoid opioids that possess active metabolites or a long half-life: opioids that have active toxic metabolites (e.g., propoxyphene and meperidine) should not be used on a long-term basis. Morphine does have active metabolites, so it should be administered with caution. In addition, opioids with extended T½ (half-life) should not be prescribed for elders who are opioid-naïve.

- Consider combination opioid preparations for relief of mild to moderate pain: combination opioid products (e.g., codeine + acetaminophen [Tylenol #3, #4], hydrocodone + acetaminophen [Vicodin, Lortabs, Lorcet], oxycodone + acetaminophen [Percocet, Roxicet, Endocet]) should be prescribed on a short-term basis for mild to moderate pain. Overuse of these medications can lead to acetaminophen hepatotoxicity.

- Consider lower doses of short-acting opioid without combination products: short-acting oxycodone (Oxy IR, OxyFast) or hydromorphone (Dilaudid) may be appropriate for patients experiencing severe pain as these preparations can be titrated to pain relief with-

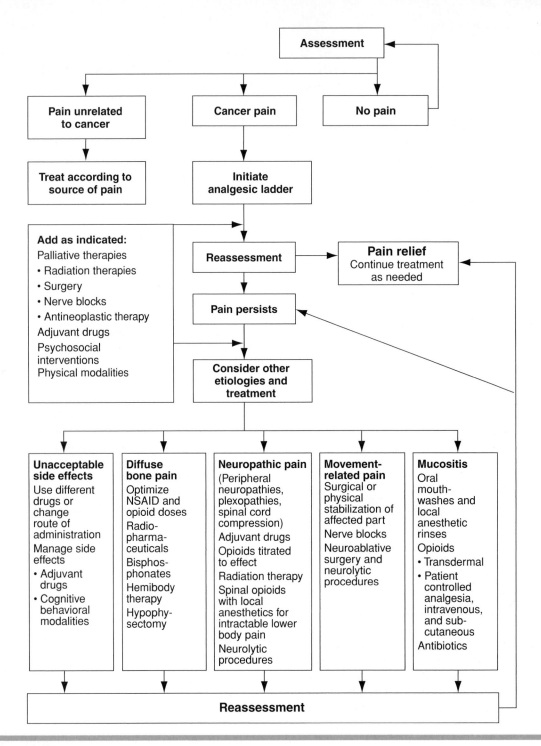

Figure 19–5
Flowchart for continuing pain management in patients with cancer.[23]

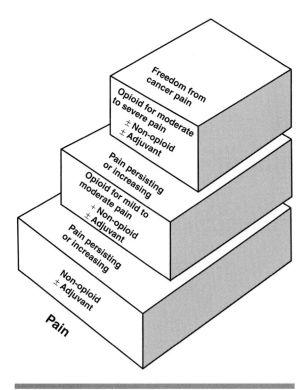

Freedom from
cancer pain
Opioid for moderate
to severe pain
± Non-opioid
± Adjuvant

Pain persisting
or increasing
Opioid for mild to
moderate pain
± Non-opioid
± Adjuvant

Pain persisting
or increasing

Non-opioid
± Adjuvant

Pain

Figure 19–6
The WHO three-step analgesic ladder.[23]

out the concern of added toxicity from combination products. Unlike short-acting morphine, these agents do not have active toxic metabolites. Morphine should be reserved for patients exhibiting tolerance to opioids.

■ Consider long-acting opioids when the response to shorter-acting agents can be evaluated: it is best to begin with a trial of short-acting opioids. Once shorter-acting opioids are tolerated, consider converting to an equianalgesic amount of oral controlled-released morphine (MSContin), oxycodone (OxyContin), or hydromorphone (Pallidone). Transdermal fentanyl system (Duragesic) provides convenient application every 72 hours. These agents are useful for the long-term management of continuous pain and can be supplemented with shorter-acting agents for breakthrough pain that is episodic or intermittent.

■ Avoid transdermal fentanyl system (Duragesic) when patients are opioid-naïve: transdermal fentanyl should never be prescribed in the absence of tolerance to less potent opioids. For example, elders should be able to tolerate a daily dose of at least 30–40 mg of short-acting oxycodone (e.g., 6–8 Percocet, Roxicet, or Endocet tablets per day), or hydrocodone (6–8 Vicodin or Lotabs or 3–4 Lorcet tablets per day) before switching to the minimum dosing patch strength (25 mcg/hr) of the transdermal fentanyl system. The common use of transdermal fentanyl, especially in long-term care facilities, is associated with several clinical problems. First, health professionals may be unaware of the equianalgesic equivalence to other opioid preparations. Second, transdermal fentanyl is intended to relieve continuous or steady-state pain, not episodic bouts of pain associated with movement or other aggravating factors. Therefore, transdermal fentanyl, if used for patients with rheumatoid arthritis, osteoarthritis, back pain, bony metastases, and other musculoskeletal conditions, should be supplemented with additional opioid medication. Clinically, transdermal fentanyl is supplemented with acetaminophen or NSAIDs alone, which may not provide adequate supplemental analgesia. Third, transdermal fentanyl is difficult to titrate in the presence of severe progressive pain, for example, pain associated with cancer. It can be extremely useful in managing pain when patients are not able to take oral medication or absorb it (e.g., chronic nausea or intermittent vomiting, noncompliance with opioid use, or mechanical obstruction in the gastrointestinal tract).

■ Assess the response to therapy: subjective pain rating scales and a pain relief scale can be used to evaluate response to opioid therapy. Clinically, other parameters such as improved function, mood, and appetite may also be indicators of decreased pain.

- Avoid the use of other psychoactive drugs: the concurrent use of other psychoactive drugs, particularly if initiated with opioids or close to the time of starting therapy with opioids, obscures assessment of the untoward effects of opioids. If adjuvant agents for pain must be initiated, it is best to introduce agents singly and allow ample time (at least several days) before giving a new agent with potential psychoactive effects.

- Manage opioid-related side effects: the major side effect of opioids in the elderly is constipation. Mild laxatives such as milk of magnesia, senna preparations (Senokot), casanthranol and docusate (Pericolace), lactulose, or bisacodyl (Dulcolax) should be started when opioids are initiated. Stool softeners alone do little or nothing to alleviate opioid-induced constipation. Unlike many other adverse effects from opioids, patients do not develop tolerance to the effects of opioids on the bowel; therefore, continued use of laxatives is necessary as long as opioid therapy is maintained. Consult the American Geriatrics Society report on the management of chronic pain in older persons for further information on analgesic dosing guidelines and strategies for treating opioid-induced side effects.[6] Published equianalgesic guidelines are often helpful in understanding opioid equivalents and potency, and essential for safe dosing when switching patients from one opioid to another.[6,23,24,37]

Nonopioid Analgesics   Nonopioid analgesics offer an acceptable alternative to opioid analgesics for both acute and chronic pain.[47,48,49] Nonopioids are indicated for cancer pain that is considered mild to moderate resulting from metastatic disease to the bones; mechanical compression of tendons, muscles, pleura, and peritoneum; and soft-tissue pain. These agents are quite effective in the management of non-cancer-related pain, such as musculoskeletal pain caused by arthritis, back pain, and orthopedic injuries. Nonopioid analgesics are classified based on their chemical structure and grouped into distinct categories—para-aminophenol derivatives (e.g.,

acetaminophen [Tylenol]), salicylic acid derivatives (e.g., aspirin and choline magnesium trisalicylate [Trilisate]), and a variety of subclasses of other non-steroidal anti-inflammatory drugs (NSAIDs). Most of these drugs have antipyretic and analgesic properties that are a result of analgesic effects that occur in the periphery. Para-aminophenol derivatives such as acetaminophen do not have anti-inflammatory properties. While nonopioid drugs are not capable of producing physical dependence, tolerance, or addiction, they do have maximum ceiling effects for their analgesic potential. Higher doses of these medications often lead to serious side effects. Acetaminophen and choline magnesium trisalicylate have no antiplatelet actions; however, the NSAIDs and aspirin do alter platelet function and coagulation. This potential hematological effect is caused by irreversible acetylation of platelet cyclooxygenase, which inhibits platelet aggregation.

Acetaminophen   Acetaminophen is recommended for mild to moderate pain. While effective for some types of pain (e.g., headache, minor arthritis, and joint and other muscular pain), it is rarely effective as a single agent for moderate to severe pain associated with disease (e.g., cancer, severe rheumatoid arthritis) or other painful conditions (e.g., herpes zoster-related pain, compression fractures, severe osteoarthritis).

Recommendations for the Use of Acetaminophen

- Daily dose should not exceed 4,000 mg in elders;[6] more prudent use of acetaminophen would restrict doses to 3,000 mg per day.

- Instruct patients about the amount of acetaminophen in combination opioid products (e.g., Tylenol #2, #3, #4, Darvocet, Vicodin, Lortabs, Lorcet, Percocet, Roxicet, and Endocet) in order to avoid acetaminophen toxicity.

- Caution patients about supplementing acetaminophen-opioid combinations with additional acetaminophen.

- Acetaminophen alone is not an adequate "rescue" drug for supplementing long-acting opioid preparations such as transdermal fentanyl (Duragesic), controlled-release morphine (MSContin), or controlled-release oxycodone (OxyContin).

NSAIDs and Salicylates

The mechanism of action for these drugs has been well described. The NSAIDs inhibit cyclo-oxygenase in peripheral tissues, which prevents arachidonic acid from converting to prostaglandin.[50] Prostaglandins are associated with pain that results from injury or inflammation, and they can sensitize pain receptors to mechanical and chemical stimulation. The action of these drugs alters the effects of prostaglandins on the nociceptors or pain receptors of primary afferents that transmit pain. NSAIDs, alone or in combination with opioids, can be helpful in the management of pain from bony metastases. As tumors invade the bone, prostaglandins are released that sensitize nociceptors and increase pain. The combination of nonopioids and opioids administered simultaneously may enhance analgesia.[49]

The benefits of NSAIDs must be weighed against their risk. Commonly, NSAIDs are prescribed for pain that may not have inflammation as its etiology, resulting in unnecessary use and lack of analgesic efficacy. NSAIDs have been linked to serious side effects in the elderly, including gastrointestinal toxicity.[51,52,53] Elderly women are twice as likely to develop gastrointestinal problems from NSAIDs as men; furthermore, the elderly in general are at much greater risk for adverse effects from these drugs. Extreme caution must also be used with concurrent use of oral anticoagulants and steroids, as these drugs pose additional risks for serious gastrointestinal side effects. A 13-fold increase in hemorrhagic peptic ulcer disease was found when NSAIDs were prescribed to elders on oral anticoagulants.[52] Hyperkalemia, renal insufficiency, and altered cognition have been frequently observed in elders.[54] Celecoxib (Celebrex) and rofecoxib (Vioxx), which are relatively new agents marketed for arthritis pain, are specific cyclo-oxygenase-2 inhibiting NSAIDs exerting reduced effects on the gastrointestinal system. Buffum and Buffum provide a comprehensive review of the properties of NSAIDs, indications, dosing guidelines, and precautions with use in elders.[55] They stress that there

are no acceptable criteria to predict which agents will work best in patients with pain. Whatever NSAID is selected, it is recommended the lowest dose possible be prescribed to elders and the duration of therapy be short. It is often necessary to allow one to three weeks of therapy for a maximum effect, before doses are escalated.[55]

Recommendations for Use of NSAIDs

- Avoid high-dose long-term use.
- For chronic pain, administer on a prn basis.
- Short-acting agents are preferred to avoid accumulation.
- Do not administer with renal dysfunction.
- Avoid concurrent use with other anti-inflammatory agents (e.g., steroids, other NSAIDs).
- Use one agent at a time.
- Avoid concurrent use with anticoagulants such as warfarin (Coumadin), as the risk for hemorrhagic ulcer disease is increased.
- Do not administer with a history of peptic ulcer disease.
- Remain within the recommended dosing guidelines; increased doses may not have added efficacy and may be associated with significant toxicities.

Steroids

Corticosteroids can be useful for treating certain pain syndromes caused by cancer, such as bony metastases and nerve compression. They may also provide short-term pain relief and allow more time to increase opioid analgesic doses. Dexamethasone in doses of 4–6 mg q 6 hr can be initiated for 1–3 days, followed by a slow taper over 7–10 days.[23] Low-dose steroid therapy can be an effective adjuvant agent for pain from bony metastases.[49]

Steroids can also be used to treat pain from rheumatoid arthritis. A recent meta-analysis of the literature on short-term low-dose steroids and NSAIDs in the treatment of rheumatoid arthritis showed that a short course of low-dose, daily prednisolone (15 mg or less) was superior to NSAIDs in relieving pain and joint tenderness.[56] Ten studies were analyzed which revealed that measurable gains in pain relief and alleviation of joint tenderness were achieved with prednisolone compared to NSAID therapy.

Other Adjuvant Agents

Tricyclic Antidepressants   Tricyclic antidepressants have demonstrated efficacy in the treatment of neuropathic pain syndromes. The subclass of tricyclic antidepressants that are tertiary amines (e.g., amitriptyline) are typically associated with greater anticholinergic effects, sedation, and orthostatic hypotension. The secondary amines (e.g., nortriptyline, desipramine) tend to produce less-severe adverse effects and may be safer in the frail elderly.[11,37,49] If tricyclic antidepressants are used for pain, it is often necessary to titrate up to doses of 75 mg per day or greater before a substantial benefit for neuropathic pain is observed. This is often difficult, as the adverse effects from these agents often limit adequate dosing. Table 19–3

outlines important information about the use of tricyclic antidepressants for neuropathic pain.[31]

Providing a safe environment is paramount when any psychoactive drug is prescribed for the elderly. In a case-control study of tricyclic antidepressant use, a 60% increase in hip fractures in persons over the age of 65 was reported.[57] Body mass, problems with ambulation, functional status, and dementia did not affect the results; thus, caution is warranted when prescribing and administering any psychoactive agents. Elders living alone or in independent assisted-living settings may require close supervision if tricyclic therapy is initiated.

Anticonvulsants   Anticonvulsant agents, such as carbamazepine (Tegretol), gabapentin (Neurontin), phenytoin (Dilantin), valproate and clonazepam (Klonopin), are particularly effective for neuropathic pain syndromes associated with shooting, electric shock-like, or lancinating sensations.[11] Table 19–4

Table 19–3   Properties of Common Tricyclic Antidepressants Used as Analgesics for Neuropathic Plan

Drugs	Relative Anticholinergic Effects	Relative Sedative Effects	Usual Starting Dose	Usual Daily Therapeutic Dosing Range	Half-Life (hr)	Comments
Tertiary amine agents						
Amitriptyline	++++	++++	10–25 mg at hs	50–150 mg	30–45	Lower initial doses and gradual titration for elders. Risk for orthostatic hypotension moderate to high. Increased risk for constipation.
Doxepin	++	+++	10–25 mg at hs	50–150 mg	8–25	
Secondary amine agents						
Desipramine	+	+	25 mg at hs	100–150 mg	12–25	Lower toxicity profile. Recommended for elderly patients.
Nortriptyline	++	++	25 mg at hs	100–150 mg	18–45	

Table 19–4   Anticonvulsants for Pain Management

Drug	Dose	Indications	Adverse Effects
Carbamazepine	100–200 mg PO bid Increase every other day to 800 mg/day in divided doses.	Useful for paroxysmal and lancinating, shooting, electric shock-like pains	Sedation, drowsiness, diplopia, ataxia, hematological toxicity
Clonazepam	0.5–1.5 mg/day PO Maximum 3–4 mg/day in divided doses.	Same as above Useful for preexisting anxiety	Sedation, ataxia, behavioral disturbances, mood or mental changes
Gabapentin	300–900 mg tid (900–2400 mg) PO Initial dose 100 mg tid, then increase by 100 mg/day as tolerated. May titrate up to 3600 mg/day. For elders, increase slowly: 100 mg/day q3–5 days.	Same as above	Sedation, ataxia, dizziness, difficulty concentrating, visual abnormalities
Phenytoin	300–500 mg/day PO.	Same as above	Sedation, drowsiness, ataxia, diplopia, nausea, skin rash, or hypertrichosis
Valproic acid	15–60 mg/kg/day PO in divided doses.	Same as above	Behavioral, mood, or mental changes; hepatotoxicity, visual disturbances, coagulopathy or thrombocytopenia, bleeding

provides dosing guidelines and clinical information on the use of some of these agents.[31] Gabapentin (Neurontin) may have significant advantages over other anticonvulsants because of its relatively low toxicity. Unlike carbamazepine and clonazepam, gabapentin is less sedating. In addition, gabapentin does not have the hematological effects that are a concern with carbamazepine and phenytoin. Somnolence, dizziness, ataxia, fatigue, and cognitive dysfunction have been linked to gabapentin, but many of these adverse effects can be prevented with careful upward titration of the drug. Begin with 100 mg at hs for 3–5 days. If no adverse effects, increase the dose to 100 mg in AM and PM for 3–5 days, then 100 mg tid for 3–5 days. Continue escalating the dose by 100 mg per day every 3–5 days. Typically, patients require at least 900–1,200 mg per day; however, higher daily doses of 2,400–3,600 mg have been suggested to maximize pain control.[58,59,60]

Topical Agents   Capsaicin, manufactured from hot peppers, is a safe and effective analgesic agent offering a wide range of uses for the treatment of pain from arthritis, herpes zoster, diabetic neuropathy, and mastectomy.[61] Capsaicin reduces inflammation and the cutaneous hypersensitivity accompanying musculoskeletal pain and neuralgias and neuropathies. When applied regularly to the skin over painful areas, capsaicin depletes the nerve terminals of substance P, a peptide responsible for pain transmission. The first few applications often increase pain, but over time (typically a few days), pain and hypersensitivity of the skin may subside. A topical anesthetic used with a lower concentration of capsaicin cream or lotion may alleviate discomfort and improve compliance with initial therapy. Capsaicin is available in non-prescription strengths of 0.025% (Zostrix Cream, Capsaicin-P Cream, and Capsin Lotion) and 0.075% (Zostrix-HP Cream, Capsin Lotion). After applying capsaicin, hands must be thoroughly washed and affected areas of the skin should not be touched.

EMLA Cream (product of prilocaine and lidocaine) is a topical agent that reduces the cutaneous hypersensitivity associated with neuropathic pain. Once applied, the affected area is covered with an occlusive transparent dressing such as Tege-Derm, Op-Cite, or even plastic wrap. While the efficacy of topical NSAIDs has not been established, various preparations (e.g., ketoprofen gel) are compounded for individual use.

Combining Opioids and Adjuvant Agents for Neuropathic Pain Syndromes Neuropathic pain syndromes appear to be less responsive to opioid analgesics than somatic and visceral pain. This is an important consideration when prescribing opioid analgesics, as opioid requirements may be greater for patients with neuropathic pain. If indicated, opioid therapy can be slowly titrated upward to the point that patients get relief or experience intolerable toxicities (e.g., sedation, nausea). Selection of opioid analgesics is critical, and those without nonopioid combinations should be considered so that doses can be escalated without added toxicities from the nonopioid drug (e.g., acetaminophen). Greater benefits may be derived from combining an opioid analgesic with effective adjuvant agents such as tricyclic antidepressants and anticonvulsants that have documented efficacy in the treatment of neuropathic pain. In some cases, adjuvant therapy alone is effective in relieving neuropathic pain. Selective interventional techniques including temporary nerve blocks, neurolysis or nerve destruction procedures, and neuraxial (epidural or subarachnoid) therapy have demonstrated significant benefits.[11]

Postherpetic neuralgia, more recently classified as herpes zoster-related pain, is an example of a neuropathic pain syndrome that persists at least three months after the acute onset of herpetic skin lesions. Elders are commonly and most severely afflicted with pain following infection from the herpes zoster virus with approximately 50% of all sufferers over the age of 65.[62] Patients may be evaluated in pain clinics for injections of local anesthetic; however, the benefits are short-term. Early treatment with corticosteriods and preemptive therapy with tricyclic antidepressants have minimized the occurrence of persistent pain. In a recent randomized-controlled study comparing amitriptyline and nortriptyline, efficacy for pain control was similar, although fewer side affects were associated with nortriptyline.[63] Controlled-release oxycodone has also demonstrated significant benefits to placebo in relieving paroxysmal spontaneous pain and cutaneous hypersensitivity.[64] Topical agents, such as capsaisin and EMLA cream, are also helpful for allodynia (pain from stimuli that are not generally considered painful) of the skin along the distribution(s) of nerve involvement.

■ Nonpharmacological Approaches for Pain

Nonpharmacological approaches for pain control can be useful adjuncts to analgesic therapy, reducing the need for drug therapy and improving overall well being. Such approaches provide a sense of personal control and offer relief during times when medication is not available. Nonpharmacological approaches should not replace analgesic therapy for disease-related pain as relief may be highly variable and unlikely to be sustained long-term. Importantly, it is essential to recognize both the advantages and disadvantages of nonpharmacological pain therapies (Table 19–5).[31]

Cutaneous Stimulation

Heat and cold therapies offer short-term relief of acute or chronic musculoskeletal pain. Heat is applied with hot packs and heating pads to achieve muscle and generalized relaxation. Elders need to be aware of potential tissue damage from heat, especially if skin sensation is impaired. The application of heat on or near the area of a transdermal

Table 19–5   Selected Nonpharmacological Interventions for Pain

Technique	Examples	Advantages	Disadvantages
Cutaneous stimulation	Superficial heating or cooling, vibration, massage	Many methods; makes pain tolerable, reduces pain, patients are receptive; can apply stimulation at site of pain or other sites; can provide distraction	Not for therapeutic or curative purposes; can damage tissue if applied incorrectly
Immobilization/ mobilization	Splinting, bracing, walking, exercise, rest	Decreases pain, improves range of motion, conserves energy, improves functional status, promotes relaxation	Discomfort on physical exertion; decrease in functional status
Distraction	*Internal:* Mental images, counting, singing silently; *external:* music, reading, television, conversation	Decreased pain intensity, increased pain tolerance; more acceptable pain sensation; greater sense of control; improved mood	Not helpful for vigilant patients; may have no effect on pain intensity; may be hard to enact; may not 'look like' they are in pain resulting in doubt about pain and/or failure to medicate after distraction; awareness of pain and fatigue may increase; irritability
Relaxation	Slow breathing, progressive muscle relaxation, relaxing mental imagery, repetitive activity or thought	Reduces anxiety, may reduce pain; promotes sleep; decreases fatigue and skeletal muscle tension; increases confidence in ability to handle pain	Can be time-consuming; difficult to teach, practice, and use effectively; is an adjunct method that does not directly relieve pain; often difficult to distinguish between relaxation and imagery
Comprehensive models	Cognitive/ behavioral interventions, psychoeducational approaches	Address multiple dimensions of pain; individualized; include patient and family; problem-focused; requires interdisciplinary team	May be difficult to assemble an appropriate interdisciplinary team depending on setting and resources; can be complex and time-consuming

fentanyl system (Duragesic) is particularly dangerous. Local heat as well as elevated body temperatures can accelerate release and absorption of the transdermal fentanyl, leading to overmedication or a serious opioid overdose. In addition to heat, cold therapy with ice packs and the application of methanol offer localized relief of pain and swelling from inflammation.

Massage therapy may relieve superficial and deep musculoskeletal pain. Massage therapy has a positive effect on the perceptions of postoperative pain, with greater duration of pain relief in older patients.[65] Transelectrical nerve stimulation (TENS) is particularly useful for musculoskeletal pain.[66] Application of cutaneous electrodes may be difficult for some elderly patients, making compliance problematic.

Cognitive or Behavioral Therapy

Cognitive or behavioral therapy is aimed at changing beliefs and attitudes toward pain, promoting adaptive coping, and reducing stress. Cognitive strategies include distraction, relaxation, visual imagery, biofeedback, and hypnosis. Behavioral approaches often rely on group therapy and individual counseling in the context of a structured program. Significant benefits have been achieved with cognitive and behavioral approaches. For example, cognitive-behavioral programs have had lasting effects on adaptive coping and improvement in fatigue with rheumatoid arthritis.[67] The mechanism for pain relief with cognitive or behavioral therapies, particularly relaxation, remain unclear, and to date the evidence is insufficient to conclude that relaxation therapy reduces chronic pain.[68]

For those interested in cognitive or behavioral therapies for pain, resources must be available (e.g., access to programs or trained professionals), and motivation and emotional stamina are needed to learn and practice the techniques. Such strategies may have little benefit for elders who are suffering from pain, debilitated, or cognitively impaired and unable to concentrate. This is especially true in long-term care facilities.

Exercise

Exercise is an inexpensive way to restore muscle and joint function, while decreasing pain associated with immobility. Apparently, isokinetic muscle-strength-training programs for persons with osteoarthritis of the knees decreases pain and stiffness and improves mobility and muscle strength.[69] Exercise programs should be tailored to specific needs, abilities, and activity tolerance levels, especially in the presence of cardiac disease. Consultation with physical or occupational therapists is critical to avoid risks of exercise-induced injuries. Swimming and water aerobics are especially useful for elders with degenerative joint disease, rheumatoid arthritis, and osteoporosis who might otherwise experience significant pain with weight-bearing exercises.

The treatment of chronic nonmalignant pain is controversial, but experts agree that a multimodality approach using a combination of pharmacotherapy and physical and psychosocial interventions is better than any one alone. While there may be reluctance to treat noncancer pain with opioid analgesics, this is certainly an acceptable and effective method of treatment when the underlying cause of the pain cannot be reversed or other strategies have failed.

 ## Summary

There is substantial evidence to support that pain is a common experience among elders and that health professionals have a responsibility to evaluate pain and treat it appropriately. Evidence- and consensus-based information, which has recently become accessible through published research and clinical practice guidelines, is the best defense against the problem of pain as experienced by older people. Nurses make an enormous contribution to patients by allowing them to express their pain and implementing sound pharmacological and nonpharmacological therapies.

References

1. Liebeskind JC, Melzack R. The International Pain Foundation: meeting a need for education in pain. *J Pain Symptom Manage*. 1988;3(3):131–134.
2. Gagliese L, Melzack R. Chronic pain in elderly people. *Pain*. 1997;70:3–14.
3. Herr KA, Mobily PR. Complexities of pain assessment in the elderly. Clinical considerations. *J Gerontol Nurs*. 1991;17(4):12–19.
4. Ferrell BA. Pain in elderly people. *J Am Geriatr Soc*. 1991;39:64–73.
5. Stein M, Ferrell BA. Pain in the nursing home. *Clin Geriatr Med*. 1996;12:601–613.
6. American Geriatrics Society Panel on Chronic Pain in Older Persons. The management of chronic pain in older persons. *J Am Geriatr Soc*. 1998;46:635–651.
7. Roy R, Thomas MR. Elderly persons with and without pain: a comparative study. *Clin J Pain*. 1987;3: 102–106.
8. Desbiens NA, Mueller-Rizner N, Connors AF Jr, Hamel MB, Wenger NS. Pain in the oldest-old during hospitalization and up to one year later. *J Am Geriatr Soc*. 1997;45(10):1167–1172.
9. Ferrell BA, Ferrell BR, Osterweil D. Pain in the nursing home. *J Am Geriatr Soc*. 1990;38:409–414.
10. Parker SL, Tong T, Bolden S, Wingo PA. Cancer statistics, 1996. *CA Cancer J Clin*. 1996;46:5–27.
11. Lipman AG. Analgesic drugs for neuropathic and sympathetically maintained pain. *Clin Geriatr Med*. 1996;12:501–515.
12. Bennett GJ. Neuropathic pain. In: Wall PD, Melzack R, eds. *Textbook of Pain*, 3rd ed. New York: Churchill Livingstone; 1994:261–274.

13. Ward SE, Goldberg N, Miller-McCauley V, et al. Patient-related barriers to the management of cancer pain. *Pain*. 1993;23(4):319–324.

14. Cleeland CS, Gonin R, Hatfield AK, et al. Pain and its treatment in outpatients with metastatic cancer: the Eastern Cooperative Oncology Group's Outpatient Pain Study. *N Eng J Med*. 1994;330(9):592–596.

15. Ferrell BA, Ferrell BR, Rivera L. Pain in the cognitively impaired nursing home patient. *J Pain Symptom Manage*. 1995;10:591–598.

16. Brockopp DY, Warden S, Colclough G, Brockopp G. Elderly hospice patients' perspective on pain management. *Hospice J*. 1996;11(3):41–53.

17. Horgas AL, Tsai PF. Analgesic drug prescription and use in cognitively impaired nursing home residents. *Nurs Res*. 1998;47(4):235–242.

18. Parmelee PA, Smith B, Katz IR. Pain complaints and cognitive status among elderly institution residents. *J Am Geriatr Soc*. 1993;41:517–522.

19. Von Roenn JH, Cleeland CS, Gonin R, Hatfield AK, Pandya KJ. Physician attitudes and practice in cancer pain management: a survey from the Eastern Cooperative Oncology Group. *Ann Intern Med*. 1993;119:121–126.

20. Brunier G, Carson MG, Harrison DE. What do nurses know and believe about patients with pain? Results of a hospital survey. *J Pain Symptom Manage*. 1995; 10(6):436–445.

21. Simon JM, McTier CL. Development of a chronic pain assessment tool. *Rehabil Nurs*. 1996;21:20–24.

22. Acute Pain Management Guideline Panel. *Clinical Practice Guidelines: Acute Pain Management: Operative or Medical Procedures or Trauma*. Rockville, Md: Agency for Health Care Policy and Research, US Department of Health and Human Services; 1992. AHCPR Publication 92–0032.

23. Management of Cancer Pain Guideline Panel. Clinical Practice Guidelines Number 9: Management of Cancer Pain. Rockville, Md: Agency for Health Care Policy and Research, US Department of Health and Human Services; 1994. AHCPR Publication 94–0592.

24. American Pain Society. *Principles of Analgesic Use in the Treatment of Acute Pain and Cancer Pain*. 4th ed. Skokie, Il: American Pain Society; 1999.

25. Herr KA, Mobily P. Comparison of selected pain assessment tools for use with the elderly. *Appl Nurs Res*. 1993;6:39–46.

26. Herr KA, Mobily PR, Kohout FJ, Wagenaar D. Evaluation of the faces pain scale for use with elderly. *Clin J Pain*. 1998;14(1):29–38.

27. Bieri D, Reeve RA, Champion GD, Addicoat L, Ziegler JB. The Faces Rating Scale for self-assessment of the severity of pain experienced by children: development, initial validation, and preliminary investigation for ration scale properties. *Pain*. 1990;41:139–150.

28. Daut RL, Cleeland CS, Flanery RC. Development of the Wisconsin brief pain questionnaire to assess pain in cancer and other diseases. *Pain*. 1983;17:197–210.

29. Melzack R. The short-form McGill Pain Questionnaire. *Pain*. 1987;30:191–197.

30. Weiner D, Pieper C, McConnell E, Martinez S, Keefe F. Pain measurement in elders with chronic low back pain: traditional and alternative approaches. *Pain*. 1996;67(2–3):461–467.

31. Polomano RC, McGuire DB, Sheidler VR. Pain (part II). In: Yarbro CH, Frogge MH, Goodman M, Groenwald SL, eds. *Cancer Nursing: Principles and Practice*. 5th ed. Sulbury, Mass: Jones and Barlett; 2000:657–690.

32. Dellasega C, Keiser CL. Pharmacologic approaches to chronic pain in the older adult. *Nurse Pract*. 1997; 22(5):20–24.

33. Gloth FM. Concerns with chronic analgesic therapy in elderly patients. *Am J Med*. 1996;101(suppl 1A): 19S–24S.

34. Pope JE, Anderson JJ, Felson DT. A meta-analysis of the effects of nonsteroidal anti-inflammatory drugs on blood pressure. *Arch Intern Med*. 1993;153:477–484.

35. Ruoff G. Management of pain in patients with multiple health problems: a guide for the practicing physician. *Am J Med*. 1998;105(Suppl 1B):53S–60S.

36. Yost JH, Morgan CJ. Cardiovascular effects of NSAIDs. *J Musculoskel Med*. 1994;11:22–34.

37. United States Pharmacopeial Convention. *USP DI Drug Information for the Health Care Professional*. 19th ed. Englewood, Co: Micromedex; 1999.

38. Lynch EP, Lazor, MA, Gellis, JE, Orav J, Goldman L, Marcantonio ER. The impact of postoperative pain on the development of postoperative delirium. *Anesth Analg*. 1998;86:781–785.

39. Richardson J, Bresland K. The management of postsurgical pain in the elderly population. *Drugs Aging*. 1998;13(1):17–31.

40. Egbert AM, Parks LH, Short LM, Burnett ML. Randomized trial of postoperative patient-controlled analgesia vs. intramuscular narcotics in frail elderly men. *Arch Intern Med*. 1990;150:1897–1903.

41. Plummer JL, Owen H, Ilsley AH, Inglis S. Morphine patient-controlled analgesia is superior to meperidine patient-controlled analgesia for postoperative pain. *Anesth Analg*. 1997;84:794–799.

42. Wulf H. Epidural analgesia in postoperative pain therapy: a review. *Anaesthetist*. 1998;47(6):501–510.

43. Scott DA, Emanuelsson BM, Mooney PH, Cook RJ, Junestrand C. Pharmacokinetics and efficacy of long-term epidural ropivacaine infusion for postoperative analgesia. *Anesth Analg*. 1997;85:1322–1330.

44. Abrahm JL. Advances in pain management for older adult patients. *Clin Geriatr Med*. 2000;16(2):269–311.

45. Cleary JF, Carbone PP. Palliative medicine in the elderly. *Cancer*. 1997;80(7):1335–1347.

46. Bernabei R, Gambassi G, Lapane K, et al. Management of pain in elder patients with cancer. SAGE study group. Systematic assessment of geriatric drug use via epidemiology. *JAMA*. 1998;279(23):1877–1882.

47. Schnitzer TJ. Non-NSAID pharmacological treatment options for the management of chronic pain. *Am J Med*. 1998;105(1B):45S–51S.

48. Beaver WT. Impact of non-narcotic oral analgesics on pain management. *Am J Med*. 1988;84(5A):3–15.

49. Portenoy RK, Kanner RM. Nonopioid and adjuvant analgesics. In: Portenoy RK, Kanner RM, eds. *Pain Management: Theory and Practice*. Philadelphia: F.A. Davis; 1996:219–276.

50. Insel PA. Analgesic-antipyretic and antiinflammatory agents: drugs employed in the treatment of gout. In: Hardman JG, Gilman AG, Limbard LE, et al, eds. *Goodman and Gilman's The Pharmacological Basis of Therapeutics*. 9th ed. New York: McGraw-Hill; 1996;617–657.

51. Tamblyn R, Berkson L, Dauphinee WD, et al. Unnecessary prescribing of NSAIDs and the management of NSAID-related gastropathy in medical practice. *Ann Intern Med*. 1997;127(6):429–438.

52. Shorr RI, Ray WA, Daugherty JR, Griffin MR. Concurrent use of nonsteroidal anti-inflammatory drugs and oral anticoagulants places elderly persons at high risk for hemorrhagic peptic ulcer disease. *Arch Intern Med*. 1993;153(14):1665–1670.

53. Smalley WE, Ray WA, Daugherty JR, Griffin MR. Nonsteroidal anti-inflammatory drugs and the incidence of hospitalizations for peptic ulcer disease in elderly persons. *Am J Epidemiol*. 1995;141(6):539–545.

54. Sack KE. Update on NSAIDs in the elderly. *Geriatrics*. 1989;44:71–90.

55. Buffum M, Buffum JC. Nonsteroidal anti-inflammatory drugs in the elderly. *Pain Manage Nurs*. 2000;1(2):40–50.

56. Gotzsche PC, Johansen HK. Meta-analysis of short-term prednisolone versus placebo and non-steroidal anti-inflammatory drugs in rheumatoid arthritis. *BMJ*. 1998;316(7134):811–818.

57. Ray WA, Griffin MR, Malcolm E. Cyclic antidepressants and the risk for hip fractures. *Arch Intern Med*. 1991; 151:754–756.

58. Wetzel CH, Connelly JF. Use of gabapentin in pain management. *Ann Pharmacother*. 1997;31(9): 1082–1083.

59. Backonja M, Beydoun A, Edwards KR, et al. Gabapentin for the symptomatic treatment of painful neuropathy in patients with diabetes mellitus: a randomized controlled trial. *JAMA*. 1998;280(21): 1831–1836.

60. Rowbotham M, Harden N, Stacey B, Bernstein P, Magnus-Miller L. Gabapentin for the treatment of postherpetic neuralgia: a randomized controlled trial. *JAMA*. 1998;280(21):1837–1842.

61. Hautkappe M, Roizen MF, Toledano A, Roth S, Jeffries JA, Ostermeier AM. Review of the effectiveness of capsaicin for painful cutaneous disorders and neural dysfunction. *Clin J Pain*. 1998;14(2):97–106.

62. Bowsher D. The management of postherpetic neuralgia. *Postgrad Med J*. 1997;73(864):623–629.

63. Watson CP, Vernich L, Chipman M, et al. Nortriptyline versus amitrityline in postherpetic neuralgia: a randomized study. *Neurology*. 1998;51(4):1166–1171.

64. Watson CP, Babul N. Efficacy of oxycodone in neuropathic pain: a randomized trial in postherpetic neuralgia. *Neurology*. 1998;50(6):1837–1841.

65. Nixon M, Teschendorff J, Finney J, Karnilowicz W. Expanding the nursing repertoire: the effects of massage on post-operative pain. *Austr J Adv Nurs*. 1997;14(3):21–26.

66. Griffin MR, Brandt KD, Liang MH, Pincus T, Ray WA. Practical management of osteoarthritis: integration of pharmacologic and nonpharmacologic measures. *Arch Fam Med*. 1995;4(12):1049–1055.

67. Sinclair VG, Wallston KA, Dwyer KA, Blackburn DS, Fuchs H. Effects of cognitive-behavioral intervention for women with rheumatoid arthritis. *Res Nurs Health*. 1998;21(4):315–326.

68. Carroll D, Seers K. Relaxation for the relief of chronic pain: a systematic review. *J Adv Nurs*. 1998;27(3): 476–487.

69. Schilke JM, Johnson GO, Housh TJ, O'Dell JR. Effects of muscle-strength training on the functional status of patients with osteoarthritis of the knee joint. *Nurs Res*. 1996;45(2):68–72.

20

Palliative Care

Howard Tuch
Neville E. Strumpf

To die of old age is a death rare, extraordinary, and singular—a privilege rarely seen.

Montaigne, *Of Age*, 1575

A Profile of Dying Older Adults

Dying has changed over the centuries, and Americans typically can expect to live until an old age. In 1995, the average life expectancy reached 75.8 years[1] compared to less than 50 years of age in 1900.[2] On average, women live until age 79 and men until age 73.[1] While the increase in life expectancy has come primarily from declines in infant and child mortality, death rates across the age spectrum have been falling for decades.[3] Women who reach age 75 are likely to live an additional 11.9 years and men an additional 9.7 years. The fastest growing segment of the population is over the age of 85 and more people will enter old age than at any prior time in history.[4]

There remain, however, significant racial differences in life expectancy. Black females live an average of 74 years and black males an average of 65.4 years. Age-adjusted mortality rates for black women are more than 1.5 times that of white women, while black males have nearly twice the age-adjusted mortality rates as white men.[1] Social and racial differences also exist for the leading causes of mortality, with injuries, HIV infection, homicides, and suicides relatively more important in minority populations.[5]

Despite the dramatic changes in mortality rates, nearly 2.5 million Americans die each year.[1] Although everyone eventually dies, the experience of dying, both its suffering and its potential, has not, until recently, been the subject of much discussion in the health-care literature.[6]

A century ago, communicable diseases (influenza, tuberculosis, and diphtheria) were leading causes of death.[2] Death came quickly, often unexpectedly, and little could be done to extend life in the seriously ill or disabled. Today, most adults live for significant periods of time with the illnesses that eventually cause or accompany their death. The three leading causes of death for the population as a whole are heart disease, cancer, and stroke.[1]

The end of life is a profound experience for patients and care providers. According to a longitudinal British community-based study, common clinical symptoms in the last year of life were: pain (72% of people), dyspnea (49%), loss of appetite (47%), sleeplessness (44%), drowsiness (44%), constipation (36%), depression (36%), and vomiting or feeling sick (36%). Along with these symptoms, older people also experience confusion, dizziness, and incontinence in the last stages of life.[7] Multiple symptoms are the rule, especially in cancer patients, where, on average, end-stage cancer patients report 11 concurrent distressing symptoms.[8]

Much recent interest in end-of-life care in this country stems from the results of a major study documenting care of patients dying in U.S. medical centers. The Study to Understand Prognoses and Preferences for Outcomes and Risks of Treatments (SUPPORT)[9] followed more than 9,000 severely ill patients and demonstrated important gaps in the delivery of care. Patients were likely to die in pain, in intensive care units, on ventilators, and with fewer than half of their physicians aware of their advance directives. Decisions to withdraw or to withhold medical intervention came very late in the hospital course, typically within 48 hours of death and after more than a week in an intensive care unit. Interventions of a nurse educator reporting to physicians on predicted mortality, level of pain, or patient/family preference for care did not result in significant improvement in outcomes. The ability of health-care providers to predict mortality accurately in most clinical circumstances, especially with chronic, non-cancer conditions, was also very limited. SUPPORT was the first systematic, population-based study of dying in health care since Osler's original treatise in 1906.[10] In persons dying in other health-care environments (nursing home, assisted living, or home health care), little is known of symptom experiences, preferences for care, or utilization of health-care resources.[11]

Where people die has also undergone significant change over the course of the century. The location of death may reflect societal attitudes toward death as much as the nature of the medical problems encountered. Death used to occur at home, an event that was intimately familiar to the multiple generations present. Today, death occurs out of sight of most family members. Currently, approximately 74% of all deaths occur in health-care institutions (60% in hospitals and 20% in nursing homes). These patterns vary considerably, however, by age and geographic region of the country.[12] Older people die more often in nursing homes, a trend that increased after the introduction of the Medicare prospective payment system in 1983[13] and the growth of hospice services.[14] An increasing number of deaths are occurring in assisted-living environments. More recent trends suggest that death will increasingly occur, once again, outside of health-care institutions. Nevertheless, the single most important determinant of the location of death is the number of available hospital beds in any geographic area.[15] Public surveys, by contrast, consistently demonstrate that the overwhelming majority of Americans prefer to die at home.[16]

The unique clinical, ethical, and policy challenges of this new way of dying are just now being addressed. Our capacity to prolong the dying period is unprecedented in human history. Older people dying from advanced chronic illness may have profoundly different needs from those who die younger and with shorter disease trajectories. Thus far, the training of health-care professionals and the priorities of the health-care system have not addressed these concerns well. This chapter reviews basic principles and emerging approaches of "palliative care."

Definition of Palliative Care

Definitions of palliative care are evolving, but two are widely circulated. According to the major text, *The Oxford Textbook of Palliative Medicine*, published in 1998, palliative care is "the study and management of patients with active, progressive, far advanced disease for whom the prognosis is limited and the focus of care is on the quality of life."[17] The definition identifies the stage of illness (progressive, far advanced) that is of interest as well as the main goal of care (enhanced quality of life) to be promoted. This definition does not, as recently noted, truly clarify what we mean by palliative care or how it distinguishes itself from other aspects of health care,[18] especially geriatrics, which shares similar populations and goals.

A second definition of palliative care, promoted by the World Health Organization (WHO), is "active, total care of patients whose disease is no longer responsive to curative treatment."[19] The WHO definition goes on to specify areas of interest in palliative care: "Control of pain and of other symptoms, as well as social and spiritual problems, is paramount. The goal of palliative care is the best possible quality of life for patients and their families. Many aspects of palliative care are also applicable earlier in the course of the illness."[19] The WHO definition delineates major domains of palliative care and recognizes the importance of family. It promotes a system of care designed to attend to social, spiritual, and emotional needs. It also emphasizes that palliative care has relevance to all stages of illness, not only the final phases.

The following Core Principles for End-of-Life Care have been widely adopted:[20]

1. Respect the dignity of both patient and caregivers.

2. Be sensitive to and respectful of the patient's and family's wishes.

3. Use the most appropriate measures that are consistent with patient choices.

4. Encompass alleviation of pain and other physical symptoms.

5. Assess and manage psychological, social, and spiritual/religious problems.

6. Offer continuity (the patient should be able to continue to be cared for, if so desired, by his/her primary-care and specialist providers).

7. Provide access to any therapy which may realistically be expected to improve the patient's quality of life, including alternative or nontraditional treatments.

8. Provide access to palliative care and hospice care.

9. Respect the right to refuse treatment.

10. Respect the physician's professional responsibility to discontinue some treatments when appropriate, with consideration for both patient and family preferences.

11. Promote clinical evidence-based research on providing care at the end-of-life.

Palliative care is emerging out of its hospice roots as a model of care designed to meet the growing challenges of end-of-life care. While palliative care embraces the hospice philosophy, it is currently characterized by an emphasis on academic development, research, and an intention to serve a wider group of patients than those currently seen in hospices. Palliative care becomes relatively more important as illness progresses and death approaches, but has relevance at all stages of illness. Hospices are still seen as a system of care reserved for a more or less definable end-stage of illness and as part of a broader range of potential services and interventions at the end of life.

Modern hospice care began in England in the 1960s and has grown as a movement and as a challenge to traditional medical care in the United States. A hospice demonstration project sponsored by the Health Care Financing Administration (HCFA) in 1980 led to the establishment of the Medicare Hospice Benefit in 1982. Since then, the number of hospice programs and number of patients cared for by hospices has grown dramatically. More than 2,500 Medicare-certified hospice programs in the country serve over 450,000 patients (about 17% of annual U.S. deaths) each year.[21] "Hospice" in the United States refers primarily to a program, philosophy of care, or system of reimbursement rather than a physical location. The hospice focus on patient comfort, interdisciplinary approaches, and provision of social and bereavement support for families and caregivers is a unique and essential component of U.S. health care. The great majority of hospice patients live in their own homes or in nursing homes.

Nearly 60% of hospice patients have cancer diagnoses. To receive Medicare hospice benefits, Medicare beneficiaries must be terminally ill (defined as a life expectancy of six months or less based on normal disease progression) and must waive the right to receive standard Medicare benefits, including all curative treatment. The uncertainty of clinical prognosis, especially with non-cancer conditions and the requirement to forgo all curative treatment upon acceptance into a hospice program, often results in very late referral to hospice. The median length of stay for patients admitted to hospice care is now less than 20 days and has actually been declining for the last several years.[22]

The National Hospice Organization has published guidelines to identify individuals who may be eligible for hospice care.[23] Nevertheless, identification of the most appropriate geriatric patients for hospice care remains a challenge for practitioners. Except in the extreme, it is usually difficult to predict with acceptable accuracy how long an individual will survive with most advanced chronic conditions.[23,24] This inability to predict when death will occur complicates decisions about forgoing interventions and may contribute to late hospice referrals.

Clinical Competence in Palliative Care

Assessment

The focus of palliative care is on the relief of suffering. Since suffering itself is multidimensional, a comprehensive and individualized patient assessment must be performed. Ideally, palliative care should be delivered in an interdisciplinary fashion.

The nurse practitioner may not be responsible for all aspects of this assessment, but should be aware of its importance in overall patient care. There are several domains of palliative care[25] that must be addressed during the course of an assessment:

- General history and current physical examination
- Disease status
- Psychological assessment
- Spiritual assessment
- Social assessment
- Practical assessment

A detailed history and description of the primary diagnosis, treatment history, likely prognosis, and comorbid conditions are essential starting points in the assessment of a palliative-care patient. Older patients are sometimes referred to a hospice prior to adequate consideration for aggressive or curative intervention. Knowledge of the disease, its individual presentation, and likely progression are essential to ensure that older patients are appropriately evaluated and receive interventions when indicated.

Physical assessment should focus on manifestations of end-stage illnesses and their functional impact. Symptoms can be related to the underlying condition or its management, medications, or coexisting conditions. Standardized and validated assessment tools are available for many of the most common clinical symptoms encountered at the end of life.[26,27] The use of these instruments assures attention to important issues and provides the means to track progress and effectiveness of different interventions. The management of several common end-of-life symptoms is described later. Most patients in the last stages of advanced illness have multiple symptoms. Each must be evaluated and managed separately.

Psychological problems can contribute greatly to patient distress at the end of life. A psychological assessment should include an evaluation of cognitive status (emphasis on depression, delirium, and dementia), anxiety, emotional state, coping mechanisms, fears (loss of control, dignity, social roles, financial concerns) and unresolved concerns (last wishes, reconciliation). Evaluation of decision-making capacity is a critical part of the psychological assessment. Many patients with advanced illness have some cognitive impairment. Loss of decision-making capacity can be global in that the individual is unable to participate meaningfully in any decision about care. More often, however, individuals may lose the capacity to make some, but not all, decisions. The capacity to execute a health-care proxy may be maintained even with mild to moderate dementia.[28]

Decisional capacity is based on a mental status evaluation with input from care providers and family. The determination of patient competence, on the other hand, is a legal determination. To the extent possible, all individuals should be encouraged to participate in important decisions regarding care. Even participation in decisions regarding more routine aspects of care can be exceedingly important to the patient who is aware of losing control in other areas. Opinions of health-care surrogates and health-care professionals often differ from those of the patient with regard to use of life-prolonging interventions.[29] A patient has the capacity to make a health-care decision if he/she:

- Understands that a decision is being made regarding care
- Makes rational inferences from the information provided
- Demonstrates a general understanding of the likely consequences of the decisions and the options for care
- Is noncoerced

Spiritual assessment should focus on the importance of faith, nonreligious spiritual practices, meaning of underlying illness, and loss of self. Rituals can be particularly important. A willingness to address spiritual concerns and ability to be present and nonjudgmental can be among the most valuable contributions made by a practitioner.

Simple spiritual assessment tools are available. One such tool[30] uses the following mnemonic: F.I.C.A. The practitioner asks each patient about his or her:

- Faith or spiritual practice: ask whether the patient considers himself/herself to be a religious or spiritual person. Inquire as to those things that are meaningful in their lives.

- Importance of the religious or spiritual practice at this time, the role that beliefs play in understanding illness or personal care.
- Community: ask about participation in a religious or spiritual community and its contribution to the patient and family.
- Assist: determine how health-care providers can assist in meeting spiritual needs at this time.

Addressing these four areas can yield much valuable information in a brief clinical encounter. People often attach profound meaning to their illnesses. An exploration of those meanings can be essential to effective management, decision making, and ultimately to the relief of suffering.

Social assessment should include an evaluation of family support, community resources, and financial concerns. Data from SUPPORT[9] reveal the tremendous family burdens that can accompany advanced illness. Nearly 30% of families caring for terminally ill patients face loss of life savings and work opportunities or disruption of support systems.[31,32]

Uncertainty about how to manage practical issues regarding caregivers (availability and capabilities), domestic needs, housing, transportation, dependents (children, spouse, and pets) can also cause great distress. Planning for the moment of death (whether to call 911, preparation of the body) and ensuring that funeral arrangements are consistent with patient wishes should be addressed with most patients and family members.

Management of Common Clinical Symptoms

Distressing symptoms often accompany advanced stages of illness, as well as longstanding chronic illness. Few texts have addressed symptom management,[33] yet effective management can greatly ease the physical suffering of patients. The op≠portunity for patients and families to address important spiritual and social concerns is greatly enhanced when physical suffering is minimized. Some general guidelines apply, regardless of symptoms:

- Perform a thorough history and physical exam

- Determine the likely cause of the symptom and the need for, or appropriateness of, further diagnostic evaluation
- Determine benefits/burdens of each treatment option
- Provide patient/family education and involve them in decision making
- Reevaluate and modify treatment approaches as needed
- Develop strategies to prevent symptom distress whenever possible

Symptoms associated with advanced illnesses can be caused by the underlying disease, comorbid illness, treatments, medications, psychosocial or spiritual factors, or any combination. Interventions should be specific and directed toward the underlying cause of the symptom when feasible. As discussed in chapter 19 on pain management, if a symptom is continuous, it should be managed with round-the-clock medications with an eye toward prevention as well as treatment. Several common clinical symptoms and their management are discussed in the sections that follow. The reader is referred to several extensive reviews for more detailed information.[17,25,34,35]

Breathlessness (Dyspnea)   Dyspnea is reported by many patients with advanced illness. The prevalence is highly variable (21–75%), depending on the diagnosis and stage of the illness. Nearly half of all palliative-care patients describe breathlessness as being of moderate to severe intensity.[36] As such, it can greatly diminish quality of life and functional capacity. Like pain, breathlessness is subjective and patient report of its presence and severity is the gold standard. Neither the respiratory rate, blood gas levels, O_2 saturation, nor clinical perception necessarily correlate with the patient's subjective report.[37] There are many potential causes of breathlessness, and underlying conditions often can be treated effectively, even in advanced illness. Antibiotics for pneumonia, diuretics for congestive heart failure, transfusions for severe anemia, and thoracocentesis for pleural effusions are examples. Specific interventions should be considered, if appropriate, for the individual patient.

Medical approaches for symptomatic management of breathlessness in palliative care include oxygen, opioids, and anxiolytics. Additionally, corticosteroids (inflammation, asthma, tracheal impingement, superior vena cava obstruction) and bronchodilators (bronchospasm, asthma) may be helpful in some patients.

Oxygen is frequently used in palliative care, and therapeutic trials in the setting of breathlessness are usually warranted. Oxygen is a potent symbol of therapeutic intervention and may produce a significant placebo effect. The relief of breathlessness may not be related to any objective improvement in O_2 saturation.

Opioids are the predominant means of symptomatic management of dyspnea, regardless of etiology. Exactly how opioids provide relief of dyspnea is not clear, but relief occurs frequently without demonstrable change in respiratory rate or oxygen saturation levels. Favorable effects on cardiac function and systemic effects have been postulated. Careful initiation and titration of opioids are safe and effective and should be considered the standard for treating breathlessness associated with terminal illness. Morphine can be administered orally, rectally, subcutaneously, intravenously, or with a nebulizer. There are no definitive reports on the optimal route, dose, or timing of administration to best manage breathlessness. The best route for administration depends on the needs and desires of the patient. The best dose is determined by individual titration to comfort. Initial recommendations for dosing in opioid-naive patients are listed below:[25]

- Hydrocodone 5 mg every 5 hours by mouth
- Morphine (elixir or tablets) 2.5–5 mg every 4 hours
- Morphine sub-q or IV 1–2 mg every 3–4 hours
- Oxycodone 2.5–5 mg every 4 hours
- Hydromorphone 0.5–2 mg every 4 hours

All doses must be individualized to the patient's needs, history, and responses. Anxiety often accompanies or contributes to dyspnea.[38] A search for the underlying cause of the anxiety is often important in revealing both physiological and psychosocial factors.

Regardless of the cause of the anxiety, however, benzodiazepines can be helpful by inducing global sedation (allowing rest) and potentially diminishing respiratory drive and the work of breathing. Lorazepam (0.5–2 mg PO every hour until settled, then routinely q 4–6 hours) is the drug of choice due to its short duration and sublingual absorption. Caution should be used in the ambulatory patient as fall risk is increased. Midazolam, titrated to patient response, is useful when a sub-q or IV medication is indicated.

Nonpharmacological Approaches   A variety of nonpharmacological approaches may be helpful in alleviation of breathlessness.[39] Providing support and education to the patient and family is helpful. Behavioral approaches of relaxation, distraction, guided imagery, and supportive counseling are often beneficial. Eliminating environmental irritants, providing fans, humidity, positioning, and cooler temperatures may also bring relief.

Constipation   Constipation, defined as discomfort associated with an increase in stool consistency or reduced bowel movements (less than usual, less than every three days), occurs in 40–90% of terminally ill patients. If not carefully assessed, prevented when possible, and managed effectively, it can cause great distress to patients (pain, nausea and vomiting, overflow incontinence, tenesmus, fecal impaction). Assessment should focus on history of elimination habits, recent changes in elimination patterns, and abdominal and rectal exams. Prevention of constipation should be the primary goal. At the time that patients are started on opioids, an effective bowel regimen to prevent constipation also needs to be in place.

Common Causes of Constipation

- Medications: opioids, NSAIDs, calcium-channel blockers, anticholinergics
- Metabolic abnormalities: hypercalcemia, dehydration
- Comorbid conditions: inactivity, weakness, autonomic dysfunction, spinal cord compression
- Obstruction: ileus, malignancy

Treatment   General measures:

- Encourage elimination routine
- Ensure privacy
- Encourage ambulation and fluids
- Discontinue constipating medications

Specific measures:

- Laxative therapy (stimulants: senna or bisacodyl, prune juice; osmotic laxatives: lactulose, sorbitol, or milk of magnesia)
- Stool softeners: usually used in combination with a laxative or stimulant
- Bulk-forming agents should generally be avoided
- Prokinetic agents: cisapride or metoclopramide are often useful
- Lubricants: mineral oil, peanut oil, glycerin suppository
- Large-volume warm water enema

Anorexia/Cachexia   Anorexia (loss of appetite) and cachexia (loss of weight) are common in advanced illnesses (> 80% of those with advanced cancer and AIDS).[40] Wasting syndromes seen with certain malignancies, heart and pulmonary diseases, chronic infections, and kidney and hepatic diseases can cause great patient and family distress. Weight loss in institutional settings may also be seen as evidence of inadequate care, abuse, or neglect. In many cultures, the refusal to eat may be misconstrued as a rejection of caring and cause great family distress. Common causes of anorexia include:

- Medications (cardiac drugs, antibiotics, antihypertensives, anticonvulsants, pain medications)
- Pain, anxiety, depression, fear of nausea/vomiting, aversion to food (sight, smells, consistency)
- GI disturbances: infection, ulceration, constipation, autonomic dysfunction, reflux, oral infections, and hygiene
- Malignancy: tumor or tumor products
- Biochemical disturbances: hypercalcemia, uremia

Anorexia is a common symptom at the end of life. Management should be guided by the patient and aimed at underlying causes when possible. "Forcing" intake beyond that which the patient will comfortably accept may actually increase suffering, both physically and emotionally. Enteral and parenteral feeding in terminal illness should be carefully evaluated and usually avoided. Decisions about therapy should always be individualized. In the frail older patient, the burdens of aggressive nutritional evaluation and intervention can be significant. Cachexia is generally not reversed by aggressive nutritional intervention.[40] General measures include:

- Offering small frequent and favorite meals (ask about preferences)
- Liberalizing or eliminating any dietary restrictions
- Minimizing odors
- Managing comorbid conditions and medications
- Attending to emotional and social implications of not eating
- Discontinuing as many routine medications as possible

Specific measures include:

- Appetite stimulants: alcohol, cryptoheptadine
- Prokinetic agents: cisipride, metacopramide
- Progestational agents: megestrol acetate
- Steroids: prednisone, dexamethasone
- Cannabinoids: dronabinol

Fatigue/Weakness   Fatigue is one of the most disturbing symptoms for patients with advanced illness.[41] Fatigue commonly accompanies anorexia and malnutrition and can be a major impediment to acceptable quality of life for a terminally ill patient. Moreover, an individual's strength is often felt to be under personal control. Families sometimes feel that fatigue means the patient has "given up," as even the smallest of functions can no longer be performed. The underlying cause of the weakness is often not clearly understood and/or due to multiple factors. At present, there are no definitive treatments. Management must be individualized. Common causes include:

- Nerve or muscle damage or atrophy from underlying cancer or treatment
- Electrolyte disturbances, dehydration, organ failure
- Medications: opioids, diuretics, antihypertensives, antidepressants
- Anemia, hypothyroidism
- Psychosocial and spiritual distress, depression
- Insomnia, immobility

General approaches:

- Encourage and train in energy conservation techniques
- Physical or occupational therapy techniques to improve mobility
- If possible, discontinue any medication which may worsen fatigue
- Encourage fluid and electrolyte intake
- Address psychosocial and spiritual concerns

Specific approaches:

- Address and correct laboratory abnormalities
- Steroids: dexamethasone may increase energy and sense of well being (effects may wane after 4–6 weeks)
- Psychostimulants: methylphenidate, dextroamphetamine, and pemoline methyphenydate have been used most commonly, even in very debilitated patients.

The Final Hours of Life

Patients often enter into a more or less well-defined terminal phase of illness, a period of "active dying." Many physiological changes take place during this time.[42] The signs and symptoms of these changes can be very distressing to patients and their families. If not prepared, last minute panic can disrupt even the most careful advance-care planning efforts. Meticulous attention to hygiene, prevention of symptoms when possible, and aggressive intervention in distressing symptoms are keys to a more comfortable dying. Among the important clinical changes that may occur are the following:

- Fatigue and weakness
- Decreased food and fluid intake

- Decreased blood perfusion
- Changes in level of consciousness
- Neurologic dysfunction
- Respiratory changes
- Dysphagia
- Incontinence
- Restlessness/myoclonus
- Delirium
- Pain

Weakness and fatigue often increase as death approaches. Problems associated with immobility can become more apparent at this time. Skin breakdown, contractures, pain, and risk of aspiration increase. Appropriate attention to positioning, turning, pressure-reducing surfaces, passive range of motion, and food consistency are important. The decline in food and fluid intake may also contribute to weakness. Food intake above that which the patient will comfortably accept may contribute to nausea, vomiting, and aspiration risk. Patients rarely complain of being hungry during this time. Anorexia may also be protective (ketosis can diminish pain and provide for a greater sense of well being).

Likewise, decreasing fluid intake may diminish edema, incontinence, breathlessness, and respiratory secretions. Thirst can be managed by careful attention to mucosal surfaces, artificial saliva, and lubricating gels for lips, eyes, and nares. Aggressive attempts at hydration and nutrition may thus increase discomfort and have the potential to prolong the dying process. Educating families about these events can relieve guilt and allow time to focus on other aspects of caregiving. It is important to consider the need for reduction in medication when oliguria and anuria occur. Lower doses of opiates, in particular, may be necessary to prevent accumulation of toxic metabolites normally excreted by the kidney. There is some controversy over the use of hydration in the dying patient. Some authors feel that aggressive hydration may prevent delirium.[43]

Changes in neurologic function are also common. Declines in level of consciousness progressing to lethargy, obtundation, and death may occur. Families should be reminded that there is a possibility that the semicomatose patient may still be able to hear and understand. Encourage families to continue to interact with the patient as if he/she could understand all that is being said.

Patients may also become more distressed, tremulous, agitated, and delirious as death approaches. Hallucinations, myoclonic jerking, and seizures can also occur. Increasing agitation is often interpreted as evidence of pain. While this may be true, pain infrequently emerges for the first time as an important problem in the last days or hours of life. Delirium from many potential sources may be a more likely explanation of the agitation. Aggressive management and prevention of distressing symptoms is indicated. Medical management includes benzodiazepines (lorazepam, midazolam), neuroleptics (haloperidol, respirdol), anticonvulsants (phenotoin, phenobarbital), and possible IV hydration.

Circulatory changes can result in reflex tachycardia, hypotension, and mottling of skin as blood is shunted away from the periphery. Preparing families for these very visible and tactile changes, along with a reassurance that these are a normal part of the body's attempt to "shut down," is important.

Loss of ability to swallow and to manage secretions can increase aspiration risk and cause an audible gurgling or rattle. Positioning, postural drainage, and attempts to dry secretions (scopolamine) can increase comfort. Vigorous suctioning should be avoided in most patients as it is frequently ineffective and can be very distressing to patient and family.

Changes in breathing patterns, apnea, shallow breathing, and Cheyne-Stokes respiration are often signs of impending death. Families often perceive these events as indices of discomfort and impending suffocation. The family needs education and reassurance that the patient is probably not feeling any discomfort with the altered breathing patterns.

Advance Care Planning

Advance care planning (ACP) is the process of planning for future health care in the event one is unable to make or communicate decisions. Most patients will, at some point in the trajectory of dying, lose the capacity to communicate. Patients have the right to accept or refuse any medical care that they specify. Statutory documents are recognized in all 50 states and include the living will and the durable power of attorney for health care.

Forms are available from appropriate state agencies and many other private groups. Older patients should be encouraged to complete both a living will and to designate a health care proxy or durable power of attorney for health care. In most states, a proxy designated by the patient has greater authority to make decisions than a surrogate appointed for the patient.

Discussions of ACP should be a routine part of all clinical care.[22] ACP is a process and ongoing dialogue,[43] not just an event or a document to be completed. It is an important opportunity to clarify knowledge of existing conditions, expectations, goals, values, fears, and conflicts. A systematic approach toward ACP should be adopted:

1. Initiate dialogue:
   - Determine familiarity with ACP and explain its importance
   - Determine capacity to make health-care decisions
   - Review state-specific regulations and forms, if any
   - Determine extent of understanding and desire for information of the terminal illness
   - Encourage appointment of health-care proxy in the event of incapacity

2. Structured discussion:
   - Describe options for care, benefits, and burdens of different interventions
   - Review underlying values and goals for medical intervention
   - Explore any inconsistencies between goals for care and desire for specific interventions
   - Consider any underlying ethical conflicts

3. Document preferences:
   - Review and formulate directives and preferences
   - Use worksheet or summary sheet to record decisions
   - Enter directives into medical record
   - Alter plan of care
   - Revise and update as needed

4. Implement directives:
   - Review current clinical conditions and regulations regarding implementation of advance directives

- Consult with proxy and family
- Carry out treatment plan
- Revise treatment plan as necessary

Multiple levels of decisions should be made (concerning resuscitation, hospitalization, invasive procedures, artificial hydration and nutrition, use of anitibiotics, and laboratory studies) in anticipation of decline. Treatment decisions should generally be based on their potential to decrease suffering, as well as the use of any invasive interventions.

It is important to understand that advance directives completed at one point in time may no longer truly reflect patient wishes at a later time. Patients and their families often approach end-of-life decision making with great ambivalence. Complex clinical situations are not always foreseen or planned for; this may be the prime reason why advance directives do not seem to influence medical decision making in many studies.[9] Directives often lack flexibility in clinical situations and common pitfalls include unclear patient statements and uninvolved proxy decision makers. Advance planning discussions cannot anticipate all possible clinical conditions. Allow patients to discuss their wishes and to designate an individual with whom wishes will be discussed and by whom decisions will be made in accordance with those wishes. Be sure that documentation is complete, widely communicated, and consistent with state statutes.

Role of the Nurse Practitioner

The multidisciplinary and patient-centered approaches of palliative care fit well with current models of geriatric care. In many populations, the nurse practitioner is best positioned to foster dialog and education on end-of-life issues and clinical management. The experience of caring for a dying older adult is often difficult. However, the extraordinary power and transformative nature of this experience for many patients and families makes such care exceptionally rewarding. The last stage of life has great potential, as well as great challenges.[44] Skillful application of palliative care principles in accordance with patient wishes can ensure a peaceful death and leave everyone involved strengthened, despite the personal suffering associated with the loss of a loved and valued human being.

References

1. Rosenberg HM, Ventura SJ, Mauer JD. Births and deaths in the United States, 1995. *Nat Center Health Statistics*. 1996;45(3)(Suppl 2).
2. Brim OG, Friedman HE, Levine S, et al, eds. *The Dying Patient*. New York: Russell Sage Foundation; 1970.
3. Singh GK, Dochanek DK, MacDorman MF, et al. Advance report and final statistics, 1994. *Month Vital Statistics Rep*. 1996;45(3) (Suppl).
4. U.S. Bureau of the Census. *Current Population Reports, Special Studies, 65 plus in the United States*. Washington, DC: US Bureau of the Census; 1996.
5. *Health United States, 1995*. Rockville, Md: U.S. Dept of Health and Human Services, 1996. PHS publication 96–1232.
6. Field MJ, Cassel CK. Institute of Medicine Committee on Care at the End of Life. *Approaching Death: Improving Care at the End of Life*. Washington, DC: National Academy Press; 1997.
7. Seale C, Cartwright A. *The Year Before Death*. Aldershot, Hauts, England: Ashgate Publishing; 1994.
8. Donnelly S, Walsh D. The symptoms of advanced cancer. *J Pall Care*. 1995;11:27–32.
9. SUPPORT Principal Investigators. A controlled trial to improve care for seriously ill hospitalized patients. *JAMA*. 1995;274:1591–1598.
10. Osler W. *Science and Immortality*. London: Constable; 1906.
11. Schonwetter RS, ed. Care of the terminally ill patient. *Clin Geriatr Med*. 1996;12.
12. Weinberg JE, Cooper M, eds. *The Dartmouth Atlas of Health Care*. Chicago: American Hospital Publishing; 1998.
13. Lubitz JD, Riley GF. Trends in medicare payments in the last year of life. *N Engl J Med*. 1993;332:1092–1096.
14. National Hospice Organization. *Hospice Fact Sheet*. Arlington, Va: National Hospice Organization; 1996.
15. Teno JM, Lynn J, Wenger N, et al. Advance directives for seriously ill hospitalized patients. *J Am Geriatr Soc*. 1997;45:500–507.
16. Seidlitzl, Duberstein PR, Cox C, et al. Attitudes of older people toward suicide and assisted suicide: an analysis of Gallop poll findings. *J Am Geriatr Soc*. 1995;43:993–998.
17. Doyle D, Hanks G, McDonald N, eds. *Oxford Textbook of Palliative Medicine*, 2nd ed. Oxford: Oxford University Press; 1998.
18. Billings JA. What is palliative care? *J Pall Med*. 1998;1:73–81.
19. World Health Organization. *Cancer Pain Relief and Palliative Care. Technical Report Series 804*. Geneva, Switzerland; 1990.
20. Cassel CK, Foley KM. *Principles for Care of Patients at the End-of-Life: An Emerging Consensus Among the Specialties of Medicine*. New York: Milbank Memorial Fund; 1999.

21. Stuart B, Kinzbrunner B. *National Hospice Organization Guidelines for the Determination of Prognosis in Selected Non-Cancer Diagnoses.* Arlington, Va: National Hospice Organization; 1995.

22. National Hospice Organization. *Fact Sheet: Hospice in America: A Statistical Profile.* Arlington, Va: National Hospice Organization; 1998.

23. Fox E, Landrum-McNiff K, Zhoug Z, et al. Evaluation of pronostic criteria for determining hospice eligibility in patients with advanced lung, heart or liver disease. *JAMA.* 1999;282:1638–1645.

24. Finucane TE. How gravely ill becomes dying. A key to end-of-life care. *JAMA.* 1999;282:1670–1672.

25. Emananuel LL, von Gunten CF, Ferris FD. *The Education for Physicians on End of Life Care.* Chicago: American Medical Association; 1999.

26. Bruera E, Kuehn N, Miller MJ, et al. The Edmonton symptom assessment system (SAS): a simple method for the assessment of palliatve care patients. *J Pall Care.* 1991;7:6–9.

27. Portnoy RK, Thaler HT, Kornblith AB, et al. The Memorial Symptom Assessment Scale. *Eur J Cancer.* 1994;30:1326–1336.

28. Mezey M, Teresi J, Ramsey G, et al. Decision-making capacity to execute a health care proxy: development and testing of guidelines. *J Am Geriatr Soc.* 2000;48: 179–187.

29. Suhl J, Simons P, Reedy T, et al. Myth of substituted judgment: surrogate decision making regarding life support is unreliable. *Arch Int Med.* 1994;154: 190–196.

30. Pulchalski CM, Romer AL. Taking a spiritual history allows clinicians to understand patients more fully. *J Pall Med.* 2000;3(1):129–137.

31. Covinsky KE, Landerfield C, Teno J. Is economic hardship on the families of the seriously ill associated with patients and surrogate care preferences? *Arch Int Med.* 1996;156:1737–1741.

32. Ferrell B, Virani R, Grant M. Analysis of symptom assessment and management content in nursing textbooks. *J Pall Med.* 1999;2:161–172.

33. Cooley M, Pickett M, eds. Palliative care. *Sem Oncol Nurs.* 1998;14(2):86–94.

34. Wrede-Seaman L. *Symptom Management Algorithms. A Handbook for Palliative Care.* 2nd ed. Yakima, Wa; Intellicard; 1999.

35. Ahmedzai S. Palliation of respiratory symptoms. In: Doyle D, Hanks G, McDonald N, eds. *Oxford Textbook of Palliative Medicine.* 2nd ed. Oxford University Press; 1998:583–616.

36. Ripamonti C, Bruera E. Dyspnea: pathophysiology and assessment. *J Pain Symptom Manage.* 1997;13: 220–232.

37. Tobin MJ. Dyspnea: pathophysiologic basis, clinical presentation and management. *Arch Int Med.* 1990; 150:1604–1990.

38. Hansen-Flaschen J. Advanced lung disease: palliation and terminal care. *Clin Chest Med.* 1997;18:645–662.

39. Ma G, Alexander HR. Prevalence and pathophysiology of cancer cachexia. In: Bruera E, Portnoy RK, eds. *Topics in Palliative Care.* 2nd ed. Oxford University Press; 1998:91–129.

40. Neuenschwander H, Bruera E. Pathophysiology of cancer asthenia. In: Bruera E, Portnoy RK, eds. *Topics in Palliative Care.* 2nd ed. Oxford University Press; 1998:57–75.

41. Twycross R, Lichter I. The Terminal Phase. In: Doyle D, Hanks G, McDonald N: (eds). Oxford Textbook of Palliative Medicine , 2nd ed., Oxford University Press, 1998:977–992.

42. Emanuel LL, Danis M, Pearlman RA, et al. Advance care planning as a process: structuring the discussion in practice. *J Am Geriatr Soc.* 1995;43:440–448

43. Byock I. *Dying Well. The Prospect for Growth at the End of Life.* New York: Riverhead Publishers; 1997.

■ INDEX

A

abdominal assessment
  for cardiac dysrhythmias, 56
  for heart failure, 49
  for hypertension, 34
abuse. *See* elder mistreatment
acarbose, 112, 113
acetaminophen (Tylenol)
  as osteoarthritis treatment, 240
  as pain treatment, 352–353
  as upper respiratory infections treatment, 73
acetazolamide (Diamox), 274
acetylcholinesterase (AchE) inhibitors, 195
achalasia, 293
acid-fast bacillus (AFB), 78
active neglect, 321
activities of daily living (ADLs), 9–10
activity. *See* exercise; physical activity
Actos, 113
acupuncture, 240
acute atrial fibrillation, 57
acute confusion. *See* delirium
acute pain
  chronic pain, distinction from, 337
  management of, 344, 348
acute sinusitis, 71
acyclovir (Zovirax), 227
addiction, 336
adenocarcinoma, 213, 214
adnexal structures, 13
adult protective services (APS), 319, 327, 328–329,
  330
advance care planning (ACP), 369–370
advance directives, 8
advanced activities of daily living (AADLs), 10
advanced practice gerontological nurses, 3–4, 5–6
adverse drug reactions (ADRs), 19

Advisory Committee on Immunization Practices
  (ACIP), 78
afterload, 47
age, functional, biological, and chronological, 312
age-associated memory impairment (AAMI), 183–184
age-related macular degeneration (AMD), 273
age-related physiology. *See* physiology, age-related
Agency for Health Care Policy and Research
  (AHCPR), 94
albuterol (Proventil, Ventolin)
  as asthma treatment, 76
  as bronchitis treatment, 72
alcohol
  as palliative care anorexia/cachexia treatment, 367
  risk factor reduction, 180
  squamous cell carcinoma and, 213
alcoholism screening, 254
aldosterone, 15
alendronate
  esophageal injury and, 293
  as osteoporosis treatment, 232
Alitraa, 306
allodynia, 335
allopurinol, 287
aloe, 212
alpha-adrenergic blockers
  as benign prostatic hyperplasia symptoms treatment,
    96–97
  as overflow urinary incontinence treatment, 89
alpha-sympathomimetic agonists, 88
alpha-tocopherol (vitamin E), 195
alphaglucosidase inhibitors (Acarbose, Miglitol), 113
alternative therapies, 241
alveolar duct, 16
Alzheimer's Association, 197
Alzheimer's disease (AD), 152, 184–186
amantadine (Symmetrel), 70